ACSM's
Resources for
Clinical Exercise Physiology
Musculoskeletal, Neuromuscular, Neoplastic,
Immunologic, and Hematologic Conditions
SECOND EDITION

SENIOR EDITORS

Jonathan Myers, PhD, FACSM
Clinical Professor
Cardiology Division
Veterans Administration Palo Alto Health Care System
Stanford University
Palo Alto, California

David Nieman, PhD, FACSM
Professor
Department of Health, Leisure, and Exercise Science
Appalachian State University
Boone, North Carolina

SECTION EDITORS

Georgia Frey, PhD, FACSM
Associate Professor
Department of Kinesiology
Indiana University
Bloomington, Indiana

Kenneth Pitetti, PhD, FACSM
Professor
College of Health Professions
Wichita State University
Wichita, Kansas

David Nieman, PhD, FACSM
Professor
Department of Health, Leisure, and Exercise Science
Appalachian State University
Boone, North Carolina

William Herbert, PhD, FACSM
Professor
Department of Human Nutrition, Foods, and Exercise
Virginia Tech
Blacksburg, Virginia

Anthony S. Kaleth, PhD
Associate Professor
Department of Physical Education
Indiana University—Purdue University Indianapolis
Indianapolis, Indiana

ACSM's
Resources for
Clinical Exercise Physiology
Musculoskeletal, Neuromuscular, Neoplastic,
Immunologic, and Hematologic Conditions

SECOND EDITION

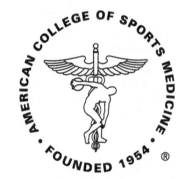

AMERICAN COLLEGE
OF SPORTS MEDICINE

Wolters Kluwer | Lippincott Williams & Wilkins
Health

Philadelphia · Baltimore · New York · London
Buenos Aires · Hong Kong · Sydney · Tokyo

Acquisitions Editor: Emily Lupash
Managing Editor: Andrea M. Klingler
Marketing Manager: Christen D. Murphy
Project Manager: Debra Schiff
Designer: Doug Smock
Production Services: Aptara, Inc.

ACSM Publication Committee Chair: Jeffrey L. Roitman, EdD, FACSM
ACSM Group Publisher: D. Mark Robertson

Printed in China

Library of Congress Cataloging-in-Publication Data

ACSM's resources for clinical exercise physiology : musculoskeletal,
neuromuscular, neoplastic, immunologic, and hematologic conditions /
American College of Sports Medicine. – 2nd ed.
   p. ; cm.
 Includes bibliographical references and index.
 ISBN 978-0-7817-6870-2 (alk. paper)
 1. Exercise therapy. I. American College of Sports Medicine. II.
Title: Resources for clinical exercise physiology.
 [DNLM: 1. Exercise Therapy–Practice Guideline. 2.
Exercise–physiology–Practice Guideline. WB 541 A1875 2010]
 RM725.A34 2010
 615.8'2--dc22

                    2008047172

Preface

The application of exercise as a preventive and therapeutic medium was once largely limited to patients with pulmonary or cardiovascular disease, mainly those who had recently sustained a myocardial infarction. Over the last three decades, many resources and guidelines have been published that have been directed toward the application of exercise evaluation and therapy in cardiovascular and pulmonary disease. The range of individuals for whom appropriately prescribed exercise has documented benefits has broadened considerably in recent years. This text was written in response to the need for guidance among exercise clinicians working with patients with a broad range of chronic diseases and disabilities beyond cardiovascular and pulmonary disease, including orthopedic, neurologic, metabolic, musculoskeletal, neoplastic, and immunodeficiency conditions—populations that have been largely underserved. It is intended to complement and extend existing ACSM publications, including *ACSM's Guidelines for Exercise Testing and Prescription* and *ACSM's Resource Manual for Exercise Testing and Prescription*.

The ACSM Registered Clinical Exercise Physiologist (RCEP) pilot examination, initiated in 1999, was designed to establish the existence of appropriate knowledge, skills, and abilities for healthcare professionals working with individuals with a broad range of chronic diseases and disabilities. Ten years later, the RCEP has become established as a standard certification for individuals working in clinical settings among patients with chronic diseases and disabilities. The ACSM has defined the RCEP as a *"healthcare professional who works in the application of exercise and physical activity for those clinical and pathological situations where it has been shown to provide therapeutic or functional benefit. Patients for whom services are appropriate may include, but are not limited to, those with cardiovascular, pulmonary, metabolic, musculoskeletal, neuromuscular, neoplastic, immunologic, and hematologic diseases and conditions. The RCEP applies exercise principles to groups such as geriatric, pediatric, or obstetric populations, and to society as a whole in preventive activities. The RCEP performs exercise evaluation, exercise prescription, exercise supervision, exercise education, and exercise outcome evaluation."* For each of the conditions covered in this text, the chapters are therefore organized by epidemiology, pathophysiology, diagnosis, medical and surgical treatments, exercise/fitness/functional testing, and exercise prescription and programming. Where appropriate, case studies are included to underscore the role of exercise in managing individuals with a particular condition.

Although this text is intended to be a resource for individuals preparing for the RCEP examination, it is also an appropriate resource for any individual trained in the exercise sciences working in the clinical setting among persons with chronic conditions and disabilities beyond cardiovascular and pulmonary disease. It should serve as a reference for physical therapists, nurses, physicians, and other rehabilitation specialists who deal with the conditions addressed in these chapters. These resources generally apply to patients with chronic disease who, in the opinion of their physician provider, are clinically stable and have sufficient functional capabilities to participate in individually prescribed exercise that is aimed at improving fitness, function, physical work potential, and quality of life, and which reduces exercise-related risk factors that have an impact on progression of their disease. Much recent research has been performed related to the benefits of exercise for patients with the wide variety of conditions described in this text. Many physicians and other health professionals have embraced the use of exercise in the diagnosis, prevention, and treatment of various chronic health problems. However, similar to cardiovascular disease, exercise as an intervention is greatly underutilized for most of these conditions. The multitude of disorders associated with a sedentary lifestyle applies to individuals with chronic disabilities just as it applies to those without such disabilities. An important goal must be to better convey the value of appropriately applied exercise therapy for these patients so that it is an integrated part of the healthcare paradigm. This text represents another step, however small, in bringing this research to the public and the medical community to foster a greater appreciation of the value of the therapeutic benefits of exercise across a broad spectrum of patients.

In this new edition of the RCEP resources, chapters from the first edition have been updated and a section has been added on *Clinical Practice Issues for the RCEP*. The Clinical Practice Issues section includes chapters on the evolution of the clinical exercise physiologist, demonstrating functional outcomes for health and fitness, legal and ethical considerations, and client referral and consulting relations with allied professions. The latter section was included to help provide the RCEP and other healthcare professionals with a better the understanding of their role and how they can have an important and integral place in today's healthcare environment. Included in the Appendix are the updated knowledge, skills, and abilities that have been developed to address the role of the clinical exercise physiologist in the exercise management of patients with chronic diseases and disabilities. We hope that this text serves not only as resource for credentialing by ACSM, but also to help further define the important role of the exercise physiologist in the clinical setting, as well as to extend the principles and recommendations of exercise programming to a broader spectrum of the population.

Jonathan Myers, PhD
David Nieman, PhD

Contributors

Mark A. Anderson, PT, PhD, ATC
Department of Rehabilitation Sciences
University of Oklahoma Health Sciences Center
Oklahoma City, Oklahoma

Yagesh Bhambhani, PhD
Professor
Department of Occupational Therapy
University of Alberta
Edmonton, Alberta, Canada

Thomas J. Birk, PhD, MPT, FACSM
Associate Professor
Department of Physical Therapy, Physical Medicine
   and Rehabilitation
Wayne State University
Detroit, Michigan

Louise Burke, MD
Head, Department of Sports Nutrition
Australian Institute of Sport
Belconnen, Canberra, Australia

Kerry S. Courneya, PhD
Professor
Department of Physical Education
University of Alberta
Edmonton, Alberta, Canada

Timothy J. Doherty, MD, PhD, FRCPc
Associate Professor
Departments of Clinical Neurological Sciences and
   Rehabilitation Medicine Schulich School of Medicine
   and Dentistry
The University of Western Ontario
London, Ontario

Kieran Fallon, PhD
Associate Professor
Head, Department of Sports Medicine
College of Medicine and Health Sciences
The Australian National University
Canberra, Australia

Stephen F. Figoni, PhD, RKT, FACSM
Research Health Scientist
Physical Medicine and Rehabilitation Service
Veterans Administration West Los Angeles
Los Angeles, California

Nadine M. Fisher, EdD
Assistant Professor
Department of Occupational Therapy
State University of New York at Buffalo
Buffalo, New York

Lisa Fleisher, MS, PT
School of Physical Therapy
Texas Women's University
Dallas, Texas

Richard Glazier, MD, MPH
Associate Professor
Health Policy, Management and Evaluation
Faculty of Medicine
University of Toronto
Toronto, Ontario, Canada

D. Shaun Gray, MD, PhD, CCFP, FRCPC
Associate Professor
Division of Physical Medicine and Rehabilitation
University of Alberta
Edmonton, Alberta, Canada
Department Chief
Halvar Johnson Centre for Brain Injury
David Thompson Health Region
Ponoka, Alberta, Canada

David Herbert, JD
Senior Partner
David L. Herbert and Associates, LLD
Canton, Ohio

Kurt Jackson, PhD, PT, GCS
Neurology Coordinator
Doctor of Physical Therapy Program
Department of Health and Sports Science
University of Dayton
Dayton, Ohio

Anthony S. Kaleth, PhD
Associate Professor
Department of Physical Education
Indiana University—Purdue University Indianapolis
Indianapolis, Indiana

Jennifer Kaleth, PT
Department of Rehabilitation
The Shelbourne Knee Center at Methodist Hospital
Indianapolis, Indiana

Steven J. Keteyian, PhD, FACSM
Division of Cardiovascular Medicine
The Henry Ford Heart and Vascular Institute
Henry Ford Hospital
Detroit, Michigan

Carl N. King, EdD
President and CEO
Cardiovascular Consultant
Hickory, North Carolina

B. Jenny Kiratli, PhD
Research Health Scientist
Spinal Cord Injury Center
Veterans Administration Palo Alto Health
    Care System
Palo Alto, California

Cliff Klein, PhD, MA, BA
Assistant Professor
Department of Physical Therapy
University of Toronto
Toronto, Ontario, Canada

John J. LaManca, PhD
Research Coordinator/ Exercise Physiologist
Heart Failure and Cardiac Transplantation
New York Presbyterian Hospital
New York, New York

James J. Laskin, PT, PhD
Department of Physical Therapy
University of Montana
Missoula, Montana

Laurel T. MacKinnon, PhD, FACSM
Freelance Writer and Editor
Queensland, Australia

Robert C. Manske, MPT, CSCS
Associate Professor
Department of Physical Therapy
Wichita State University
Wichita, Kansas

Margaret L. McNeely, PT, MSc, PhD
Professor
Department of Physical Education and Recreation
University of Alberta
Edmonton, Alberta, Canada

Janet A. Mulcare, PhD, PT, FACSM
Professor of Physical Therapy
Department of Health Sciences
College of Mount St. Joseph
Cincinatti, Ohio

David L. Nichols, PhD
Assistant Research Professor
Institute for Women's Health
Texas Women's University
Denton, Texas

Terry Nicola, MD, FACSM
Director of Sports Medicine and Rehabilitation
Department of Orthopedics
University of Illinois Medical Center
Chicago, Illinois

David Nieman, PhD, FACSM, Section Editor
Professor
Department of Health, Leisure, and Exercise Science
Appalachian State University
Boone, North Carolina

Stephanie Nixon, PhD, MSc, BHSc(PT), BA
Assistant Professor
Department of Physical Therapy
University of Toronto
Toronto, Ontario, Canada

Kelly O'Brien, BSc, BScPT
Lecturer
Department of Physical Therapy
University of Toronto
Toronto, Ontario, Canada

Robin Parisotto, BAppSci
Laboratory Manager
Sports Haematology and Biochemistry Laboratory
Australian Institute of Sport
Leverrier Crescent
Bruce, Australian Capitol Territory, Australia

Jonathan Peake, PhD
School of Human Movement Studies
The University of Queensland
Queensland, Australia

Carolyn J. Peddle, MS
Department of Physical Education and Recreation
University of Alberta
Edmonton, Alberta, Canada

Mark T. Pfefer, RN, MS, DC
Cleveland Chiropractic College
Overland Park, Kansas

Kenneth Pitetti, PhD, FACSM, Section Editor
Professor
College of Health Professions
Wichita State University
Wichita, Kansas

Elizabeth J. Protas, PT, PhD, FACSM, FAPTA
Interim Dean and Ruby Decker Endowed Professor
Senior Fellow, Sealy Center on Aging
School of Allied Health Sciences
University of Texas Medical Branch
Galveston, Texas

James H. Rimmer, PhD, Professor
Director, National Center on Physical Activity
and Disability and Rehabilitation Engineering
    Research Center RecTech
Department of Disability and Human Development
University of Illinois at Chicago
Chicago, Illinois

Gary Rowland, MScOT, OT(c)
Faculty of Rehabilitative Medicine
University of Alberta
Edmonton, Alberta, Canada

Roy Sasaki, MD
Spinal Cord Injury Center
Veterans Administration Palo Alto Health Care System
Palo Alto, California

Christopher Sellar, MS
Department of Physical Education
    and Recreation
University of Alberta
Edmonton, Alberta, Canada

Maureen J. Simmonds, PT, PhD
Professor and Director
School of Physical & Occupational Therapy
McGill University
Montreal, Quebec, Canada

Sue Ann Sisto, PT, MA, PhD
Professor, Physical Therapy
Research Director, Division of Rehabilitation Science
School of Health Technology and Management
Stony Brook University
Stony Brook, New York

Susan Smith, PT, PhD
Associate Professor and Director
Physical Therapy and Rehabilitation Services
Drexel University
Philadelphia, Pennsylvania

Rhonda K. Stanley, PT, PhD
Associate Professor, Physical Therapy
Arizona School of Health Sciences
A.T. Still University
Mesa, Arizona

Mark Tarnopolsky, MD, PhD, FRCPc
Professor of Pediatrics and Medicine
Hamilton Hospitals Assessment Center Endowed
    Chair in Neuromuscular Disorders
Director of Neuromuscular and Neurometabolic
    Clinic
McMaster University Medical Center
Hamilton, Ontario, Canada

Elaine Trudelle-Jackson, MS, PT
School of Physical Therapy
Texas Women's University
Dallas, Texas

Anne-Marie Tynan, BA
Research Coordinator
St. Michael's Hospital
Centre for Research on Inner City Health
Toronto, Ontario, Canada

David E. Verrill, MS, RCEP, FAACVPR
Program Coordinator
Presbyterian Hospital Pulmonary Rehabilitation
    Program
Presbyterian Novant Heart and Wellness
Charlotte, North Carolina

Reviewers

Anthony A. Abbott, Ed.D., FACSM, FNSCA
President
Fitness Institute International, Inc.
Boca Raton, Florida

Susan A. Bloomfield, Ph.D., FACSM
Director, Bone Biology Laboratory
Member, Intercollegiate Faculty of Nutrition
Professor
Health & Kinesiology
Texas A&M University
College Station, Texas

Eileen Collins RN, PhD
Research Health Scientist
Edward Hines Jr., VA Hospital, Chicago
Associate Professor
UIC College of Nursing
Chicago, Illinois

Dino G. Costanzo, FACSM, RCEP
Administrative Director
Health Promotion, Bariatrics, and Cardiology
The Hospital of Central Connecticut
New Britain, Connecticut

Brian J. Coyne, M.Ed., RCEP
Instructor
Department of Kinesiology
University of Louisiana at Monroe
Monroe, Louisiana

Cathryn R. Dooly, FACSM
ACSM Exercise Specialist Certified
Chair and Associate Professor
Lander University,
Department of Physical Education & Exercise Studies
Greenwood, South Carolina

Julianne Frey, MS, RCEP
Senior Clinical Exercise Physiologist
Cardiovascular Testing Department
Internal Medicine Associates
Bloomington, Indiana

Dennis J. Guillot, MS, RRT, CSCS, RCEP
Assistant Professor
Human Performance Education Teacher Education
    Nicholls State University
Thibodaux, Louisiana

Chris Kemnitz, PhD
Associate Professor
Department of Nursing
University of Wisconsin–Superior
Superior, Wisconsin

Tom LaFontaine, PhD, FACSM, FAACVPR, CSCS, NSCA-CPT, RCEP
Owner, PREVENT Consulting Services, LLC
Clinical Exercise Physiologist
Co-Director, Optimus: The Center for Health
Columbia, Missouri

James J. Laskin, PT, PhD
Associate Professor
School of Physical Therapy and Rehabilitation Sciences
University of Montana
Missoula, Montana

Randi S. Lite, MA, RCEP
Senior Instructor of Biology
Simmons College
Boston, Massachusetts

Jacalyn J. McComb, PhD, FACSM
Professor in the Department of Health Exercise
    and Sport Sciences
Texas Tech University
Lubbock, Texas

Peter M. Magyari, PhD
Assistant Professor of Exercise Physiology
Brooks College of Health
University of North Florida
Jacksonville, Florida

Jeanne F. Nichols, PhD, FACSM
School of Exercise & Nutritional Sciences
San Diego State University
San Diego, California

Mark A. Patterson, MEd, RCEP
Clinical Exercise Physiologist
Cardiovascular Services/Vascular Surgery
Kaiser Permenante Colorado
Denver, Colorado

Elizabeth J. Protas, PT, PhD, FACSM
Interim Dean and Ruby Decker Endowed Professor
Senior Fellow, Sealy Center on Aging
School of Allied Health Sciences
University of Texas Medical Branch
Galveston, Texas

Jeffrey L. Roitman, EdD, FACSM
Associate Professor, Director Exercise Science Program
Rockhurst University
Exercise Science
Kansas City, Missouri

Peter Ronai, MS, NSCA CSCS-D, NSCA-CPT
Exercise Physiologist
Ahlbin Rehabilitation Centers
Bridgeport Hospital
Bridgeport, Connecticut

William F. Simpson, PhD, FACSM
Associate Professor/Director, Exercise Physiology
    Laboratory
University of Wisconsin–Superior
Department of Health and Human Performance
Superior, Wisconsin

Paul Sorace, MS, RCEP
Clinical Exercise Physiologist
Hackensack University Medical Center
Hackensack, New Jersey

David E. Verrill, MS, RCEP, FAACVPR
Clinical Exercise Physiologist
Presbyterian Hospital Pulmonary Rehabilitation
    Program
Presbyterian Novant Heart and Wellness
Charlotte, North Carolina

Karen Wallman (BEd, BSc (hons), PhD)
School of Sport Science Exercise and Health
Senior Lecturer
University of Western Australia
Perth, Western Australia

Contents

Neuromuscular Disorders

GEORGIA FREY, *Section Editor*

Stroke

EPIDEMIOLOGY AND PATHOPHYSIOLOGY

DEFINITION AND PREVALENCE

The primary cause of stroke is an interruption of blood flow and oxygen delivery to the brain (1,2). Some experts refer to it as a brain attack to relate its symptoms and sequelae with a heart attack. It is also known as a cerebrovascular accident or CVA. Because of the significant improvements in stroke emergency medicine and acute management of stroke, most individuals survive, recover, and experience only a modest decrease in life expectancy (3).

Stroke is the most common cause of adult disability in the United States as well as in many other industrialized nations throughout the world, with the incidence approximately doubling each decade after the age of 55 (4). In the United States alone, the annual rate of stroke prevalence is approximately 700,000; 500,000 of these are first stroke and 200,000 are recurrent stroke (2). Stroke is the second most common cause of death worldwide and the third most common cause of death, behind coronary heart disease and cancer, in Europe and the United States (5). However, most strokes are not fatal and the common occurrence is physical and cognitive impairment that affect daily functioning (6). The health and economic consequences of stroke impose a substantial economic burden on the individual, family, and society at large. In 2004, the medical costs in the United States alone was estimated at $33 billion (1).

Current estimates are that there are 4 million stroke survivors living in the United States (2). Although all segments of the population are affected by stroke, blacks have nearly twice the risk than whites or Hispanics and are more likely to be disabled from a stroke (2). Men have a 30% greater risk of stroke than women in earlier life, whereas women have a greater risk in later life. Despite advances in medical treatment for stroke, it remains the leading cause of disability in adults (2). Although the incidence of severe stroke has decreased, milder stroke incidence has increased, reflecting the important need to maintain health and function through exercise training programs after rehabilitation (7,8).

CLASSIFICATION

A stroke is considered a heterogeneous disorder that can involve the rupturing of a large blood vessel in the brain, or the occlusion of a tiny blood vessel that may affect a certain area of the brain (9). Cell damage and impaired neurologic function associated with strokes result from a restricted blood supply (ischemia) or by bleeding (hemorrhage) into the brain tissue. As such, strokes are classified as *hemorrhagic* or *ischemic*. The injury to the brain affects multiple systems, depending on the site of injury and the amount of damage sustained during the event. These include motor and sensory impairments and language, perception, affective, and cognitive dysfunction (10). Strokes can cause severe limitations in mobility and cognition or can be very mild with only short-term consequences that are often not permanent.

Hemorrhagic strokes are subclassified as intracerebral (bleeding directly into the brain) or subarachnoid (bleeding into the spaces and spinal fluid around the brain), depending on where the injury occurs. Ischemic strokes are usually divided into two types: thrombotic and embolic. Hemorrhagic strokes constitute approximately 15% of all strokes, whereas the ischemic type make up the remainder of strokes (10–12). Risk factors for stroke are listed in Table 1.1.

PATHOPHYSIOLOGY

A hemorrhagic stroke results in blood leaking into the extravascular space within the cranium or into the brain tissue itself. This bleeding damages the brain by cutting off connecting pathways and by causing localized or generalized pressure injury to brain tissue. Biochemical substances released before and after the hemorrhage can also adversely affect vascular and brain tissues (9).

Ischemic strokes result from some type of thrombosis or embolus. *Thrombosis* refers to an obstruction of blood flow owing to a localized occlusion within one or more blood vessels (9). *Thrombotic infarction* occurs when a thrombus or clot forms on an atherosclerotic plaque. *Embolic infarction* results when a material (embolus) formed elsewhere in the vascular system occludes an artery or arteriole (10). Infarcts resulting from occlusion of the carotid artery or proximal middle artery have the worst prognosis (10).

TABLE 1.1. RISK FACTORS FOR STROKE

Ischemic Stroke
- Atherosclerosis—associated with the following risk factors: hypertension, cigarette smoking, hyperlipidemia, diabetes, sedentary lifestyle
- Hypothyroidism
- Use of oral contraceptives
- Sickle cell disease
- Coagulation disorders
- Polycythemia vera
- Arteritis
- Dehydration combined with any of the previous conditions
- Atrial fibrillation

Hemorrhagic Stroke
- Hypertension
- Arteriovenous malformation
- Anticoagulant therapy
- Drug abuse with cocaine, amphetamines, or alcohol

Atrial fibrillation and stroke is a common cause of stroke manifested by a rapid uncoordinated generation of electrical impulses by the atria of the heart. This condition often precedes a stroke and must be controlled with medication to reduce the risk of recurrent stroke.

Clinical features of stroke depend on the location and severity of the injury. Signs of a hemorrhagic stroke include altered level of consciousness, severe headache, and usually elevated blood pressure (13). Cerebellar hemorrhage usually occurs unilaterally and is associated with dysequilibrium, nausea, and vomiting. Hemorrhage into the brainstem is often fatal (10).

Cerebral blood flow (CBF) is the primary marker for assessing ischemic strokes. When CBF drops below 18 mL/100 g/min (normal CBF is 50–55 mL/100 g/min), synaptic transmission failure occurs. When CBF drops below 8 mL/100 g/min, cell death results. The *ischemic cascade* refers to a complex series of biochemical events that result from ischemic stroke (13). Acidosis, altered calcium homeostasis, transmitter dysfunction, free radical production, cerebral edema, and microcirculatory obstruction are all involved in the injury phase. Diagnostic tests used to assess stroke include computed tomography (CT) and magnetic resonance imaging (MRI) (13).

FUNCTIONAL CONSEQUENCES OF STROKE

The injury that occurs as a result of a stroke affects multiple systems, depending on the site of injury and the amount of damage sustained during the event. These include motor and sensory impairments and language, perception, affective, and cognitive dysfunction (10). Strokes can cause severe limitations in mobility and cognition or can be very mild with only short-term consequences that are often not permanent.

COMORBIDITY, SECONDARY CONDITIONS, AND ASSOCIATED CONDITIONS[1]

The loss in function that often accompanies a stroke affects both physical and psychological function (14,15). The magnitude of impairments or activity limitations will vary depending on the severity of stroke. Poststroke depression (PSD) is a very common condition experienced by approximatly 30% of stroke survivors (11). Those with PSD have increased risk of second strokes, cardiovascular events, increased mortality, and increased healthcare costs (11). In efforts to decrease the risk of recurrent stroke, it is critical that risk factor modification, lifestyle modification, and compliance with prescribed pharmacologic therapy are adopted (8).

Many stroke survivors require moderate to extensive care after rehabilitation (16). *Comorbid conditions*, which occur independent of the primary condition, include coronary artery disease (CAD), obesity, hypertension, type 2 diabetes, and hyperlipidemia (17). Secondary conditions, which occur as a direct or indirect result of the primary condition, include a higher incidence of injury from falls, pain, fatigue, stress, depression, and social isolation. Associated conditions, which occur simultaneously with the stroke and directly result from it, include spasticity, weakness (hemiparesis, quadriparesis), paralysis (hemiplegia, tetraplegia), impaired balance, memory loss, aphasia, and sleep apnea (17).

The combination of a loss in physical function and an exacerbation of one or more comorbidit conditions or secondary conditions severely compromises the functional independence and quality of life of many stroke survivors (18). Additionally, persons dealing with the combination of physical limitations and fatigue are even less likely to participate in social and leisure-time activities (19). These conditions add complexity to the design of the exercise prescription for this population. A list of comorbid conditions, and secondary and associated conditions can be found in Table 1.2.

CLINICAL EXERCISE PHYSIOLOGY

ACUTE RESPONSES TO EXERCISE

Many factors associated with stroke negatively affect daily living and functioning (20–23). These factors may be classified as direct medical consequences impacting function, such as the ability to walk or dress independently, or as secondary responses to the degree of impairment or disability, including reduced functional aerobic capacity and activity intolerance (24–29). At discharge

---

[1]A comorbidity exists before having a stroke (e.g., obesity, hypertension). A secondary condition is the direct result of having a stroke (e.g., pain, fatigue).

TABLE 1.2. COMMON ASSOCIATED, SECONDARY, AND CHRONIC CONDITIONS IN STROKE SURVIVORS[a]

ASSOCIATED	SECONDARY	CHRONIC
Spasticity	Depression	Coronary artery disease
Muscle weakness	Social isolation	Hypertension
Balance impairments	Falls	Hyperlipidemia
Paralysis	Memory loss	Diabetes mellitus
Paresis	Low self-esteem	Obesity
Aphasia	Low self-efficacy	Peripheral vascular disease
Visual disturbance	Emotional lability	
Cognitive impairment	Fatigue	

[a]An associated condition is a direct result of a having a stroke and is not preventable; a secondary condition occurs after a stroke and is considered preventable; chronic conditions affect the the general population and do not occur at a higher occurrence in individuals with stroke.

from rehabilitation, most stroke survivors regain their ability to walk independently, but only a small percentage have sufficient functional (aerobic) capacity to ambulate outside of their homes and function effectively within their community (30–33). Furthermore, multiple comorbid conditions associated with stroke, including hypertension, CAD, diabetes, depression, and obesity, worsen recovery and compound the loss in movement and overall function (27–29,34).

Most strokes are caused by vascular disease resulting in physiologic limitations during acute exercise (35,36). The few studies that have assessed the peak oxygen uptake ($\dot{V}O_2$) of stroke survivors have reported very low peak $\dot{V}O_2$ levels in this cohort (37). Most studies reported cardiorespiratory fitness levels (peak $\dot{V}O_2$) in stroke populations between 12.0 $mL\,kg^{-1} \cdot min^{-1}$ and 17.0 $mL\,kg^{-1} \cdot min^{-1}$ (37–39). As a comparison, nondisabled, sedentary but otherwise healthy individuals in a similar age group generally have peak $\dot{V}O_2$ levels that range between 25 and 30 $mL\,kg^{-1} \cdot min^{-1}$ (38).

In randomized, controlled trials involving aerobic exercise training with stroke survivors, changes in peak $\dot{V}O_2$ ranged from 9.0% (40) to 22.5% (41). Potempa et al. (42) reported changes in peak $\dot{V}O_2$ values after 10 weeks of training ranging from 0% to 35.7%. Rimmer et al. (43) used a more severely disabled stroke population and reported a mean improvement of 8.2% after a 12-week intervention. The relatively low baseline aerobic capacity is associated with a number of factors, including multiple comorbid conditions (e.g., CAD, obesity) and lifestyle-related behaviors (e.g., lack of regular physical activity).

Peak heart rate during acute exercise will vary for persons with stroke, depending on their age, level of disability (extent of muscle atrophy on hemiparetic side), number and severity of comorbid conditions (e.g., hypertension, CAD); associated conditions (e.g., spasticity, cognitive impairment); secondary conditions (e.g., pain, fatigue, depression); and medication use (e.g., β-blockers). Potempa et al. (44) noted that some stroke survivors may reach near-normal peak heart rates, whereas others may attain significantly lower peak heart rates for a similar bout of exercise. Although this will vary for each individual, in general, peak heart rates for stroke survivors during acute exercise will be lower than those for persons of the same age and gender who do not have a disability (8). The relatively low aerobic capacity reported in stroke survivors is likely attributed to a reduction in the number of motor units capable of being recruited during dynamic exercise, the reduced oxidative capacity of paretic muscle, and the sedentary lifestyle of most stroke survivors.

Improving functional capacity in stroke survivors can reduce the physiologic burden of performing basic activities of daily living (BADL) and instrumental activities of daily living (IADL), thus increasing the likelihood that individuals with stroke will be able to perform a greater volume of daily physical activity at a lower percentage of their maximal functional capacity (45–47). The 3.77 $\dot{V}O_2$ peak metabolic equivalent (MET) level reported in one study (48) is well below the threshold (energy cost) required to perform various BADL and IADL. This suggests that a given task will require a higher percentage of peak oxygen uptake, making it difficult or impossible to perform these common household chores necessary for independent living.

Muscular strength and endurance are also deficient in stroke survivors. Rimmer et al. (43) evaluated the strength levels of a relatively young group of male and female stroke survivors (Mean age = 53 yr). Mean strength scores 10 repetitions maximum (10-RM) on two LifeFitness machines were 26 lb on the bench press and 147 lb on the leg press. Grip strength on the nonaffected side was 30.7 lb, and on the affected side, 20.4 lb. Considering the average weight of the subjects (M = 200 lb), scores on both of these measures would be less than the tenth percentile according to data reported on nondisabled individuals of the same age and gender (49). Other studies have confirmed low strength scores in this population (50).

PHYSICAL EXAMINATION

The extent of damage occurring from a stroke can be physical and cognitive. Left-hemisphere lesions are typically associated with expressive and receptive language deficits compared with right-hemisphere lesions. The motor impairment from stroke usually results in hemiplegia (paralysis) or hemiparesis (weakness). When damage occurs to the descending neural pathways, an abnormal regulation of spinal motor neurons results in adverse changes in postural and stretch reflexes and difficulty with voluntary movement. Deficits in motor control can involve muscle weakness, abnormal synergistic organization of movements, impaired regulation of force, decreased reaction times, abnormal muscle tone, and loss of active range of motion (ROM) (51).

EXERCISE TESTING AND SCREENING CRITERIA

SCREENING PROTOCOL

Before conducting a graded exercise test, persons with stroke should be screened by their primary care physician. Although no published guidelines exist on the type of screening that should be conducted before a graded exercise test, taking the utmost precaution is critical because many stroke survivors are older and have cardiovascular disease. The screening should include a fasting blood draw, resting electrocardiogram (ECG), resting heart rate, resting blood pressure (standing, seated, supine), and basal temperature. To be approved for peak $\dot{V}O_2$ testing, participants' blood screening tests (i.e., complete blood count [CBC], enzymes, protein levels) should be within normal limits. If the preliminary blood work is acceptable, the participant can be scheduled for testing. Participants who successfully complete the graded exercise test can be recommended for an exercise program. Individuals who have adverse cardiovascular changes during exercise testing should be advised for further follow-up and may need to begin an exercise program in a closely supervised setting, such as cardiac rehabilitation.

EXERCISE TESTING

Peak Oxygen Uptake (Cardiorespiratory Fitness)

Cycle ergometer testing with stroke survivors is considered safe and feasible when a medical prescreening is performed and the participant's exercise response is closely monitored to minimize risk (52). Determination of aerobic exercise capacity is an important component for developing appropriate exercise programs and evaluating the effectiveness of the programming (52). Because of a significant loss of muscle function resulting from hemiparesis or hemiplegia, stroke survivors have a severely reduced maximal or peak oxygen uptake (37,52). Because many stroke survivors also have cardiovascular comorbidity (e.g., hypertension, CAD), graded exercise tests are often symptom-limited, thus not allowing the person to achieve high peak capacities. Additionally, limited

data are available on the test-retest reliability of peak exercise testing among stroke survivors and it is recommended that at least one preliminary testing trial be performed to minimize the possible practice effect (53). In the postacute stage, a symptom-limited graded exercise test (peak $\dot{V}O_2$) can be performed on a stationary bike or treadmill, or in persons with severe hemiplegia, with an arm ergometer. Although it may be necessary to perform the exercise test with an arm ergometer, performance will be limited because of the limited amount of muscle recruitment and a greater strain on the cardiac system per unit of peripheral muscle mass recruited (53). Typically, arm-cranking yields a peak $\dot{V}O_2$ 30%–35% less than treadmill performance. The two most preferred exercise modes are the stationary cycle and treadmill. For individuals with balance difficulties or severe hemiplegia where walking on a treadmill is difficult or not possible, the stationary cycle is preferred because it eliminates the risk of falls.

Ramp Cycle Protocol

There are several different testing protocols that have been used with persons with stroke. Rimmer et al. (43) measured peak $\dot{V}O_2$ in 35 stroke survivors using a ramp cycle ergometer testing protocol. Participants began cycling at a workload of 20 W at a target cadence of 60 revolutions per minute (rpm) and increased by 10 W every minute until maximal effort was achieved. Heart rate and blood pressure were recorded every 2 minutes. Tests were terminated if one of the following criteria was observed: (a) respiratory exchange ratio (RER) ≥ 1.1, (b) peak heart rate within ± 10 beat per min^{-1} of age-predicted maximal value, (c) abnormal blood pressure or ECG response, or (d) unable to continue pedaling above 50 rpm. Potempa et al. (22) used a similar ramp cycle ergometer protocol with stroke survivors. Testing began at 10 W and increased 10 W each minute until maximal effort was attained.

Macko et al. (26) performed several exercise testing and training studies with stroke survivors using a treadmill protocol. They recommended that a treadmill test at 0% incline be conducted before the maximal exercise test to assess gait safety and walking velocity. As a safety measure, individual wore a gait support belt. Participants who successfully completed at least 3 consecutive minutes of treamill walking at .22 m/s or faster (0.5 mph) were allowed to have a maximal exercise stress. After a 15-minute rest, the participants performed a constant velocity, progressively graded treadmill test to volitional fatigue or peak effort and were continuously monitored (ECG and vital signs) during testing.

Tang et al. (52) conducted exercise testing on stroke survivors who were in the subacute (<3 months) stage of recovery. They used a semirecumbent cycle ergometer (Biodex) to perform the exercise test. The ramp protocol included a 2-minute warm-up at 10W at a cadence of 50 rpm, followed by progressive 5 W increases in work rate every minute. The test lasted 8–10 minutes and heart rate, blood pressure, and ECG were monitored during testing. The investigators reported that 89% (31 of 35 participants; 2 participants were excluded because of blood pressure or ECG abnormalities) completed the graded exercise test without incident. Details on criteria for stopping the test are reported in the study and included such things as participant choice, breathing effort, generalized fatigue, or nonaerobic issues such as leg discomfort. Based on the successful completion rate by most of the subjects, the investigators stated that exercise testing is feasible and safe in those in a subacute stage provided pretest medical screening is conducted and ongoing monitoring is performed during testing. It is also recommended that at least one practice trial is conducted before testing to familiarize individuals with the protocol and minimize the potential for confounding training-related benefits.

Based on the studies that have been conducted with this population, several recommendations can be made. First, blood pressure should be measured on the unaffected (nonparetic) arm. Testing time in most of the studies ranged from 4 to 12 minutes. The use of the American College of Sports Medicine (ACSM) test termination guidelines with a more conservative blood pressure endpoint (systolic ≤210 mm Hg) is considered appropriate for patients in the subacute and postacute stages (52).

Strength

Strength testing has been shown to be reliable in stroke populations. Weiss et al. (54) and Ouellette et al. (55) both used 1-RM testing in stroke survivors and found it to be a safe procedure with this population. Rimmer et al. (43) used the 10-RM method on two exercise machines, one measuring upper body strength and one measuring lower body strength in stroke survivors. A handgrip dynamometer was also used to measure grip strength on the affected and nonaffected sides. Strength can be assessed in a number of ways using standard exercise machines, free weights, or dynamometers. Instruction on proper lifting technique must be conducted before testing. Persons with cognitive impairments or severe mobility limitations may require more time to perform the test correctly. Adaptive gloves or Velcro may be necessary to secure a hand to the weight or bar. During the strength assessment, it is important to evaluate each limb separately to determine the disparity in strength between the hemiparetic and nonhemiparetic side. It is also important to ascertain whether the affected limb(s) has sufficient residual innervation to allow strength gains. This is typically determined by manual muscle test of the muscles to be strengthened to see that they can contract and cause

movement against gravity or greater than 'fair grade' strength. If that is the case, then the individual can begin gradual use of weights or related resistance devices. Surface electromyography (EMG) may be helpful as well.

Flexibility

Hamstring and low back flexibility are important muscle groups to evaluate in stroke survivors participating in exercise testing because of the increased spasticity on the hemiparetic side. These muscle groups can be assessed using a modified version of the sit-and-reach test. If sitting on the floor is difficult, a modified version can be performed using a bench. The patient is asked to sit on a bench with legs fully extended and feet placed against the sit-and-reach box. Participants extend their arms and reach in the direction of their feet. The distance from the middle finger to the center of the box is recorded.

A good measure of functional shoulder flexibility is to have the person put one hand over the shoulder (slide the hand down the back) and the other hand behind the back (slide the back of the hand up the middle of the back). The participant is asked to bring the fingers as close as possible to each other. The distance between the two middle fingers of each hand is recorded. Record scores on both sides of the body by reversing the position of the arms. A more comprehensive evaluation of flexibility can be performed with a goniometer.

Body Composition

Body composition measurements should include height, weight, skinfold measures, body mass index (BMI), and waist-to-hip ratio (WHR). The sum of skinfold measurements can be used in place of an estimated percent body fat if the skinfold calipers do not open sufficiently wide to obtain the entire skinfold. Some stroke survivors are severely obese (56) and it may not be possible to obtain an accurate skinfold measure at certain sites (e.g., thigh). Because it is sometimes difficult to distinguish between subcutaneous fat and muscle tissue on the hemiparetic side, it is recommended that skinfold measurements be taken on the noninvolved side.

PRESCRIPTION AND PROGRAMMING

The emphasis in working with stroke survivors traditionally has been directed at rehabilitation during the first 6 months of recovery (16,57). Relatively few studies have been conducted on improving the fitness in stroke survivors after rehabilitation (58). The small number of training studies that have been completed, however, have supported the use of exercise in improving mobility and functional independence and in preventing or reducing further disease and functional impairment in persons with stroke (38,55,59–65). Research data provide evidence that physical activity for stroke survivors is beneficial by documenting reduced risk factors and reduced risk for mortality from cardiovascular disease and stroke (8,66).

Most people with stroke go through a significant recovery period during the first 6 months after having had a stroke, whereas others will see significant recovery for up to a year or longer (8). The goal of resistance training is to maximize recovery and sustain and improve fitness throughout the lifespan (55). The clinical exercise physiologist should work closely with the client's physician or therapist in developing a safe and effective program. Stroke survivors who return home from a hospital or rehabilitation facility shortly after their injury will need greater attention to ensure that cardiovascular adaptations are conducted in a safe environment with timely and appropriate supervision.

CARDIORESPIRATORY ENDURANCE TRAINING

Cardiorespiratory fitness training is of critical importance to stroke survivors. Cardiovascular-related morbidity and mortality remains high after stroke and cardiovascular deconditioning places added risk on the individual (38). Stroke survivors often vary widely in age, severity of disability, motivational level, and number and severity of comorbid conditions, secondary conditions, and associated conditions (Table 1.2). Although gait training and use of the affected side (arm, leg) are major components of stroke rehabilitation, several important studies have suggested that aerobic exercise training should be a critical part of the recovery process (26,38,44,63). Aerobic exercise training can result in improved tolerance performing ADL and allow more physical activity to be completed at a lower submaximal threshold, thus reducing myocardial oxygen demand (67).

FREQUENCY AND DURATION

The goal of the exercise program for stroke survivors should be to have each participant engage in a tolerable level of physical fitness depending on their overall health and function. Thirty to 60 minutes a day most days of the week is ideal, but if the individual has substantial barriers to participating in physical activity (68,69), a lower volume of exercise is also beneficial given their high rate of deconditioning. If the individual is at a higher risk because of cardiovascular comorbidity or falls, suggestion is that the person exercise under the supervision of a qualified staff person, preferably trained in rehabilitation or clinical exercise physiology. Hospital wellness centers are excellent places for stroke survivors to exercise because staff are usually trained in working with individuals who have various types of disabilities. These programs, however, are usually located in only a few select communities.

The cardiovascular exercise program should consist of a warm-up and cool-down. Participants should have their blood pressure checked at regular intervals before, during, and after the training session. The cardiovascular exercise can be continuous or accumulated over the day to total 20–60 minutes (8). Obviously for individuals who are older and more severely deconditioned, smaller doses of physical activity may be necessary (i.e., 5–20 min/day). After the comprehensive screening has been completed according to ACSM guidelines (49), the first 2–4 weeks of the program should be used to train participants in using the equipment and becoming accustomed to the program. Individual goals should be established for each participant to ensure that he or she is exercising within his or her comfort zone and achieving the desired training effect.

INTENSITY LEVEL

When possible, the intensity level of the cardiovascular exercise should be established for each participant from the graded exercise test. The American Heart Association scientific statement on physical activity and exercise recommendations for stroke survivors recommends training at an intensity of 40%–70% of peak $\dot{V}O_2$ or heart rate reserve (HRR) while also monitoring rating of perceived exertion (RPE) (8). In the few studies that have been conducted on stroke survivors, intensity was set at different levels. Rimmer et al. (43) based the intensity level on the participants' peak $\dot{V}O_2$ measure. The heart rate that the participant reached at a respiratory quotient (RQ) of 1.00 was used to set the target heart rate range (THRR). Five beats per minute was subtracted from this value, and the THRR for the participant was then set from this heart rate to 10 bpm below this heart rate. For example, if a participant's heart rate was 130 bpm at an RQ = 1.00, subtracting 5 bpm from this value would put the THRR at 115–125 bpm.

In the work by Potempa et al. (42), initial training for stroke survivors was set at 40%–60% of measured peak $\dot{V}O_2$ for a duration of 30 minutes of continuous or discontinuous exercise. The emphasis during the early stages of the program was on duration as opposed to intensity. Once the person was able to exercise for 30 minutes, training intensity was progressively increased to the highest workload tolerance without cardiac symptoms. It is important to note that the investigators used telemetry monitoring with their subjects and were thus able to be more aggressive in their training intensity.

Macko et al. (26,36,63,67) have done a substantial amount of treadmill training with stroke survivors. Their training protocol started at low intensity (40%–50% HRR) for 10–20 minutes and increased approximately 5 minutes every 2 weeks as tolerated until participants were able to train at 60%–70% of HRR. Teixeira-Salmela et al. (50) used an intensity of 70% of the maximal heart rate attained from an exercise test with a higher functioning group of stroke survivors. Chu et al. (41) developed an 8-week, water-based program for 12 poststroke survivors using shallow water walking, mild running, and various other activities and increased training intensity from 50%–70% HRR (weeks 1–2), to 75% (weeks 3–5), and finally to 80% HRR (weeks 6–8). This is the only study in the published literature that trained stroke survivors at such a high intensity level (80%), although it was only for a couple of weeks. Interestingly, they reported the highest increases in peak $\dot{V}O_2$ (22%) after an exercise intervention with stroke subjects.

In the study by Rimmer et al. (43), participants who had an abnormal blood pressure response during the exercise test (systolic $\geq$220 mm Hg, diastolic $\geq$110 mm Hg) had a modification to their exercise prescription. They were instructed not to exceed a rate pressure product (RPP) of 200. The RPP was calculated by multiplying heart rate times systolic blood pressure, divided by 100. For example, if a participant's blood pressure response during an exercise session was 180 mm Hg at a heart rate of 130 bpm, the RPP would be 180 $\times$ 130/100 or 234. Because the value is more than 200, the participant would not be allowed to exercise on that day or had to wait until RPP dropped below 200.

Resting diastolic blood pressure (DBP) should be less than 100 mm Hg to begin exercising. If resting DBP is greater than 100 mm Hg, ROM exercises should be performed until the DBP drops below 100. Exercise should be terminated if blood pressure is elevated to 220/110 mm Hg or higher and should only be resumed when blood pressure drops below this value.

Participants should begin with intermittent exercise during the first 4 weeks of the program. At the end of 4 weeks, most participants should be able to complete 30 minutes of continuous or discontinuous exercise in their THRR. However, it is important that participants have approval from their physician before participating in the training program and that physicians are updated on their patient's performance at regular intervals.

TRAINING MODALITIES

Examples of cardiovascular training modalities for stroke survivors include stationary cycling (recumbent and upright), over-ground walking, or walking on a treadmill (provided the patients have adequate balance, are closely supervised, and do not experience joint pain), elliptical crosstraining, and recumbent stepping (especially useful for those with severe hemiplegia). Participants should be given the opportunity to select their own equipment as long as it is considered safe and does not cause adverse cardiovascular (i.e., excessive rise in blood pressure or heart rate) or musculoskeletal complications (i.e., pain, injury). Individuals with balance difficulties and a high risk of falls should use a sitting modality such as the recumbent stepper or stationary or recumbent cycle.

Several training advantages are seen to using a treadmill for improving cardiorespiratory fitness, gait, and strength (70). Treadmill training allows the individual to practice walking, which is critical to overall function; handrails and body weight support (BWS) system (i.e., harness) allow professionals to load or unload some of the body weight, depending on the patient's strength and balance; and grade can be used to adjust intensity, allowing a comfortable speed to be maintained (63).

STRENGTH TRAINING

Muscle weakness has been recognized as a major symptom following stroke (71). Research has also demonstrated that the torque generated by the knee extensors, ankle plantar flexors, and hip flexors is correlated to gait performance in stroke survivors (72). Poor levels of strength can also be a major factor contributing to significant functional limitations, reduced walking speed and endurance, impaired stability, and increased postural sway (73–75). The primary goal of strength training is to increase independence in function, which can include walking, prevention of falls, and performing BADL and IADL (76).

TRAINING INTENSITY

No published guidelines exist for developing resistance training programs for persons with stroke. Based on the research, several studies have demonstrated significant improvements in strength using various levels of resistance (73). Training intensity varied from 30%–50% of maximal strength (77), to as high as 80% of 1-RM after a 2-week adjustment period (50,78). One study also found significant improvements in strength using a circuit training program that involved persons with stroke using their body weight as the overload by performing sit-to-stand from various chair heights; stepping forward, backward, and sideways onto blocks of various heights; and performing heel raises.

Rimmer et al. (43) initiated a strength training protocol for stroke survivors at 70% of each participant's 10-RM for one set of 15–20 repetitions. When participants were able to complete 25 repetitions for 2 consecutive sessions with proper lifting technique (i.e., proper biomechanical motion, without Valsalva maneuver), the weight was increased by 10% of their 10-RM. Participants trained using a variety of exercises, including the bench press, leg press, leg curl, triceps push-down, seated shoulder press, seated row, lateral pull-down, and biceps curl.

A general strength training prescription should use a minimum of one set of 8–10 lifts using the large muscle groups of the body, lighter weights, and higher repetitions (e.g., 10–15 repetitions), and perform them 2–3 days a week. Blood pressure and RPE should be recorded at the completion of each set until the person adjusts to the program. Adaptive gloves and other types of assistive aids may be necessary to ensure that the participant can safely hold or grasp the weight.

TRAINING VOLUME

A major determinant of training volume is the amount of muscle mass that is still *functional*. Persons with paralysis, hemiplegia, impaired motor control, or limited joint mobility have less functional muscle mass and, therefore, will only tolerate a lower training volume. For individuals who cannot lift the minimal weight on certain machines, resistance bands or cuff weights are recommended. If bands and cuff weights are too difficult, use the person's own limb weight as the initial resistance. For example, lifting an arm or leg against gravity for 5–10 seconds may be the initial starting point for those with very low strength levels.

Training volume will also depend on the patient's health status. Many individuals with stroke have been inactive for much of their lives and will need only a small amount of resistance exercise during the *initial* stage of the program to obtain a training effect. How responsive individuals with stroke will be to resistance exercise during the *conditioning* stage depend on their current health status and the severity of their stroke. For individuals who start out at very low levels of strength, significant improvements can be made with very light resistance.

TRAINING MODALITIES

Certain muscle groups need strengthening in persons with physical disabilities (including stroke survivors) to maintain the ability to perform BADL (e.g., dressing and undressing) and IADL (e.g., lifting and carrying items, walking up and down stairs). Lifting any type of resistance requires good trunk stability and may be difficult to perform for individuals who have severe limitations in motor control and coordination. Modes of resistance exercise fall into four general categories: free weights, portable equipment (i.e., elastic bands, tubing), machines, and person's own body weight. Any of these modalities is acceptable for improving strength levels in stroke survivors, provided the person is not at risk for injury. When an instructor feels that the resistance mode presents a concern to the person, the exercise routine should be either adapted (e.g., securing the weight to the hand, changing the movement) or substituted with a safer piece of equipment.

In persons with very low strength levels, *gravity-resistance* exercise (lifting limbs against gravity) may be all that the person is capable of performing. Abducting an arm or extending a leg for several repetitions may be a good entry point. These exercises can be used for persons who are extremely weak after a stroke, whereas other modes of resistance exercise can be used those who are stronger. Once an individual is able to complete 8–12 repetitions of a gravity-resistance exercise, the person could progress to free weight, bands, or machines. If an individual is unable to move a limb against gravity because of extreme weakness, the instructor could place the limb in a certain position (e.g., shoulder abduction) and have that person hold the position isometrically for a few

seconds, gradually increasing the time. Horizontal movements and aquatic exercises can be performed with gravity eliminated, thus allowing the limb to move more freely.

Rehabilitation professionals are also recommending the use of treadmill training for improving functional strength in stroke participants. A recent study found that BWS treadmill training increased gait speed and strength in individuals with stroke (70).

Active-assistive exercise may be required for certain individuals who do not have sufficient strength to overcome the force of gravity. The instructor can assist that person in performing the movement by providing as much physical assistance as necessary. At various points in the concentric phase, the instructor may have to assist the person in overcoming the force of gravity. During the eccentric phase, the instructor may need to control the movement so that the weight or limb is not lowered too quickly. In many instances, active-assistive exercise can be used with severely weak musculature whereas *active* exercise can be used with stronger muscle groups.

FLEXIBILITY TRAINING

Participants should be taught a variety of stretching exercises targeting both upper and lower body muscle groups. Participants should stretch at the beginning of each exercise session, at the end of the cardiovascular exercise session, between strength exercises, and at the end of the exercise session. Stretches should held with mild tension for 15–30 seconds, being careful not to cause pain. A particular emphasis should be made to stretch the tight (spastic) muscle groups on the hemiparetic side, which include the finger and wrist flexors, elbow flexors, shoulder adductors, hip flexors, knee flexors, and ankle plantar flexors. The primary goal of flexibility training for stroke survivors is to increase ROM and prevent joint contractures (8).

GENERAL PROGRAM GUIDELINES

STAFF SUPERVISION

Exercise sessions should be supervised by a clinical exercise physiologist with guidance and support from the patient's physician. It is helpful to have an assistant who can be trained to monitor blood pressure, heart rate, and vital signs, especially if several stroke survivors are exercising in the facility at the same time. A recommended staff-to-client ratio will depend on the functional level of the client, number and type of comorbid conditions, associated or secondary conditions, and the expertise of the fitness professional in working with stroke participants.

FACILITY PREPARATION

An emergency contact number should be posted in the exercise facility. If possible, physician pager numbers of stroke survivors should be available. An automated external defibrillator is a good safety device to keep in the fitness center. An infectious waste container for blood specimens should be available for clients who must check their blood glucose level. Blood specimens should be performed in a sterile setting away from equipment and high-volume traffic areas.

CLIENT MONITORING

Given the higher level of comorbid and secondary conditions associated with stroke, it is important for the clinical exercise physiologist to monitor the exercise session closely until the client adjusts to the exercise bout and does not show signs of discomfort or exhibit any unusual symptoms (e.g., fluctuations in blood pressure, dyspnea, light-headedness). One way that many clinical exercise physiologists monitor their client's progress is with a SOAP form. S stands for *Subjective*, which is a client self-report of his or her current state (e.g., how much sleep they had, do they feel well, did they eat breakfast, did they take their medication(s), symptoms). O stands for *Objective*, which is the clinical staff's evaluation of the participant's current state and quantitative performance during the exercise session (i.e., modality, workload, blood pressure response, physiologic signs). A stands for *Assessment*, which is how the clinician interprets S and O. P stands for *Plan*, which refers to the prescribed or recommended treatment plan, including modifications that need to be made to the exercise prescription in the next session (e.g., trying a new exercise, increasing resistance). At the end of each session, blood pressure and heart rate should be recorded to ensure that the participant returns to resting values before departure from the fitness center.

The instructor should attempt to provide a program that is appropriate in intensity, mode, duration, frequency, and progression to minimize the likelihood of developing prolonged or unusual *fatigue* and *delayed-onset muscle soreness*. Although this occasionally can be a common side effect of any new training regimen, it could present a problem for persons with stroke if the soreness prevents them from conducting their normal BADL or IADL. Although a client with stroke may aspire to make rapid gains in strength and can train at a moderate-to-high intensity level, the clinical exercise physiologist should be cautious not to overwork the muscle groups. Use light resistance for at least the first 2 weeks of the program (50% of 1-RM), and only proceed to higher training loads if muscle soreness and fatigue are not evident and no other side effects are evident. A verbal evaluation of the previous session should be conducted with the patient on return for the next session. If it is determined that some soreness in certain muscle groups prevented the person from performing routine daily activities, the exercise should be discontinued until the soreness improves. On continuation of the program, the clinical exercise physiologist may need to reduce the training volume or

avoid certain exercises that result in pain or fatigue. If prolonged bouts of pain or soreness occur 24–48 hours after exercise, the client should consult with his or her physician to determine the cause.

It is worth repeating that blood pressure must be monitored closely in persons with stroke. Because hypertension is a common comorbidity, follow the guidelines in ACSM's *Guidelines for Exercise Testing and Prescription* for working with persons with hypertension (49). It is especially important for the person's blood pressure to be under control before initiating the program. During the first 4 weeks of the program, monitor blood pressure frequently to ensure that complications or adverse changes are not occurring. If blood pressure continually fluctuates, contact the patient's physician. Under no circumstances should a person who has had a stroke and continues to have difficulty maintaining a stable blood pressure be allowed to exercise.

Persons with type 1 diabetes should bring their own portable glucometer to the fitness center and take a blood glucose measurement before and after each exercise session. Orange juice and other high carbohydrate snacks should be available for those who become hypoglycemic (<50 mg $\cdot$ dL^{-1}). Participants should be encouraged to drink adequate amounts of water during the exercise session to avoid dehydration.

Many individuals with stroke will exhibit asymmetrical weakness or will have a disproportionately greater degree of weakness to the flexor or extensor muscle groups. It is important to evaluate individual muscle groups on both sides of the body, including both agonists and antagonists, to isolate the degree of weakness in key muscle groups. Individuals with asymmetric weakness will often "hike" their body toward the weaker side to compensate for this weakness while performing resistance training. Make sure that each person is performing the activity with proper form. If there is a tendency to "hike" the body, lower the resistance and emphasize good form.

An important goal of the clinical exercise physiologist is to teach the client how to measure his or her own RPE, how to use the equipment safely, and to understand the warning signs when to stop exercising. A sample checklist of safety guidelines for self-regulating exercise is shown in Table 1.3. Stroke survivors should also be taught the warning signs for when they should stop exercising. Table 1.4 provides a list of items that should be reviewed with each person. Once the persons understands these warning signs and can repeat them back to the instructor, both parties should sign the form. This assures the instructor that the client has a basic understanding of how to exercise safely.

EDUCATION AND COUNSELING

The clinical exercise physiologist has an important responsibility to teach stroke survivors the importance of good

TABLE 1.3. SAMPLE CHECKLIST FOR TEACHING CLIENTS TO PERFORM EXERCISE SAFELY

Client Name: _____ Staff Name: _____ Date:_____

Before participation in an exercise program, you must be able to competently execute the tasks listed below. If you have difficulty performing any of these tasks, you will receive additional training before participating in the program.

Able to monitor target heart rate.	
Able to use the rating of perceived exertion (RPE) scale.	
Knows the warning signs to stop exercising.	
Able to safely operate the treadmill.	
Able to program the treadmill.	
Able to safely operate the upright bike.	
Able to program the upright bike.	
Can record aerobic and strength activities on assigned log sheet.	
Display knowledge of the goals of strength training.	
Know what a set is.	
Know what a repetition is.	
Can adjust the bench press to fit him or her.	
Can display proper form when using the bench press.	
Can display proper breathing (lack of Valsalva maneuver) when using the bench press.	
Can adjust the leg press to fit him or her.	
Can display proper form when using the leg press.	
Can display proper breathing (lack of Valsalva maneuver) when using the leg press.	
Can adjust the shoulder press to fit him or her.	
Can display proper form when using the shoulder press.	
Can display proper breathing (lack of Valsalva maneuver) when using the shoulder press.	
Can adjust the triceps push-down to fit him or her.	
Can display proper form when using the triceps push-down.	
Can display proper breathing (lack of Valsalva maneuver) when using the triceps push-down.	
Can adjust the biceps curl to fit him or her.	
Can display proper form when using the biceps curl.	
Can display proper breathing (lack of Valsalva maneuver) when using the biceps curl.	
Can adjust the front row to fit him or her.	
Can display proper form when using the front row.	
Can display proper breathing (lack of Valsalva maneuver) when using the front row.	
Can adjust the lat pull-down to fit him or her.	
Can display proper form when using the lat pull-down.	
Can display proper breathing (Lack of Valsalva maneuver) when using the lat pull-down.	
Can adjust the hamstring curl to fit him or her.	
Can display proper form when using the hamstring curl.	
Can display proper breathing (lack of Valsalva maneuver) when using the hamstring curl.	

health promotion practices (mind–body relationship) where clients and their caregiver can learn about various strategies to enhance their health. Limited access to healthcare and healthcare follow-up, combined with lack of health education and health awareness, presents formidable barriers to effective health promotion in this population. Subsequently, many stroke survivors do not understand the importance of good health maintenance (e.g., diet, exercise, health behavior) in preventing a recurrent stroke and the educational component is an extremely important part of the exercise plan.

Structured lectures that address questions and misconceptions should be an integral part of the program. Participants must learn new ways to think about changes in their lives following a stroke and thus facilitate healthier living. Group discussions about stressful events related to stroke (e.g., change in family roles) can be an important part of the educational component and can be used to facilitate development of peer support relationships. Through these peer relationships, participants can help each other develop new ways to think about coping and adapting following their stroke and identify ways to incorporate exercise, healthier

TABLE 1.4. GUIDELINES FOR SELF-REGULATING EXERCISE IN STROKE PARTICIPANTS

You understand that you are being asked to exercise within your own comfort level. During exercise, your body may give you signs that you should stop exercising.

These signs Include:

Lightheadedness or dizzyness
Chest heaviness, pain, or tightness; angina
Palpitations or irregular heart beat
Sudden shortness of breath **not due to increased activity**
Discomfort or stiffness in muscles and joints persisting for several
    days after exercise

Call your doctor if you experience any of these sensations.

Please call your exercise instructor at (111-1111) if you experience any of the following signs:

A change in your medication.
A change in your health, such as:
    An increase or change in blood pressure, resting heart rate (just
        sitting around), or other symptoms related to your heart
    Hospitalization for any reason
    Cold/flu
    Emotional stress or upset at work or at home
    Any other change that you feel is important
    Your doctor advises you to stop exercising for any reason

I realize that it is my responsibility to report any of these signs/symptoms to my **DOCTOR**. Once the situation is resolved, I must contact **MY INSTRUCTOR, Clinical Exercise Physiologist, at 111-1111.**

Signature of Participant	Date
Signature of Instructor	Date

cooking and eating habits, and new approaches to adjusting to life changes living with a disability.

BARRIERS TO EXERCISE

Rimmer et al. (79) examined barriers to exercise in persons with stroke and other physical disabilities. Data were collected through an in-depth telephone interview using an instrument that addressed issues related to physical activity and the subjects' disability (*Barriers to Physical Activity and Disability Survey*–B-PADS). Sub-

jects were asked questions pertaining to their participation or interest level in structured exercise. The four major barriers were cost of the exercise program (84.2%), lack of energy (65.8%), transportation (60.5%), and did not know where to exercise (57.9%). Barriers commonly reported in nondisabled persons (e.g., lack of time, boredom, too lazy) were not observed in this cohort. Interestingly, only 11% of the subjects reported that they were not interested in starting an exercise program. Most subjects (81.5%) wanted to join an exercise program, but were restricted by the number of barriers reported. The investigators noted that black women with stroke and other physical disabilities were interested in joining exercise programs, but were limited in doing so because of their inability to overcome several barriers to increased physical activity participation.

In a more recent study (69), researchers reported that the five most common barriers reported by a cohort of stroke survivors in rank order were (1) cost of the program (61%), (2) lack of awareness of fitness center in the area (57%), (3) no means of transportation to get to a facility (57%), (4) don't know how to exercise (46%), (5) don't know where to exercise (44%). Least common barriers were (1) lack of interest (16%), (2) lack of time (11%), and (3) exercise will make my condition worse (1%).

To increase exercise adherence among stroke survivors, the clinical exercise physiologist must first assess and subsequently work with the individual and other support systems to problem-solve removing as many of the actual (i.e., transportation) and perceived (i.e., exercise will not improve condition) barriers as possible. Available resources should be utilized, such as the National Center on Physical Activity and Disability (www.ncpad.org, 800/900-8086), which is a federally funded information center that contains many useful physical activities for people with stroke, including ways to reduce or remove barriers to participation by providing home exercise videos and a listing of organizations and facilities that provide specialized programs for people with disabilities. The website also provices access to the aforementioned B-PADS instrument, which a useful way to sytematically identifyand remove barriers to particiption for stroke survivors.

CASE STUDIES

It should be noted that in all cases, physical, occupational, and speech therapists had seen these patients and completed programs in these allied healthcare disciplines. Physician care included primary management by an internist and a neurologist, with other specialty consults, as needed. A psychiatrist, cognitive psychologist, or both were also involved in patient care where needed for depression and deficits in task processing were noted.

CASE 1

RM: 55-year-old married businessman, retired because of a cerebrovascular accident, which left him with partial left hemiplegia (hemiparesis). Chief complaint at the time of visit was tightness of the left shoulder and reduced grip strength, especially notable when golfing. There was also a longstanding history of recurrent low back pain with x-rays showing degenerative joint disease in the spine. Medications: Plavix, Bayer ASA, Procardia, Zocor, MVI, vitamins B_6, B_{12}, and folic acid. With patient upright, his posture showed a left shoulder droop relative to the right side. Rhomberg sign was negative. Gait up to 2 miles/hour was normal. He was unable to walk on a narrow straight line for 10 feet without making a side balance error. He was able to do a partial squat. Spine ROM showed blocking of movement with side tilt to the right side. The shoulder ROM was limited to 90 degrees for abduction and 100 degrees for forward flexion, 50 degrees of 90 degree abducted-external rotation. There were no one-sided sensory, position sense, or one-sided sensory neglect deficits detected. Babinski sign was absent and muscle stretch reflexes were normal. Cranial nerves showed a mild left facial paresis. A program with the exercise physiologist was conducted for 20 sessions over a 9-month period. Initially, he was able to walk 2 mph for 10 minutes, and reached a heart rate of 130 bpm. He could hold a 2 lb. weight in the left hand, although was unable to use the thumb. He could not control a coffee cup full of fluid without spilling it. Exercises to establish a neutral spine posture were initiated. Isometric program for the left scapular muscles was initiated with feedback from a take-home electrical muscle stimulation device. He was able to progress to diagonal pattern upper extremity exercises and some grip movements of the left thumb. His endurance improved to 4 mph for 20 minutes at a heart rate of 140 bpm. The low back pain became more evident as the patient became more active and played golf 3 times per week, completing 18 holes, using a golf cart for transportation. X-rays showed osteophytes and degenerative joint changes in the facets, sacroiliac, symphysis pubis, and hip joints, no change since x-rays taken 5 months earlier. Fluoroscopically guided injection was done to the left sacroiliac joint, which reduced pain and interference from guarding of that area during sessions with the exercise physiologist.

Problems to Consider

Left hemiparesis primarily involved the left upper extremity, the most common form of hemiparesis. Usually some muscles are spared, but it is rare to see complete sensorimotor hemiplegia of every muscle group on the left side. Deficits on the left side sometimes are more obvious with fatigue after a period of ambulation at a given speed, or after an increased challenge to coordination, such a line-walking

Low back pain, which may lateralize to the side of poorest function, but the presence of pain alerts the healthcare practitioner that the individual is aware of affected side. The biomechanical deficits associated with low back pain in this case are questionable. X-rays show a long history of low back cumulative wear that probably extends before the onset of the stroke. X-rays without findings of unstable conditions, such as stress fracture

(spondylolysis), osteoporotic fracture, or tumors, will not interfere with the exercise program. It is important to address motor control of the oblique muscles of the lumbopelvic girdle, emphasizing spine posture and avoiding fatigue to those muscles. Isometric exercises, while maintaining the neutral spine (the most relaxed midposition between full spine flexion and full spine extension), will be beneficial. Weakness and increased tone of the muscles on the hemiplegic side should be noted.

Golfer. The fact that the client is still able to golf demonstrates an ability to swing right-handed. Assistive devices, such as the tube device hooked to a glove for the left hand, may minimize grip deficits and optimize the individual's ability to coordinate the movements of the upper extremity. He was also able to sometimes golf in the 90s score range because of focus on ball direction instead of distance. The emphasis in this program was first normal trunk control, then head position and retraining of the scapular movement with the golf swing.

The electromuscle stimulation machine was prescribed to increase muscle contraction beyond the individual's ability to do it simply by his own volition. Such devices are used in disorders of the central nervous system to (*a*) compensate for loss of maximal contraction owing to loss of central nervous system input and (*b*) provide increased feedback to the brain by the sensory input from the electrical impulse to the muscle. It is important to know the difference between this device and other devices, such as a transcutaneous stimulation machine. The latter only stimulates skin sensors to try to block pain, but does not have the proper electrical settings to reach muscle.

CASE 2

DK: 46-year-old woman with juvenile onset diabetes mellitus (type 1), smoker, suffered a cerebrovascular accident at age 17 and has a history of seizures. This left her with a spastic type of hemiparesis of the right upper and lower extremities and aphasia (expressive type). Her chief complaint is of difficulty with sustained daily activities and exercise because of the hemiplegia. In addition, she complains of tender points in the left hand over the thenar (thumb) muscle pad in the palm along with pain and numbness into her fingers of that hand, the left tensor fascia lata, and the left heel. Her lifestyle was basically self-care, community errands, and a long-term relationship with a boyfriend. She finished high school, but never developed a career. She smoked one-half pack per day. Medications: Tegretol, Dilantin, Provera, Valium, metoprolol, gabapentin, cyclobenzaprine, alendronate, and Insulin pump (implantable device for infusion of insulin instead of injection needles). On physical examination, she was an alert, oriented person who understood and obeyed either simple or multistep instructions. Her speech was markedly limited by nonfluent use of single words and phrases and she often corrected herself. Naming of simple objects, such as a pen or watch, resulted in mispronunciations and nonwords. She could communicate during most routine conversation if allowed to self-correct. Sensation was decreased, but present for the right side, no neglect or sensory extinction was noted. The presence of the trigger points in the areas of tenderness supported the absence of neglect on the right side. Increased tone was noted in the right lower extremity with a knee-extended gait. Posturing of the foot was partially masked by previous ankle/tendon surgery for equinovarus ankle posturing. Increased tone was noted in the right hand in the form of a grip posture. Range of motion was otherwise, normal. Pressure over any of the trigger points would cause a sudden spastic response. Reflexes were increased for the right upper and lower extremities, Babinski sign was positive on the right, but negative on the left side. Strength and motor control were evaluated. Volitional movements tended to follow flexion or extension synergy patterns on the right side. Movement could be isolated for the scapulothoracic and hip muscles. The individual could assume upright posture with cuing. The individual entered a clinical exercise physiology program for a period of 6 months. The first 3 months involved every-other-week visits for endurance and a home exercise program. She was independent and safe in the community at the time of initial visit, however her speed of gait was approximately 1.5 mph and very labor intensive with aerobic level heart rates greater than 130 bpm. She was unable to progress in the program initially, owing to the painful trigger points described. Phenol blocks were performed twice over the treatment period, which provided marked relief of symptoms and reduction in spasticity. The second 3 months of the program was done in an exercise class setting. She made marked progress in the ability control the right lower extremity during the swing phase of gait. She also was prescribed a plastic ankle-foot brace. The right upper extremity function improved with the combined effect of improved scapular control with electrical muscle stimulation and the use of a wrist-hand brace to help positioning for gross grip of objects during daily activity and weight training. She initially avoided use of the right upper extremity, but by the end of the treatment session she was able to use it as an assist in two-handed activities with the left upper extremity. Throughout the program, blood glucose levels were monitored and low blood sugars less than 60 mg · dL^{-1} were treated with a high glucose content beverage. High blood sugars were addressed with increased water ingestion. Dietary adjustments and insulin pump (physician or nurse adjusted) dosage changes were made in response to increased physical activity, blood glucose and glucometer readings, and physical symptoms. The program is now focusing on help toward further education and career pursuits.

Problems to Consider

In insulin-dependent diabetes, even with an implantable device, wide fluctuations of blood sugar can occur, resulting in loss of consciousness or lethargy. Lethargic mood can be misinterpreted as fatigue, lack of enthusiasm, or poor ability to follow instructions.

Aphasia is a broad family of classifications to describe communication deficits in relationship to organic brain disorders. They can be considered most simply as primarily disorders of comprehension or disorders of expression. Disorders of comprehension aphasias are the most difficult to address during exercise programs. This individual was primarily in the expressive disorders category. Aphasia should not be confused with *apraxia*, in which the individual can appropriately name objects and converse, but has difficulty with the formation of words. Also, *paralysis* of facial muscles or the tongue, such as an injury to a nerve, is not aphasia. If a patient has an aphasia, then communication through a very few written words and pictures can improve exercise comprehension and compliance.

Spasticity and increased tone in the spine and extremities must be addressed by first working with muscles that do have near normal function. Then, progression extends to the next group of muscles, usually spine-related muscles first, followed by more distal muscles, in the hope of sequential spread of motor control. Spasticity is usually stimulated an undesirable increase in response to fast movements or sudden large loads for resistance training. Single sustained submaximal contractions, rather than fast repetitions may be better. *Proprioceptive neuromuscular facilitation* is used to describe various forms of feedback through either tapping or light pressure during use of the muscle desired. The individual should be positioned in a lying or sitting position to avoid excessive spasticity response. Electrical muscle stimulation may have a biofeedback effect in combination with a voluntary contraction of a given muscle.

Contracture of the hemiplegic ankle received *tendon lengthening surgery* to relieve the contracture. Contractures can respond at least in part to single prolonged stretching, sometimes in excess of 2 minutes. If surgery is done, then the contracture will be relieved, but anticipate weakening of that muscle as a side effect of the surgery.

Tender points and trigger points are specific mapped out areas where tenderness can be greatest in a muscle. The tenderness can cause a noxious (pain) response that may lead to muscle guarding and spasticity. Phenol blocks either to a trigger point or to the actual nerve or its junction in the muscle may reduce the spasticity and pain.

One-sided neglect was not present in this individual. This is important in stroke because brain injury can affect sensory processing areas. The patient can sometimes feel the paralyzed side; however, neglect is when both sides are stimulated at the same time with the individual stating that she can only feel one side.

Smoking history is part of the risk factor profile that accompanies stroke. In this case, her pulmonary function may be a limiting factor during exercise. An inquiry regarding her pulmonary function is important, especially if she is short of breath.

Pharmacologic issues: Be aware of reduced patient arousal because of the somnolence side effects of her medications (e.g., muscle relaxant [cyclobenzaprine], antiseizure medications [carbamazepine]). Metoprolol is a β-blocker that reduces maximal heart rate and may limit her exercise endurance.

Nerve conduction studies and needle electromyography testing were used to discover the slowed median nerve conduction across the wrist called carpal tunnel syndrome, explaining the numbness and pain in the nonhemiplegic left hand. Electrical stimulation by a recording device measures the speed and size (amplitude) of nerve conduction to determine if the nerve is healthy or injured. She has both a nerve pinch (i.e., carpal tunnel syndrome) and diabetes, which will also show abnormal results on nerve conduction study. The needle form of electromyography is also used to assess for loss of motor nerve function or muscle disease by observing the electrical muscle membrane and muscle contraction potentials heard and viewed on a screen.

CASE 3

JP: 72-year-old man suffered a cerebrovascular accident 2 years before his visit. He was a depressed gentleman, a retired successful businessman, and he had a history of participation in competitive sports. His chief complaint was lack of improvement from a left hemiparesis after the stroke and lack of energy. Extensive medical work-up uncovered sleep apnea and a home airway (CPAP) device was implemented through an affiliated sleep laboratory. He needed help in bathing, dressing, and for community walks greater than household distances (i.e., 50 feet). He could eat, but not cut his own food. A wheelchair was used for community mobility pushed usually by his wife. His wife would state that he had several falls at home while ambulating, none with any injury. Medications: Dilantin, Coumadin, Synthroid, Prozac, Zocor, MVI, Digoxin. The physical examination noted a tall slender man with clear speech and communication, but with wandering of thoughts during his responses and slowed responses. He showed a left facial hemiparesis. He could repeat five of seven numbers in forward order, but was unable to repeat them in reverse order. He also would tend to avoid looking over to his left side and would not pay attention to his left arm hanging off of the wheelchair. He displayed minimal movement of the proximal scapula-related muscles and no voluntary motor response in the more distal upper extremity. The lower extremity strength was graded fair in the proximal muscle of the hip and knee and poor in more distal muscles of the ankle and foot. Sensation was

partially decreased on the left side, with sensory extinction on simultaneous (left and right tested at the same time) light touch. Grafesthesia was also impaired but present on the left side. Reflexes were decreased on the left side, with a positive Babinski sign on the left and right sides. Cranial deficits were noted in facial muscles on the left side. No aphasia was present. He needed several attempts to arise from a sitting to a stand position. However, with a quad cane he did ambulate at less than 1 mph with no deviations at that speed on noncarpeted surface. He had a foot drop and would have difficulty clearing his toe during swing phase of gait. He entered the clinical exercise physiology program to improve both safety in ambulation and focus on details as they related to a home exercise program. The goal was also to facilitate maximal use of the left upper extremity and attention to his left side. Throughout the program he displayed interruption in ambulation, reaching tasks, and therapeutic exercises, accompanied by random conversations about issues that concerned him. He would also periodically bump his left side in the doorway or other obstacles. The program was adjusted to raise his awareness by having him navigate various obstacle courses and objects to reach another point. He was noted to not bump into these obstacles when asked specifically to walk around them. He also gradually responded to verbal cues to the left side. Resistance exercise for the right side involved lifting the left extremities. Electrical muscle stimulation pulsed to turn on every 5 seconds for 5 seconds duration was used to cue muscles of the left shoulder, and left hip- and knee-related muscles. No gait training was done on the treadmill, because his speed of ambulation was initially 0.6 mph and never faster than 1.5 mph. He was successful in the cessation of any falls at home. His speed of ambulation increased, and he could discontinue his left plastic ankle foot orthosis without a foot drop at the end of 6 months of the program, on an every-other-week basis. His left upper extremity became functional for arm swing during ambulation. He was successfully connected with psychological support care, as well as support counseling for him and his wife.

Problems to Consider

One-sided neglect is a problem most common to individuals who have had a stroke to the right (or dominant side) hemisphere with left hemiplegia. They will ignore the left side of the body, often as if it did not exist. Setting up safe challenges that requires the individual to become aware of that side, such as an obstacle course, is one form of cuing to that side. Other strategies are to use the recognized extremities to find and use the neglected side in bilateral two-extremity exercises. Biofeedback, such as electrical stimulation with activities, can be useful.

Sensory extinction is the absence of recognition of a sensory stimulus to one extremity when both are touched. For example, if both extremities recognize a sensory stimulus when touched or pin-pricked one at a time, one side will not be recognized if both are simultaneously touched. This sensory extinction is considered a sign of a one-side brain injury or disease. *Grafesthesia*, or the recognition of numeric signs gently traced (no marker or inks), is another organic brain function test.

Depression and distractibility appear the same, but are different in the underlying cause. Depression is a disorder of the mind, with feelings of helplessness and hopelessness. People with depression may not be very arousable and will appear distractible. Organic brain diseases will often have distractibility without depression because of lack of arousal. In this case, depression played a significant role in the individual's distraction.

Flaccid hemiparesis is distinct from the *spastic hemiparesis* in that the muscles show decreased activity, both with voluntary and sudden involuntary movement. The hemiparesis described above was of the flaccid type. For muscles that do function, repetitive movement exercises are not a problem as they would be with the spastic form.

Domestic falls are considered a functional concern, even if the individual is noted to have strength and coordination adequate for ambulation and arising from a sitting position. The problem may be distractibility, fatigue, or desire to move to another location faster than is safe to move with a hemiparesis. Challenges in the clinic, such as fast ambulation and obstacle courses, help to deter further falls. Other causes, such as vertigo, heart failure, medication side effects, and an unsafe household with throw rugs, uneven surfaces, and slippery bathrooms must be addressed as well.

REFERENCES

1. Mackay J, Mensah GA, Mendis S, Greenlund K. World Health Organization. *The Atlas of Heart Disease and Stroke*. Geneva: World Health Organization; 2004.
2. Rosamond W, Flegal K, Friday, G, et al. Heart disease and stroke statistics—2007 update. A report from the American Heart Association Statistics Committee and Stroke Statistics Subcommittee. *Circulation* 2007;115:e69–e171.
3. Lopez-Yunez A. The management of stroke patients by neurologists: Common questions and new observations. *Semin Neurol* 2002,;22(1):53–61.
4. Feigin V, Lawes CM, Bennett DA, et al. Stroke epidemiology. A review of population-based studies of incidence, prevalence, and case-fatality in the late 20th century. *Lancet Neurol* 2003;2:43–53.
5. Pendlebury S. Worldwide under-funding of stroke research. *Int J Stroke* 2007;2:80–84.
6. Wolfe C. The impact of stroke. *Br Med Bull* 2000;56:275–286.
7. Khadilkar A, Phillips K, Jean N, Lamothe C, Milne S, Sarnecka J. Ottawa panel evidence-based clinical practice guidelines for post-stroke rehabilitation. *Top Stroke Rehabil* 2006;13(2):1–269.
8. Gordon N, Gulanick M, Costa F, et al. Physical activity and exercise recommendations for stroke survivors: An American Heart Association scientific statement from the Council on Clinical Cardiology, Subcommittee on Exercise, Cardiac Rehabilitation, and Prevention; the Council on Cardiovascular Nursing; the Council on Nutrition, Physical Activity, and Metabolism; and the Stroke Council. *Circulation* 2004;109(5):2031–2041.
9. Caplan L. *Stroke. A Clinical Approach*, 3rd ed. Boston: Butterworth-Heinemann; 2000.
10. Collins C. Pathophysiology and classification of stroke. *Nurs Stand* 2007;21(28):35–39.
11. Williams LS, Kroenke K, Bakas T, et al. Care management of post-stroke depression: A randomized, controlled trial. *Stroke* 2007; 38(3):998–1003.
12. Rich DQ, Gaziano JM, Kurth T. Geographic patterns in overall and specific cardiovascular disease incidence in apparently healthy men in the United States. *Stroke* 2007;38(8):2221–2227.
13. Stewart DG. Stroke rehabilitation. 1. Epidemiologic aspects and acute management. *Arch Phys Med Rehabil* 1999;80(5 Suppl 1):S4–S7.
14. Kwok T, Lo RS, Wong E, Wai-Kwong T, Mok V, Kai-Sing W. Quality of life of stroke survivors: A 1-year follow-up study. *Arch Phys Med Rehabil* 2006;87(9):1177–1182; quiz 1287.
15. Lai SM, Studenski S, Richards L, et al. Therapeutic exercise and depressive symptoms after stroke. *J Am Geriatr Soc* 2006;54(2): 240–247.
16. Teasell R, Foley N, Bhogal S, Bagg S, Jutai J. Evidence-based practice and setting basic standards for stroke rehabilitation in Canada. *Top Stroke Rehabil* 2006;13(3):59–65.
17. Black-Schaffer RM, Kirsteins AE, Harvey RL. Stroke rehabilitation. 2. Co-morbidities and complications. *Arch Phys Med Rehabil* 1999;80(5 Suppl 1):S8–S16.
18. Rimmer JH, Shenoy SS. Impact of exercise on targeted secondary conditions. In: Field MJ, Jette AM, Martin L, eds. *Workshop on Disability in America*. Washington, DC: National Academies Press; 2006.
19. Roth EJ, Lovell L. Community skill performance and its association with the ability to perform everyday tasks by stroke survivors one year following rehabilitation discharge. *Top Stroke Rehabil* 2007; 14(1):48–56.
20. Ebrahim S. *Clinical Epidemiology of Stroke*. New York: Oxford University Press; 1990.
21. Gordon NF. Stroke. Your Complete Exercise Guide. The Cooper Clinic and Research Institute fitness series. Champaign, IL: Human Kinetics; 1993.
22. Kelly JF. Stroke rehabilitation for elderly patients. In: Kemp B, Brummel-Smith K, Ramsdell JW, eds. *Geriatric Rehabilitation*. Boston: Little, Brown and Company; 1990: 61–89.
23. Pauls JA, Reed KL. *Quick Reference to Physical Therapy*. Gaithersburg, MD: Aspen; 1996.
24. Ramasubbu R, Robinson RG, Flint AJ, Kosier T, Price TR. Functional impairment associated with acute poststroke depression: the Stroke Data Bank Study. *J Neuropsychiatry Clin Neurosci* 1998;10(1): 26–33.
25. Alberts MJ, Easton JD. Stroke best practices: A team approach to evidence-based care. *JAMA* 2004;96(4 Supplement):5S–20S.
26. Macko RF, DeSouza CA, Tretter LD, et al. Treadmill aerobic exercise training reduces the energy expenditure and cardiovascular demands of hemiparetic gait in chronic stroke patients. A preliminary report. *Stroke* 1997;28(2):326–330.
27. Wolf PA, Claggett GP, Easton JP, et al. Preventing Ischemic Stroke in Patients With Prior Stroke and Transient Ischemic Attack: A Statement for Healthcare Professionals From the Stroke Council of the American Heart Association. *Stroke* 1999, 30: 1991–1994.

28. Niemi ML, Laaksonen R, Kotila M, Waltimo O. Quality of life 4 years after stroke. *Stroke* 1988;19:1101–1107.

29. Black-Schaffer RM, Kirsteins AE, Harvey RL. Stroke rehabilitation: Co-morbidities and complications. *Arch Phys Med Rehabil* 1999; 80:S8–S16.

30. Corr S, Bayer A. Poor functional status of stroke patients after hospital discharge: Scope for intervention? *Br J Occup Ther* 1992;55:383–385.

31. Dean CM, Richards CL, Malouin F. Task-related circuit training improves performance of locomotor tasks in chronic stroke: A randomized controlled pilot trial. *Arch Phys Med Rehabil* 2000;81(4): 409–417.

32. Hill K, Ellis P, Berhnardt J, Maggs P, Hull S. Balance and mobility outcomes for stroke patients: A comprehensive audit. *Aust J Physiother* 1997;43:173–180.

33. Goldie PA, Matyas TA, Evans OM. Deficit and change in gait velocity during rehabilitation after stroke. *Arch Phys Med Rehabil* 1996; 77:1074–1082.

34. Duncan PW, Samsa GP, Weinberger M, et al. Health status of individuals with mild stroke. *Stroke* 1997;28:740–745.

35. Mackay-Lyons MJ, Makrides L. Exercise capacity early after stroke. *Arch Phys Med Rehabil* 2002;83:1697–1702.

36. Macko RF, Katzel LI, Yataco A, et al. Low-velocity graded treadmill stress testing in hemiparetic stroke patients. *Stroke* 1997;28(5): 988–992.

37. Rimmer JH, Wang E. Aerobic exercise training in stroke survivors. *Top Stroke Rehabil* 2005;12(1):17–30.

38. Ivey F, Macko RF, Ryan AS, Hafer-Macko CE. Cardiovascular health and fitness after stroke. *Top Stroke Rehabil* 2005, 12(1):1–16.

39. Pang M, Eng JJ, Gylfadottir S, et al. The use of aerobic exercise training in improving aerobic capacity in individuals with stroke: A meta-analysis. *Clin Rehabil* 2006;20:97–111.

40. Duncan P, Studenski S, Richards L, et al. Randomized clinical trial of therapeutic exercise in subacute stroke. *Stroke* 2003;34(9): 2173–2180.

41. Chu KS, Eng JJ, Dawson AS, Harris JE, Ozkaplan A, Gylfadottir S. Water-based exercise for cardiovascular fitness in people with chronic stroke: A randomized controlled trial. *Arch Phys Med Rehabil* 2004;85(6):870–874.

42. Potempa K, Braun LT, Szidon JP, Fogg L, Tincknell T. Physiological outcomes of aerobic exercise training in hemiparetic stroke patients. *Stroke* 1995;26:101–105.

43. Rimmer JH, Riley B, Creviston T, Nicola T. Exercise training in a predominantly African-American group of stroke survivors. *Med Sci Sports Exerc* 2000;32(12):1990–1996.

44. Potempa K, Braun LT, Tinknell T, Popovich J. Benefits of aerobic exercise after stroke. *Sports Med* 1996;21:337–346.

45. Binder EF, Burge SJ, Spina R. Peak aerobic power as an important component of physical performance in older women. *J Gerontol Med Sci* 1999;54A(M353–M356).

46. Malbut-Shennan K, Young A. The physiology of physical performance and training in old age. *Coron Artery Dis* 1999;10:37–42.

47. Rimmer JH, Nicola T. Stroke and exercise. In: *ACSM's Resources for Clinical Exercise Physiology for Special Populations*. Baltimore: Lippincott Williams & Wilkins; 2002.

48. Rimmer JH, Riley B, Creviston C, Nicola T. Exercise training in a predominantly African-American group of stroke survivors. *Med Sci Sports Exerc* 2000;32:1990–1996.

49. American College of Sports Medicine. *ACSM's Guidelines for Exercise Testing and Prescription*, 7th ed. Baltimore: Lippincott Williams & Wilkins; 2006.

50. Teixeira-Salmela LF, Olney SJ, Nadeau S, Brouwer B. Muscle strengthening and physical conditioning to reduce impairment and disability in chronic stroke survivors. *Arch Phys Med Rehabil* 1999, 80(10):1211–1218.

51. Duncan PW. Synthesis of intervention trials to improve motor recovery following stroke. *Top Stroke Rehabil* 1997;3:1–20.

52. Tang A, Sibley KM, Thomas SG, McIlroy WE, Brooks D. Maximal exercise test results in subacute stroke. *Arch Phys Med Rehabil* 2006;87(8):1100–1105.

53. McArdle W, Katch FI, Katch VL. *Exercise Physiology: Energy, Nutrition and Performance*. Baltimore Lippincott Williams & Williams; 2006.

54. Weiss A, Suzuki T, Bean J, Fielding RA. High intensity strength training improves strength and functional performance after stroke. *Am J Phys Med Rehabil* 2000;79(4):369–376.

55. Ouellette M, LeBrasseur NK, Bean JF, et al. High-intensity resistance training improves muscle strength, self-reported function, and disability in long-term stroke survivors. *Stroke* 2004;35:1404–1409.

56. Rimmer JH, Wang E. Obesity prevalence among a group of Chicago residents with disabilities. *Arch Phys Med Rehabil* 2005;86(7): 1461–1464.

57. Duncan PW, Lai SM, Keighley J. Defining post-stroke recovery: Implications for design and interpretation of drug trials. *Neuropharmacology* 2000;39(5):835–841.

58. Meek C, Pollock A, Potter J, et al. A systematic review of exercise trials post stroke. *Clin Rehabil* 2003;17:6–13.

59. Ivey FM, Hafer-Macko CE, Macko RF. Exercise rehabilitation after stroke. *NeuroRx* 2006;3(4):439–450.

60. Pang MY, Eng JJ, Dawson AS, et al. A community-based fitness and mobility exercise program for older adults with chronic stroke: A randomized, controlled trial. *J Am Geriatr Soc* 2005;53(10): 1667–1674.

61. Patten C, Lexell J, Brown HE. Weakness and strength training in persons with poststroke hemiplegia: rationale, method, and efficacy. *J Rehabil Res Dev* 2004;41(3A):293–312.

62. Rimmer J. Exercise and physical activity in persons aging with a physical disability. *Phys Med Rehabil Clin N Am* 2005;16(1): 41–56.

63. Macko RF, Ivey FM, Forrester LW, et al. Treadmill exercise rehabilitation improves ambulatory function and cardiovascular fitness in patients with chronic stroke. A randomized, controlled trial. *Stroke* 2005;26:2206–2211.

64. Macko RF, Ivey FM, Forrester LW, et al. Treadmill exercise rehabilitation improves ambulatory function and cardiovascular fitness in patients with chronic stroke: A randomized, controlled trial. *Stroke* 2005;36(10):2206–2211.

65. Ivey FM, Ryan AS, Hafer-Macko CE, Goldberg AP, Macko RF. Treadmill aerobic training improves glucose tolerance and indices of insulin sensitivity in disabled stroke survivors: a preliminary report. *Stroke* 2007;38(10):2752–2758.

66. Rimmer JH, Rauworth AE, Wang E, Nicola TL, Hill B. A preliminary study to examine the effects of aerobic and therapeutic (non-aerobic) exercise on cardiorespiratory fitness and coronary risk reduction in stroke survivors. *Arch Phys Med Rehabil*. In press.

67. Macko RF, Smith GV, Dobrovolny CL, Sorkin JD, Goldberg AP, Silver KH. Treadmill training improves fitness reserve in chronic stroke patients. *Arch Phys Med Rehabil* 2001;82(7):879–884.

68. Rimmer J. The conspicuous absence of people with disabilities in public fitness and recreation facilities: Lack of interest or lack of access? *Am J Health Promot* 2005;19:327–329.

69. Rimmer J, Wang E, Smith D. Barriers associated with exercise and community access for individuals with stroke. *J Rehab Res Develop* 2008;45:315–322.

70. Sullivan K, Brown DA, Klassen T, Mulroy S, Winstein CJ. Effects of task-specific locomotor and strength training in adults who were ambulatory after stroke: Results of the STEPS randomized clinical trial. *Phys Ther*. 87:1580–1602.

71. Yang Y, Wang R, Lin K, Chu M, Chan R, : Task-oriented progressive resistance strength training improves muscle strength and functional performance in individuals with stroke. *Clin Rehab* 2006;20: 860–870.

72. Sharp S, Brouwer BI. Isokinetic strength training at the hemiparetic knee: effects on function and spasticity. *Arch Phys Med Rehabil* 1997;78:1231–1236.

73. Morris S, Dodd KJ, Morris ME. Outcomes of progressive resistance strength training following stroke: A systematic review. *Clin Rehabil* 2004;18:27–39.

74. Kim C, Eng JJ. The relationship of lower-extremity muscle torque to locomotor performance in people with stroke. *Phys Ther* 2003;83: 49–57.

75. Tihanyi T, Horvath M, Gazekas G, Hortobagyi T, Tihanyi J. One session of whole body vibration increases voluntary muscle strength transiently in patients with stroke. *Clin Rehabil* 2007;21: 782–793.

76. Patten C, Lexell UJ, Brown HE. Weakness and strength training in persons with poststroke hemiplegia: Rationale, method, and efficacy. *J Rehabil Res Dev* 2004;41(3A):293–312.

77. Badics E, Wittman A, Rupp M, Stabauer B, Zifko UA. Systematic muscle building exercises in the rehabilitation of stroke patients. *J Neurorehabil* 2002;17:211–214.

78. Texeira-Salmela L, Nadeau S, McBride I, Olney SJ. Effects of muscle strengthening and physical conditioning training on temporal, kinematic and kinetic variables during gait in chronic stroke survivors. *J Rehabil Med* 2001;33:53–60.

79. Rimmer JH, Rubin SS, Braddock D. Barriers to exercise in African American women with physical disabilities. *Arch Phys Med Rehabil* 2000;81(2):182–188.

Cerebral Palsy

EPIDEMIOLOGY AND PATHOPHYSIOLOGY

In 1959, cerebral palsy (CP) was viewed as an unchanging disorder of movement and posture that appeared early in life and was caused by a nonprogressive brain lesion (1). With advancements in the understanding of CP, the view has expanded and it is now considered an umbrella term that encompasses a group of nonprogressive, but changing motor impairments that affect muscle tone and occur secondary to early development lesions or anomalies in the motor control areas of the brain (2). It is important to note that, although the brain lesion is static, the resultant movement disorder many times is not, and symptoms may improve or become worse (3). Nelson and Ellenberg (4) found that half of all children diagnosed with CP and two-thirds of those diagnosed with spastic diplegia by their first birthday had "outgrown" the motor signs of the condition by age 7. Other studies have shown that the motor skills of children diagnosed with dystonic and athetoid CP can continue to worsen for years (4,5).

The overall incidence of CP in the United States is 1.5–2.5 per 1,000 live births (3). The incidence is higher among black children in the United States (7) and among ethnic minority children in other parts of the world (8,9). The Metropolitan Atlanta Developmental Disabilities Surveillance Program reported in 2000 that the prevalence of CP in the five-county metropolitan area of Atlanta was 3.1 per 1,000, with a higher prevalence among males and blacks (10). Sinha et al. (11) reported incidences of CP among Asian families in the Yorkshire region of Britain of between 5.48 and 6.42 per 1,000 live births. The Surveillance of Cerebral Palsy in Europe reported an increasing trend in the prevalence of CP in Europe from 1.7 per 1,000 live births in the 1970s to 2.4 per 1,000 live births in the 1990s. Also, a strong association was noted between socioeconomic status and the occurrence of CP. In the United Kingdom, the prevalence of CP was 3.33 per 1,000 in the poorest socioeconomic quartile compared with 2.08 per 1,000 in the most affluent quartile. This was true for both children of normal birth weight as well as low birth weight children (12).

The most readily identified cause of CP is the combination of prematurity and low birth weight (13). The diagnosis of CP has been associated with several prenatal factors, including viral infections, maternal substance abuse, multiple births, congenital brain malformations, and certain genetic conditions. In addition, certain perinatal factors, such as anoxia from traumatic delivery, hemorrhage with direct brain damage from birth trauma, and kernicterus, may all cause CP. Postnatal factors occurring before the age of 2, such as viral and bacterial meningitis, traumatic head injury, anoxia, and toxin-induced encephalopathy, are also considered risk factors for CP (13). According to Stanley et al. (14), CP is the result of a causal pathway rather than a single event. This pathway identifies multiple causal factors that lead to the child developing CP. For example, multiple births may lead to preterm delivery, and preterm delivery can lead to neonatal cerebral damage and, ultimately, CP. These factors increase the child's vulnerability to other causal factors, such as intrauterine growth restriction, which may decrease the child's capacity to cope with intrapartum stress.

Classification of CP may be done using physiologic (Table 2.1) or anatomic (Table 2.2) categorization, or by predominant movement disorder (Table 2.3). Classification allows the categorization of CP into subtypes that display certain specific characteristics. For each person with CP, the type and degree of motor impairment, combined with other effects of diffuse brain damage, ultimately determines functional level and the need for a variety of intervention services, regardless of classification.

The prevalence of other conditions related to CP has also been noted in the literature. Saito et al. (15) reported a 68% incidence of scoliosis in those diagnosed with spastic CP. Scoliosis usually started before the age of 10 and progressed rapidly during the growth period. Risk factors for progression of scoliosis in this population included having a spinal curve of 40 degrees before the age of 15 years, having spasticity which involved the total body, being bedridden, and having a thoracolumbar curve.

Odding et al. (12) also reported an increased incidence of CP-related impairments. Motor impairment in some form was found in 100% of children with CP. The incidence of musculoskeletal impairments increased in those with spastic type of CP and included hip luxations (75%), joint contractures (73%), and scoliosis (72%).

TABLE 2.1. PHYSIOLOGIC CLASSIFICATION OF CEREBRAL PALSY (13,79)

TYPE	SITE OF INJURY	PRESENTATION
Pyramidal	Cortical system	Spastic, hyperreflexia, "clasp-knife" hypertonia, susceptible to contractures
Extrapyramidal	Basal ganglia and cerebellum	Athetosis, ataxia, "lead-pipe" rigidity, chorea
Mixed	Combination of above	Combination of above

TABLE 2.2. ANATOMIC CLASSIFICATION OF CEREBRAL PALSY (13,79)

TYPE	PRESENTATION
Hemiplegia	Unilateral involvement; upper extremity generally more involved than lower extremity
Diplegia	Bilateral involvement; legs generally more involved than arms
Tetraplegia	Total body involvement, including cranial nerves; frequently with mental retardation
Monoplegia	Single limb involvement
Paraplegia	Legs only involved; arms normal
Triplegia	One limb unaffected

They also reported cognitive impairments in 23%–44% of cases. Sensory impairments included decreased stereognosis and proprioception, speech impairments, and dysarthria. Ophthalmic abnormalities were seen in 62% of children with CP. Urogenital impairments were also noted in 25% of children with CP having primary urinary incontinence. Endocrine impairments noted in this population included feeding problems, silent aspiration, growth disturbances, body mass issues, and reduced bone mineral density. Del Giudice et al. (16) reported that 92% of children with CP in their sample had clinically significant gastrointestinal (GI) symptoms. These included swallowing disorders, regurgitation and vomiting, abdominal pain, chronic pulmonary aspiration, and chronic constipation. They concluded that most of these GI clinical manifestations were the result of motility disorders and were not related to any specific brain damage.

CLINICAL EXERCISE PHYSIOLOGY

Limited research has been conducted on exercise responses in individuals with CP. This may be related to the fact that participation in exercise programs has been limited in this population. This lack of participation should not be construed as a lack of desire to participate. In many instances, lack of participation is related to a paucity of programs designed for, or accessible to, persons with disabilities.

In some individuals with CP, impaired motor function can cause a decrease in daily activity and diminished function associated with physical activity (17–18). Persons with CP have also been reported to have increased adiposity (17), low muscle force (19), lower aerobic and anaerobic power (18,20), decreased mechanical efficiency (20), and decreased respiratory function (21). All of these factors are signs of poor overall fitness. This may be related to poor exercise habits, difficulty in performing skilled movements, muscle imbalances, or overall poor functional strength. It has also been reported that fatigue and stress associated with a strenuous exercise program can cause a transient increase in spasticity and discoordination in persons with CP (22).

Exercise testing of individuals with CP may be difficult because of their spasticity and dyskinesia, and the inefficient nature of their mobility often leads to higher than expected exercise response values. Studies examining

TABLE 2.3. CLASSIFICATION OF CEREBRAL PALSY BASED ON MOVEMENT DISORDER (3,47)

CLASSIFICATION	PRESENTATION
Spastic cerebral palsy	Present in ~65 % of those with CP; diplegia most common; typically greater lower extremity involvement than upper (diplegia, hemiplegia, extremity; involves flexors, adductors, and internal rotators greater than their antagonists; hypotonia at birth progressing tetraplegia, paraplegia, to spasticity after infancy; increased DTR; clonus; abnormal postural reflexes.monoplegia, triplegia)
Dyskinetic cebebral palsy	*Athetosis*—slow, writhing motions of the appendicular musculature; present in ~25% of those with CP; impairment of dystonia, chorea, ataxia) postural reflexes; nonrhythmic involuntary movement; dysarthria; dysphagia; signs increase with anxiety, absent during sleep.
	Dystonia—sustained muscle contractions that result in twisting and repetitive movement or abnormal posture; present in 15%–25% of those with CP; persists throughout life, but no joint contractures or deformities owing to continuous movement.
	Chorea—state of excessive, spontaneous movements, irregularly timed; nonrepetitive and abrupt; unable to maintain voluntary muscle contraction; present in ~25% of those with CP.
	Ataxia—uncoordinated, voluntary movements; wide-based gait with genurecurvatum; mild intention tremors; in the infant, generalized hypotonia; normal DTR; in its mildest form, called *apraxia,* which is an inability to perform coordinated voluntary gross and fine motor skills.
Mixed cerebral palsy	Present in ~20% of those with CP; both spastic and dyskinetic components

CP, cerebral palsy; DTR, deep tendon reflex.

heart rate, blood pressure, expired air, and blood lactate have shown that individuals with CP respond with higher heart and respiratory rates, as well as elevated blood pressures and blood lactate levels for a given submaximal work rate than those without CP. Peak physiologic responses are also lowered (10%–20%) in persons with CP. Physical work capacity has been shown to be 50% that of able-bodied subjects (22). Bowen et al. (23), however, reported no statistically significant differences in the percentage of variability of oxygen cost, oxygen consumption, or physiologic cost index between subjects with and without CP at free-walking velocity.

PHARMACOLOGY

Pharmacotherapy for the movement disorders of CP has focused on the dyskinesia that most affects the person's functional level. Several main drugs are used to treat the types of involuntary movements found in CP, specifically dystonia, myoclonus, chorea and athetosis, and spasticity (24).

The main categories of drugs used to treat dystonia, myoclonus, chorea, athetosis, and spasticity are listed in Table 2.4. Up to 50% of patients with dystonia positively respond to anti-Parkinsonian drugs and less than 25% respond positively to antispasticity, dopaminergic, or anticonvulsant drugs. Anticholinergic drugs may be helpful in controlling the drooling in CP and may be delivered via a transdermal patch. Drugs used for myoclonus typically are anticonvulsants which facilitate the action of γ-aminobutyric acid (GABA), the principal inhibitory neurotransmitter in mammalian brain. Benzodiazepines are often used to treat chorea and athetosis, but are subject to development of tolerance. Neuroleptics, which block dopamine receptors, are effective drugs for chorea and athetosis, but they are also associated with the most permanent side effects and are the most problematic with chronic use. Spasticity may be of either cerebral or spinal origin, and each requires a specific drug therapy. Baclofen, however, has been shown to be effective in controlling both cerebral and spinal spasticity (24).

Continuous intrathecal baclofen is perhaps the first highly effective medical treatment of spasticity in persons with CP (25) and it has been used for more than 15 years (26). The first double-blind study on the use of intrathecal baclofen for spinal spasticity reported that lower extremity spasticity was significantly reduced and that muscle tone on the Ashworth scale was decreased from 4.0 (considerable increased tone–passive movement difficult) before treatment to 1.2 (slight increased tone) after treatment (27). Baclofen has no direct effect on improving function, although it improves the effectiveness of other treatments, such as physical therapy (28).

General indications for continuous intrathecal baclofen infusion are to improve function, to facilitate care, and to retard or prevent the development of contractures. Another uncommon indication is to decrease pain associated with involuntary muscle spasms. According to Albright (26) and Bodensteiner (29), continuous intrathecal baclofen is indicated for treating spasticity in four distinct groups: (a) those whose gait and lower extremity movements are impeded by spasticity, but whose underlying strength is poor; (b) individuals older than age 16 with spasticity of the lower or both the upper and lower extremities that is interfering with gait or lower extremity function; (c) nonambulatory persons with spastic quadriparesis whose spasticity interferes with their activities of daily living (ADLs), comfort, and endurance; and (d) nonfunctional persons in whom the goal is to enable their care.

Almeida et al. (30) described a case study in which the reflex status, range of motion (ROM), strength, and motor performance of an 11-year-old boy with spastic diplegia were assessed before and following implantation

TABLE 2.4. PHARMACOLOGIC MANAGEMENT OF CEREBRAL PALSY (24,79)

DISORDER	CATEGORY	EXAMPLES	SIDE EFFECTS
Dystonia	Anti-Parkinsonian, anticholinergic, anticonvulsants, dopaminergic, antispasmotics, antidopaminergic and antidepressants	Baclofen, carbamazepine, clonazepam, levadopa/, carbidopa lorazepam, reserbine tetrabenazine, trihexyphenidyl	Drowsiness, dizziness, weakness fatigue, skin rash, bone marrow suppression, ataxia, nausa, hepatotoxicity, depression, psychosis, dry mouth, blurred vision, and nervousness
Myoclonus	Anticonvulsants	Clonazepam, valproate, phenobarbital, baclofen, piracetam, lorazepam	Drowsiness, dizziness, weakness, ataxia, fatigue, sedation, dry mouth, and hyperactivity
Chorea/ Athetosis	Anticonvulsants, neuroleptics	Baclofen, clonazepam, fluphenazine, haloperidol, pimozide, reserbine, tetrabenazine, valproate	Drowsiness, dizziness, weakness, dizziness, weakness, fatigue, skin rash, bone marrow suppression, hepatotoxicity, ataxia, sedation, extrapyramidal reactions, and depression
Spasticity	Muscle relaxants, antispasmotics	Baclofen, dantrolene, diazepam	Drowsiness, fatigue, hepatotoxicity, ataxia, and diarrhea

of an intrathecal baclofen pump. They showed that spasticity, Babinski reflexes, clonus, strength, and coactivation of antagonist muscles during voluntary movement were decreased following baclofen administration. They also reported an increase in hip and ankle ROM and upper extremity movement speed, as well as improved independence in dressing and transfers and elimination of orthoses. Gerszten et al. (31) reported that continuous intrathecal baclofen for the treatment of spastic CP reduces the need for subsequent orthopedic surgery for the effects of lower extremity spasticity. They further recommended that in people with spastic CP, spasticity should be treated before orthopedic procedures are performed.

Continuous intrathecal baclofen has no affect on athetosis, ataxia, and chorea, and is contraindicated for choreathetoid CP, ataxic CP, and for individuals with severe contractures. It may be effective in treating extensor rigidity that occurs after anoxic episodes and appears to improve generalized dystonia. Children receiving continuous intrathecal baclofen have demonstrated insignificant increases in plasma baclofen (32). Excessive dosages of baclofen result in patient listlessness, apathy, urinary hesitancy, or leg weakness, but these symptoms respond readily to lowering the dosage (25). Complications owing to the intrathecal catheter occur in approximately 20% of patients, and infection requiring the removal of the pump occurs in approximately 5% of patients (33).

Physicians have used neuromuscular blocking agents, such as 45% ethyl alcohol, 4%–6% phenol, local anesthetics, or botulinum A toxin to treat the muscle imbalance, spasticity, and joint deformities associated with CP for over 30 years. The neuromuscular blockade may be used to interrupt the function of the nerve, the neuromuscular junction, or the muscle. The blockade is used to balance agonist–antagonist muscle forces by (*a*) diminishing stretch reflexes through neural destruction and blocking of nerve transmission (phenol, alcohol, local anesthetic); (*b*) preventing or decreasing muscle fiber contraction by direct muscle fiber destruction (alcohol or phenol); or (*c*) blocking neuromuscular junction activity (botulinum A toxin). The goal is complete or partial paralysis of the agonist muscle while leaving antagonist muscles unaffected. All neuromuscular blockade procedures are contraindicated in the presence of fixed contractures (34).

Local anesthetics can be used diagnostically to differentiate between dynamic deformity and fixed contracture or to evaluate the performance of antagonist muscles and to determine the potential functional effects of longer-acting agents. Injection of the drugs within the target muscle in the vicinity of the myoneural junction produces the maximum blockade effect. No well-controlled studies have documented the effectiveness of alcohol injection in modifying spasticity in those with CP. Reports in peer-reviewed literature indicate that the clinical effects of alcohol vary in duration and that there are occasional complications, including the need for anesthetic because of the pain. Phenol, which produces a functional and clinical effect for 3–18 months, depending on the concentration and duration of exposure, may also be extremely painful if injected in the vicinity of a sensory nerve. However, phenol has been reported as safe, simple, and economically advantageous in children with CP (34).

The use of botulinum A toxin, although widely used as a neuromuscular blockade, is a bit more controversial. Botulinum A toxin was first introduced to treat strabismus and blepherospasm and is now being used in an increasing number of conditions, including involuntary tremor, focal dystonias (e.g., spasmodic torticollis), and autonomic disorders (e.g., focal hyperhydrosis of the palms) (35). Botulinum A toxin has been used in persons with CP to diminish paravertebral spasticity, to facilitate positioning and hygiene, to improve ambulation, as an alternative to serial casting, diagnostically to determine the efficacy of surgery, as an adjunct to further therapy, to facilitate or replace bracing, to delay surgery, and to improve upper extremity function (34–38). Following injection, the onset of weakness is usually detectable in 2 or 3 days. Generally, weakness wears off by 3 months, but functional improvement may last considerably longer (37). Treatment may be given at periodic intervals, as long as continued efficacy is documented. A positive response rate of 70% has been reported in appropriately selected ambulatory patients (34). Massin and Allington (39) demonstrated that botulinum A toxin was effective in reducing the energy cost of movement and in improving the endurance of spastic muscles in children with CP.

Postoperative pain in children with CP is often a problem and may be difficult to manage with traditional analgesics, such as opiates and benzodiazepines. Barwood et al. (40) conducted a double-blind, randomized, placebo-controlled clinical trial looking at the analgesic affect of botulinum A toxin in children with CP following surgery. They found that botulinum A toxin reduced mean pain scores by 74%, reduced mean analgesic requirements by 50%, and reduced mean length of hospital stay by 33%. They concluded that an important part of postoperative pain in this population was caused by muscle spasm, which can be effectively managed by preoperative injection of botulinum A toxin.

Few adverse effects from botulinum A toxin injection have been reported, and when they have occurred, they are generally mild. The most common complaints were excessive weakness in the injected muscle or unwanted weakness in adjacent muscles (37). Other side effects may include pain around the injection site, frequent falls from balance problems, and generalized fatigue (41). Contraindications for the use of botulinum A toxin include fixed contracture, the presence of certain neuromuscular diseases (e.g., myasthenia gravis), treatment with medications that may exaggerate the neuromuscular blockade response, muscles that fail to respond to alcohol or phenol injections, the absence of objective benefit, or the presence of botulinum A toxin antibodies (34). The presence of such antibodies may contribute to a phenomenon known as *secondary unresponsiveness*, where an individual fails to respond to botulinum A toxin on a subsequent administration, after an earlier successful treatment. The presence of these antibodies is reported to be 3%–10% in adults, but thus far the incidence has not been established in children (42). Disadvantages include the requirement of repeated treatment at regular intervals and cost (35).

The controversy that exists regarding the use of botulinum A toxin relates to a perceived lack of scientifically rigorous studies on the efficacy of the treatment. Forssberg and Tedroff (43) reviewed the literature on botulinum A toxin and found scientific rigor lacking in the published studies. Lannin et al. (44) conducted a systematic review of the effectiveness of therapy for children with CP after botulinum A toxin injections and concluded that insufficient evidence existed to either support or refute the use of therapy interventions after this treatment. Reeuwijk and Van Schie (45) also concluded that insufficient evidence existed to support the use of botulinum A toxin injections to reduce spasticity or increase ROM and upper limb function in people with CP. In addition, a Cochrane review published in 2007 (46) reported that there was not strong evidence to either support or refute the use of botulinum A toxin injections for the treatment of leg spasticity in children with CP. However, consensus is that more, well-designed and well-controlled studies are needed to better evaluate the efficacy of botulinum A toxin, inducing functional improvements in people with CP.

PHYSICAL EXAMINATION

In children with CP, movement disorders become apparent as the nervous system matures and new motor skills are learned. This produces what appears to be a progressive rather than a static disorder. The extent of the disorder may not be recognized until the child reaches age 2 or 3 years or even later. A definitive diagnosis of CP is rarely made before age 6 months and many times much later, but certain clinical findings should arouse suspicion of the diagnosis (47).

Children with CP commonly exhibit tonal abnormalities, such as hypotonia, hypertonia, or a combination of both. Hypotonia may be identified by increased ROM of the shoulders and hips. Hypertonicity of the lower extremities may be present if the infant displays a scissoring posture of the legs. Asymmetry of movement or posture between the right and left sides of the body should be evaluated for possible dysfunction (47). Prechtl (48) reported that even at very early infancy, distinct movement patterns called general movements are predictive of neu-

rologic outcome over 2 years, in particular the presence of CP.

Persistence of primitive reflexes and the delayed appearance of postural reflexes are consistent with a diagnosis of CP. Asymmetry of reflex response should also be regarded as significant. Both hyperreflexia of the deep tendon reflexes and ankle clonus should signal further evaluation. Abnormal behavioral characteristics, such as irritability, irregular sleep patterns, continuous gross motor activity, delayed speech, and diminished attention span, are more subtle, but may signify central nervous system dysfunction. Additional behavioral signs include delayed achievement of motor milestones, which is often the first recognized sign and primary complaint (47).

MEDICAL AND SURGICAL TREATMENTS

Conservative treatment of people with CP is directed at improving overall function and facilitating care. Besides traditional physical and occupational therapy, a number of different approaches have been used. Traditional therapy has focused on improving strength and ROM to promote improved function through a combination of therapeutic exercise, neurodevelopmental treatment (NDT), and motor learning approaches (49). The efficacy of such treatments alone has been questioned. Law et al. (50) found no significant differences in upper extremity function, quality of movement, or parents' perception of functional performance in children with CP between a group receiving intensive NDT and casting, and a group receiving regular occupational therapy programs. Weindling et al. (51) found no difference in functional outcomes between infants at high risk for CP receiving NDT and a group whose therapy was delayed until abnormal signs were present. Bower et al. (52) reported that, in children with CP, the use of specific measurable goals directed at motor skill acquisition was more strongly associated with the actual skill acquisition than either conventional amounts or intensive amounts of physical therapy alone.

Several studies have demonstrated the positive effects of various conservative interventions. Normal movement with emphasis on weight bearing in children with spastic CP has been shown to significantly increase femoral neck bone mineral content and volumetric bone mineral density (53). Carlson et al. (54) showed that using an ankle-foot orthosis during gait training provided biomechanical benefits with more efficient gait in children with spastic diplegia, whereas using supramalleolar orthoses appeared to have little measurable effect. No differences in walking speed, energy cost, and perceived exertion have been shown when using anterior versus posterior walkers among children with CP who were familiar with both walkers, and most children preferred the posterior walker (55).

Exercise can also be viewed as a treatment to improve physical functioning in this population. Damiano and

Abel (56) showed that children with spastic diplegia and spastic hemiplegia could have significant strength gains in targeted muscles following a 6-week strength training program. In addition, they demonstrated that, with increased strength, these children had higher gait velocities with increased cadence, as well as an increase in the Gross Motor Function Measure with no increase in energy expenditure. Swimming has been shown to improve baseline vital capacity in children with CP (21). Van den Berg-Emons et al. (18) looked at the effects of two 9-month sports programs on level of daily physical activity, fat mass, and physical fitness in children with spastic CP. They found that the children involved in the training had no increase in fat mass compared with the control group who showed an increase. Also noted, were a favorable increase in muscle strength and peak aerobic power in those involved in the training program.

Surgical intervention in persons with CP is designed to improve function by relieving spasticity or by correcting deformity. Selective dorsal (posterior) rhizotomy (SDR) is the surgery used to treat spastic diplegia and quadriplegia in children with spastic CP. Numerous studies have demonstrated the effectiveness of this procedure (57). Wright et al. (58), Steinbok et al. (59,60) found that SDR in combination with physical, occupational therapy, or both leads to significantly greater functional improvement at 1 year following surgery than either physical therapy or occupational therapy alone. The functional improvement was achieved through reduced knee and ankle tone, increased ankle dorsiflexion ROM, and more normal foot-floor contact during gait. Buckon et al. (61) compared SDR and orthopedic surgery outcomes using the Gross Motor Performance Measure, the Gross Motor Function Measure, and the Pediatric Evaluation and Disability Inventory. They found that both surgical interventions demonstrated multidimensional benefits for ambulatory children with spastic diplegia. Subramanian et al. (62) reported that SDR alleviated spasticity resulting in lasting functional benefits as measured by improved gait in children with spastic CP.

Postoperative weakness following SDR has been reported (63), but it is not consistently confirmed. For example, Engsberg et al. (64,65) found no loss of hamstring or ankle plantar flexor strength following SDR.

Abbott (63) reported various complications, either immediately postoperative or at long term follow-up after SDR. Besides postoperative hypotonia, other complications include persistent sensory loss, postoperative urologic dysfunction, cerebrospinal fluid leakage around the wound, subdural hematomas, and headache. Long-term complications include changes in postural spinal alignment, low back pain, spondylolisthesis, soft tissue contractures, hip dislocation, and persisting neurogenic bladder. Buckon et al. (61) found no significant decrease in upper extremity muscle tone at 1 year following SDR in ambulatory children with spastic CP.

Stereotactic surgery of the basal ganglia for the improvement of rigidity, choreoathetosis, and tremor in persons with CP is another option (66). The surgery involves placing a well-planned lesion either in the ventrolateral nucleus of the thalamus or ventroposterior pallidum and the site is chosen based on the predominance of individual symptoms. Speelman and van Manen (67) conducted a 21-year follow-up on people who received stereotactic surgery for CP and found subjective improvement in function in 44% of the sample, with 64% reporting side effects, such as hemiparesis and speech impairments. In persons with unilateral dystonia, tremor, and choreathetoid symptoms, it is the consensus that this surgery is very successful (66).

Surgery to correct upper and lower extremity deformity in persons with CP generally falls into one of three categories: (a) soft tissue releases; (b) tendon transfers; or (c) bone/joint stabilization. Table 2.5 describes these procedures with specific examples of how each is used in the upper and lower extremity (68,69).

Hip problems, such as subluxation or dislocation, are commonly seen in children with CP and they are usually related to the severity of involvement. The incidence of hip displacement ranges from 1% in those with spastic hemiplegia to 75% in those with spastic quadriplegia (70). These hip problems can lead to significant morbidity in terms of pain, soft tissue contractures, and problems with sitting, standing, or walking; fractures, skin ulceration, difficulty with perineal care, pelvic obliquity, or scoliosis (71). Soft tissue release, such as adductor, iliopsoas tenotomy, or psoas release has been shown to be effective in preventing hip dislocation, particularly in those children who were ambulatory before surgery and in those with spastic diplegia (72,73). Dobson et al. (74) and Hagglund et al. (71) reported that early screening through radiological hip examination of all children with bilateral CP is an effective way to prevent future hip problems in this population. Screening should begin at 18 months of age and be performed at 6- to 12-month intervals thereafter, with appropriate surgical or pharmacologic management implemented to reduce the chance of hip dislocation.

Van Heest et al. (68) observed significant improvement with regard to upper limb function following surgical intervention for upper extremity dysfunction in people with CP over a 25-year period. Subjects were rated before and after surgery on a Classification of Upper Extremity Functional Use Scale from 0 (does not use) to 8 (spontaneous use, complete) developed by House et al. (75). The average functional use score was 2.3 before surgery (range, 0–7) and 5.0 after surgery (range, 2–8). The average change of 2.7 levels of improvement in functional use scores was significant (68).

Davids et al. (76) suggest that orthopedic clinical decision-making regarding surgery to optimize the walking ability of children with CP should be based on

TABLE 2.5. COMMON SURGICAL PROCEDURES TO CORRECT DEFORMITIES ASSOCIATED WITH CEREBRAL PALSY (68,69,79)

PROCEDURE	TYPE	UPPER EXTREMITY	LOWER EXTREMITY
Soft-tissue releases	Tendon lengthening; tendon release; aponeurosis release	Biceps lengthening for elbow flexion contracture; Biceps aponeurosis release for pronation contracture; Adductor pollicis flexion and first dorsal interosseous release for thumb in palm	Achilles tendon lengthening for equinus deformity; Fasciectomy of medial and lateral hamstrings for knee contracture; Long head of the rectus femoris release for hip flexion contracture
Tendon transfers	Tendon rerouting; tendon transfer for muscle substitution	Pronator teres rerouting for pronation contracture; Flexor carpi ulnaris transfer to extensor digitorum communis for finger deformity	Distal rectus femoris tendon transfer to sartorius to assist knee flexion during gait; Posterior tibial tendon rerouting for supination/varus deformity of forefoot
Bone/Joint stabilization	Rotational osteotomies; arthrodesis; capsulodesis	Rotational osteotomy of the radius for pronation contracture; Wrist arthrodesis with proximal row carpectomy for wrist flexion/ulnar deviation deformity; Palmar plate capsulodesis for finger deformity	External rotation osteotomy of the femur for femoral anteversion; Extra-articular subtalar arthrodesis for valgus deformity of the foot; Palmar plate capsulodesis for hammer toe deformity

five sources of information, which are then plugged into a diagnostic matrix. These include clinical history, physical examination, diagnostic imaging, quantitative gait analysis, and examination under anesthesia. Their indications for common orthopedic surgical interventions (iliopsoas recession, femoral rotational osteotomy, medial hamstring lengthening, rectus femoris transfer, and gastrocnemius lengthening) are presented in Table 2.6.

Persons with CP commonly develop deformities of the spine, such as scoliosis, kyphosis, and lordosis. Kyphosis and lordosis are usually treated conservatively unless tendon lengthening of the hip flexors or extensors is required to correct the deformity. Conservative management of scoliosis in persons with CP is usually ineffective in stopping the progression of the deformity. Surgical intervention is indicated if the scoliosis curve exceeds 40%–50% and the spine will not be severely shortened by arrest of its further growth. Spinal arthrodesis with internal fixation is the definitive treatment of progressive scoliosis in persons with CP. This procedure should produce a balanced spine over a level pelvis to facilitate sitting balance, improve sitting endurance, facilitate care and personal hygiene, and improve patient outlook (69). Both Teli et al. (77) and Vialle et al. (78) report positive outcomes following surgical stabilization for scoliosis in those with CP, including a reduction of the scoliosis with correction of the pelvic obliquity, as well as an improvement in quality of life.

DIAGNOSTIC TECHNIQUES

Along with the risk factors of prematurity, low birth weight, and maternal history of smoking or drug abuse, delayed motor milestones are often the first recognized signs and primary complaint that eventually may lead to the diagnosis of CP (79). The Early Motor Pattern Profile is an effective instrument to identify children in their first year of life who are at greatest risk for the development of CP. This profile, consisting of 15 items related to variations in muscle tone, reflexes, and movement and organized into a standardized format, may be incorporated into a routine health screening. The format only adds minutes to the routine screening and has high sensitivity and specificity (80). A number of tests and measures are useful in documenting and quantifying the outcomes of intervention for children with CP. These tests may be categorized in a variety of ways, including tests for assessing ADLs (e.g., Canadian Occupational Performance Measure and Pediatric Evaluation of Disability Inventory); tests of motor function (e.g., Pediatric Evaluation Disability Inventory, Gross Motor Function Measure, and Peabody Developmental Motor Scales); and measures of functional ability (Table 2.7) (81,82).

TABLE 2.6. INDICATIONS FOR THE SELECTION OF SPECIFIC ORTHOPEDIC SURGICAL INTERVENTIONS TO OPTIMIZE THE GAIT OF CHILDREN WITH CEREBRAL PALSY (13,47,76)

	CLINICAL HISTORY	PHYSICAL EXAMINATION	QUANTITATIVE GAIT ANALYSIS
Iliopsoas Recession	Inability to stand and walk with upper body erect	Hip flexion contracture >30°	• Anterior pelvic tilt with "double bump" waveform during stance phase • ↓ Hip external in terminal stance with ↓ dynamic range throughout gait cycle • ↑ Internal or external moment in midstance with delayed crossover to an int. flexion moment in terminal stance
Femoral Rotational Osteotomy	In-toeing, genu valgum, tripping	• ↑ Femoral anteversion • ↑ Hip internal rotation • ↓ Hip external rotation	• ↑ Hip internal rotation throughout gait cycle
Medial Hamstring Lengthening	Inability to stand up straight, walks with knees bent Anterior knee pain, fatigue with prolonged walking	• Straight leg raise limited <60° • ↓ Popliteal V angle <130° • Spastic response to fast stretch of hamstrings	• ↑ Knee flexion during loading response • Variable knee alignment during mid- and terminal stance • ↓ Knee extension in terminal swing • ↑ Internal or external moment during stance • Prolonged medial hamstring activity into midstance
Rectus Femoris Transfer	Stiff knees, toe dragging, tripping	(+) prone rectus test (Duncan-Ely)	• ↓Dynamic ROM <80% normal • Delayed and ↓ peak flexion in swing phase • Activation of rectus femoris during midswing • (+) coactivation of vastus lateralis during midswing
Gastrocnemius Lengthening	Walks on toes, toe dragging, tripping, in-toeing	• ↓ Passive ankle dorsiflexion • Clonus • ↑ Achilles DTR	• Excessive plantarflexion in stance and swing phase • Disruption of all 3 ankle rockers in stance phase • Absence of internal dorsiflexion moment in loading response • ↑ Internal plantarflexion moment in midstance • Premature activation of the gastrocnemius in stance phase, beginning at initial contact

DTR, deep tendon reflex; ROM, range of motion.

EXERCISE/FITNESS/FUNCTIONAL TESTING

Given the varied presentations of CP in terms of physical attributes, cognitive abilities, communication abilities, visual and hearing deficits, and chronological age, it not possible to provide a simple recipe for exercise testing in this population. In addition, limited research is available to support the application of the able-bodied exercise adaptation model, testing protocols, principles, and techniques among people with CP (22,83–85). Therefore, it is up to clinicians to use their experience, common sense, the details provided in this chapter, and the basic principles of exercise testing as published by the American College of Sports Medicine (86,87) to devise the most appropriate individualized exercise testing. To assist in the assessment of needs, goals, and objectives, it is suggested that the clinician utilize the Cerebral Palsy—International Sports and Recreation Association's Functional Classification System (see Table 2.8) (84,88). This classification system, although developed for sports, can be used as a tool to help the clinician gain insight into a person's functional abilities. With this information, the clinician will be better prepared to recommend specific exercise test protocols and recognize the need for adaptations that will help ensure the success of the testing session.

CARDIOVASCULAR

Cardiovascular fitness can be evaluated in wheelchair uses with CP using a wheelchair or arm-crank ergometer. In wheelchair ergometry, allowing persons to push their own chair on a roller system provides the most functional assessment. A disadvantage of the wheelchair

TABLE 2.7. MEASUREMENTS OF FUNCTIONAL ABILITY (81,82)

IMPAIRMENT	MEASUREMENT TOOL
Involuntary Movement	**Motion analysis** Position and orientation of multiple joints and body segments Biofeedback training to reduce unwanted movements or to measure changes following intervention
Speed/Progression of Movement	**Motion analysis** Position and orientation of multiple joints and body segments Measure changes following intervention
Spasticity	**Ashworth scale** Measure resistance to passive movement following intervention
Postural Control/Alignment	**Gross motor performance measure** Quantifying impairment in postural alignment, weightshifting, coordination, and select activation of specific joints or segments during gross motor skill performance **Assessment of behavioral components** Capture disordered postural alignment in children with cerebral palsy (CP) using illustrated criterion referenced postures in children **Sitting assessment scale** Ratings of postural control of the head, trunk, and feet during performance of reaching and various functional tasks in addition to functional performance measures of these skills **Melbourne assessment of unilateral upper limb function** Quality-of-movement scale addressing trunk control and alignment, fluence and range of movement, and quality of grasp and release during 12 fine motor and reaching activities **Examination of a child with mild neurological dysfunction** Measures balance, coordination, posture, and motor function
Force	**Hand-held dynamometry or isokinetic dynamometry** Useful measures of outcomes of strength training programs for children with CP
Range of Motion	**Goniometry or electrogoniometry** Goniometry lacks satisfactory reliability in the presence of spasticity; electrogoniometry shown to be more reliable than traditional approaches
Balance	**Functional reach test** Assess ability to reach forward in standing without losing one's balance—simple, fast, and reliable
Energy Cost	**Physiological cost index** Indicates biological cost of ambulation using heart rate during walking minus resting heart rate divided by speed of walking; owing to inefficient gait of persons with CP, this measure is only an estimate of energy cost

TABLE 2.8. OVERVIEW OF THE CEREBRAL PALSY—INTERNATIONAL SPORTS AND RECREATION ASSOCIATION'S FUNCTIONAL PROFILES FOR ATHLETES WITH NONPROGRESSIVE BRAIN INJURIES (22,84,88)

CLASS	FUNCTIONAL PROFILE
1	Moderate to severe spasticity—severe involvement of all four limbs. Poor trunk control and functional strength in upper extremities (UE).
2 (Lower)	Moderate to severe spasticity—severe involvement of upper extremities and trunk. Poor functional strength and control of UE. Propels wheelchair with legs.
2 (Upper)	Moderate to severe spasticity—severe involvement of lower extremities and trunk. Poor functional strength and control of lower extremities. Propels wheelchair poorly with arms.
3	Fair functional strength and moderate control in UE. Almost full functional strength in dominant UE. Propels wheelchair slowly with one or both arms.
4	Moderate to severe involvement of lower limbs. Functional strength and minimal control problems in UE.
5	Good functional strength; minimal control problems in UE. Usually ambulates with an assistive device.
6	Moderate to minimal involvement of all four limbs and trunk (typically athetoid); competes without an assistive device.
7	Moderate to minimal hemiplegia. Good functional ability on nonaffected side. Ambulates well.
8	Minimally affected or monoplegic. Good coordination and balance.

roller ergometer is the difficulty in accurately calculating, controlling, and progressing the rolling resistance. Often, the persons are asked to wheel at progressively faster cadences during each stage of the test protocol. Spasticity and athetosis may be aggravated, however, by the increased speed of movement. Ultimately, coordination and, therefore, performance may be limited.

Various forms of arm-crank ergometers have been used to assess cardiovascular function in this population (83). Starting power outputs range from 0–15 W at 30–50 rpm and increasing in 5–10W increments every 2 minutes during typical arm-crank ergometry tests to volitional exhaustion (83,89), but the specific resistance or cadence will depend on the person's functional abilities and the presence of any concomitant secondary conditions. Individual should be positioned so that during the pedaling action their forearms do not rise above the horizontal plane and their elbows do not fully extend. Their stability in the seated position is critical. An axiom in rehabilitation is that one cannot achieve distal mobility without proximal stability. Participants with CP typically present with increased muscle tone in the extremities and decreased tone in the trunk. Using the patient's own wheelchair or some other stable seating system, with or without strapping of the trunk, pelvis, and lower extremities may be necessary.

The clinician must also consider the handle position of the ergometer. It is preferable to use handles that are in the vertical versus the horizontal plane. If the handles are grasped in the horizontal plane, the shoulder is forced into marked internal rotation, thereby increasing the risk for impingement and rotator cuff overuse syndromes (22). Caution is warranted when considering strapping the client's hand to the handle. This type of strapping is most commonly done for those with hemiplegia or marked weakness of the hands. If the affected limb that is strapped does not have sufficient ROM to complete the same pedal stroke as the unaffected side, serious injury could result to the wrist, elbow, or shoulder. A final consideration is the distance between the individual and the arm-crank ergometer. The typical setup described above works primarily the upper-extremity musculature, with the trunk muscles co-contracting for proximal stability. The clinician may choose to increase the distance between the ergometer and the patient to force the trunk to move through a greater ROM during the exercise (22).

Many wheelchair users, although not functional for ambulation, will have some level of lower extremity use. Exercise modalities, such as the Schwinn Air-Dyne and the NuStep Recumbent Stepper, both allow for the use of all four extremities. Utilization of all four limbs in a dynamic rhythmic movement pattern will help control the spasticity or athetosis experienced by the patient. This form of exercise will also maximize the number of muscle groups involved in the exercise. The clinician may choose to perform a graded exercise test on a Schwinn

Air-Dyne; however, the only way to increase the resistance is to increase the cadence. Increasing the cadence often increases the spasticity in the participant with moderate to severe resting spasticity, thus significantly increasing both the person'sr perceived effort and absolute energy expenditure at any given workload. The NuStep Recumbent Stepper allows the user to maintain a constant cadence while resistance is increased, minimizing the velocity of movement-related increases in spasticity (22).

The treadmill will optimize the exercise test response for those with CP who are ambulatory (22,88,90). The clinician should note that, as the participant fatigues, the spasticity of the hip adductors might increase (22,88), leading to an increase in the genu valgus (knocked knees). This may cause the individual to hit his or her knees together and fall. Using a treadmill protocol that allows the participant to choose a self-selected pace and increase only the incline has been demonstrated to be the most appropriate for those with mild to moderate spasticity or athetosis. Because of the increased risk of falls in this population (even those experienced with treadmill use), a spotter should always be in place. For persons with minimal motor deficits, any of the typical able-bodied treadmill protocols would be appropriate (22,83,88).

Limitations in balance and coordination among ambulatory individuals with CP may dictate use of a cycle ergometer or some other form of ergometry (e.g., arm-crank), or use of an unweighting system (90). Studies on cycle ergometry in this population have employed power outputs varying from an initial 25–50 W at 50–60 rpm and increases in resistance from 15–25 W every 2 minutes until volitional fatigue (22,83). The clinician will find that cage-type toe clips are invaluable for keeping the participant's feet on the pedals of a cycle ergometer, especially with moderate to high resistances and cadences. As previously mentioned, fatigue can lead to an increase in the genu valgus (knocked knees) and cause the individual's knees to hit against the frame of the ergometer.

Research has documented high reliability coefficients for testing maximal aerobic capacity using wheelchair, arm-crank, and cycle ergometry in people with CP (88,91–93). Determination of anaerobic threshold in wheelchair athletes with CP using a discontinuous protocol has demonstrated poor reliability. Bhambhani et al. (92) suggested that the poor reliability in this type of exercise may be owing to the protocol used or inconsistencies related to the effect of spasticity and lactate diffusion from the working muscles into the blood.

Clinicians who elect to collect metabolic data should be aware that the mouth often develops abnormally in a person with CP. The long-term effects of increased tone of the facial muscles and tongue result in a very acute mandibular angle. This results in oral deformities that may make the use of the typical mouthpiece difficult in terms of fit, comfort, and the assurance of an airtight seal. Also, a spastic tongue typically thrusts outward, thus making it difficult for the cpatient to keep the mouthpiece in place (22). Clinicians who resort to using a mask must be careful to ensure that the seal remains unbroken at rest and during exercise.

MUSCULAR STRENGTH AND ENDURANCE

Muscular strength and endurance testing in individuals with spasticity or athetosis has often been considered inappropriate and invalid (94–96), but this is not well substantiated and several researchers have found these tests to be appropriate in people with CP (95, 97–99). Strength testing is a measurement of the capacity of the person to activate a specific muscle or group while inhibiting the antagonist. Bohannon et al. (95,97,100) present a body of evidence that not only highlights the appropriateness of muscular strength and endurance testing in this population, but also demonstrates the predictive traits between the initial and final clinical evaluations. Other research has documented high test–retest reliability coefficients for both upper and lower extremity one repetition maximal (1-RM) strength testing (83). The clinician must remember that, as a result of spasticity, the involuntary contraction of the opposing muscle group during a manual muscle test may result in a situation of co-contraction. The co-contracting muscle groups may both be "strong," but net little functional muscle strength during the manual muscle testing procedure.

Before muscular strength and endurance testing, the appropriate ROM measurements should be performed. These measurements will help the clinician determine if there are substantial side-to-side differences and if contractures exist. With substantial side-to-side differences, the case can be made to test muscle strength and endurance unilaterally versus bilaterally. Both active and passive measurements should be made. If the passive ROM is substantially greater than the active ROM, then the difference is likely caused by increased tone or spasticity of the antagonist or weakness of the agonist. If both the passive and active ROM are equally clinically less than the expected normal limits, then the loss is most likely owing to a permanent contracture (79,82,101).

The main considerations for muscular strength and endurance testing are stability, coordination, ROM, and timing (75,96,101). The forms and protocols for testing do not necessarily need to be modified from the able-bodied model. Typically, an 8-RM muscular strength testing protocol can be used. This protocol will adequately estimate approximately 80%–85% of the individual's 1-RM. Using a protocol that utilizes moderate resistances will help to minimize the risk of increased spasticity resulting in decreased coordination and functional movement. The goal for this protocol is to reach volitional fatigue (6–10 repetitions) in no more than three sets. When assessing

muscular endurance, a resistance in the order of 50%–60% of the predicted 1-RM should be used (83). The clinician must pay particular attention to the participant's technique. Any deviation from the prescribed technique or cadence would be reason to discontinue the test even if the patient does not reach volitional fatigue. Fatigue-related increases in spasticity and in coordination should be expected (22,79,101).

As mentioned previously, proximal (trunk) stability is critical for the optimal performance of the extremity movements. Wide benches, low seats (so the participant's feet can rest on the floor), and trunk and pelvic strapping are potentially necessary adaptations for the person with CP. Given the potential for altered coordination and balance, it would be preferable to use selectorized weight machines for this population. With the movements guided, the participant can focus on muscular effort, the learning curve of the task is diminished, and ultimately the participant's performance is optimized. Persons with athetosis can especially benefit from the guided movement that the weight machines offer. Free weights, although more functional, may pose a safety threat to all but the most experienced individual (79).

Using a metronome or other timing system to ensure slow, controlled movements will help optimize the participant's performance. Slow, controlled movements will facilitate coordination of movement and lessen the impact of spasticity. Another consideration when testing for muscular strength and endurance is the use of large, nonslip hand grips to help those individuals with weak or dysfunctional handgrip. The clinician may also consider the use of gloves, tension wraps, or other hand-strapping systems to augment grip.

It is not uncommon for participants with CP to report short-term increases in spasticity, athetosis, and incoordination during testing (79,82,101). After the testing session, provide them with plenty of time to recover and be prepared to assist those whose function has been significantly impaired. Individuals often express that one of the most profound changes that they observe when performing a regular exercise program is a decrease in their long-term neurologic symptoms (83). When documenting the testing session, be sure to record this and other behavioral observations, such as changes in gait pattern and function or independence.

Regardless of the exercise mode and test protocol used, provide adequate practice and make the necessary adaptations to the equipment to help ensure a successful testing session. At the very least, the clinician must provide participants with adequate time to familiarize themselves with the equipment and testing protocol. This learning period may be substantially longer than the time needed for the able-bodied population because of differences in cognitive ability, previous experience, and the amount of spasticity or athetosis and incoordination (79,82,96).

EXERCISE PRESCRIPTION AND PROGRAMMING

People with CP typically have low levels of physical fitness and are at extremely high risk for secondary conditions (83,102–104). These low levels of physical fitness relate to perceptions of poor quality of life, difficulties with ADLs, and limited abilities to gain and retain employment. Although the research is limited, it has been documented that people with CP incur positive adaptations to both muscular strength and cardiovascular exercise programs (22,83,85,88,102). There are resources to help guide the clinician in developing exercise programs for this population (86,87). Selection of the specific exercise modes, frequency, intensity, duration, and progressions will be individualized and will require the clinician to be observant and request client feedback on a regular basis. As discussed in the exercise testing section, a comprehensive initial evaluation will help identify the needs or goals of clients, their activity preferences, specific precautions, potential barriers to the exercise program, as well as considerations for equipment modification and setup.

In general, the exercise program should be simple and easy to follow. Initially, it is better to underestimate the capabilities to the client. The clinician must remember that the exercise program is just one component of the person's day and if unable to complete daily activities because of an exercise program that was too demanding, that person might stop participating in the program (83,85).

The detrained ambulatory client will be used as an example of an initial exercise program. This initial exercise program should start with a cardiovascular activity such as 10–15 minutes on the treadmill or cycle ergometer at a self-selected cadence. The activity should be at a conversational pace (50%–65% of the maximal age-predicted heart rate) and the desired health benefits may be gained by continuous and discontinuous exercise (86). Because many ambulatory persons with CP have limited dorsiflexion owing to spasticity of the plantar flexors, it is best to keep the inclination of the treadmill relatively flat. A few generalized stretches (3–5 repetitions for 15–20 seconds each) for the upper and lower extremities should be completed after the cardiovascular component of the program. The clinician must be aware that spastic muscles respond best to slow, controlled movements, therefore, stretching is best performed once the perspm has completed a warm-up and is in a stable, safe seated or supine position. After stretching, strength training can be undertaken and typically 1–2 sets of 10–12 repetitions per exercise are sufficient. To help the participant's technique and to maximize the functional nature of strength exercises, an emphasis is placed on a slow, controlled eccentric phase (count of two concentrically and a count of four eccentrically) (22,83,85–86). Initial

strength exercises could include chest press, seated row, lateral pull-down, seated leg press, seated leg curl, and abdominal curls. Progression of these exercises and the addition of new exercises would be at the discretion of the clinician and the desire of the participant.

Another consideration when trying to determine the appropriate resistance for a given strengthening exercise is whether or not the antagonistic muscle presents with increased muscle tone. If this is the case, then the working muscle must not only overcome the resistance provided by the exercise, but also the resistance to movement being created by the spastic antagonist. To minimize this effect, ensure that the participant is well supported and the exercise is being performed in a relatively slow, controlled manner. Many people with CP present with altered or nonfunctional movement patterns. These movement patterns have developed because of the neurologic involvement of the condition or the client has developed substitution strategies. When using strapping, avoid direct contact with the skin and watch for reddened areas.

Because CP is a condition that must be addressed across the lifespan, the clinician must take into account the client's chronological age, and activities should be age-appropriate and related to the individual's interests, needs, and goals. In addition, we have found that these persons often have limited opportunities for social engagement, therefore, group-oriented programs that facilitate social interaction are helpful in maintaining adherence to the program. Frequent positive feedback and routine supervision are also important to promote exercise adherence (56,79,82–83,85).

EDUCATION AND COUNSELING

Clinicians can educate people with CP by developing a rapport with each patient and facilitating adherence to a program. The congenital nature of CP results in a population that often has a long history of contact with the medical and allied health professions. They may also have lived very sheltered, protected lives. For many, instead of a childhood of play-related recreation and sport, their experience with exercise is one of regimented stretching, positioning, and rehabilitation. This scenario has dramatically changed with the advent of early intervention programs and the Individuals with Disabilities Education Act legislation (79,82,88). However, the adult population may have a very jaded and negative opinion of exercise and health professionals, hence the need for patient education and participant-driven, goal-oriented programming. The participant may need to be educated in areas such as role of exercise in preventing secondary chronic disease, the effects of exercise on depression, exercise as a component of weight management, and the ways in which exercise may facilitate improvements in

TABLE 2.9. PRIMARY BENEFITS OF AN EXERCISE PROGRAM FOR PEOPLE WITH CEREBRAL PALSY (22,79,83,88)

1 Risk reduction for secondary chronic diseases
2 Maintain and improve bone health
3 Maintain and improve muscular strength
4 Maintain and improve cardiovascular fitness
5 Maintain and improve flexibility and mobility
6 Maintain and improve balance and coordination
7 May facilitate a decrease in spasticity or athetosis
8 Facilitate weight management
9 Reduce anxiety and stress
10 Provide a sense of well-being
11 Increased participation in individual pursuits and community engagement

ADLs and quality of life. Table 2.9 summarizes some of the primary reasons why a person with CP might be motivated to exercise. Because of communication disorders, this information may have to be provided in a variety of formats and repeated numerous times. In addition, education can be reinforced by introducing participants with CP to an appropriate support network that includes other involved healthcare professionals (79,82).

The primary educational objective of the clinician is to inform the participant about the benefits of a lifelong health-oriented exercise program. The clinician could also present information regarding the recreational and sporting opportunities that are available to those with CP. Besides the obvious easily integrated recreational activities of walking, cycling, and swimming, numerous sporting opportunities are available to people with CP. Clinicians should familiarize themselves with the variety of local, regional, statewide, national, and international organizations that provide sporting opportunities for these individuals (79,82). DePauw and Gavron (88) published an excellent resource that provides an overview of the variety of options and the appropriate contact organizations. Rehabilitation centers, school districts, community fitness facilities, and city parks and recreation departments are also potential sources for information regarding recreation and sporting opportunities for people with disabilities (79).

A variety of barriers, including communication, physical limitations, medications, limited prior exposure to participating in an exercise program, social and environmental isolation, embarrassment to be in public, difficulty with accessing and using public transportation, unsupportive caregivers, and financial considerations are potential barriers to exercise that must be taken into consideration when working with participants with CP. As such, attendance at the initial evaluation may be a significant step for the participant (22,79,82) and this is an important opportunity for the clinician to use his or her knowledge, experience, and creativity to encourage and motivate the participant.

REFERENCES

1. Club L. Memorandum on terminology and classification of 'cerebral palsy.' *Cerebral Palsy Bulletin* 1959;1:27–35.
2. Mutch L, Alberman E, Hagberg B, et al. Cerebral palsy epidemiology: Where are we now and where are we going? *Dev Med Child Neurol* 1992;34:574–551.
3. Albright AL. Spasticity and movement disorders in cerebral palsy. *J Child Neurol* 1996;11(Suppl 1):S1–S4.
4. Nelson KB, Ellenberg JH. Children who "outgrew" cerebral palsy. *Pediatrics* 1982;69:529–536.
5. Arvidsson J, Hagberg B. Delayed onset dyskinetic 'cerebral palsy': A late effect of perinatal asphyxia? *Acta Pediatr Scand* 1990;79:1121–1123.
6. Lesny I. The development of athetosis. *Dev Med Child Neurol* 1968; 10:441–446.
7. Murphy CC, Yeargin-Allsopp M, Decoufle P, et al. Prevalence of cerebral palsy among ten year old children in metropolitan Atlanta, 1985 through 1987. *J Pediatr* 1993;123:S13–S19.
8. Arens LJ, Molteno CD. A comparative study of postnatally-acquired cerebral palsy in Cape Town. *Dev Med Child Neurol* 1989;31: 246–254.
9. Al-Rajah S, Bademosi O, Awada A, et al. Cerebral palsy in Saudi Arabia: A case-control study of risk factors. *Dev Med Child Neurol* 1991;33:1048–1052.
10. Bhasin TK, Brocksen S, Avchen RN, Braun KVN. Prevalence of four developmental disabilities among children aged 8 years—Metropolitan Atlanta developmental disabilities surveillance program, 1996–2000. *MMWR* 55(SS-1) 2006:1–9.
11. Sinha G, Corry P, Subesinghe D, et al. Prevalence and type of cerebral palsy in a British ethnic community: the role of consanguinity. *Dev Med Child Neurol* 1997;39:259–262.
12. Odding E, Roebroeck ME, Stam HJ. The epidemiology of cerebral palsy: Incidence, impairments and risk factors. *Disabil Rehabil* 2006;28(4):183–191.
13. DeLuca PA. The musculoskeletal management of children with cerebral palsy. *Pediatr Clin North Am* 1996;43(5): 1135–1150.
14. Stanley F, Blair E, Alberman E. *Cerebral Palsies: Epidemiology and Causal Pathways. Clinics in Developmental Medicine.* Number 87. London: Mac Keith Press; 2000:1–51.
15. Saito N, Ebara S, Ohotsuka K, et al. Natural history of scoliosis in spastic cerebral palsy. *Lancet* 1998;351:1687–1692.
16. Del Giudice E, Staiano A, Capano G, et al. Gastrointestinal manifestations in children with cerebral palsy. *Brain Dev* 1999;21: 307–311.
17. Bandini LG, Schoeller DA, Fukagawa NK, et al. Body composition and energy expenditure in adolescents with cerebral palsy or myelodysplasia. *Pediatr Res* 1991;29:70–77.
18. Van den Berg-Emons RJ, van Baak MA, Speth L, et al. Physical training of school children with spastic cerebral palsy: Effects on daily activity, fat mass and fitness. *Int J Rehabil* 1998;21:179–194.
19. Damiano DL, Kelly LE, Vaughn CL. Effects of quadriceps femoris muscle strengthening on crouch gait in children with spastic cerebral palsy. *Phys Ther* 1995;75:658–671.
20. Bar-Or O, Inbar O, Spira R. Physiological effects of a sports rehabilitation program on cerebral palsied and post-poliomyelitic adolescents. *Med Sci Sports Exerc* 1976;8:157–161.
21. Hutzler Y, Chacham A, Bergman U, et al. Effects of a movement and swimming program on vital capacity and water orientation skills of children with cerebral palsy. *Dev Med Child Neurol* 1998; 40: 176–181.
22. Laskin JJ. Cerebral palsy. In: *ACSM's Exercise Management for Persons with Chronic Diseases and Disabilities,* 2nd ed. Champaign, IL: Human Kinetics; 2003.
23. Bowen TR, Lennon N, Castagno P, et al. Variability of energy-consumption measures in children with cerebral palsy. *J Pediatr Orthop* 1998;18:738–742.

24. Pranzatelli MR. Oral pharmacotherapy for the movement disorders of cerebral palsy. *J Child Neurol* 1996;11(Suppl 1):S13–S22.

25. Albright AL. Intrathecal baclofen in cerebral palsy movement disorders. *J Child Neurol* 1996;11(Suppl 1):S29–S35.

26. Penn RD, Kroin JS. Intrathecal baclofen alleviates spinal cord spasticity. *Lancet* 1984;1:1078.

27. Penn RD, Savoy SM, Corcos D, et al. Intrathecal baclofen for severe spinal spasticity. *N Engl J Med* 1989;320:1517–1521.

28. Goldstein M. The treatment of cerebral palsy: What we know, what we don't know. *J Pediatr* 2004;145:S45–S46.

29. Bodensteiner JB. The management of cerebral palsy: Subjectivity and conundrum. *J Child Neurol* 1996;11(2):75–76.

30. Almeida GL, Campbell SK, Girolami GL, et al. Multidimensional assessment of motor function in a child with cerebral palsy following intrathecal administration of baclofen. *Phys Ther* 1997; 77(7): 751–764.

31. Gerszten PC, Albright AL, Johnstone GF. Intrathecal baclofen infusion and subsequent orthopedic surgery in patients with spastic cerebral palsy. *J Neurosurg* 1998;88:1009–1013.

32. Albright AL, Shultz BL. Plasma baclofen levels in children receiving continuous intrathecal baclofen infusion. *J Child Neurol* 1999; 14: 408–409.

33. Albright AL. Baclofen in the treatment of cerebral palsy. *J Child Neurol* 1996;11:77–83.

34. Koman LA, Mooney JF, Smith BP. Neuromuscular blockade in the management of cerebral palsy. *J Child Neurol* 1996;11(Suppl 1): S23–S28.

35. Gordon N. The role of botulinus toxin type A in treatment—With special reference to children. *Brain Dev* 1999;21:147–151.

36. Gouch JL, Sandell TV. Botulinum toxin for spasticity and athetosis in children with cerebral palsy. *Arch Phys Med Rehabil* 1996;77: 508–511.

37. Carr LJ, Cosgrove AP, Gringras P, et al. Position paper on the use of botulinum toxin in cerebral palsy. *Arch Dis Child* 1998;79: 271–73.

38. Hazneci GB, Vurucu, S, Örs, F, Tan AF, Gençdoğan, S, Alp, T. Factors affecting the functional level in children with cerebral palsy. *Turk J Phys Med Rehab* 2006;52:105–109.

39. Massin M, Allington N. Role of exercise testing in the functional assessment of cerebral palsy children after botulinum A toxin injection. *J Pediatr Orthop* 1999;19:362–365.

40. Barwood S, Baillieu C, Boyd R, Brereton K, Low J, Nattrass G, Graham HK. Analgesic effects of botulinum toxin A: A randomized, placebo-controlled clinical trial. *Dev Med Child Neurol* 2000;42: 116–121.

41. Jefferson RJ. Botulinum toxin in the management of cerebral palsy. *Dev Med Child Neurol* 2004;46:491–499.

42. Ubhi T, Bhakta BB, Ives HL, Allgar V, Roussounis SH. Randomised double blind placebo-controlled trial of the effect of botulinum toxin on walking in cerebral palsy. *Arch Dis Child* 2000;83: 481–487.

43. Forssberg H, Tedroff KB. Botulinum toxin treatment in cerebral palsy: Intervention with poor evaluation? *Dev Med Child Neurol* 1997;39:635–640.

44. Lannin N, Scheinberg A, Clark K. AACPDM systematic review of the effectiveness of therapy for children with cerebral palsy after botulinum toxin A injections. *Dev Med Child Neurol* 2006;48: 533–539.

45. Reeuwijk A, van Schie PEM. Effects of botulinum toxin type A on upper limb function in children with cerebral palsy: A systematic review. *Clin Rehabil* 2006;20:375–387.

46. Ade-Hall RA, Moore AP. Botulinum toxin type A in the treatment of lower limb spasticity in cerebral palsy. The Cochrane Database of Systemic Reviews, The Cochran Library 2007;(2).

47. Davis DW. Review of cerebral palsy. Part II: Identification and intervention. 1997;16(4):19–25.

48. Prechtl HFR. State of the art of a new functional assessment of the young nervous system. An early predictor of cerebral palsy. *Early Hum Dev* 1997;50:1–11.

49. Barry MJ. Physical therapy interventions for patients with movement disorders from cerebral palsy. *J Child Neurol* 1996;11(Suppl 1): S51–S60.

50. Law M, Pollock N, Rosenbaum P, et al. A comparison of intensive neurodevelopmental therapy plus casting and a regular occupational therapy program for children with cerebral palsy. *Dev Med Child Neurol* 1997;39:664–670.

51. Weindling AM, Hallam P, Gregg J, et al. A randomized controlled trial of early physiotherapy for high-risk infants. *Acta Paediatr* 1996;85:1107–1111.

52. Bower E, McLellan DL, Arney J, et al. A randomised controlled trial of different intensities of physiotherapy and different goal-setting procedures in 44 children with cerebral palsy. *Dev Med Child Neurol* 1996;38:226–237.

53. Chad KE, Bailey DA, McKay HA, et al. The effect of a weight-bearing physical activity program on bone mineral content and estimated volumetric density in children with spastic cerebral palsy. *J Pediatr* 1999;135:115–117.

54. Carlson WE, Vaughan CL, Damiano DL, et al. Orthotic management of gait in spastic diplegia. *Am J Phys Med Rehabil* 1997;76: 219–225.

55. Mattsson E, Andersson C. Oxygen cost, walking speed, and perceived exertion in children with cerebral palsy when walking with anterior and posterior walkers. *Dev Med Child Neurol* 1997;39:671–676.

56. Damiano DL, Abel MF. Functional outcomes of strength training in spastic cerebral palsy. *Arch Phys Med Rehabil* 1998;79:119–25.

57. Morton R. New surgical interventions for cerebral palsy and the place of gait analysis. *Dev Med Child Neurol* 1999;41:424–428.

58. Wright FV, Sheil EM, Drake JM, et al. Evaluation of selective dorsal rhizotomy for the reduction of spasticity in cerebral palsy: A randomized controlled trial. *Dev Med Child Neurol* 1998;40:239–247.

59. Steinbok P, Reiner AM, Beauchamp R, et al. A randomized clinical trial to compare selective posterior rhizotomy plus physiotherapy with physiotherapy alone in children with spastic diplegic cerebral palsy. *Dev Med Child Neurol* 1997;39:178–184.

60. Steinbok P, Reiner A, Kestle JRW. Therapeutic electrical stimulation following selective posterior rhizotomy in children with spastic diplegic cerebral palsy: A randomized clinical trial. *Dev Med Child Neurol* 1997;39:515–520.

61. Buckon CE, Thomas SS, Aiona MD, et al. Assessment of upper extremity function in children with spastic diplegia before and after selective dorsal rhizotomy. *Dev Med Child Neurol* 1995;38: 967–975.

62. Subramanian N, Vaughan CL, Peter JC, et al. Gait before and 10 years after rhizotomy in children with cerebral palsy spasticity. *J Neurosurg* 1998;88:1014–1019.

63. Abbott R. Sensory rhizotomy for the treatment of childhood spasticity. *J Child Neurol* 1996;11(Suppl 1):S36–S42.

64. Engsberg JR, Olree KS, Ross SA, et al. Spasticity and strength changes as a function of selective dorsal rhizotomy. *J Neurosurg* 1998;88:1020–1026.

65. Engsberg JR, Ross SA, Park TS. Changes in ankle spasticity and strength following selective dorsal rhizotomy and physical therapy for spastic cerebral palsy. *J Neurosurg* 1999;91:727–732.

66. DeSalles AAF. Role of stereotaxis in the treatment of cerebral palsy. *J Child Neurol* 1996;11(Suppl 1):S43–S50.

67. Speelman JD, van Manen J. Cerebral palsy and stereotatic neurosurgery: Long term results. *J Neurol Neurosurg Psychiatry* 1989;52: 23–30.

68. Van Heest AE, House JH, Cariello C. Upper extremity surgical treatment of cerebral palsy. *J Hand Surg* 1999;24A:323–330.

69. Renshaw TS, Green NE, Griffin PP, et al. Cerebral palsy: Orthopaedic management. *Instr Course Lect* 1996;45:475–490.

70. Lonstein JE, Beck K. Hip dislocation and subluxation in cerebral palsy. *J Pediatr Orthop* 1986;6:521–526.

71. Hagglund G, Andersson S, Duppe H, Lauge-Pedersen H, Nordmark E, Westbom L. Prevention of dislocation of the hip in children with cerebral palsy: The first ten years of a population based prevention program. *J Bone Joint Surg* (Br) 2005;87-B:95–101.

72. Terjesen T, Lie GD, Hyldmo AA, Knaus A. Adductor tenotomy in spastic cerebral palsy. *Acta Orthop* 2005;76(1):128–137.

73. Presedo A, Oh C, Dabney KW, Miller F. Soft-tissue releases to treat spastic hip subluxation in children with cerebral palsy. *J Bone Joint Surg* 2005;87-A(4)832–841.

74. Dobson F, Boyd RN, Parrot J, Nattrass GR, Graham HK. Hip surveillance in children with cerebral palsy: Impact on the surgical management of spastic hip disease. *J Bone Joint Surg* (Br) 2002;85-B(5):720–726.

75. House JH, Gwaathmey FW, Fidler MO. A dynamic approach to the thumb-in-palm deformity in cerebral palsy. *J Bone Joint Surg* 1981;63A:216–225.

76. Davids JR, Ounpuu S, DeLuca PA, Davis RB. Optimization of walking ability of children with cerebral palsy. *J Bone Joint Surg* 2003;85-A(11):2224–2234.

77. Teli MG, Cinnella P, Vincitorio F, Lovi A, Grava G, Brayda-Bruno M. Spinal fusion with Cotrel-Dubousset instrumentation for neuropathic scoliosis in patients with cerebral palsy. *Spine* 2006;31(4):E441–E447.

78. Vialle R, Delecourt C, Morin C. Surgical treatment of scoliosis with pelvic obliquity in cerebral palsy. *Spine* 2006;31(13): 1461–1466.

79. Onley, SJ , Wright MJ. Cerebral palsy. In: Campbell SK, Vander Linden DW, Palisano RJ, eds. *Physical Therapy for Children*. Philadelphia: Saunders Elsevier; 2006:625–664.

80. Morgan AM, Aldag JC. Early identification of cerebral palsy using a profile of abnormal motor patterns. *Pediatrics* 1996;98:692–697.

81. Campbell SK. Quantifying the effects of interventions for movement disorders resulting from cerebral palsy. *J Child Neurol* 1996;11(Suppl 1):S61–S70.

82. Tecklin JS. *Pediatric Physical Therapy*. 4th ed. Philadelphia: Lippincott Williams & Wilkins; 2007.

83. Laskin JJ. Physiological adaptations to concurrent muscular strength and aerobic endurance training in functionally active people with a physical disability. Unpublished doctoral dissertation, University of Alberta, 2001.

84. Carroll KL, Leiser J, Paisley TS. Cerebral palsy: Physical activity and sport. *Curr Sports Med Rep* 2006;5(6):319–322.

85. Damiano DL. Activity, activity, activity: Rethinking our physical therapy approach to cerebral palsy (III STEP Series). *Phys Ther* 2006;86(11):1534–1537.

86. American College of Sports Medicine. *ACSM's Guidelines for Exercise Testing and Prescription*, 7th ed. Baltimore: Lippincott Williams & Wilkins; 2005.

87. American College of Sports Medicine. *ACSM's Resource Manual for Guidelines for Exercise Testing and Prescription*, 5th ed. Philadelphia: Lippincott Williams & Wilkins; 2005.

88. DePauw KP, Gavron SJ. *Disability Sport*, 2nd ed. Champaign, IL: Human Kinetics; 2005.

89. Shinohara T, Suzuki N, Oba M, Kawasumi M, Kimizuka M, Mita K. Effect of exercise at the AT point for children with cerebral palsy. *Bull NYU Hosp Jt Dis* 2002;61(1/2):63–67.

90. Unnithan VB, Kenne EM, Logan L, Collier S, Turk M. The effect of partial body weight support on the oxygen cost of walking in children and adolescents with spastic cerebral palsy. *Pediatr Exerc Sci* 2006;18(1):11–22.

91. Bhambhani YN, Holland LJ, Steaward RD. Maximal aerobic power in cerebral palsied wheelchair athletes: Validity and reliability. *Arch Phys Med Rehabil* 1992;73(3):246–252.

92. Bhambhani YN, Holland LJ, Steaward RD. Anaerobic threshold in wheelchair athletes with cerebral palsy: Validity and reliability. *Arch Phys Med Rehabil* 1993;74(3):305–311.

93. Suzuki N, Oshimi Y, Shinohara T, Kawasumi M, Mita M. Exercise intensity based on heart rate while walking in spastic cerebral palsy. *Bull NYU Hosp Jt Dis* 2001;60(1):18–22.

94. Bohannon RW. Is the measurement of muscle strength appropriate in patients with brain lesions? A special communication. *Phys Ther* 1989;69(3):225–229.

95. Bohannon RW, Walsh S. Nature, reliability, and predictive value of muscle performance measures in patients with hemiparesis following stroke. *Arch Phys Med Rehabil* 1992;73:721–725.

96. Allen J, Dodd K, Taylor N, McBurney H, Larkin H. Strength training can be enjoyable and beneficial for adults with cerebral palsy. *Disabil Rehabil* 2004;26(19):1121–1128.

97. Bohannon RW, Larkin PA, Smith MB, et al. Relationship between static muscle strength deficits and spasticity in stroke patients with hemiparesis. *Phys Ther* 1987;67(7):1068–1071.

98. Bohannon RW. Relative decreases in knee extension torque with increased knee extension velocities in stroke patients with hemiparesis. *Phys Ther* 1987;67(7):1218–1220.

99. Bohannon RW, Smith MB. Assessment of strength deficits in eight paretic upper extremity muscle groups of stroke patients with hemiplegia. *Phys Ther* 1987;67(4):522–525.

100. Bohannon RW, Smith MB. Upper extremity strength deficits in hemiplegic stroke patients: Relationship between admission and discharge assessment and time since onset. *Arch Phys Med Rehabil* 1987;68:155–157.

101. Bennett SE, Karnes JL. *Neurological Disabilities: Assessment and Treatment*. Philadelphia: Lippincott Williams & Wilkins; 1998.

102. Fernandez JE, Pitetti KH, Betzen MT. Physiological capacities of individuals with cerebral palsy. *Hum Factors* 1990;32(4):457–466.

103. Parker DF, Carriere L, Hebestreit H, et al. Anaerobic endurance and peak muscle power in children with spastic cerebral palsy. *Am J Dis Child* 1992;146(9):1069–1073.

104. Parker DF, Carriere L, Hebestreit H, et al. Muscle performance and gross motor function of children with spastic cerebral palsy. *Dev Med Child Neurol* 1993;35(1):17–23.

Multiple Sclerosis

EPIDEMIOLOGY/ETIOLOGY

Multiple sclerosis (MS) is a common neurologic disease that affects women at a rate two to three times greater than men (1). It is estimated that approximately 400,000 individuals in the United States have MS, with a worldwide estimate of 2.5 million (1). Studies of migrating populations have indicated that where a person resides in relation to the equator before the age of 15 appears to determine the likelihood of developing MS (2). The incidence of MS is nearly 3/100,000 in temperate zones, and below 1/100,000 in tropical areas (3). The initiation of MS, either propensity for the disease or the disease itself, begins in childhood. A variety of mild viral infections, such as measles and upper-respiratory infections, are thought to be etiological (4). A threefold increase in the incidence of exacerbations of MS is seen following an upper-respiratory infection (5,6). Exacerbation rate is reduced during pregnancy and is increased threefold in the postpartum period up to approximately 3 months (7). The onset of MS usually occurs between the ages of 20 and 40; however, it is often possible to obtain a history of transient neurologic deficits, such as numbness of an extremity, weakness, blurring of vision, and diplopia, in childhood or adolescence before the development of more persistent neurologic deficits. The latter often lead to a definitive diagnosis (8,9). It is possible that viruses causing upper-respiratory infections may be responsible for sensitizing the brain to subsequent autoimmune insult, producing inflammatory demyelination.

Several distinct courses of the disease are now recognized, as well as the prevalence rate associated with each type: Relapsing-remitting MS (RRMS; 85%), primary progressive MS (PPMS; 10%), and progressive relapsing MS (PRMS; 5%). After an initial period of RRMS, many develop a secondary-progressive (SPMS) disease course, characterized by a more steady decline in function with or without flare-ups and remissions. Of the 85% of those initially diagnosed with RRMS, more than 50% will go onto to develop SPMS within 10 years. Furthermore, 90% of patients with RRMS will develop SPMS within 25 years. These statistics, however, are based on data collected before the widespread use of newer disease-modifying agents that may delay or reduce the progression of RRMS to SPMS. An overview of the course of each pattern and related disability is presented in Figure 3.1 (10).

For decades scientists have speculated about a "genetic predisposition" for MS; however, only recently has the presence of two specific genes been identified that could be related to the increased susceptability (11). Patients who have a definite diagnosis of MS are more likely to have a variety of other illnesses of an autoimmune nature, such as systemic lupus erythematosus (SLE), rheumatoid arthritis (RA), polymyositis, myasthenia gravis, and so forth (12). Studies have shown that if a first-degree relative has MS, there is a 12- to 20-fold increase in the likelihood of having MS (13). In monozygotic twins there is a 33% increase in the incidence of MS, whereas in dizygotic twins the incidence is about 8%, or that found in the normal population (14,15).

PATHOPHYSIOLOGY

Multiple sclerosis is a disease of the central nervous system in which there are multiple areas of inflammatory demyelination with a predilection for distribution around the ventricles and vascular spaces. Multiple mechanisms are involved in producing damage to central nervous system myelin, as well as axons (16,17). An immune reaction to myelin (myelin basic protein [MBP]) and myelin oligodendrocyte glycoprotein (MOG) occurs. Activated T cells attach to the endothelium of capillaries within the brain and migrate into the brain parenchyma, where activated macrophages attack and digest myelin. A number of cytokines, including tumor necrosis factor (TNF), and interferons, as well as IgG, are involved in the immune attack. B cells produce IgG directed at MOG. There is increased production of IgG and an increased prevalence of specific IgG moieties, some of which represent antiviral IgG. Recent studies of total brain N-acetylaspartate (NAA)-to-creatine ratios have provided evidence for loss of axons, as well as evidence for membrane damage (demyelination) as an increase in choline-to-creatine ratio (18).

Lesions representing focal areas of inflammatory demyelination can be present in the cerebral hemispheres, brainstem, and spinal cord. For a definite diagnosis to be established, two or more areas of demyelination (white matter lesions) must be established. Furthermore, there must be two or more remissions of neurologic deficits.

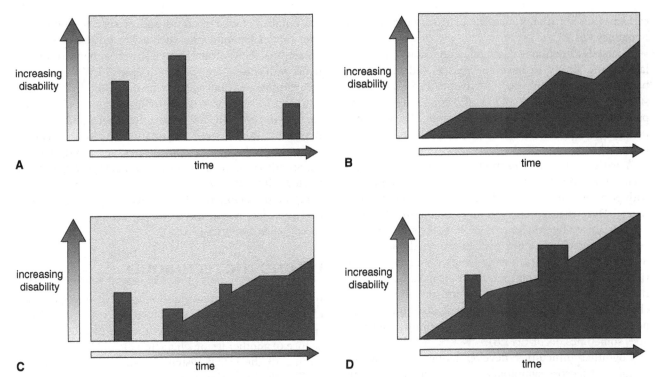

FIGURE 3.1. Graphic illustration of the four clinical subtypes of MS. **A.** Relapsing-remitting. **B.** Primary progressive. **C.** Secondary progressive. **D.** Progressive relapsing (10).

This must be accompanied by paraclinical evidence of disease seen as the presence of magnetic resonance imaging (MRI) T2-weighted lesions in white matter, as well as evidence of increased IgG synthesis with positive oligoclonal bands (OCBs) in the spinal fluid (20). OCBs result from a reduction in the number of different migrating species of IgG obtained on electrophoresis. Other conditions, such as bacterial or viral infection, autoimmune diseases, such as SLE, and vasculitis, may also produce increased IgG or oligoclonal bands.

CLINICAL FEATURES

Long-fiber pathways or tracts are more likely to be involved in the process of demyelination. For example, it is very common for patients to have posterior column signs, such as loss of vibration sense, and pyramidal signs early in the course of the disease when the disease is virtually asymptomatic. A common feature of MS is profound fatigue often with a diurnal pattern. This is characterized as malaise or a lack of motivation for the performance of any physical activity, as well as motor fatigue, which develops with continued physical inactivity (19,20). Another extremely interesting phenomenon is a marked decrease in heat tolerance (internal and external), which is sometimes accompanied by the development of neurologic signs (21). Blurring of vision in one or both eyes may occur with physical exertion (Uhthoff's phenomenon). Demyelination reduces the efficiency of axonal conduction so that

less current is available for depolarization at nodes of Ranvier. With demyelination and reduction of current density, the safety factor for conduction can be exceeded

Common signs and symptoms of MS include painful blurring or loss of vision in one eye with evidence of deafferentation (the Marcus-Gunn pupil) occurring as the result of optic neuritis. Eventually, there will be marked loss of visual acuity. Most patients will begin to recover vision within 6 weeks, with more rapid recovery and reduced pain when treated with methylprednisolone (22,23). Various other visual complaints include blurring of vision with rapid eye movements, difficulty with visual fixation, diplopia (double vision), decreased night vision, and an inability to ascertain contrast. The patient may complain of facial numbness or pain typical of trigeminal neuralgia. Numbness of the tongue and loss of taste may occur. Patients rarely complain of difficulty swallowing, although the prevalence of dysphagia is higher than commonly appreciated. Often, weakness and loss of coordination affect first the lower extremities and then the upper extremities, sometimes in a typical hemiparetic pattern. Spastic paraparesis along with ataxia is a common combination referred to as the "spastic ataxic syndrome." Early in the illness, neurogenic bladder manifests itself as an inability of the bladder to hold an adequate volume of urine. Consequently, urinary frequency and urgency exceeds six times per day, often with incontinence. Nocturia is common. There is a high incidence of urinary tract infections. Greater than 50% of early diagnosed patients complain of urinary urgency and frequency (24,25).

Sexual dysfunction is common, with loss of sensation, lack of the ability to have an orgasm, and impotence being very common (26). Adynamia (i.e., a loss of strength or vigor) of the colon is also common with most patients experiencing severe constipation (25). Some patients require partial colectomy secondary to obstipation (intractable constipation).

A variety of skin sensations and loss of sensation occur, most commonly vibration sense loss in both feet with position sense preserved until vibration sense loss is severe. Dysesthesias, characterized as abnormal sensations produced by touching or stroking the skin, are also very common. These sensory disturbances do not occur in a distribution characteristic of involvement of a peripheral nerve. Abnormal sensation over the trunk, particularly a bandlike sensation around the abdomen or chest, is also characteristic. Most patients, however, do not complain of severe pain in the extremities, but this does sometimes occur (27,28).

Cognitive difficulties develop along with cranial, motor, and sensory symptoms (29–31). The patient may complain of an inability to function in the workplace when he or she is required to monitor two or more activities at the same time. Attentiveness is decreased so that the patient may be unable to register information accurately in memory. Emotional lability is also common in association with subfrontal demyelination, which produces a pseudobulbar palsy. Studies have shown that cognitive deficit is greater in individuals with prominent signs of pseudobulbar palsy or excessive emotional lability (32).

MEDICAL AND SURGICAL TREATMENTS

Exacerbations of MS are usually treated with high-dose adrenocortical steroids customarily administered intravenously at a dose of 1000 mg/day for 3 to 5 days, followed by a prednisone taper over approximately 6 weeks (22,23). It has been demonstrated that patients with monosymptomatic MS initially treated with methylprednisolone defer the development of more typical MS when they are treated with methylprednisolone (22). Development of two or more deficits, marked weakness and incoordination, loss of sensation in both lower extremities, or all of those are indication for treatment with adrenocortical steroids.

Prophylactic treatments include interferon beta-1a (Rebif, Avonex) and -1b (Betaseron), which reduce lymphocytic invasion of the brain, induce a suppressor immune reaction, provide an antiviral action, reduce the number of exacerbations over time, and preserve brain mass (32–34). Glatiramer (copolymer I or Copaxone), a peptide consisting of four amino acids—glycine, alanine, lycine, and tyrosine—act by inducing immune tolerance to myelin basic protein (35). This is also effective in reducing

the number of exacerbations and preserving brain mass over time. Chemotherapy, such as methotrexate and mitoxantrone (Novantrone), are also recommended for patients with chronic progressive disease (36,37).

Symptomatic management includes the treatment of neurogenic bladder with anticholinergic medications, such as oxybutynin, for urinary frequency and urgency. Regimens for treating obstipation include psyllium preparations, laxatives, suppositories, and physical activity. Spasticity, particularly flexor and extensor spasms, is treated with either γ-aminobutyric acid (GABA-b-ergic) compound (baclofen), which increases spinal inhibition, or Tizanidine, which increases supraspinal inhibitors of spinal reflex activities (38,39).

DIAGNOSTIC TECHNIQUES

If the patient's history is highly suggestive of MS, then an MRI of the brain, often combined with imaging of the spinal cord are obtained. Sometimes, to establish the existence of another lesion characteristic of MS, evoked potentials of the visual systems (visual evoked potential [VEP]), the brainstem, or somatosensory (SSEP) systems are obtained. In MS, there is a marked delay in conduction of the action potential. Evaluation of the spinal fluid during an exacerbation early in the disease may reveal a mild pleocytosis of usually less than 100 cells consisting predominantly of lymphocytes and a mild elevation of protein, usually less than 100 mg%. An increase in IgG synthesis and decreased variability of the different moieties of IgG are also characteristic. In the first few months of the disease, spinal fluid findings may be normal, but repeat examination a year or so later may reveal increased IgG synthesis and OCBs. Early definitive diagnosis is important so that prophylactic treatment can be instituted to prevent injury to the central nervous system (40).

CLINICAL EXERCISE PHYSIOLOGY

ACUTE EXERCISE RESPONSE

Studies have shown that persons with MS have a lower maximal aerobic capacity than the average age- and gender-matched, nondisabled adult without MS (38,39). Furthermore, maximal aerobic capacity appears to be inversely related to level of disability (39) as measured on the Kurtzke Expanded Disability Status Scale (EDSS) (40). Individuals with a higher EDSS score, indicative of more neurologic impairment as derived from a clinical examination, have a lower maximal and submaximal aerobic exercise capacity. Despite the variability in peformance, one common effect of acute exercise in individuals with MS is an overwhelming sense of fatigue during postexercise recovery. No scientific evidence, however, suggests that the postexercise fatigue is reflective of an exacerbation of existing or new MS symptom. Furthermore, recent evidence shows that the level of self-reported postexercise fatigue as measured by the Modified Fatigue Impact Scale (MFIS) can be reduced following training (40,41).

To understand basic physiologic responses to an acute bout of exercise, it is helpful to use the two directions commonly taken in the literature: (a) as it relates to muscle performance (i.e., strength and endurance) and (b) cardiovascular responses (i.e., heart rate, blood pressure, oxygen utilization).

MUSCLE PERFORMANCE

In the absence of documented spasticity or use of antispasmodic drugs, several studies have reported that muscle endurance for persons with MS during a sustained isometric contraction (e.g., 30% of maximal voluntary contraction [MVC]) is similar to that of a nondisabled, healthy adult (42). Although these findings are in direct conflict with other studies of acute muscle response (43–47), it is important to consider that in none of the these other studies was the presence of spasticity or the use of antispasmodic drugs controlled in the design. Both Chen et al. (46) and Ponichtera et al. (44) hypothesized that spasticity of antagonistic muscles may decrease concentric agonist force production. In contrast, antagonists are not stretched during an eccentric contraction, whereas the agonist receives additional stretch to facilitate its contraction. Ponichtera et al. (44) suggested that, although spasticity in 44% of their sample may have contributed to a significantly lower force production during concentric knee extension, force production during eccentric knee extension for the MS patients was normal. Thus, spasticity and or co-contraction of opposing muscle groups may be one factor that can reduce concentric muscle performance in this population.

To believe that spasticity is the sole contributor to differences in muscle performance observed between MS and non-MS persons would be naïve. Other contributors to observed differences have been attributed to conduction block of demyelinated fibers (48), reduced muscle metabolic responses during voluntary exercise (49), muscle weakness owing to fiber atrophy (50,51), as well as sensory deficits, which have been discussed previously.

Maximal muscle force during isokinetic exercise at various velocities has also been shown to be consistently lower for persons with MS when matched to controls (43–46). Furthermore, maximal aerobic power (PO_{max}) using leg cycling or combination leg–arm cycling protocols have shown that most persons with MS are likely to generate 20%–68% less power (38,39) than healthy individuals. More recently, similar findings have confirmed that persons with MS have lower PO_{max} than healthy, sedentary adults. Performance during arm cranking and combined arm–leg cycling shows similar findings: 31% lower during arm cranking and 24% lower during combined arm–leg cycling (39). However, when disability level (i.e., EDSS) is taken into account and power output is expressed in terms of body weight (watts/kilogram), it appears that individuals with an EDSS of 4.0 or less (i.e., fully ambulatory) are not significantly weaker than ablebodied, matched controls (52). Thus, documentation of disability level in both research and clinical practice is important to understanding the potential work capacity in this population and to setting realistic therapeutic goals.

ACUTE CARDIORESPIRATORY RESPONSES

Physiologic responses to an acute bout of submaximal aerobic exercise appear to be normal for many persons with MS. Heart rate (HR), blood pressure (BP), and oxygen uptake (VO_2), and minute ventilation (V_E) have been shown to increase in a linear fashion to increments in workload (38,39). Normal metabolic and cardiovascular responses are consistent over a wide range of impairment levels (i.e., EDSS). In contrast, when HR response to incremental exercise is examined in the context of metabolic cost (i.e., oxygen pulse-VO_2/HR), Tantucci et al. (53) reported a significantly lower oxygen pulse for those with MS compared with healthy controls. These findings are consistent during both submaximal and maximal aerobic exercise. A higher HR at a given $\dot{V}O_2$ might imply that stroke volume is insufficient to support the metabolic demand. However, in a case study by Vaz Fragoso and associates (54), right and left ventricular ejection fraction were recorded at rest and at anaerobic threshold showed normal cardiac output and O_2 saturation levels; implicating an abnormality in peripheral O_2 distribution or utilization. A reduction in O_2 distribution could be related to a diminished sympathetic outflow to arterial smooth muscle. Cardiovascular autonomic dysfuction, both sympathetic and parasympathetic, has been well-documented in the MS population (55–58). A deficiency in O_2 utilization is suggestive of peripheral muscle pathology, which has already been supported in earlier research findings (49–51). Future research should focus on the question of peripheral issues, such as oxygen extraction during exercise. Furthermore, whether oxygen pulse (i.e, reduced HR) can be improved with increased stroke volume following training is certainly an important question to be answered.

From a clinical perspective, using HR as an index of exercise intensity presents a twofold problem. First, if oxygen pulse is significantly lower in this population, then absolute workloads will need to be lower during training. With exercise intensity being lower, smaller absolute gains in aerobic capacity are probable. Second, in the presence of diminshed cardioacceleration, the application of either the Karvonen method or the standard practice of calculating HR_{max} as 220–age, from which a training HR is calculated, should be done so with caution. Percieved exertion scales would be better suited for this population with the use of the Category-Ratio Rating of Perceived Exertion (59) possibly being the best choice. This scales uses perceived stress level in three categories: peripheral, central, and integrated. This alternative scale appears to represent a potentially useful tool for obtaining information in lieu of a the presences of unreliable input from "central" (e.g., HR) sources and has been used successfully with the MS population (38).

Maximal aerobic power (VO_2max), when measured using indirect calorimetry, varies greatly based on the degree of physical impairment and neurologic symptoms present (38,39,52–55,60). When compared with that of healthy adults, even minimally impaired MS clients will perform more poorly (i.e., lower VO_2max), regardless of whether the test is performed using leg, arm, or combined arm–leg exercise (39,53). Comparison of VO_2max (mL/kg/min) of 20 minimally to moderately impaired sedentary persons with MS against normative fitness standards showed that 75% fell into the "low fitness" range, whereas 15% and 10% were "fair" and "average," respectively (61).

Aerobic exercise endurance (i.e., time to fatigue) has been measured using various modes of ergometry, and does not appear to be directly related to the level of physical impairment. At a moderate level of exercise (i.e., 50% VO_2max) patients have been able to exercise for as little as 15 minutes to as long as 60 minutes (38). Correlational analysis found no relationship between endurance time and the level of physical impairment (EDSS).

CHRONIC EXERCISE RESPONSE

The body of research documenting the effects of training on muscle performance in persons with MS has grown over the past decade. Current literature confirms that MS patients have the capacity to improve muscle strength following a supervised program of resistance (i.e., weights) and aerobic training. Preliminary studies by Petajan et al. (62) and Ponichtera-Mulcare et al. (63) reported modest improvements (e.g., 11%–17%) following 15 weeks of training and more substantial improvements (29%) after 24 weeks of training in muscle performance, respectively.

Resistance Training

Early resistance training research focused primarily on documenting absolute muscle performance in the MS population. More recent data focus on gait kinematics (64) and mobility (65,66). Training regimens have varied between 8 and 10 weeks in duration, most requiring a minimum of two sessions per week, and have based resistance levels on 60%–80% of one repetition maximum (1-RM) (66,67). Improvements in walking distance, walking speed, endurance, and perceived levels of fatigue have been reported. Common among all these studies is the use of fairly mobile subjects (EDSS ≤5.5). When a more severely-impaired sample has been used (e.g., EDSS >5.5), the level of improvement has been less dramatic (63). Thus, when developing realistic expectations based on the available literature two specific factors must be considered. First, subtle neurologic changes that may not be observable to the clinician may affect exercise training outcomes. Therefore, it is important to carefully monitor neurologic changes by periodically interviewing the client regarding subjective impressions of their disease status. The Kurtzke Expanded Disability Status Scale, which is most commonly used in qualifying disability in research, requires physical examination by a trained clinician, most often a neurologist. However, The Guy's Neurologic Disability Scale offers a valid means for documenting baseline disability and subsequent levels of disability based on patient interview (69). Second, when applying current research findings to patients it should be remembered that training outcomes observed under strict supervision may not be similar to unsupervised, uncontrolled environments, as would be the case of a home exercise program.

AEROBIC TRAINING

Similar to the new breed of resistance training studies, aerobic training research is focusing more on indices of endurance, such timed walking tests, walking speeds, self-reports of fatigue, percieved vitality and activity level, and even changes in anaerobic threshold. Most studies have incorporated the use of cycle ergometry, for as few as 4 weeks (68,70) and as long as 24 weeks (71). Although direct comparison among studies is impossible because of the numerous differences in protocols, there appears to be a trend toward greater levels of improvement in functional outcome measures as the length of the training protocols increased (68,70–74).

EXERCISE/FITNESS/ FUNCTIONAL TESTING

General principles of fitness testing as outlined by the American College of Sports Medicine (67) can be appropriately applied to many persons in this population. When evaluating fitness in the person with MS, it is important, however, to consider special needs related to the specific symptoms experienced by the client.

FLEXIBILITY

Because many MS patients experience lower-extremity spasticity, flexibility may be restricted in the hip, knee, and ankle joints. Hip flexor, hamstring, and gastrocsoleus tightness is particularly problematic and should be evaluated in the sitting position (e.g., Sit-and-Reach Test). Use of this particular test will serve to eliminate any problem with balance during testing. Lateral trunk flexibility should also be evaluated from a sitting position or, if standing, the clinician may place his or her hands on the client's waist to prevent loss of balance.

BALANCE

To truly appreciate how balance deficits might affect the MS client's ability to perform exercise safely, balance should be evaluated under both static and dynamic conditions. A fairly short and easy battery of tests can be found using the Berg Balance Scale (75). This test is valid for neurologic conditions such as MS and takes approximately 15 minutes to administer. The results of this test will provide a better understanding of the client's ability to exercise safely using standard equipment. A home-based program of balance training that challenges sensory systems as well as dynamic and static postural control has been shown to result in significant improvements (76).

AEROBIC FITNESS

Often persons with MS experience problems with balance as well as foot drop. The latter is commonly associated with weakness of the tibialis anterior, which can be improved with appropriate resistance training (77,78). Foot drop can appear during both weight-bearing and non-weight-bearing exercise. For safety purposes, aerobic fitness is best eevaluated using a bicycle ergometer. Even so, this mode of exercise testing can also present challenges. Ankle clonus (i.e., spasmodic alternation of contraction and relaxation of muscles) and sensory abnormalities (e.g., numbness, tingling, deficits in joint proprioception) can make it difficult for the client to keep his or her feet on the pedals. The use of standard toe clips and Velcro-secured heel straps can reduce or eliminate this problem.

The general procedures for submaximal testing of cardiorespiratory endurance using a cycle ergometer published by the American College of Sports Medicine can be applied to this population; however, workloads suggested in standard tests, such as the YMCA Cycle Ergometry Protocol or the Astrand-Rhyming Test, may need to be reduced. Modification of these protocols can be accomplished simply by beginning with a warm-up phase of no-load pedaling, followed by fixed rate pedaling (determined by the patient's ability level) at 50 W for 6 minutes or by proceeding with increments of 0.25 kp at 50 rpm until the appropriate HR response is achieved. Of these two protocols, the latter may be more appropriate with extremely sedentary MS clients (male and female), who may have maximal workload capacities less than 50 W. Treadmill testing and training has been used in fairly nondisabled MS clients (68,73), but harness support is recommended with more severely disabled individuals (74).

MUSCULAR STRENGTH AND ENDURANCE

The general procedures for measuring muscle strength and endurance suggested by the American College of Sports Medicine can be applied to this population (67). Again, to proceed safely, any reduction in joint range of motion, sensory loss (upper and lower extremity), coordination deficits, ataxia, and spasticity needs to be considered before testing. Suggestions for activities and special considerations during testing, training, and counseling are summarized in Tables 3.1 and 3.2, respectively.

TABLE 3.1. GENERAL GUIDELINES FOR PRESCRIBING PHYSICAL ACTIVITY AND EXERCISE PROGRAMING

MODE OF EXERCISE/ ACTIVITY	GENERAL GOALS	INTENSITY/FREQUENCY/ DURATION	SPECIAL CONSIDERATIONS
Physical Activity • Activities of daily living • Built-in inconveniences • Leisure activities and hobbies	• Increase daily activity energy expenditure	• 30 minutes of accumulated physical activity each day on most days	• Strategies for energy conservation may be necessary
Aerobic and Endurance Exercise • Stationary cycling • Walking • Water or chair aerobics • Weight supported treadmill	• Increase cardiovascular function reduce risk for coronary artery disease (CAD)	• 60%–70% heart rate (HR) peak/50%–65% $\dot{V}O_2$peak • 3 sessions/week • 1, 30-min session or 3, 10-min sessions per day	• Air temperature should be kept cool; fans are helpful; therapeutic swimming pool water is often too warm
Strength Training • Resistance training • Therabands • Free weights • Weight machines • Pulley weights • Pilates	• Increase general muscle strength • Improve muscle tone • Equalize agonist/antagoist strength • Reduce spasticity	• Perform on nonendurance training days • 2 sessions/week • 8–15 repetitions • 60%–80% 1-RM • Minumum of 1 min rest between sets/exercises	• With upper-extremity sensory deficit, free weights should not be used. • Training should be performed in seated position if balance impaired.
Flexibility (Stretching) • Passive range of motion (ROM) • Active ROM • Yoga • Tai Chi	• Increased joint ROM • Counteracts spasticity • Improved balance	• Perform 1–2 × daily • Hold stretch 30–60 sec for mild/mod tightness • Positional stretching with assistance of gravity up to 20 min for contracture	• Should be performed from a seated or lying position.

TABLE 3.2. SPECIAL CONSIDERATIONS WHEN PRESCRIBING PHYSICAL ACTIVITY EXERCISE

CONSIDERATION	DESCRIPTION
Heat Sensitivity	There is ample research documenting the presence of heat sensitivity in most persons with multiple sclerosis (MS). The exact mechanism of how either external (e.g., environmental) or internal (e.g., metabolic) heat affects these individuals remains unknown. The resulting sequelae, however, can include any one or all of the following: general or severe fatigue, loss of balance, foot drop, visual changes (e.g., blurred vision), speech changes (e.g., slurred speech), and muscle weakness or paralysis. Sweating has also been shown as being abnormal in as much as 50% of the population (52). The absence of sweating may contribute to a perception of being overheated as capillary skin blood flow increases in an effort to dissipate heat generated from exercising muscles. As such, the perception of overheating coupled with heat-related fatigue may preempt the exercise session before the desired time. Use of fans, wet neck wraps, and spray bottles may help reduce the perception of overheating. Surface cooling has been shown to improve aerobic endurance slightly (84). Others have shown that precooling before exercise also has a beneficial effect on performance (85). Exercise is also recommended to occur early in the day. This is when circadian body temperature is at its lowest. Subjective reports from most individuals with MS indicate a decline in energy level occurs during the afternoon hours, with the occurrence of fatigue and other MS-related symptoms.
Bladder Dysfunction	Bladder dysfunction is an MS symptom that can indirectly affect exercise performance. Because of symptoms such as bladder urgency and exertional incontinence, clients with MS may limit their daily intake of liquids. This is also a common practice observed during exercise. Recommendations for proper hydration before exercise and rehydration following should be addressed when working with this population.
Sensory Deficits	Subtle losses in tactile and proprioceptive sensation may make using some equipment difficult and even dangerous. Deficits may be reflected in an inability to grasp and control free weights, as well as to perceive muscle and joint position. Visual feedback by training in front of a mirror or performing rhythmic counting during repetitions can provide alternate forms of input to ensure proper performance. When possible, the use of machines, such as the LifeCycle Series, is recommended because it reduces the amount of control and coordination needed by the client and provides visual feedback regarding range of motion and force produced for each repetition.
Incoordination	Safety is also an issue for persons who have coordination deficits. The presence of spasticity, ataxia, or tremor can result in uncoordinated movement patterns in the affected extremities. Therefore, use of equipment that requires coordinated movement (i.e., free weights) is contraindicated. Use of synchronized arm or leg ergometers may improve exercise performance by allowing the arms to assist the less-coordinated legs.
Cognitive and Memory Deficits	Subtle cognitive changes and memory deficits may require a modified approach to instructing the client with MS. This might include providing information in both written and diagrammatic format, and reminders of proper form, repetitions, and use of equipment. In addition, providing an easy form of recording exercises will eliminate the need for accurate recall.
Neurologic Impairment Level	Depending on the level of neurologic impairment, it may take longer for some persons with MS to experience notable improvements in muscle strength, endurance, and aerobic fitness. In more extensively impaired clients, this may be related to any or all of the following: the need to (a) begin with very low levels of resistance, (b) reduce the number of weekly sessions because of a protracted recovery time, and (c) disperse the daily exercise time into two to three smaller bouts.

EDUCATION AND COUNSELING

Many people with disabilities (79), particularly those with MS (80), *believe* that they do not possess the knowledge and skills needed to exercise safely. Because of these beliefs, it is not surprising to find that preliminary evidence shows that persons with MS are less active than the average, nondisabled American (81). However, before the person with MS can be counseled regarding exercise and physical activity, it is important to understand the perceived barriers that may be present.

In disabled populations, the major barriers to participation in an exercise program have been reported as financial cost, lack of energy, transportation, and not knowing where to exercise (82). Other barriers that have been cited include not having someone to exercise with, childcare responsibilities, lack of confidence, and lack of encouragement from healthcare providers (81,82). These factors, some more than others (e.g., lack of energy, lack of confidence), are more than likely real issues for the person with MS. Such barriers need to be overcome before successful participation in a program of regular exercise can be facilitated.

At the foundation, counseling should focus on the basic principles of training (i.e., frequency, intensity, duration, and mode). Special emphasis on how to modify each principle specific to the client's lifestyle and physical impairments is very important. Advice related to dealing with spasticity, tremor, incoordination, balance deficits, and general fatigue, when appropriate, will set a tone of "understanding" that will help to promote a level of confidence for these individuals. These issues have been outlined in the section "Special Considerations."

Although evidence related to the efficacy of surface cooling for improving exercise performance is equivocal, previous research has shown that persons with MS perceive exercise to be less stressful when surface cooling is present (38,52). As such, strategies to promote surface cooling may improve exercise tolerance and adherence. These include (*a*) selecting water exercise instead of land, (*b*) using a bicycle ergometer with a fan-style flywheel, (*c*) wearing a presoaked neck scarf, (*d*) ingesting ice chips before exercise, and (*e*) skin surface misting with cool water. Prehydration and drinking during exercise should also be discussed.

Providing information to the client regarding cost, accessibility, and scheduling of local exercise opportunities sponsored by community recreational facilities, senior citizen centers, universities, and hospital outreach programs can reduce or eliminate several other barriers. However, if clients feel sufficiently confident in their general knowledge base, they may prefer to exercise at home. This will require the clinician to provide basic information regarding appropriate choices of home equipment, particularly as it relates to safety, cost, and ease of use.

Finally, an important key to successful counseling and education for persons with MS, or any other disability, is the building of confidence to practice self-advocacy. A candid and comprehensive discussion of basic exercise responses, training principles, modifications related to symptomatology, safety issues, and programming can provide a solid foundation for this to occur.

CASE STUDY

HISTORY

Patient is a 67-year-old woman with a 30-year history of relapsing-remitting and secondary progressive MS. Her current medications include Rebif and Baclofen. She is retired, and uses a four-wheeled walker for mobility in the home setting but has begun using an electric scooter outdoors following a recent fall. This patient was referred to a hospital-based wellness center after formal physical therapy for instruction in a community-based exercise program.

EVALUATION FINDINGS

Height: 5'4"; **Weight:** 152 lb; **BMI:** 26; **BP:** 128/83; **RHR:** 85 **Muscle Performance:** Manual muscle testing reveals the following; both upper extremities and the right lower extremity are grossly 4/5. Left ankle dorsiflexion and knee flexion are 2+/5, left knee extension and hip flexion 3+/5. **Endurance:** 6-Minute Walk—90 m (normal 512–640 m) with an ending HR of 124 bpm. **Functional Measures:** *30-Second Sit to Stand Test*—four repetitions (normal 12–18). *Timed Up-an-Go*—47 sec (normal <10 sec), *Berg Balance Test*—37 (normal 54–56). **Range of Motion:** Mild hip flexion contractures of 10° bilaterally and a 5° plantarflexion contracture in the left ankle. **Tone:** Moderately increased extensor tone in left lower extremity with two to three beat clonus in the left ankle. **Sensation:** Moderate loss of vibration sense in the left LE distal to the knee, light touch and sharp dull are mildly impaired. **Gait:** The patient ambulates with a four-wheel walker with excessive trunk flexion with decreased step length and occasional toe drag on the left. She also demonstrates knee hyperextension on the left during stance.

INTERPRETATION OF FINDINGS

This patient demonstrates deficits in muscle performance as evidenced by her manual muscle grades and her *30-Second Sit to Stand Test*. The results of her *6-Minute Walk Test* demonstrate a significant impairment in walking endurance and speed. Her *Berg Balance* and *Timed Up-and-Go* indicate a higher risk for falls and her lack of sensation and increased tone will have an impact on selection of appropriate and safe exercises.

EXERCISE PRESCRIPTION

Cardiorespiratory Endurance

Use of NuStep recumbent stepper beginning with 5–10 minutes at 60%–75% of predicted max heart rate and progressing to 30 minutes, 3–5 days a week.

Rationale: Provides reciprocal upper and lower extremity movement similar to walking while distributing work to all four extremities to reduce chances of local muscle fatigue limiting exercise time. Seated position is safe for persons with balance deficits and large platform pedals are easier to use for persons with coordination and sensory deficits.

Strength and Muscular Endurance

Circuit training of leg press, seated knee flexion, standing hip and knee flexion, latissimus pull-downs and seated rows starting with 1 set of 12–15 repetitions at 60%–70% 1-RM progressing to 2 sets of 8–12 repetitions at 70%–80% 1-RM twice a week.

Rationale: Seated leg press will improve strength of muscles used for activities such as sit to stand transfers. Seated knee flexion to increase hamstring strength and counter extensor tone bias. Standing hip and knee flexion to improve toe clearance during swing phase of gait. Lateral pull-downs and seated rows to increase strength of postural extensor muscles to reduce effects of prolonged sitting and improve antigravity muscle control during functional activities.

Flexibility

- Stretching of pectoralis major or minor and illiopsoas to improve trunk and hip extension.
- Stretching of gastocnemius or soleus to improve ankle dorsiflexion. Perform two repetitions holding each stretch for 60 seconds twice a day.

REFERENCES

1. Web site home page-National Mulitple Sclerosis Society [Internet]. New York, NY. National MS Society; [cited 2007]. Avaiblable from: http://www.nmms.org.
2. Rosati G. Descriptive epidemiology of MS in Europe in the 1980's: A critical overview. *Ann Neurol* 1994;36:5164–5174.
3. Weinshenker BG. Epidemiology of MS. *Neurol Clin* 1996;14:291–308.
4. Sibley WA, Bamford CR, Clark K. Clinical viral infections and MS. *Lancet* 1985;1:1313–1315.
5. Panitch HS. Influence of infection on exacerbation of MS. *Ann Neurol* 1994;36:525–528.
6. Korn-Labetzki I, Khana E, Cooper G, et al. Activity of MS during pregnancy and puerperium. *Ann Neurol* 1984;16:229–231.
7. Carriere, W, Baskerville J, Ebers, GC. The natural history of MS: A geographically based study. Applications to planning and interpretation of clinical and therapuetic trials. *Brain* 1991;114:1057–1067.
8. Wynn DR, Rodriguez M, O'Fallon M, Kurland LT. A reappraisal of the epidemiology of MS in Olmstead County, Minnesota. *Neurology* 1990;40:780–786.
9. Lublin FD, Reingold SC. Defining the clinical course of multiple sclerosis: Results of an international survey. National Multiple Sclerosis Society (USA) Advisory Committee on Clinical Trials of New Agents in Multiple Sclerosis. *Neurology* 1996;46:907–911.
10. The International Multiple Sclerosis Genetics Consortium. Risk alleles for multiple sclerosis identified by a genomewide study. *N Engl J Med* [Internet]. 2007 [cited 2007, July 29. Available from: http://www.nejm.com.
11. Haegert DG, Marrosu MG. Genetic susceptibility to MS. *Ann Neurol* 1994;36:2S04–S210.
12. Mumford CJ, Wood NW, Kellar-Wood H, Thorpe JW, Miller DH, Compston, DA. The British Isles survey of MS in twins. *Neurology* 1994;44:11–15.
13. Sadovnick AD, Armstrong H, Rice GP, et al. A population-based study of MS in twins: Update. *Ann Neurol* 1993; 33:281–285.
14. Prineas JW. Pathology of MS. In: Cook SD, ed. *Handbook of MS.* New York: Marcel Dekker. 1990:187–218.
15. Sobel RA. The pathology of MS. *Neurol Clin* 1995;13:1–21.
16. Waxman SG. Pathophysiology of MS. In: Coo DS, ed. *Handbook of MS.* New York: Marcel Dekker. 1990:219–249.
17. Prineas JW, Barnanrd RD, Revesz T, Kwon EE, Sharer L, Cho E-S. MS: Pathology of recurrent lesions. *Brain* 1993;116:681–693.
18. Gonen O, Patalace I, Babb JS, et al. Total brain N-acetylaspartate, a new measure of disease load in MS. *Neurology* 2000;54:15–19.
19. Poser CM, Paty DW, Scheinberg L, et al. New diagnostic criteria for MS: Guidelines for research protocols. *Ann Neurol* 1983;13:227–231.
20. Krupp LB, Alvarez LA, LaRocca NG, et al. Fatigue in MS. *Arch Neurol* 1988;45:435–437.
21. Freal JE, Kraft GH, Coryell JK. Symptomatic fatigue in MS. *Arch Phys Med Rehabil* 1984;65:165–168.
22. Thompson AJ, Kennard C, Swash M, et al. Relative efficacy of intravenous methylprednisolone and ACTH in the treatment of acute relapse in MS. *Neurology* 1989;39:696–971.
23. Beck RW, Cleary PA, Anderson MM, et al. A randomized controlled trial of corticosteroids in the treatment of acute optic neuritis. *N Engl J Med* 1992;326:581–588.
24. Blaivas JG. Management of bladder dysfunction in MS. *Neurology* 1980;30:12–18.
25. Bradley WE, Logothetis JL, Timm GW. Cystometric and sphincter abnormalities in MS. *Neurology* 1973;23:1131–1139.
26. Valleroy ML, Kraft G. Sexual dysfunction in MS. *Arch Phys Med Rehabil* 1984;65:125–128.
27. Svendsen, KB, Jensen, TS, Hansen, HJ, Bach, FW. Sensory function and quality of life in patients with multiple sclerosis and pain. *Pain* 2005;114:473–481.
28. Osterberg, A, Boivie, J, Thuomas, K-A. Central pain in multiple sclerosis—prevelance and clinical characteristics. *Eur J Pain* 2005; 9:531–542.
29. Herholz, K. Cognitive dysfunction and emotional-behavioural changes in MS: The potential of positron emission tomography. *J Neurol Sci* 2006;245(1–2);9–12.
30. The IFNB MS study group and the University of British Columbia MS/MRI analysis group. Interferon beta-1b in the treatment of MS: Final outcome of the randomized controlled trial. *Neurology* 1995;45:1277–1285.
31. Gold R, Rieckmann P, Chang P, Abdalla J; the PRISMS Study Group. The long-term safety and tolerability of high-dose interferon β-1a in relapsing-remitting multiple sclerosis: 4-year data from the PRISMS study. *Eur J Neurol* 2005;12:649–656.
32. Johnson KP, Brooks BR, Cohen JA, et al. Copolymer-1 reduces relapse rate and improves disability in relapsing-remitting MS: Results of a phase III multicenter double-blind placebo-controlled trial. *Neurology* 1995;45:1268–1276.
33. Thompson AJ, Noseworthy JH. New treatments for MS: Clinical perspective. *Curr Opin Neurol* 1996;9:187–198.
34. Fidler JM, DeJoy SQ, Smith FR 3rd, Gibbons JJ Jr. Selective immunomodulation by the antineoplastic agent mitoxantrone. Nonspecific adherent suppressor cells derived from mitoxantrone-treated mice. *J Immunol* 1986;136:2747–2754.
35. Katz R. Management of spasticity. *Am J Phys Med Rehabil* 1988; 67:108–116.
36. Nance DW, Sheremata WA, Lynch SG, et al. Relationships of the antispasticity effect of Tizanidine to plasma concentration in patients with MS. *Arch Neurol* 1997;54:731–736.
37. Rudick RA, Goodman A, Herndon RM, Panitch HS. Selecting relapsing-remitting MS patients for treatment: The care for early treatment. *J Neuroimmunol* 1999;98:22–28.
38. Ponichtera-Mulcare JA, Glaser RM, Mathews T, Camaione, DN. Maximal aerobic exercise in persons with MS. *Clin Kinesiol* 1983; 46(4):12–21.
39. Ponichtera-Mulcare JA, Mathews T, Glaser RM, Mathrews T Gupta SC. Maximal aerobic exercise of individuals with MS using three modes of ergometry. *Clin Kinesiol* 1995;49:4–13.
40. White LJ, McCoy SC, Castellano V, Guiterrez G, Stevens JE, Walter GA, Vandenborne K. Resistance training improves strength and functional capacity in persons with multiple sclerosis. *Mult Scler* 2004;10:668–674.
41. Surakka J, Romberg A, Ruutiainen J, Aunola S, Virtanen A, Karppi SL, Maentaka K. Effects of aerobic and strength exercise on motor fatigue in men and women with multiple sclerosis: A randomized controlled trial. *Clin Rehabil* 2004;18(7):737–746.

42. Ng AV, Dao HT, Miller RG, Gelina DF, Kent-Braun JA. Blunted pressor and intramuscular metabolic responses to voluntary isometric exercise in MS. *J Appl Physiol* 2000;88:871–880.

43. Lambert CP, Archer RL, Evans WJ. Muscle strength and fatigue during isokinetic exercise in individuals with multiple sclerosis. *Med Sci Sport Exerc* 2001;33(10):1613–1619.

44. Ponichtera JA, Rodgers MM, Glaser RM, Mathews, T. Concentric and eccentric isokinetic lower extremity strength in persons with MS. *J Orthop Sport Phys Ther* 1988;16(3):114–122.

45. Armstrong LE, Winant DM, Swasey PR, Seidle ME, Carter AL, Gehlsen GM. Using isokinetic dynamometry to test ambulatory patients with MS. *Phys Ther* 1983;63:1274–1279.

46. Chen W-Y, Peirson FM, Burnett CN. Force-time measurements of knee muscle function in MS. *Phys Ther* 1987;67:934–940.

47. Rice CL, Volmer TL, Bigland-Ritchie B. Neuromuscular responses of patients with MS. *Muscle Nerve* 1992;15:1123–1132.

48. McDonald WI, Sears TA. Effect of a demyelinating lesion on conduction in the central nervous system studied in single nerve fibers. *J Physiol (London)* 1970;207:53–54P.

49. Kent-Braun JA, Sharma KR, Miller RG, Weiner MW. Postexercise phosphocreatine resysntheis is slowed in multiple sclerosis. *Muscle Nerve* 1994;17(8):835–841.

50. Kent-Braun JA, Sharma KR, Weiner MW, Miller RG. Effects of exercise on muscle activation and metabolism in MS. *Muscle Nerve* 1994;17(10):1162–1169.

51. Sharma KR, Kent-Braun J, Mynhier MA, Weiner MW, Miller RG. Evidence of an abnormal intramuscular component of fatigue in MS. *Muscle Nerve* 1995;18(12):1403–1411.

52. Mulcare JA, Webb P, Mathews T, Gupta, SC. Sweat response in persons with multiple sclerosis during submaximal aerobic exercise. *International Journal of MS Care* 2001;3(4):26–33.

53. Tantucci, C Massucci M, Piperno R, Grassi V, Sorbini CA. Energy cost of exercise in MS patients with low degree of disability. *Mult Scler* 1996; 2(3):161–167.

54. Vaz Fragoso C, Wirz D, Mashman J. Establishing a physiological basis to multiple sclerosis-related fatigue: A case report. *Arch Phys Med Rehabil* 1995;76:583–586.

55. Linden D, Diehl RR, Kretzschmar A, Berlit P. Autonomic evaluation by means of standard tests and power spectral analysis in multiple sclerosis. *Muscle Nerve* 1997;20(7):809–814.

56. Flachenecker P, Wolf A, Krauser M, Hartung HP, Reiners K. Cardiovascular autonomic dysfunction in multiple sclerosis: Correlation with orthostatic intolerance. *J Neurol* 1999;246(7):578–586.

57. Bonnett M, Mulcare J, Mathews T, Gupta SA, Ahmed N, Yeragani V. Heart rate and QT interval variability in multiple sclerosis: Evidence for decreased sympathetic activity. *J Neurol Sci* [Turkish] 2006;23(4):248–256.

58. Pepin EB, Hicks RW, Spencer MK, Tan ZC, Jackson CGR. Pressor response to isometric exercise in patients with multiple sclerosis. *Med Sci Sports Exerc* 1996;23:656–660.

59. Noble BJ, Roberton RJ. *Perceived Exertion.* Champaign, IL: Human Kinetics; 1996.

60. Pariser G, Madras D, Weiss E. J Outcomes of an aquatic exercise program including aerobic capacity, lactate threshold, and fatigue in two individuals with multiple sclerosis. *Neur Phys Ther* 2006; 30(2):82–90.

61. Nieman DC. *Fitness and Sports Medicine: An Introduction.* Palo Alto, CA: Bull Publishing Company. 1990:500.

62. Petajan JH, Gappmaier E, White AT, Spencer JK, Mino L, Hicks RW. Impact of aerobic training on fitness and quality of life in MS. *Ann Neurol* 1996;34:432–441.

63. Ponichtera-Mulcare JA, Mathews T, Barrett PJ, Gupta SC. Change in aerobic fitness of patients with MS during 6-month training program. *Sports Medicine, Training, and Rehabilitation* 1997;7:265–272.

64. Gutierrez GM, Chow JW, Tillman MD, McCoy SC, Castellano V, White J. Resistance training improves gait kinematics in persons with multiple sclerosis. *Arch Phys Med Rehabil* 2005;86:1824–1929.

65. White LJ, McCoy SC, Castellano V, Guiterrez G, Stevens JE, Walter GA, Vandenborne K. Resistance training improves strength and functional capacity in persons with multiple sclerosis. *Mult Scler* 2004;10:668–674

66. Taylor NF, Dodd KJ, Prasad D, Denisenko S. Progressive resistance exercise for people with multiple sclerosis. *Disabil Rehabil* 2006; 28(18):1119–1126.

67. American College of Sports Medicine. Progression models in resistance training for healhty adults. *Med Sci Sports Exerc* 2002;34(2): 364–380.

68. van den Berg M, Dawes H, Wade DT, Newman M, Burridge J, Izadi H, Sackley CM. Treadmill training for individuals with multiple sclerosis: A pilot randomised trial. *J Neurol Neurosurg Psychiatry* 2006;77:531–533.

69. Hoogervorst ELJ, Eikelenboom MJ, Uitdehaag BMJ, Polman CH. One year changes in disability in multiple sclerosis: Neurlogical examination compared with patient self report. *J Neurol Neurosurg Psych* 2003;74(4):439–442.

70. Mostert S, Kesselring J. Effect of a short-term exercise training program on aerobic fitness, fatigue, health perception and activity level of subjects with multiple sclerosis. *Mult Scler* 2002;8:61–168.

71. Romberg A, Virtanen A, Ruutiainen J. Long-term exercise improves functional impairment but not quality of life in multiple sclerosis. *J Neurol* 2005;252:839–845.

72. Kileff J, Ashburn A. A pilot study of the effect of aerobic exercise on people with moderate disabilty multiple sclerosis. *Clin Rehabil* 2005;19:165–169.

73. Newman MA, Dawes H, van den Berg M, Wade DT, Burridge J, Izadi H. Can aerobic treadmill training reduce the effort of walking and fatigue in people with multiple sclerosis: A pilot study. *Mult Scler* 2007;13:113–119.

74. Giesser B, Beres-Jones J, Budovitch A, Herlihy E, Harkema S. Locomotor training using body weight support on a treadmill improves mobility in persons with multiple sclerosis: A pilot study. *Mult Scler* 2007;13:224–231.

75. Berg KO, Wood-Dauphine SL, Williams JI, Maki B. Measuring balance in the elderly: Validation of an instrument. *Can J Public Health* 1992;83[Suppl 2]:S7–S11.

76. Jackson KJ, Mulcare JA, Donahoe-Fillmore B, Fritz HI, Rodgers MM. Home balance training intervention for people with multiple sclerosis. *Int J MS Care* 2007;9:111–117.

77. Gutierrez GM, Chow JW, Tillman MD, McCoy SC, Castellano V, White LJ. Resistance training improves gait kinematics in persons with multiple sclerosis. *Arch Phys Med Rehabil* 2005;86:1824–1829.

78. White LJ, McCoy SC, Castellano V, Guiterrez G, Stevens JE, Walter GA, Vandenborne K. Resistance training improves strength and functional capacity in persons with multiple sclerosis. *Mult Scler* 2004;10:668–674.

79. Stuifbergen A. Health promoting behaviors and quality of life among individuals with MS. *Scholarly Inquiry for Nursing Practice* 1995;9:31–50.

80. Stuifbergen A, Becker H. Predictors of health promoting lifestyles in persons with disabilities. *Res Nurs Health* 1994;17:3–13.

81. Ng AV, Kent-Braun J. Quantification of lower physical activity in persons with MS. *Med Sci Sports Exerc* 1997;29(4):517–523.

82. Rimmer JH, Rubin SS, Braddock D. Barriers to exercise in African American women with physical disabilities. *Arch Phys Med Rehabil* 2000;81(2):182–188.

83. Abramson S, Stein J, Schaufele M, et al. Personal exercise habits and counseling practices of primary care physicians: A national survey. *Clin J Sport Med* 2000;10(1):40–48.

84. Mulcare JA, Webb P, Mathew T, Gupta SC. The effect of body cooling on the aerobic endurance of persons with MS following a 3-month aerobic training program. *Med Sci Sports Exerc* 1997; 29(5):S83.

85. White AT, Wilson TE, Petajan JH. Effect of pre-exercise cooling on physical function and fatigue in MS patients. *Med Sci Sports Exerc* 1997;29(5):S83.

CHAPTER 4

Parkinson's Disease

EPIDEMIOLOGY

Parkinsonism is a progressive, degenerative neurological disorder. The pathology of Parkinson's disease (PD) is associated with the dysfunction of the central nervous system resulting in the decrease, or abnormal activity, of neurotransmitter systems. The resulting neurotransmitter imbalance is exhibited by abnormal movements of the body.

Parkinsonism is ranked as one of the most common neurological syndromes affecting individuals older than age 50 and includes a variety of disorders that consist of varying degrees of resting tremor, bradykinesia (slowness of movement), rigidity, and impaired postural reflexes (15,64,146)(Marttila, 1983). Primary or idiopathic Parkinson's disease (IPD) is the most common type of parkinsonism with the median age of onset being 56 years (119) and most often presents itself between the ages of 50 and 79 years (75,104).

IPD is thought to occur worldwide, and to date, no population has been found immune to the disease (15,85). It is the most common neurodegenerative movement disorder in the world and effects 1% of individuals older than age 60 and increases in prevalence with increasing age (105,119). Races are affected differently by the disease; crude prevalence ratios in the Caucasian population vary from 84 to 270 per 100,000 people (85), while African Americans and Asians appear to have lower prevalence rates, ranging from 4 to 85.7 per 100,000 (Marttila, 1983). The ratio of African Americans to Caucasians is reported to be 1:4 (85). In the United States alone, based on a population of 250 million and using an average prevalence ratio of 160 per 100,000, the number of persons affected by IPD would be approximately 400,000 (104). In the United States, it is also estimated that 1 million Americans are impacted by PD (119).

The incidence of PD has been studied less often than prevalence, with rates varying from 5 to 24 per 100,000 (85). Because the incidence of PD increases with age, after the age of 50, age-specific incidence is said to sharply increase varying from 53 to 229 per 100,000 (Marttila, 1983; 82).

Because prevalence and incidence are closely related, changes in one can affect the other. Prevalence is "the proportion of individuals in a population who have the disease at a specific instant" (45), whereas "incidence quantifies the number of new events or cases of disease that develop in a population of individuals at risk during a specified time interval" (45). Since the advent of levodopa (L-dopa) therapy in the late 1960s, the incidence of PD has remained relatively constant, although the prevalence has increased. This increase in prevalence has been attributed to an increase in the age at time of death—the result of the success of L-dopa therapy (Marttila, 1983; 75). Consequently, individuals with IPD are living longer with the disease.

Prevalence and/or incidence rates between males and females vary depending on whether crude or sex-specific calculations are determined. In studies where sex-specific prevalence and incidence calculations were used, no differences between the sexes in PD affliction have been shown (80,103). Other studies have found that the prevalence and incidence are lower in women versus men (60–62,116).

As with prevalence and incidence, mortality rates associated with PD vary between studies. Prior to L-dopa therapy, mortality related to PD was reported to be 2.9 times higher than in the general population (50). With the advent of L-dopa therapy, this rate has decreased to 1.3 to 1.9 times higher than that in the general population (Marttila, 1983; 21,81,129,145). Because coding and reporting of diseases on death certificates can be inconsistent and often times inaccurate, the underlying cause of death due to complications related to the PD is thought to be underestimated (45). Respiratory and urinary infections are the leading causes of death in individuals having PD (116,123).

CLASSIFICATION

Parkinsonism is a complex of neurological syndromes characterized by clinical symptoms consisting of varying degrees of tremor, bradykinesia, rigidity, and impaired postural reflexes (64). Idiopathic Parkinson's disease (IPD) is classified as such because the damage to the dopaminergic nigrostriatal pathway is unknown and because there is the distinct presence of Lewy body inclusions found in the substantia nigra and locus ceruleus (39,54,102). In contrast, secondary parkinsonism is a neurological syndrome displaying similar motor symptoms as IPD, but the cause of damage to the nigrostriatal system has been identified (40). This secondary classification includes postencephalitic, drug-induced, toxic, traumatic, metabolic, and neoplastic causes (40,54). A third classification includes parkinsonism due to multiple system degenerations or atrophies and has also been labeled parkinsonism-plus syndromes (40). This classification includes striatonigral and pallidonigral degenerations, olivopontocerebellar atrophy, progressive supranuclear palsy, and Shy-Drager syndrome (40,64). This category also includes various degenerative diseases and disorders of the nervous system that are inherited, all of which can present with or cause parkinsonianlike symptoms (54). Approximately 10% of all patients with parkinsonism have "secondary" parkinsonism, and 15% of all patients seen in specialized clinics are diagnosed with multiple system degenerations (54).

For purposes of this chapter, emphasis will be placed on IPD. As much as 75% to 90% of parkinsonian syndromes are thought to be IPD (54,116). Within this classification, distinct clinical pictures occur with the descriptive subgroups labeled depending on which authority one reads (40,54,64).

Clinical symptoms for IPD may be categorized within three subgroups (64): (i) tremor predominant; (ii) postural instability-gait difficulty (PIGD), and (iii) akinetic-rigidity predominant. In addition, there are differentiating features dependent upon age of onset, mental status, and clinical course of the disease. The age of onset is typically broken down into juvenile, younger than 40 years, between 40 and 75 years, or older than 75 years. Classification of mental status is dependent upon dementia being present or absent. The clinical course of the disease can be classified as benign, progressive, or malignant.

As a means to classify the severity of the disease, one of the historical scales, which continues to be used by neurologists today, is the Hoehn and Yahr Staging Scale (50). This original scale stages the progression or severity of the disease from I to V. The scale is based upon symptoms being unilateral or bilateral (I), one's impairment of balance (II), one's functional capability in relation to normal activities (III), employment status (IV), and level of independence (V). In the original version, the descriptives under each stage lack congruity and allow for extreme subjectivity when trying to rate an individual (Table 4.1). Although modified scales have been developed that are more congruent and less ambiguous (such as the United Parkinson's Disease Rating Scale [32]), they still allow for subjectivity when rating an individual. The latter scale is frequently used clinically and in research as a means of classifying patients according to the severity of their disease. Despite its measurement limitations, when reference is made to a particular stage these scales, permit some concept of where an individual is in the possible progression of the disease.

TABLE 4.1. HOEHN AND YAHR STAGING OF PARKINSON'S DISEASE

Stage 1
1. Signs and symptoms on one side only
2. Symptoms mild
3. Symptoms inconvenient but not disabling
4. Usually presents with tremor of one limb
5. Friends have noticed changes in posture, locomotion, and facial expression

Stage 2
1. Symptoms are bilateral
2. Minimal disability
3. Posture and gait affected

Stage 3
1. Significant slowing of body movements
2. Early impairment of equilibrium on walking or standing
3. Generalized dysfunction that is moderately severe

Stage 4
1. Severe symptoms
2. Can still walk to a limited extent
3. Rigidity and bradykinesia
4. No longer able to live alone
5. Tremor may be less than earlier stages

Stage 5
1. Cachectic stage
2. Invalidism complete
3. Cannot stand or walk
4. Requires constant nursing care

PATHOPHYSIOLOGY

As stated previously, IPD is a neurodegenerative process that can result in movement disorders. In addition, these symptoms of dysfunctional movement are often accompanied by nonmotor abnormalities, such as cognitive changes and mood disturbances. The anatomical structure within the central nervous system known to be a primary area affected by the disease is the basal ganglia. Collectively, the basal ganglia are thought to control the more complex aspects of motor planning. In addition, parts of the thalamus and reticular formation work in close association with the above structures and are, therefore, considered to be part of the basal ganglia system for motor control. Furthermore, the basal ganglia is anatomically linked to other parts of the brain that control not only motor and sensory programs, but cognitive and motivational aspects of the human body and psyche as well. Therefore, any disease of the basal ganglia can result in various movement disorders as well as nonmotor abnormalities.

Although it is not the only area affected by the disease, the structure within the basal ganglia most vulnerable to the pathological process of IPD is the substantia nigra. Widespread destruction of the pigmented neurons in the substantia nigra pars compacta is associated with IPD, and as a result of this destruction, the nigrostriatal tract degenerates. The degeneration of the dopaminergic nigrostriatal pathway has been recognized as the primary pathological event resulting in parkinsonian syndromes (40,42,144). This degeneration results in the loss of dopamine normally secreted in the caudate nucleus and putamen, resulting in the classic motor symptoms. The cause of the destruction within the substantia nigra in IPD remains to be answered.

As mentioned previously, there are numerous nonmotor difficulties that can be equally debilitating for those with IPD. These include autonomic dysfunctions, neuropsychiatric problems, sleep disorders, and sensory disorders (119). Some of these problems are thought to be associated with the length of time having had the disease, the severity of the disease, and/or the use of antiparkinsonian medications.

The presentation of autonomic dysfunction appears to be associated with the duration and severity of the disease or the use of antiparkinsonian medications. Structurally, there have been lesions found within the hypothalamus and the locus ceruleus that are both involved in the central control of the autonomic nervous system (74). In addition, abnormalities within the dorsal nucleus of the vagus nerve, a disturbed metabolism of catecholamines, as well as Lewy bodies found within the enteric system have been implicated in autonomic nervous system dysfunction (79,99,129,140–142).

ETIOLOGY

Although the cause of IPD is currently unknown, there are two main theories that have been frequently studied and debated. These involve genetic predisposition and of environmental etiology.

Early twin studies lead researchers to believe that genetics did not provide a significant contribution in the cause of IPD (25,65,78,84,143). Even as recent as the mid-1990s, it was thought that there was no genetic link in the development of PD. Re-examinations of some of the old studies as well as design of newer studies have brought investigators back to reconsidering IPD as a genetically inherited disease. The results of more recent research indicate that genetics may indeed be a causative factor in the development of PD (43). Although the links between the genetic markers to sporadic cases of PD are still unclear, it has generated a significant increase in research examining a genetic cause to PD. The goals of this research have been to determine whether there is indeed a connection and then to determine whether early genetic testing and counseling will impact the development and prognosis of PD, if detected.

As support for an environmental cause, a bizarre outbreak of parkinsonism in northern California in 1983 led to the theory that environmental factors play a role in the etiology of IPD. The victims of this outbreak were drug abusers and had been inadvertently exposed to 1-methyl-4-phenyl-1,2,3,6-tetrahydropyridine (MPTP). MPTP can result as a by-product during the synthesis of the narcotic,1-methyl-r-phenyl-r-proprionorypiperidine (MPPP), a synthetic form of heroine. The drug abusers were exposed to the MPTP as a result of injecting contaminated MPPP and later developed rapid and severe parkinsonian symptoms that included bradykinesia, rigidity, weakness, severe speech difficulties, tremor, masked faces, seborrhea, festinating gait, drooling, flexed posture, as well as a fixed stare and decreased blinking (121). L-dopa/carbidopa treatment was initiated in all patients and improved symptoms, but within a few weeks drug-related side effects of dyskinesias and clinical fluctuations ensued. Thus, an earnest endeavor to search for an environmental cause of IPD began.

Currently, there are no definitive data clearly supporting a genetic or environmental cause. Some believe that it is likely a combination of both. Consequently, the search goes on.

Two other theories that have been suggested as possible mechanisms contributing to the pathogenesis of the disease include mitochondrial dysfunction and free-radical toxicity. Several studies currently suggest that nigral mitochondrial Complex I is abnormal in those with IPD (11,12,108,130). This abnormality appears to be specific to the brain because other studies looking at tissues, such as platelets and muscle (as well as other components of the electron transport chain), have been less consistent in their results. Consequently, more research is needed in this area.

Another body of evidence that is growing suggests that free-radical toxicity causes nigral cell degeneration in those with IPD (27,47,56). This theory suggests that free radicals are produced in the basal ganglia and lead to the progressive degeneration and eventual cell death of neurons in the substantia nigra, although more research is also needed in this area. Unfortunately, there are currently no definitive recognizable risk factors for the development of IPD.

FUNCTIONAL IMPACT

The functional problems that a person with PD displays are dependent upon the symptoms with which they present. Some of the common motor problems related to function in those with PD include gait and balance deficits and difficulty getting out of bed, out of a car, or arising from a chair. Other problems include difficulties with getting dressed (especially fastening buttons), writing, and speech or swallowing problems. Nonmotor problems that can result in functional difficulty and decline include sleep disorders, sensory disorders, and neuropsychiatric problems. In general, the person with PD has trouble doing more than one task at a time. As the disease progresses, these problems usually become more pronounced and the person will eventually lose their ability to perform activities of daily living (ADL). In the last stage of the disease, the person is usually wheelchair- and/or bed-bound.

FUNCTIONAL DIFFICULTY RELATED TO MOTOR SYMPTOMS

In general, problems associated with PD can be categorized into either motor or nonmotor problems. The classic gait pattern displayed by the person with PD is a decrease in step length and foot clearance. The heel-toe pattern is lost, and there is a tendency to shuffle the feet. Posture is flexed forward out of the base of support, which causes the person to take quicker and quicker steps with an inability to stop. This propulsion forward with quick steps is called festination. The person often has difficulty stopping and may eventually fall. In addition, the natural arm swing with gait is greatly decreased or absent.

Balance deficits are also common in those with PD. Because postural reflexes are absent (if the person is perturbed outside the base of support), he or she is often unable to recover and will fall. Falls are a major concern in those with PD and should be kept in mind when prescribing any kind of exercise program.

In addition to gait and balance deficits, segmental movements in the joints (especially in the vertebrae) are greatly decreased if rigidity is present. As a result, the person will have difficulty isolating movements such as rolling from side-to-side as is required when getting out of bed, or being able to rotate the trunk when getting out of a car. In general, movement can be very difficult due to the rigidity and bradykinesia.

Another phenomenon that can greatly impact function is called "freezing." This most typically occurs during gait. The person will be unable to initiate gait or while walking will suddenly become "frozen" in place, as if the person's feet have become glued to the floor. Various techniques such as taking a step backward, marching in place, or visualizing stepping over a line on the floor can bring the person out of the "freeze."

It is important to remember that the functional problems experienced by those with PD are extremely variable from person to person. This requires that an individualized approach be taken with each person afflicted with PD.

FUNCTIONAL DIFFICULTY RELATED TO NONMOTOR SYMPTOMS

As mentioned previously, there are numerous nonmotor problems associated with PD. These include autonomic dysfunctions, neuropsychiatric problems, sleep disorders, and sensory disorders (119). These problems are linked to increased morbidity and mortality, decreased independence, and increased cost of care for those having PD (1,34).

Associated difficulties linked with autonomic nervous system dysfunction include drooling, gastrointestinal problems (constipation, dysphagia), urinary problems (urinary frequency), orthostatic hypotension, erectile dysfunction, dysphagia, excessive sweating, and hypohydrosis (119).

The neuropsychiatric problems linked to PD include mood disorders, anxiety disorders, psychotic hallucinations or delusions, cognitive decline, and dementia. Depression is thought to be relatively common in those having PD although the exact estimate varies widely (13). The estimated range of those suffering from depression is reported to be 7% to 76% (67,119). In addition to depression, mood fluctuations and anxiety are also common and appear to be associated with motor fluctuations, most frequently occurring in the "off" state (3). The presentation of psychosis is most commonly in the form of hallucinations or delusions. These disturbances are thought to be due to secondary illness, medications, underlying dementia, or all of these (119). Many individuals, especially the elderly, experience visual hallucinations that are most common during the evening hours. When asked about these hallucinations, many individuals say they see people or animals and recognize them for what they are and are not usually threatened by them. The importance of recognizing psychosis is that has been associated with nursing home placement and increased mortality (31).

Sleep disorders are estimated to exist in 67% to 88% of individuals having PD (19,92). The cause of these problems is not known, but seems to be linked to how long one has had the disease. Sleep problems occur most frequently in the later stages of the disease process (119). These problems include difficulty falling asleep, difficulty in maintaining sleep or sleep fragmentation, hypersomnolence (especially during the day), rapid eye movement sleep disorders, restless leg syndrome, and obstructive sleep–breathing disorders (76,120).

Sensory disorders experienced by those with PD include pain, akathisia, anosmia, and hyposmia. A common musculoskeletal disorder associated with PD is adhesive capsulitis of the shoulder ("frozen shoulder"). Frozen shoulder can cause extreme pain with or without movement of the involved arm and most often occurs in the upper extremity most affected by the associated motor symptoms rigidity and bradykinesia. In addition, pain is often associated with dystonia, which occurs most frequently in the feet or toes during the "off" state. This pain with dystonia can be so severe that the individual may not be able to walk until it subsides.

FUNCTIONAL PROBLEMS ASSOCIATED WITH COGNITIVE DECLINE AND DEMENTIA

Dementia is common in those with PD. Although the etiology is unclear, dementia is associated with a more rapid functional decline compared to those who do not experience dementia (77). In addition, dementia in those with PD is associated with greater caregiver burden, increased likelihood of nursing home placement and increased mortality. Research has found that in those individuals having even mild cognitive impairment of memory, language, or executive function have a greater likelihood of developing dementia (49,55). In addition, individuals having more severe motor symptoms, as seen in those having the PIGD subtype, have been found to have a greater risk of a more rapid cognitive decline and the eventual development of dementia (4,14). Both have a significant impact on quality of life for the PD patient, as well as for family and friends.

OTHER PROBLEMS THAT MAY AFFECT FUNCTION

Other problems that are less well-studied in those with PD are weight loss and subjective complaints of fatigue. It was suggested by a series of studies spanning 5 years that one-third or more of individuals participating in these studies complained of fatigue (2,30,37,38,46,58,73,113,114). These complaints were found to be more frequent than in age matched healthy controls. The specific impact of this fatigue factor on function for those with PD is not yet clear.

CLINICAL EXERCISE PHYSIOLOGY

Research on the effects of exercise for individuals with PD has been directed toward interventions that would most likely impact the motor control problems associated with the disease. Typical treatment protocols that might be used include range of motion (ROM) and flexibility exercises, balance and gait training, mobility, and/or co-ordination exercises (7,18,41,35,52,85,97,124). Little research has been conducted assessing the aerobic capacity of, or the impact that aerobic exercise might have on, those with IPD. Likewise, there have been few studies assessing strength or using strength training as the intervention for IPD patients.

Most studies have found no difference in maximum or peak oxygen consumption $\dot{V}O_{2peak}$ in those with IPD compared to healthy normals. Stanley et al. (122) had 20 men and women with IPD and 23 healthy men and women perform a one-time exercise bout using a stationary bicycle. It was determined that there was no difference in $\dot{V}O_{2peak}$ between those with IPD and the healthy group. The only significant difference found was in time to maximum exercise in the male subjects. Those with IPD reached $\dot{V}O_{2peak}$ sooner than the healthy group. An additional notable finding between groups was a different response to submaximal exercise. Men and women with IPD appeared to have higher submaximal $\dot{V}O_2$ levels for each stage of exercise. These authors concluded that those with IPD might be less efficient during exercise.

Canning et al. (17) assessed exercise capacity in those with IPD during cycle ergometry to determine if exercise capacity was affected by abnormalities in respiratory function and gait. These researchers did not compare their subjects to healthy individuals, but rather compared actual values to predicted values. No differences were found in peak work or $\dot{V}O_{2peak}$ during exercise. However, they did find certain respiratory abnormalities at rest and during

exercise. Koseoglu et al. (66) also found an impairment in maximum voluntary ventilation and exercise tolerance in those with IPD when compared to a healthy control group. Following a 5-week exercise program involving unsupported upper-extremity exercises (specifics not explained), they found improvement in some respiratory measures as well as an increase in exercise tolerance and a decrease in rating of perceived exertion.

In a study by Reuter et al. (105), patients with PD and age-matched healthy controls were tested using a ramped cycle ergometer protocol. Heart rate variability and lactate levels were measured during exercise with the assumption that these would be impaired if a deficit in the respiratory chain was present. Other variables measured included systolic and diastolic blood pressure and heart rate. They found that heart rate variability was abnormal in those with PD compared to the control group for all tests. The increase in heart rate during exercise was not significantly different between groups, nor was diastolic blood pressure. Systolic blood pressure was lower in those with PD at submaximal and maximal levels of exercise and lactate levels tended to be lower at higher rates of exercise for those with PD but were not statistically significant. These researchers concluded that those with PD can be tested for aerobic capacity and would be expected to achieve changes in aerobic capacity with appropriate exercise intervention.

As with studies addressing aerobic capacity, the research looking at strength issues in those with PD is also limited. Kakinuma et al. (57) found that lower-extremity strength in those with PD was lower on the affected side compared to the unaffected side and that this difference increased as the speed of movement increased. Nogaki et al. (89) have also shown that muscle weakness increases as performance velocity increases. Other studies that have compared strength when the IPD patient has been either on or off antiparkinsonian medications have shown strength to be significantly less when the patient was off their medications (20,69,96).

PHARMACOLOGY

Pharmacologic treatment is the primary therapeutic intervention for the problems associated with IPD. This treatment is based on what is currently known about the neurochemical imbalances that exist in the neurotransmitter concentrations within the basal ganglia of individuals having IPD. Treatment modes have been classified into two general categories by Berg et al. (9), which are: (i) a reduction of the functional excess of acetylcholine with anticholinergics, and (ii) an alleviation of the pathological deficiency of dopamine with drugs that act on the dopaminergic system. In more recent years, protective therapy aimed at slowing the progression of this disease has been introduced (86).

The most common drug classifications used for treatment of IPD include dopaminergics, anticholinergics, monoamine oxidase type "B" (MAO-B) inhibitors, and catechol-O-methyltransferase (COMT) inhibitors. In addition, there are various other drugs that are often prescribed depending on signs and symptoms of the disease (i.e., baclofen, clozapine). The most common medications for each of the above classifications include the following:

1. Dopaminergics (levodopa, levodopa/carbidopa, amantadine, pergolide, bromocriptine)
2. Anticholinergics (benztropine, trihexyphenidyl)
3. MAO-B inhibitors (selegiline)
4. COMT inhibitors (entacapone, tolcapone)

The acute and long-term side-effects can be considerable for all medications taken for PD. Peripheral side effects include gastrointestinal upset, orthostatic hypotension, bradycardia, tachycardia, arrhythmia, dry mouth, blurred vision, and headaches. Central side effects include motor disturbances, insomnia, ataxia, vivid dreams, cognitive/psychiatric disturbances, and edema.

Some of the most debilitating side-effects are those that occur after long-term use of L-dopa. These side-effects are motor disturbances that include dyskinesias, dystonias, and clinical fluctuation (end-of-dose wearing off and predictable or unpredictable "off time"). These frequently appear approximately 5 to 7 years after L-dopa therapy was initiated, although more recent studies suggest that these side-effects may occur as early as 1 to 2 years (94,95). Consequently, newer drugs have been introduced in efforts to address some of the side-effects related to long-term use of levodopa. These include the combination drug Stalevo (levodopa/carbidopa/entacapone) and drugs that utilize different delivery modes, such as Rotigotine (transdermal patch) and Selegiline orally disintegrating tablets. Clinical trials have shown that all of these medications can potentially reduce end-of-dose wearing off and/or "off time" (44,59,69,70,117).

Consideration should be taken when exercising an individual who exhibits any of the above mentioned side-effects. The abnormal movements may interfere in any physical activity that the person attempts to perform. For considerations to be taken during exercise testing and training, please refer to Protas (102).

PHYSICAL EXAMINATION

When examining an individual with PD, it is important to take a thorough history, as well as perform a complete neurological exam and an orthopedic screen. It is also important to determine how the individual is responding to the antiparkinsonian medications, especially if they are beginning to experience any of the long-term side effects.

During the neurological exam, rigidity, tremor, bradykinesia, and postural reflexes must be examined. To illicit rigidity, the examiner can grasp one or both wrists and shake the hand(s) up and down. Looseness and ease of the movement is normally observed. Flexing and extending the forearm repetitively while feeling the ease of movement can also be done to assess rigidity. The same can be done with examination of the lower extremities at the hip, knee, and ankle. The neck and trunk must also be examined by moving the body segment through all planes of movement. Ease of movement and the degree of range will determine the extent of the rigidity. When assessing for rigidity, the movement should be passive, with the individual relaxed. Unlike spasticity, rigidity is not affected by speed of movement (91).

To assess for resting tremor, one should have the patient sit with his/her hands resting in the lap. Then, have the individual recite a specific sentence or count backwards by 2s or 7s. The stress of this activity will allow the tremor to become obvious. The movement is often seen in the hands and is similar to rolling a pill between the fingers (referred to as "pill rolling"). Although resting tremor is the most recognized type of tremor associated with IPD, it is not uncommon that postural tremor and/or intention tremor will present as the disease progresses. Postural (static) tremor can be elicited by having the individual hold a limb against gravity, such as holding one or both arms out in front of the body parallel to the floor. Look for slow up-and-down movement of the arm(s) as the individual maintains this position. In addition, postural tremor can be seen when the individual is asked to maintain a standing position. A slow oscillatory back-and-forth movement will be seen (112). Intention tremor is elicited by having the individual move a limb voluntarily, such as reaching for a cup of water on a table, picking it up, bringing it to the mouth to take a drink, and then returning the cup to the table. An alternative action is to have the individual repetitively bring the forefinger from resting in the lap to his/her nose and then watching for tremor during the course of the movement.

One can assess bradykinesia by having the individual sit with both hands in his or her lap. Ask the patient to supinate and pronate the forearm as fast as possible for at least 30 seconds. If bradykinesia is present, the quality of the movement will begin to break down after a few seconds. There may be a slowing of the movement, a decrease in range of motion, or decreased coordination of the movement.

Postural reflexes can be examined by having the individual stand with his/her back to the examiner. The individual is told to keep their eyes open while the examiner reaches around to the front of the shoulders and pulls quickly and firmly posteriorly. The examiner is observing for recovery from the pull test. Does the individual: (i) stay in place, (ii) step or stagger backwards but recover independently, (iii) step or stagger backwards requiring assistance from the examiner to recover, or (iv) fall straight back without any attempt to recover? It is important that the examiner be behind the individual during this test in order to prevent the individual from falling.

In addition to these tests, a general coordination, sensory, and cognitive examination should also be performed. The Unified Parkinson's Disease Rating Scale (UPDRS) is a comprehensive examination administered by a health professional (32). The UPDRS examines cognition, ADL, motor behaviors, complications of therapy, and also provides a disability rating.

Because the person with IPD can have significant postural changes, a postural screen should be performed. This should be done in both sitting and standing positions. The examiner observes for a forward head, rounded shoulders, kyphosis/scoliosis, decreased lordosis, and/or excessive hip and knee flexion.

To determine responsiveness to the antiparkinsonian medications, certain questions should be asked. To determine whether the individual is having dyskinesias or dystonias, the examiner should ask whether the patient is having any abnormal involuntary movements or postures. If the answer is yes, they should ask when these movements occur in relation to taking his/her dose of medication. The examiner should also ask if there are times after taking his/her dose that the medication does not seem to work and if their symptoms worsen. If this is the case, the individual may be having clinical fluctuations, also known as "on/off" phenomenon. All of this information can be important in determining the best time for the person to exercise.

Numerous outcome measures have been developed that can be used to evaluate the above mentioned problems associated with IPD and the impact that the disease has on the individual's quality of life. These tools can be helpful in being able to objectively document the problems and how they impact one's daily life. Some of the tools that have been developed specifically for those with IPD or have been psychometrically tested with those having the disease include the UPDRS mentioned above, the Parkinson's Disease Questionnaire (PDQ-39), the Timed Up and Go (TUG), Functional Reach, the Berg Balance Scale, the Tinetti Gait and Balance (POMA), the Gait and Balance Scale (GABS), the Functional Independence Measure (FIM), and the 6 Minute Walk Test (6MWT) (8,24,98,110,100,133,135,136).

MEDICAL AND SURGICAL TREATMENTS

As stated previously, drug therapy is the primary means of medical management for IPD. Secondary lines of treatment include sophisticated brain surgeries. Surgical procedures have historically included thalamotomy, pallidotomy, and deep brain stimulation (6,51). For the thalamotomy and pallidotomy, neuroablation procedures or lesions are made to specific areas in the thalamus or globus pallidus. The procedure is an irreversible disruption of the abnormal functioning structure that eliminates the undesired movement disorder such as tremor, leaving other volitional movement intact. Thalamotomy

has been performed to correct drug-resistant tremor, and pallidotomy to decrease rigidity, bradykinesia, tremor, muscular spasms, and off-state dystonias.

Currently the most common surgical procedure used for the treatment of symptoms related to IPD is deep brain stimulation (DPS). In this procedure, a programmable pulse-generating device is implanted in the brain. Like a heart pacemaker, the device can be adjusted telemetrically. The theory behind DPS is that by providing a high-frequency electrical stimulation to specific regions in the brain, it will mimic the effects of creating a lesion as done in the above mentioned surgeries. The advantages over creating permanent lesions are that it is safer, reversible, adaptable, and can be performed bilaterally. Because of these features, DPS has essentially replaced the use of ablative stereotaxy except in special cases. The most common areas within the brain that are targeted for DPS are the subthalamic nucleus (STN) and the internal segment of the globus pallidus (GPi). Studies that have applied stimulation to the STN or the GPi areas have resulted in a decrease of the cardinal motor symptoms related to IPD, improvements in ADL, a decrease in the "off" time related to medication use, and improvements in the "on" time without dyskinesias (106,139). Some studies indicate that stimulation of STN is superior over that of the GPi (132).

Those individuals considered to be candidates for DPS may experience intractable tremor or long-term complications from L-dope therapy (139). These complications include severe motor fluctuations and dyskinesias (138).

Considerable interest has been generated over the use of stem cell transplants as a means of replacing the lost dopaminergic cells in IPD. Three types of cells have been studied for neural transplantation: neural stem cells, embryonic stem cells, and other tissue-specific types of stem cells (e.g., bone marrow stem cells) (87). The strategy is to produce dopamine precursor cells for transplantation that are functional in the host brain without increasing the risk for tumor formation (87). The results so far have been disappointing. Two double-blind clinical trials have not demonstrated improvements. Some of the subjects had problems with nausea and vomiting or developed graft-related involuntary movements (87). Future work may provide greater insight into this approach and offer another treatment option for people with IPD.

DIAGNOSTIC TECHNIQUES

One important line of research related to IPD is the identification of a potential biomarker for early diagnosis of the disease. Currently, the diagnosis is based on a number of clinical symptoms. However, it is currently difficult to differentiate between IPD, various parkinsonianlike syndromes that are distinct from IPD, and other conditions, such as dementia with Lewy-body disease. Patients with IPD and their families often go years without a definitive diagnosis because of this problem. Clearly, early diagnosis would be helpful in terms of treatment alternatives and in understanding the course of the disease.

Some research has led to the identification of myocardial sympathetic denervation in individuals with IPD. A technique using a radiolabeled tracer, I-123-metaiodobenzlyguanidine–single photo emission tomography (MIBG SPECT), displays the myocardial denervation through decreased uptake of the MIBG in individuals with IPD and other Lewy-body diseases, such as dementia with Lewy-body disease. Although most people with IPD have this problem, it is not indigenous to IPD. In other words, the technique is sensitive to the condition, but not exclusive to IPD (i.e., specificity) (88). Future work in this area may improve the specificity of the test and provide an early diagnosis.

EXERCISE AND PHYSICAL PERFORMANCE TESTING

Before exercise testing is performed, it is recommended that balance, gait, general mobility, range of motion (ROM), and manual muscle testing be performed. Results of these tests will provide guidance on how to safely test the individual for functional capacity and performance.

Both static and dynamic balance while in sitting and standing positions should be performed. Clinical balance tests that can be used with those having IPD include the Functional Reach (24), the Berg Balance Scale (8), the Gait and Balance Scale (133), or sensory organization testing (72).

Gait can be observed while the individual walks a 20- to 50-foot pathway. The examiner observes step length, stride width, and heel strike. Because those with IPD have trouble turning, the examiner should observe the individual changing directions. Continuity of steps and coordination during the transition phase are noted. It is also important to observe the person coming to a sudden stop while walking and looking for ease of stopping the momentum. Does the individual stop easily, have to take several steps, stagger or stutter step, or possibly fall? Also, have the individual step over an object in the path. The examiner should take note of any freezing episodes that occur. If balance and gait are seriously compromised, it is not recommended that the treadmill be used for exercise testing without some safety devices, such as safety harnesses and support systems (101,126).

General mobility can be tested by using a tool like the Duke Mobility test (125). Although the scoring of this test uses an ordinal scale, it incorporates several of the above tasks, such as walking, turning, and stepping over an object, as well as reaching, bending down, chair transfers, stairs, and static sitting and standing. It takes only about 10 minutes to administer. Even though mobility may appear to be greatly compromised, the person may still be able to perform an exercise test using a stationary bicycle or arm ergometry protocol. The activity should be tried before assuming the individual cannot undergo exercise testing.

For the rehabilitation specialist, the standard way of testing muscle strength is by manually testing specific muscles or muscle groups. More objective measures include using devices such as hand-held dynamometers, cable tensiometers, handgrip dynamometers, and isokinetic equipment. Because this area has not been well researched, there are no recommendations as to which strength testing protocols should be used. Therefore, recommendations as outlined by the ACSM should be followed for testing muscle strength and endurance (5).

When deciding to test for aerobic endurance, the absolute and relative contraindications for exercise testing outlined by the ACSM should be followed (5). In addition, precautions should be taken if the individual is experiencing severe dyskinesias or dystonias. The results of the physical and functional exam should guide the examiner in what exercise protocol is safe to use. Further research is needed with regard to strength and aerobic testing for those with IPD.

EXERCISE PRESCRIPTION AND PROGRAMMING

When prescribing exercise for the person with IPD, an overall, individualized program should be the goal. Because the disease is chronic and progressive, an exercise program should begin early when the disease is first diagnosed and be maintained on a regular long-term basis. The program should be updated and revised as the disease progresses and the needs of the individual change. Each of the following areas should be addressed: flexibility, aerobic conditioning, strengthening, functional training, and motor control.

To address flexibility, slow static stretches should be performed for all major muscle groups. In addition, ROM exercises should be prescribed for all joints. The upper quadrant and trunk should be emphasized early because the disease affects these areas first and because frozen shoulders and loss of segmental movements in the spine are common as the disease progresses.

Although the optimal frequency for flexibility and ROM exercises for IPD has not been established, suggestions range from once a week to daily. Schenkman et al. (111) conducted a randomized, clinical trial with 51 people with IPD. Twenty-three people participated in a 10-week, 3 times per week program focused on spinal flexibility. This program resulted in improvement in trunk flexibility and functional reach (a measure of balance) but did not result in improvement in the time to move from a supine to a standing position. Even though moving from supine to standing may be limited due to reduced trunk flexibility, increased trunk movement did not result in improved function in this particular study.

Because few studies conducted have used aerobic conditioning or strength training for those with IPD, specifics for prescribing exercise are lacking. Guidelines as outlined by the ACSM should be followed for frequency, intensity, duration, and progression (5,101,102). The mode of exercise should depend on the problems the individual exhibits. As mentioned previously, caution should be taken in placing someone on a treadmill if he/she has gait or balance problems or a history of falls. A stationary bicycle, recumbent bicycle, or arm ergometer may be safer. If walking is used, a level surface with minimal obstacles, such as a walking track, is recommended. Mall walking may be feasible if the person walks when pedestrian traffic is at a minimum. Anecdotal reports from those with IPD indicate that swimming can be a good mode of exercise. Some report that the water enables them to move more easily. When prescribing a strength training program, exercise machines may be safer than the use of free weights because the movement can be better controlled. If a person has severe intention tremor or dyskinesias, free weights may not be as safe as resistive machines. Several small studies suggest that high resistance strength training is safe and effective in individuals with IPD (22,47).

Functional training often includes gait and balance training, as well as fall prevention and specific training in ADL. Again, little research supports the efficacy of these interventions. One small study suggested that gait and step perturbation training on a treadmill can improve gait and balance and reduce falls in individuals with IPD (101). A more recent study supported the use of speed-dependent treadmill training to improve gait speed in people with IPD (16). Training the patient to use visual and auditory cues demonstrates improvements in gait and a reduction in freezing (126,131). There is some evidence that treadmill walking improves walking in people with IPD because the treadmill acts as an externally cued pacemaker (36). One synopsis of the literature related to external cueing and gait in patients with IPD concluded that the best evidence showed strong support for improving walking speed with the help of auditory cues. This study also suggested that there is insufficient evidence for the effectiveness of visual and somatosensory cueing (71).

Motor control strategies emphasize slow, controlled movement for specific tasks through various ranges of motion while lying, sitting, standing, and walking. Dietz & Colombo (23) reported that using a body-weight support system while those with IPD walked on a treadmill improved some gait parameters. Another intriguing approach is training people with IPD to increase the amplitude of movements. One small, nonrandomized study demonstrated improvements in reaching and walking with a 4-week amplitude training program (33).

In a study by Viliani et al. (137), physical training was given to those with IPD that included active mobilization for the lower and upper extremities, spinal mobility exercises, limb coordination exercises, and postural and gait exercises. Specific motor tasks were measured that included supine to sitting, sitting to supine, rolling to supine, and standing from a chair. All the variables showed significant improvement following the intervention. These researchers concluded that specific motor task training can improve movements with which individuals with IPD have problems. Another study investigated the outcomes of a physical therapy program with multiple modes and also demonstrated the effectiveness of this approach (29).

Because of the potential demands of an exercise program, the participant needs to understand and follow instructions in order to safely complete the requirements of the program. Cognitive changes for those with IPD can range from mild to severe; consequently, it is important that the instructor determine whether the person is able to safely follow the program. Ways to ensure this include providing both verbal and written instructions, giving repetitive demonstrations, closely observing the individual while performing all tasks, and instructing the spouse, friend, or other caregiver so that support and direction can be given as needed when at home.

For the older person with IPD, comorbidity can be an issue. Cardiopulmonary disease as well as coexisting arthritis and related musculoskeletal abnormalities should be considered and included in patient screening. Some of the cardiac abnormalities that may be present on the electrocardiogram include frequent premature ventricular contractions, ST-segment depression, a blunted heart rate response (similar to those on β-blockade), and sinus tachycardia during peak dose–related dyskinesias.

As mentioned previously, it is important to have a clear understanding of how the individual responds to his/her medications. Although timing the medication so that the individual is at his/her best during the exercise session is important, precautions should be taken if the person is having dose-related dyskinesias during his/her peak time. Depending on the severity of the dyskinesias, exercise during this time may be contraindicated. For those having "on/off" phenomenon, exercising during an "off" time may be difficult or impossible.

Depending on the severity of the disease, supervision during exercise may or may not be required. For those more involved IPD patients or those with cognitive deficits, group exercise may be more beneficial in order to ensure safety, adherence, and socialization.

Recently published evidence-based practice guidelines suggest that four intervention strategies are based on evidence from two or more controlled trials (63). These strategies include: (i) the application of cueing strategies to improve gait, (ii) the application of cognitive movement strategies to improve transfers, (iii) specific exercises to improve balance, and (iv) training of joint mobility and muscle power to improve physical capacity. Clearly, there is much more research needed on clinical interventions for individuals with IPD.

EDUCATION AND COUNSELING

Because the person with IPD may decrease his/her activity level as it becomes more difficult to move or the tremor becomes an embarrassment, it is imperative that the individual and his/her family be educated about the importance of maintaining an active lifestyle. Parkinson's support groups are organized in larger cities. These groups can be very important in educating the individual and family about the disease, as well as encouraging continued socialization. Exercise groups are often available through these organizations and often include educational presentations. In geographical areas where support groups may not be available, the World Wide Web may be of assistance for those with personal computers in finding virtual support groups and/or information through the various PD associations.

The barriers to exercise can be many for the person with IPD, but the number one barrier may well be the inability to do the activity because of the movement difficulties. When prescribing exercise, careful consideration should be given to the ability of the person and the complexity of the program being prescribed. The more complex the program, the less likely the individual will adhere and exercise compliance may become a problem.

THE FUTURE OF PARKINSON'S DISEASE RESEARCH

GENETICS AND NEUROBIOLOGY

Rapid progress has recently occurred in our understanding of the genetics and neurobiology of IPD. Research has identified several genetic mutations, called PARK mutations, that are related to genetic rather than sporadic or idiopathic forms of IPD. One mutation to the α-syncline gene may be related to neurotoxicity and is a major constituent in Lewy bodies seen in IPD. Another mutation in PARK 2 suggests that the ubiquitin-proteosome pathway may be involved in IPD. Other mutations implicate oxidative damage and mitochondria in the pathogenesis of IPD (10). This research has led to agents that deal with oxidative stress and the mitochondria, such as coenzyme Q10 (115). New insights provided by genetic forms of IPD and the neurobiology of the disease promise to offer new directions and possible biological interventions in the future.

NEUROPROTECTION

Because IPD is a progressive neurodegenerative disease and current treatment does not stop or delay the disease progression, an important question is whether interventions can be found that will protect against the neural degeneration seen in the disease. To date, no treatment that provides neuroprotection has been found; however, research that examines the role of an intervention as a neuroprotective agent is fraught with difficulties (10). One early issue in this research is that loss of more than 80% of the dopaminergic cells in the striatum occur before clinical symptoms arise. Enrolling patients with even mild, early symptoms may provide a population who still have significant loss of neural cells. Another issue is that interventions that are currently available do offer symptomatic relief. Clinical trials can imply neuroprotection when, in fact, only symptomatic improvements occur. Improvements in clinical trail designs, such as a delayed start, have addressed some of these concerns. Other issues are the variability and the slow progression of the disease. There are insufficient methods to categorize variations in the disease. For example, those who develop IPD in their 80s often have mild symptoms that progresses very slowly, while those who have a young onset in their 30s often have more severe symptoms that progress more rapidly.

With the above limitations in mind, the Committee to Identify Neuroprotective Agents for Parkinson's (CINAPS) was established by the National Institute of Neurological Disorders and Stroke. This evidence-based assessment of various drugs and agents has identified a number of promising candidates (Ravina et al., 2003). Drugs such as amantadine, cyclooxygenase I and II inhibitors, and Ropinirole, as well as agents such as ascorbic acid, caffeine, and nicotine were included. Interestingly, epidemiologic studies have suggested that both caffeine and nicotine use may have neuroprotective effects for developing IPD.

There is also evidence from animal studies of a number of mechanisms that may be neuroprotective (147). An interesting line of this research is whether physical activity can have a neuroprotective effect (118). In an animal model that uses neurotoxin exposure to produce Parkinson-like symptoms, moderate treadmill exercise attenuated the neurochemical loss and produced behavioral sparing (134). Obviously, similar studies on the effects of moderate exercise in people with early IPD will require large clinical trials and significant resources. Indeed, we may see such a trial (or trials) in the near future.

NEURAL IMAGING

Recent advances in neural imaging techniques have allowed studies that could provide images of the brain areas affected by IPD. Clearly, these approaches are important to examine not only responses to intervention but also possible neuroprotection of these interventions. With functional magnetic resonance imaging, human locomotor centers in the brainstem and cerebellum can be studied during brain mental imagery of standing, walking, and running in healthy individuals (53). Although this technique has not been used with people with IPD, the methodology does have promise for future research. Radiotracer-based imaging of nigrostriatal dopamine function may also be a method of monitoring the progression of the disease (28). Another method, spatial covariance analysis with ^{18}F-fluorodeoxyglucose positron emission tomography, detects abnormal patterns of brain metabolism in people with IPD (28). Another radiolabeled methodology, ^{18}F-fluoropropyl-β-CIT, quantifies the dopamine transporter binding in the caudate and putamen—an index of presynaptic nigrostriatal dopaminergic function (28). These methodologies may provide a biomarker to diagnose IPD and related disorders, determine sensitive measures of neuroprotection, and/or identify mechanisms underlying some of the interventions such as exercise.

REFERENCES

1. Aarsland D, Larsen JP, Tandberg E, Laake K. Predictors of nursing home placement in Parkinson's disease: A population-based, prospective study. *J Am Geriatr Soc* 2000;48:938–942.

2. Abe K, Takanashi M, Yanagihara T. Fatigue in patients with Parkinson's disease. *Behav Neurol* 2000;12(3):103–106.

3. Adler CH. Nonmotor complications in Parkinson's disease. *Mov Disord* 2005;20(suppl 11):23–29.

4. Alves G, Larsen JP, Emre M, et al. Changes in motor subtype and risk for incident dementia in Parkinson's disease. *Mov Disord* 2006;21(8):1123–1130.

5. American College of Sports Medicine. *ACSM's Guidelines For Exercise Testing And Prescription*. 8th ed. Baltimore: Lippincott Williams & Wilkins; 2009.

6. Arle JE, Alterman RL. Surgical options in Parkinson's disease. *Med Clin North Am.* 1999;83(2):483–498.

7. Banks MA, Caird FI. Physiotherapy benefits patients with Parkinson's disease. *Clin Rehabil* 1989;3:11–16.

8. Berg K, Wood-Dauphinee S, Williams JI, et al. Measuring balance in the elderly: Preliminary development of an instrument. *Physiother Can* 1989;41(6):304–311.

9. Berg MJ, Ebert B, Willis DK, et al. Parkinsonism—drug treatment: Part I. *Drug Intell Clin Pharm* 1987;21(1):10–21.

10. Biglan KM, Ravina B. Neuroprotection in Parkinson's disease: An elusive goal. *Semin Neurol* 2007;27:106–112.

11. Bindoff LA, Birch-Machin MA, Cartlidge NEF, et al. Mitochondrial function in Parkinson's disease. *Lancet* 1989;2:49.

12. Blin O, Desnuelle C, Rascol O, et al. Mitochondrial respiratory failure in skeletal muscle from patients with Parkinson's disease and multiple system atrophy. *J Neurol Sci* 1994;125:95–101.

13. Bohnen NI, Kaufer DI, Hendrickson R, Constantine GM, Mathis CA, Moore RY. Cortical cholinergic denervation is associated with depressive symptoms in Parkinson's disease and parkinsonian dementia. *J Neurol Neurosurg Psychiatry* 2007;78:641–643.

14. Burn DJ, Rowan EN, Allan LM, Molloy S O'Brien JT, McKeith IG. Motor subtype and cognitive decline in Parkinson's disease, Parkinson's disease with dementia, and dementia with Lew bodies. *J Neurol Nurosurg Psychiatry* 2006;77:585–589.

15. Caird FI. Parkinson's disease and its natural history. In: Caird FI, editor. *Rehabilitation In Parkinson's Disease*. New York: Chapman & Hall; 1991. p. 1–7.

16. Cakit BD, Saracoglu M, Genc H, Erdem HR. The effects of incremental speed-dependent treadmill training on postural instability and fear of falling in Parkinson's disease. *Clin Rehabil* 2007;21:698–705.

17. Canning CG, Alison JA, Allen NE, et al. Parkinson's disease: An investigation of exercise capacity, respiratory function, and gait. *Arch Phys Med Rehabil* 1997;78:199–207.

18. Comella CL, Stebbins GT, Brown-Toms N, et al. Physical therapy and Parkinson's disease: A controlled clinical trail. *Neurology* 1994;44:376–378.

19. Comella C. Sleep disturbances in Parkinson's disease. *Curr Neurol Neurosci Rep* 2003;3:173–180.

20. Corcos DM, Chen CM, Quinn NP, et al. Strength in Parkinson's disease: Relationship to rate of force generation and clinical status. *Ann Neurol* 1996;39:79–88.

21. Diamond SG, Markham ChC. Present mortality in Parkinson's disease: The ratio observed to expected deaths with a method to calculate expected deaths. *J Neural Transm* 1976;36:259–269.

22. Dibble LE, Hale T, Marcus RL, Gerber JP, LaStayo PC. The safety and feasibility of high-force eccentric resistance exercise in persons with Parkinson's disease. *Arch Phys Med Rehabil* 2006;87:1280–1282.

23. Dietz V, Colombo G. Influence of body load on the gait pattern in Parkinson's disease. *Mov Disord* 1998;13(2):255–261.

24. Duncan PW, Weiner DK, Chandler J, et al. Functional reach: A new clinical measure of balance. *J Gerontol* 1990;45:M192–197.

25. Duvoisin RC, Eldridge R, Williams A, et al. Twin study of Parkinson's disease. *Neurology.* 1981;31:77–80.

26. Duvoisin RC. Genetics of Parkinson's disease. *Adv Neurol* 1986;45:307–312.

27. Ebadi M, Srinivasan SK, Baxi MD. Oxidative stress and antioxidant therapy in Parkinson's disease. *Prog Neurobiol* 1996;48:1–19.

28. Eckert T, Tang C, Eidelberg D. Assessment of the progression of Parkinson's disease: A metabolic network approach. *Lancet Neurol* 2007;6:926–932.

29. Ellis T, de Goede CJ, Feldman RG, Wolters EC, Kwakkel G, Wagenaar RC. Efficacy of a physical therapy program in patients with Parkinson's disease: A randomized controlled trial. *Arch Phys Med Rehabil* 2005;86:626–632.

30. Erdal KJ. Depressive symptom patterns in patients with Parkinson's disease and other older adults. *J Clin Psychol* 2001;57(12):1559–1569.

31. Factor SA, Feustel PJ, Friedman JH, et al. Logitudinal outcome of Parkinson's disease patients with psychosis. *Neurology* 2003;60(11):17546–1761.

32. Fahn S, Elton RL, Members of the UPDRS Development Committee. Unified Parkinson's disease rating scale. In: Stanley F, Marsden CD, Goldstein M, et al., editors. *Recent Developments In Parkinson's Disease*, volume II. Florham Park (NJ): MacMillan Healthcare Information; 1987. p. 153–303.

33. Farley B, Koshland GF. Training BIG to move faster: The application of the speed-amplitude relation as a rehabilitation strategy for people with Parkinson's disease. *Exp Brain Res* 2005;167:462–467.

34. Findley L, Aujla M, Bain PG, et al. Direct economic impact of Parkinson's disease: A research surve in the United Kingdom. *Mov Disord* 2003;18(10):1139–1145.

35. Flewitt B, Capildeo R, Rose FC. Physiotherapy and assessment in Parkinson's disease using the polarised lightgoniometer. In: Rose FC, Capildeo R, editors. *Research Progress In Parkinson's Disease*. Kent: Pitman Medical; 1981. p. 404–413.

36. Frenkel-Toledo S, Giladi N, Peretz C, Herman T, Gruendlinger L, Hausdorff JM. Treadmill walking as an external pacemaker to improve gait rhythm and stability in Parkinson's disease. *Mov Disord* 2005;20:1109–1114.

37. Friedman J, Friedman H. Fatigue in Parkinson's disease. *Neurology* 1993;43(10):2016–2018.

38. Friedman JH, Friedman H. Fatigue in Parkinson's disease: A nine-year follow-up. *Mov Disord* 2001;16(6):1120–1122.

39. Gershanik OS, Nygaard TG. Parkinson's disease beginning before age 40. In: Streifler MB, Korcqyn AD, Melamed E, et al., editors. *Advances In Neurology: Parkinson's Disease: Anatomy, Pathology, and Therapy*. New York: Raven Press, Ltd.; 1990; p. 251–258.

40. Gerstenbrand F, Poewe WH. The classification of Parkinson's disease. In: Stern G, editor. *Parkinson's Disease*. Baltimore: John Hopkins University Press; 1990. p. 315–331.

41. Gibberd FB, Page NGR, Spencer KM, et al. A controlled trial of physiotherapy for Parkinson's disease. In: Rose FC, Capildeo R, editors. *Research Progress in Parkinson's Disease*. Kent: Pitman Medical; 1981. p. 401–403.

42. Gupta M. Parkinson's disease pathology: Multineurotransmitter systems defects. In: Schneider JS, Gupta M, editors. *Current*

Concepts In Parkinson's Disease Research. Seattle: Hogufe & Haber Publishers; 1993. p. 21–40.

43. Hardy J, Cai H, Cookson MR, Gwing-Hardy K, Aingleton A. Genetics of Parkinson's disease and parkinsonism. *Ann Neurol* 2006;60:389–398.

44. Hauser RA. Levodopa/carbidopa/entacapone (stalevo). *Neurology* 2004;62(Suppl 1):S64–S71.

45. Hennekens CH, Buring JE. *Epidemiology in Medicine.* Boston: Little, Brown and Co.; 1987. p. 57.

46. Herlofson K, Larsen JP. Measuring fatigue in patients with Parkinson's disease—the Fatigue Severity Scale. *Eur J Neurol* 2002;9(6):595–600.

47. Hirsch EC. Does oxidative stress participate in nerve cell death in Parkinson's disease? *Eur Neurol* 1993;33(Suppl 1):52–59.

48. Hirsch MA, Toole T, Maitland CG, Rider RA. The effects of balance training and high-intensity resistance training on persons with idiopathic Parkinson's disease. *Arch Phys Med Rehabil* 2003; 84:1109–1117.

49. Hobson P, Meara J. Risk and incidence of dementia in a cohort of older subjects with Parkinson's disease in the United Kingdom. *Mov Disord* 2004;19(9):1043–1049.

50. Hoehn M, Yahr MD. Parkinsonism: Onset, progression, and mortality. *Neurology* 1967;17(5):427–442.

51. Honey C, Gross RE, Lozano AM. New developments in the surgery for Parkinson's disease. *Can J Neurol Sci* 1999;26(Suppl 2):S45–S52.

52. Hurwitz LJ. Improving mobility in severely disabled parkinsonian patients. *Lancet* 1964:953–955.

53. Jahn K, Deutschlander A, Stephan T, Kalla R, Wiesmann M, Strupp M, Brandt T. Imaging human suprspinal locomotor centers in brainstem and cerebellum. *NeuroImage* 2008;39:786–792.

54. Jankovic J. Parkinsonism—plus syndromes. *Mov Disord* 1989; 4(suppl 1):S95–S119.

55. Janvin CC, Larsen JP, Aarsland D, et al. Subtypes of mild cognitive imparment in Parkinson's disease: Progression to dementia. *Mov Disord* 2006;21(9):1343–1349.

56. Jenner P, Olanow CW. Oxidative stress and the pathogenesis of Parkinson's disease. *Neurology* 1996;47(suppl 3):S161–S170.

57. Kakinuma S, Hiroshi N, Pramanik B, et al. Muscle weakness in Parkinson's disease: Isokenetic study of the lower limbs. *Eur Neurol* 1998;39:218–222.

58. Karlsen K, Larsen JP, Tandberg E, Jorgensen K. Fatigue in patients with Parkinson's disease. *Mov Disord* 1999;14(2):237–241.

59. Kenney C, Jankovic J. Rotigotine transdermal patch in the treatment of Parkinson's disease and restless legss syndrom. *Expert Opin Pharmacother* 2007;8(9):1329–1335.

60. Kessler II. Epidemiologic studies of Parkinson's disease II. A hospital-based survey. *Am J Epidemiol* 1972;95(4):308–318.

61. Kessler II. Epidemiologic studies of Parkinson's disease III. A community-based survey. *Am J Epidemiol* 1972;96(4):242–254.

62. Kessler II, Diamond EL. Epidemiologic studies of Parkinson's disease I. Smoking and Parkinson's disease: A survey and explanatory hypothesis. *Am J Epidemiol* 1972;94(1):16–25.

63. Keus SHJ, Bloem BR, Hendriks EJM, Bredero-Cohen AB, Munneke M. Evidence-based analysis of physical therapy in Parkinson's disease with recommendation for practice and research. *Mov Disord* 2007;22:451–460.

64. Koller WC, Hubble JP. Classification of parkinsonism. In: Koller WC, editor. *Handbook of Parkinson's Disease.* 2nd ed. New York: Marcel Dekker, Inc.; 1992. p. 59–103.

65. Kondo K, Kurland LT, Schull WJ. Parkinson's disease, genetic analysis and evidence of a multifactorial etiology. *Mayo Clin Proc* 1973;48:465–475.

66. Koseoglu F, Inan L, Ozel S, et al. The effects of a pulmonary rehabilitation program on pulmonary function tests and exercise tolerance in patients with Parkinson's disease. *Funct Neurol* 1997;12: 319–325.

67. Leentjens AF, Van den Akker M, Metsemakers JF, Lousberg R, Verhey FR. Higher incidence of depression preceding onset of Parkinson's disease: A register study. *Mov Disord* 2003;18(4):414–418.

68. Lew MR, Pahwa R, Leehey M, Bertoni J, Kricorian G, the Sydis Selegiline Study Group. Safety and efficacy of newly formulated selegiline orally disintegrating tablets as an adjunct to levodopa in the management of "off" episodes in patients with Parkinson's disease. *Curr Med Res Opin* 2007;23(4):741–750.

69. LeWitt PA, Bharucha A, Chitrit I, et al. Perceived exertion and muscle efficiency in Parkinson's disease: L-dopa effects. *Clin Neuropharmacol* 1994;17(5):454–459.

70. LeWitt PA, Lyons KE. Pahwa R, SP 650 Study Group. Advanced Parkson disease treated with rotigotine transdermal system: PREFER study. *Neurology* 2007;68:1262–1267.

71. Lim I, van Wegen E, de Goede C, et al. Effects of external rhythmical cueing on gait in patients with Parkinson's disease: A systematic review. *Clin Rehabil* 2005;19:695–713.

72. Liston RAL, Brouwer BJ. Reliability and validity of measures obtained from stroke patient using the balance master. *Arch Phys Med Rehabil* 1996;77:425–430.

73. Lou JS, Kearns G, Oken B, Sexton G, Nutt J. Exacerbated physical fatigue and mental fatigue in Parkinson's disease. *Mov Disord* 2001;16(2):190–196.

74. Ludin SM, Steiger MJ, Ludin. Autonomic disturbances and cardiovascular reflexes in idiopathic Parkinson's disease. *J Neurol* 1987; 235:10–15.

75. Maguire GH. Occupational therapy. In: Abrams WB, Berkow R, Fletcher AJ, et al., editors. *The Merck Manual of Geriatrics.* Rathway (NJ): Merck Sharp and Dohme Research Laboratories; 1990. p. 274–278.

76. Maria B, Sophia S, Michalis M, et al. Sleep breathing disorders in patients with idopathic Parkinson's disease. *Respir Med* 2003;97(10): 1151–1157.

77. Marras C, Rochon P, Lang AE. Predicting motor decline and disability in Parkinson disease: A systematic review. *Arch Neurol* 2002;59:1724–1728.

78. Marsden CD. Parkinson's disease in twins. *J Neurol Neurosurg Psychiatry* 1987;50:105–106.

79. Martignoni E, Micieli G, Cavallini A, et al. Autonomic disorders in idiopathic parkinsonism. *J Neural Transm* 1986;22(suppl):149–61.

80. Marttila RJ, Rinne UK. Epidemiology of Parkinson's disease in Finland. *Acta Neurol Scand* 1976;53:80–102.

81. Marttila RJ, Rinne UK, Siirtola T, et al. Mortality of patients with Parkinson's disease treated with levodopa. *J Neurol* 1977;216: 147–153.

82. Marttila RJ, Rinne UK. Epidemiology of Parkinson's disease—an overview. *J Neural Trans* 1981;51:135–148.

83. Marttila RJ. Hennekens CH, Buring JE. *Epidemiology in Medicine.* Boston: Little, Brown and Co.; 1987. p. 57.

84. Martilla RJ, Kaprio J, Kistenvuo MD, et al. Parkinson's disease in a nationwide twin cohort. *Neurology* 1988;38:1217–1219.

85. Marttila RJ. Epidemiology. In: Koller WC, editor. *Handbook of Parkinson's Disease.* 2nd ed. New York: Marcel Dekker, Inc.; 1992. p. 35–57.

86. Montgomery EB, Lipsy RJ. Treatment of Parkinson's disease. In: Bressler R, Kane MD, editors. *Geriatric Pharmacology.* New York: McGraw Hill, Inc.; 1993. p. 309–328.

87. Morizane A, Li JY, Brundin P. From bench to bed: The potential of stem cells for the treatment of Parkinson's disease. *Cell Tissue Res* 2008;331:323–336.

88. Nagayama H, Hamamoto M, Ueda M, Nagashima J, Katayama Y. Reliability of MIBG myocardial scintigraphy in the diagnosis of Parkinson's disease. *J Neurol Neurosurg Psychiatry* 2005;76:249–251.

89. Nogaki H, Kakinuma S, Morimatsu M. Movement velocity dependent muscle strength in Parkinson's disease. *Acta Neurol Scand* 1999; 99:152–157.

90. Olanow CW. An introduction to the free radical hypothesis in Parkinson's disease. *Ann Neurol* 1992;32(Suppl):S2–S9.

91. O'Sullivan SB. Parkinsons disease. In: O'Sullivan SB, Schmitz TJ, editors. *Physical Rehabilitation.* 5th ed. Philadelphia: FA Davis Company; 2007. p. 853–893.

92. Pal PK, Thennarasu K, Fleming J, Schulzer M, Brown T, Calne SM. Nocturnal sleep disturbances and daytime dysfunction in patients with Parkinson's disease and in their caregivers. *Parkinsonism Relat Disord* 2004;10(3):157–168.

93. Palmer SS, Mortimer JA, Webster DD, et al. Exercise therapy for Parkinson's disease. *Arch Phys Med Rehabil* 1986;67:741–745.

94. Parkinson Study Group. Impact of deprenyl and tocopherol treatment on Parkinson's disease in DATATOP subjects not requiring levodopa. *Ann Neurol* 1996;39:29–36.

95. Parkinson Study Group. Pramipexole versus levodeopa as initial treatment for Parkinson's disease: A randomized controlled trial. Parkinson Study Group. *JAMA* 2000;284:1931–1938.

96. Pedersen SW, Oberg B, Insulander A, et al. Group training in parkinsonism: Quantitative measurements of treatment. *Scand J Rehab Med* 1990;22:207–211.

97. Pedersen SW, Oberg B. Dynamic strength in Parkinson's disease. *Eur Neurol* 1993;33:97–102.

98. Petro V et al. The development and validation of a short measure of functioning and well being for individuals with Parkinson's disease. *Qual Life Res* 1995;4:241.

99. Piha SJ, Rinne UK, Rinne RK, et al. Autonomic dysfunction in recent onset and advanced Parkinson's disease. *Clin Neurol Neurosurg* 1988;90(3):221–226.

100. Podsiadlo D, Richaardson S. The timed "Up and Go": A test of basic functional mobility for frail elderly persons. *J Am Geriatri Soc* 1991;39:142–148.

101. Protas EJ, Williams A, Qureshy H, Caroline K, Lai E. Gait and step training to reduce falls in Parkinson's disease. *Neurorehabilitation* 2005;20(3):183–190.

102. Protas EJ, Stanley R, Jankovic J. Parkinson's disease. In: Durstine JL, Moore GE, editors. *Exercise Management for Persons with Chronic Disease and Disabilities.* 3rd ed. Indianapolis: American College of Sports Medicine. 2009; p. 295–302.

103. Rajput AH, Offord, Beard CM, et al. Epidemiology of parkinsonism: Incidence classification and mortality. *Ann Neurol* 1984;16:278–282.

104. Rajput AH. Current concepts in the etiology of Parkinson's disease. In: Schneider JS, Gupta M, editors. *Current Concepts in Parkinson's Disease Research.* Seattle: Hagrefe & Huber Publishers; 1993. p. 11–19.

105. Ravina BM, Fagan SC, Hart RG, et al. Neuroprotective agents for clinical trials in Parkinson's disease: a systematic assessment. *Neurology* 2003;60(8):1234–1240.

106. Rodriguez-Oroz MC, Obeso JA, Lang AE, et al. Bilateral deep brain stimulation in Parkinson's disease: A multicentre study with 4 years follow-up. *Brain* 2005;128,2240–2249.

107. Samii A, Nutt JG, Ransom BR. Parkinson's disease. *Lancet* 2004; 363(9423):1783–1793.

108. Schapira AHV, Cooper JM, Dexter DT, et al. Mitochondrial complex I deficiency in Parkinson's disease. *Lancet* 1989;1:1269.

109. Schenkman M, Butler RB. A model for multisystem evaluation treatment of individuals with Parkinson's disease. *Phys Ther* 1989; 69(11):932–943.

110. Schenkman M, Cutson TM, Kuchibhata M, Chandler J, Pieper C. Reliability of impairment and physical performance measures for persons with Parkinson's disease. *Phys Ther* 1997;77(1):19–27.

111. Schenkman M, Cutson TM, Kuchihhatla M, et al. Exercise to improve spinal flexibility and function for people with Parkinson's disease: A randomized, controlled trial. *J Am Geriatr Soc* 1998;46:1207–1216.

112. Schmitz TJ. Examination of coordination. In: O'Sullivan SB, Schmitz TJ, editors. *Physical Rehabilitation.* 5th ed. Philadelphia: FA Davis Company; 2007. p. 199.

113. Scott B, Borgman A, Engler H, Johnels B, Aquilonius SM. Gender differences in Parkinson's disease symptom profile. *Acta Neurol Scand* 2000;102(1):37–43.

114. Shulman LM, Taback RL, Rabinstein AA, Weiner WJ. Non-recognition of depression and other non-motor symptoms in Parkinson's disease. *Parkinsonism Relat Disord* 2002;8(3):193–197.

115. Shults CW, Oakes D, Kieburtz K. Effects of coenzyme Q10 in early Parkinson disease: Evidence of slowing of the functional decline. *Arch Neurol* 2002;59:1541–1550.

116. Siderowf A, Stern M. Update on Parkinson's disease. *Ann Int Med* 2003;138(8):651–658.

117. Silver DE. Clinical experience with the novel levodopa formulation entacapone + levodopa + carbidop (stalevo®). *Expert Rev Neurother* 2004;4(4):589–599.

118. Smith AD, Zigmond MJ. Can the brain be protected through exercise? Lessons from an animal model of parkinsonism. *Exp Neurol* 2003;184(1):31–39

119. Snyder CH, Adler CH. The patient with Parkinson's disease: Part I—treating the motor symptoms. *J Am Acad Nurse Pract* 2007; 179–197.

120. Snyder CH, Adler CH. The patient with Parkinson's disease: Part II—treating the nonmotor symptoms. *J Am Acad Nurse Pract* 2007;189–197.

121. Sonsalla PK, Nicklas WJ. MPTP and animal models of Parkinson's disease. In: Koller WC, editor. *Handbook of Parkinson's Disease.* 2nd ed. New York: Marcel Dekker, Inc.; 1992. p. 319–340.

122. Stanley RK, Protas EJ, Jankovic J. Exercise performance in those having Parkinson's disease and healthy normals. *Med Sci Sports Exerc* 1999;31(6):761–766.

123. Stefaniwsky L, Bilowit DS. Parkinsonism: Facilitation of motion by sensory stimulation. *Arch Phys Med Rehab* 1973;54(2):75–77.

124. Stern PH, McDowell F, Miller JM, et al. Levodopa and physical therapy in treatment of patients with Parkinson's disease. *Arch Phys Med Rehab* 1970;(5):273–277.

125. Studenski S, Duncan PW, Hogue C, et al. Progressive mobility skills: A mobility scale with hierarchical properties. In: *American Geriatrics Society Annual Meeting,* Boston; 1989. p. 41.

126. Suteerawattananon M, MacNeill E, Protas EJ. Supported treadmill training for gait and balance: A case report in progressive supranuclear palsy. *Phys Ther* 2002;82;485–495.

127. Suteerawattananon M, Morris GS, Etnyre BR, Jankovic J, Protas EJ. Effect of visual and auditory cues on individuals with Parkinson's disease. *J Neuro Sci* 2004;219(1-2):63–69.

128. Sweet RD, McDowell FH. Five years' treatments of Parkinson's disease with levodopa. *Ann Intern Med* 1975;83:456–463.

129. Tanner CM, Goetz CG, Klawans HL. Autonomic nervous system disorders. In: Koller WC, editor. *Handbook of Parkinson's Disease.* New York: Marcel Dekker, Inc.; 1992. p. 185–215.

130. Taylor DJ, Krige D, Barnes PRJ, et al. A^{31} P magnetic resonance spectroscopy study of mitochondrial function in skeletal muscle of patients with Parkinson's disease. *J Neuro Sci* 1994;125:77–81.

131. Thaut MH, McIntosh GC, Rice RR, et al. Rhythmic auditory stimulation in gait training for Parkinson's disease patients. *Mov Disord* 1996;11(2):193–200.

132. The Deep Brain Stimulation for Parkinson's Disease Study Group. Deep-brain stimulation of the subthalamic nucleus or the pars interna of the globus pallidus in Parkinson's disease. *New Engl J Med* 2001;345:956–963.

133. Thomas M, Jankovic J, Suteerawattananon M, Wankadia S, Caroline K, Vuong KD, Protas E. Clinical gait and balance scale (GABS). *J Neuro Sci* 2004;217:89–99.

134. Tillerson JL, Caudle WM, Reveron ME, Miller GW. Exercise induces behavioral recovery and attenuates neruochemical deficits in rodent models of Parkinson's disease. *Neuroscience* 2003;119:899–911.

135. Tinetti ME. Performance-oriented assessment of mobility problems in elderly patients. *JAMA* 1986;34:119–126.

136. Uniform Data System for Medical Rehabilitation. 1997. The Guide for the Uniform Data Set for Medical Rehabilitation (Including the FIM Instrument), Version 5.1, Buffalo:UDS$_{MR}$.

137. Viliani T, Pasquetti P, Magnolfi S, et al. Effects of physical training on straightening-up processes in patients with Parkinson's disease. *Disabil Rehab* 1999;21(2):68–73.

138. Volkmann, Alleret N, Voges J, Sturm V, Schnitzler A, Freund JH. Long-term results of bilateral pallidal stimulation in Parkinson's disease. *Ann Neurol* 2004;55:871–875.

139. Volkmann J. Update on surgery for Parkinson's disease. *Curr Opin Nuerol* 2007;20:465–469.

140. Wakabayashi K, Takahashi H, Takeda S, et al. Parkinson's disease: The presence of Lewy bodies in Auerbach's and Meissner's plexuses. *Acta Neuropathol* 1988;76:217–221.

141. Wakabayashi K, Takahashi H, Takeda S, et al. Louie bodies in the enteric nervous system in Parkinson's disease. *Arch Histol Cytol* 1989;52(Suppl 1):191–194.

142. Wakabayashi R, Takahashi H, Ohama E, et al. Parkinson's disease: An immunohistochemical study of Lewy body-containing neurons in the enteric nervous system. *Acta Neuropathol* 1990;79:581–583.

143. Ward CD, Duvoisin RC, Ince SE, et al. Parkinson's disease in 65 pairs of twins and in a set of quadruplets. *Neurology* 1983;33:815–824.

144. Wichmann T, DeLong MR. Pathophysiology of parkinsonian motor abnormalities. In: Narabayashi H, Nagatau T, Yanagisawa N, et al., editors. *Advances in Neurology*. New York: Raven Press, Ltd.; 1993:60. p. 53–61.

145. Yahr MD. Evaluation of long-term therapy in Parkinson's disease. Mortality and therapeutic efficacy. In: Birkmayer W, Hornykiewicz O, editors. *Advances in Parkinsonism*. Basle: Editiones Roche; 1976. p. 435–443.

146. Yahr MD, Pang SWH. Movement disorders. In: Abrams WB, Berkow R, Fletcher AJ, et al., editors. *The Merck Manual of Geriatrics*. Rahway, NJ: Merck Sharp & Dohme Research Laboratories; 1990. p. 973–994.

147. Zigmond M. Triggering endogenous neuroprotective mechanisms in Parkinson's disease: studies with a cellular model. *J Neural Transm Suppl* 2006;(70):439–442.

Spinal Cord Dysfunction

In this chapter, the term "spinal cord dysfunction" (SCD) will represent either acquired spinal cord injury (SCI) or spina bifida (SB), both of which involve lesions on the spinal cord. It will not include poliomyelitis, postpolio, or postpolio syndrome (see Chapter 6). Also, because of the continuity of the spinal cord and cauda equina in the spine, SCD will include both injury to the spinal cord itself (part of the central nervous system) and to the cauda equina (part of the peripheral nervous system). The resulting damage to the neural elements within the spinal canal results in impairment or loss of motor and/or sensory function in the trunk and extremities. Depending on the neurologic level and severity of the lesion, SCI may result in (*a*) "tetraplegia or paresis" (formerly "quadriplegia or-paresis"—paralysis or weakness of upper and lower extremities) or (*b*) "paraplegia or paresis" (paralysis or weakness of the lower extremities).

Spinal cord injury is acquired after birth by trauma to, or disease in, the spinal cord. The resulting compression, contusion, or severance of the spinal cord or the associated spinal arteries cause spinal cord necrosis and dysfunction. This is in contrast to SB, which is a congenital neural tube defect in which the posterior arch of the spine fails to close during the first month of pregnancy. The most severe type of SB with functional consequences is "myelomeningocele," (1) where the spinal meninges and nerves herniate through an opening in the lumbar or sacral vertebrae, damaging the spinal cord (Fig. 5.1).

EPIDEMIOLOGY

SPINAL CORD INJURY

Most SCIs are acquired from trauma, with approximately 10,000 new SCIs each year in the United States. The incidence of SCI is approximately 30–40/million people in the population, with another 20/million (5,000/yr) not surviving the initial injury. The highest per capita rate of SCI occurs between ages 16 and 30. An estimated 250,000–400,000 people with SCI live in the United States, with about 80% being male. Mean age at time of injury is 33 years (median 26, mode 19).

Causes of traumatic SCI in the United States include motor vehicle accidents (44%), violence (24%), falls (22%), and sports (8%). An undetermined number also acquire SCI from diseases such as tumor, infection, and thrombosis. Approximately 50% of SCIs involve the cervical spine, 25% thoracic, 20% lumbar, and 5% sacral. About 45% of SCIs are "complete" with total loss of sensorimotor and autonomic function below the injury level. The remaining 55% are "incomplete" with partial loss. This proportion is increasing with improved emergency medical treatment. Approximately half of all SCIs result in tetraplegia, and this proportion increases with the age at onset (2,3).

SPINA BIFIDA

In the United States, SB occurs in about 0.6 per 1,000 live births and is steadily declining. At least 2,000 children with SB are born annually in the United States. Incidence is greatest among Hispanic Americans, lower among white Americans, and lowest among African Americans. About 80% of SB cases involve myelomeningocele (1).

PATHOPHYSIOLOGY

SPINAL CORD INJURY

Spinal cord injury results in impairment or loss of motor, sensory function or both in the trunk or extremities owing to damage to the neural elements within the spinal canal. Injury to the cervical segments (C1–C8) or the highest thoracic segment (T1) causes tetraplegia/-paresis, with impairment of the arms, trunk, legs, and pelvic organs (bladder, bowels, and sexual organs). Injury to the thoracic segments T2–T12 causes paraplegia/-paresis, with impairment to the trunk, legs, and/or pelvic organs. Injury to the lumbar or sacral segments of the cauda equina (L1–S4) impairs the legs and/or pelvic organs. The neurologic level and completeness of injury determines the degree of impairment. See Figure 5.2 for an illustration of spinal cord segmental innervation of muscles and other organs (4,5). The American Spinal Injury Association (ASIA) Impairment Scale in Table 5.1 is used

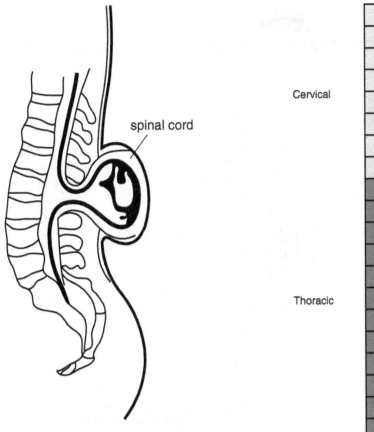

FIGURE 5.1. Lumbar myelomeingocele with spinal nerves and meninges protruding from the newborn's spine.

to grade the degree of impairment or completeness at a given level (6,7).

Physiologic impairment from either acquired or congenital SCI can include sensory loss, muscular paralysis, and sympathetic nervous system impairment. These frequently have an impact on the magnitude and quality of acute physiologic responses to exercise and the ultimate trainability of the person with SCI. Basic anatomic and physiologic impairments and residual functions are often summarized by physicians on the form shown in Figure 5.3 (6,7).

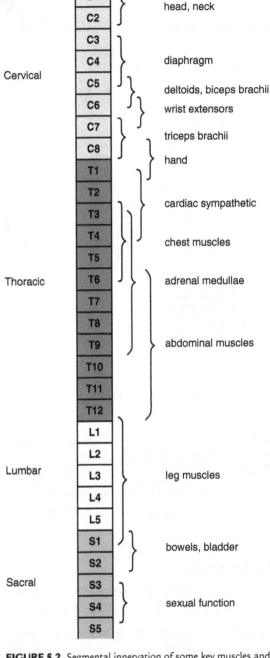

FIGURE 5.2. Segmental innervation of some key muscles and organs in spinal cord dysfunction.

TABLE 5.1. AMERICAN SPINAL INJURY ASSOCIATION (ASIA) IMPAIRMENT SCALE FOR ASSESSING THE SEVERITY OF SPINAL CORD INJURY (6,7)

CLASS	DESCRIPTION
A	Complete. No sensory or motor function is preserved in the sacral segments S4–S5.
B	Incomplete. Sensory but no motor function is preserved below the neurologic level and extends through the sacral segments S4–S5.
C	Incomplete. Motor function is preserved below the neurologic level, and most key muscles below the neurologic level have a manual muscle test grade <3 out of 5.
D	Incomplete. Motor function is preserved below the neurologic level, and most key muscles below the neurologic level have a manual muscle test grade ≥3 out of 5.
E	Normal. Sensory and motor function is normal.

ASIA. International Standards for Neurological Classification of SCI. Atlanta: American Spinal Injury Association; 2002.
ASIA. Standard neurological classification of spinal cord injury. Atlanta: American Spinal Injury Association; 2006. (accessed online, 2-17-08: http://www.asia-spinalinjury.org/publications/2006_Classif_worksheet.pdf)

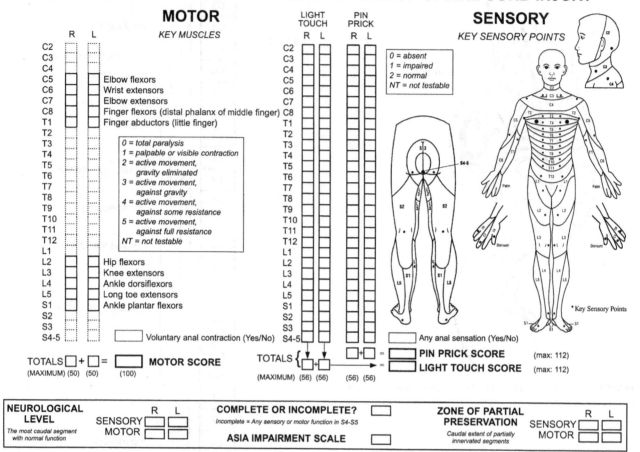

FIGURE 5.3. ASIA standard neurological classification of spinal cord injury (7).

Clinical SCI Syndromes

Six major SCI syndromes are recognized (7), usually associated with incomplete SCI or low-level paraplegia.

- **Brown-Sequard syndrome** is an incomplete spinal cord lesion resulting in relatively greater ipsilateral proprioceptive and motor loss and contralateral loss of sensitivity to pinprick and temperature.
- **Central cord syndrome** results from cervical cord lesion, spares sacral sensory function, and produces greater weakness in the upper limbs than in the lower limbs.
- **Posterior cord syndrome** is caused by a posterior lesion to the spinal cord and produces loss of pinprick and temperature sensation, but largely preserves motor function and proprioception.
- **Anterior cord syndrome** is a condition where blood supply to the anterior spinal cord is reduced and results in profound motor loss, but may spare light touch and pressure sensation.

- **Conus medullaris syndrome** is an injury to the sacral cord (conus) and lumbar nerve roots within the spinal canal, usually resulting in an areflexic bladder, bowel, and lower limbs.
- **Cauda equina syndrome** is an injury to the lumbosacral nerve roots within the neural canal, resulting in an areflexic bladder, bowel, and lower limbs.

Immediate Neurologic Consequences of SCI

1. Sensorimotor and autonomic function: (*a*) normal function above neurologic level of lesion, (*b*) impaired function (flaccid paralysis) at the level of lesion, (*c*) impaired function (spastic paralysis) below the level of lesion (spasticity in skeletal and smooth muscles)—according to myotome and dermatome diagrams (Figs. 5.2 and 5.3).
2. Expected levels of functional independence varies by level of lesion (8):
   - Tetraplegia: impaired lower and upper body function, impaired cardiac and adrenal sympathetic

innervation, vasomotor paralysis, susceptibility to hypotension and autonomic dysreflexia, impaired cough.
- Paraplegia: impaired lower body function.
3. Spastic or flaccid bladder requires catheterization or urinary collection system for emptying and management; risk of urinary incontinence.
4. Bowel constipation; risk of bowel incontinence.
5. Bone demineralization or osteopenia; risk of fracture.

Secondary Conditions and SCI

Secondary medical conditions may further compromise the health and function of persons with SCI as they age. These conditions generally increase with time since SCI. The most prevalent secondary conditions are chronic pain, problematic spasticity, depression, obesity, urinary tract infections, and pressure sores (9–12). Many years of dependence on the upper extremities for daily activities (wheelchair or crutch use, and transfers) makes the shoulders, elbows, and wrists susceptible to overuse injury, tendon inflammation, joint degeneration, and pain. Severe spasticity can cause joint contractures and loss of range of motion. Paralysis of abdominal (expiratory) musculature impairs cough and increases susceptibility to respiratory infections. Frequent bladder infections and use of antibiotics can lead to kidney damage and systemic infection. Inactivity, dyslipidemia, insulin resistance, and hypertension put long-surviving persons with SCD at risk for cardio- and cerebrovascular disease and metabolic disease (13,14).

Exercise-related Consequences of SCI

Spinal cord injury can result in two major exercise-related problems: (a) reduced ability to perform large-muscle-group aerobic exercise voluntarily (i.e., without using functional electrical stimulation leg cycle ergometry [FES-LCE] with paralyzed leg muscles), and (b) the inability to stimulate the autonomic and cardiovascular systems to support higher rates of aerobic metabolism (15,16). Therefore, catecholamine production by the adrenal medullae, skeletal muscle venous pump, and thermoregulation (17) may be impaired, which restricts exercise cardiac output (CO) to subnormal levels. Hopman et al. (18) examined the properties of the venous vasculature in the lower extremities in persons with paraplegia. Compared with non-SCI subjects, they noted lower venous distensibility and capacity and higher venous flow resistance. They attributed these to vascular adaptations to inactivity and muscle atrophy rather than the effect of an inoperable leg muscle pump and sympathetic denervation.

Common secondary complications during exercise, especially in persons with tetraplegia, may include limited positive cardiac chronotropy and inotropy, excessive venous pooling, venous atrophy, orthostatic and exercise hypotension, exercise intolerance, and autonomic dysreflexia. This latter condition is a syndrome resulting from mass activation of autonomic reflexes causing extreme hypertension, headache, bradycardia, flushing, gooseflesh, unusual sweating, shivering, or nasal congestion.

Tetraplegia usually results in a sedentary lifestyle with profound deconditioning of many physiologic systems. This exacerbates mobility impairment, bone demineralization, myocardial and skeletal muscle atrophy, and changes in body composition, such as decreased lean body mass, body water content, blood volume, and increased percentage of body fat (19).

SPINA BIFIDA

Immediate Neurologic Consequences of SB

Infants with SB generally have surgery within 24 hours of birth to close the spinal malformation to minimize the risk of infection and prevent further neurologic damage. About 80% of SB affects the lumbosacral nerve roots (1), resulting in damage to the lumbar or sacral segments of the cauda equina from L1 to S4. As with SCI at the same neurologic level, SB usually results in sensorimotor and autonomic impairment to the legs, pelvic organs (bladder, bowels, and sexual organs), or both. The exact neurologic level and completeness of injury determines the degree of impairment (Figs. 5.2 and 5.3). Also as with SCI, the ASIA Impairment Scale in Table 5.1 can be used to grade the degree of impairment or completeness in SB at a given level (6,7).

A frequent complication of SB is "hydrocephalus" (an abnormal accumulation of cerebrospinal fluid (CSF) in the cavities of the brain, which can lead to increased intracranial pressure and progressive enlargement of the head, convulsion, and mental disability) occurring in about 90% of individuals with SB (1). SB impairs proper absorption and drainage of CSF and allows excessive accumulation of CSF in the ventricles of the brain. If ineffectively treated or left untreated, hydrocephalus compresses the brain and causes brain damage and permanent cognitive impairment and learning disabilities. Most people with SB have a plastic shunt implanted to drain CSF from the ventricles of the brain under the skin into the chest or abdomen. Shunts will fail if they become obstructed; people with SB typically have their failed shunt replaced twice in their lifetime.

Presence of the Arnold-Chiari malformation, a displacement of the cerebellar tonsils and the medulla through the foramen magnum, may result in compression of the brainstem and cerebellum (1). Symptoms in children or adolescents may include neck pain, changes in sensorimotor function, or problems with swallowing, speech, or breathing. The only treatment is surgical decompression. Some may exhibit cerebellar dysfunction with dysmetria, fine motor incoordination, tremors, nystagmus, and ataxic gait. These individuals may experience difficulty with fine motor skills.

Spinal cord function must be closely monitored in people with SB. Changes in muscle tone or strength, rapidly progressing scoliosis, or changes in bowel or bladder function may indicate the presence of "hydromyelia" or "tethered cord" (1). In hydromyelia (or syringomyelia), a fluid cavity develops in the central canal of the spinal cord that further impairs neurologic function. It could develop at any time or level, requiring surgical shunting of fluid. Spinal cord tethering is stretching of the spinal cord with longitudinal growth of the spine or with movement or exercise. When this occurs, surgical correction of tethering is necessary to prevent further spinal cord damage and loss of neurologic function.

Secondary Conditions and SB

Unlike most people with SCI, SB survivors endure their condition over their entire life span. By the time children with SB reach adulthood, they usually have had multiple orthopedic and neurologic surgeries that can compromise long-term functional status. If children with SB have walked with assistive devices for years, stress and strain on spinal and lower-extremity joints may require several orthopedic surgeries to correct deformities, such as scoliosis, hip subluxation or dislocation, Achilles tendon contracture, and muscle imbalance (1). Scoliosis is reported to occur in 80% of people with SB and is treated often with spinal fusion. Similarly, lifelong wheelchair users may acquire upper-extremity overuse syndromes, such as carpel tunnel syndrome, tendinitis, and arthritis, further impairing their mobility. Osteoporosis is common in children and adults with flaccid paralysis of the lower extremities who use wheelchairs. Thus, they are vulnerable to painless fractures with symptoms, such as local redness, deformity, or fever.

As with those with SCI, many people with SB need to pay close attention to skin care and hygiene. If the skin over the ischial tuberosities, greater trochanters, or sacrum is insensitive, then frequent weight shifts, pushups, seat cushioning, pressure relief, and cleanliness are necessary to prevent pressure sores on these areas. Also, chronic urinary tract infections over a lifetime may cause renal damage and failure, especially if bacteria become antibiotic-resistant.

Obesity is particularly prevalent as children with SB reach adolescence. Many children with SB are highly mobile with weight-bearing ambulation using braces and crutches. However, during adolescence, weight gain frequently interferes with, and precludes, efficient upright ambulation, forcing the person to use a manual wheelchair for mobility. This encourages further weight gain, inactivity, and the vicious cycle of deconditioning and declining health and functional independence. Wheelchair use also exposes the person to unusually high upper-extremity stresses, increasing his or her susceptibility to upper-extremity repetitive motion disorders. Special attention should be paid to weight management throughout adolescence and adulthood.

About 30% of persons with SB frequently have mild-to-moderate cognitive and learning disabilities necessitating special education (20). Many have low self-esteem, immature social skills, lack of initiative, and depression that make independent living difficult. Lifelong guidance, support, and medical or therapeutic follow-up may be necessary to maintain independence in the community.

Exercise-related Consequences of SB

If extensive lower-extremity paralysis is present, SB can result in reduced ability to perform large-muscle-group aerobic exercise voluntarily. Consequently, FES will not reactivate flaccidly paralyzed gluteal, hamstring, and quadriceps muscle groups; therefore, FES is not usually an option unless the neurologic level of lesion is above L1. During aerobic exercise testing and training, ambulatory people with SB can probably walk or jog on a treadmill. On the other hand, people with SB who primarily use wheelchairs for mobility will require an exercise mode involving wheelchair treadmill exercise, wheelchair ergometry (WERG), arm-crank ergometry (ACE), upper body ergometry (UBE), or combined arm and leg ergometry to elicit maximal physiologic responses.

Therapeutic exercises are recommended to maintain balanced strength and flexibility in the upper extremities. These are intended to help prevent upper-extremity overuse syndromes, such as nerve entrapment syndromes and degenerative joint disease, in lifelong wheelchair or crutch users (21).

About 70% of people with SB have an allergic hypersensitivity to latex (natural rubber) (1). Therefore, they should not touch exercise, clinical, or research equipment made of, or covered with, latex (e.g., elastic bands or tubing, rubber-coated dumbbells, latex gloves, blood pressure cuffs). If latex touches their skin or mucous membranes or enters their circulation, they react with watery eyes, wheezing, hives, rash, swelling, and, in severe cases, life-threatening anaphylaxis.

Poor fitness and low physical activity have been documented among adults and youth with SCD (22,23). Compared with peers with disability, adolescents with SCD have 27% lower handgrip strength, 47% greater skinfold thicknesses (i.e., higher body fatness), 65% lower $\dot{V}O_2$ peak (16 versus 40 mL/kg/min), and very slow long-distance mobility times (24,25).

CLINICAL EXERCISE PHYSIOLOGY

ACUTE RESPONSES TO EXERCISE

Spinal Cord Injury

Table 5.2 summarizes representative physiologic responses during rest and peak arm ergometry (ACE or WERG) in two relatively large samples of adults with SCI. The data from Morrison et al. (26) are from subjects

TABLE 5.2A. MEAN ± SD PHYSIOLOGICAL RESPONSES OF 94 (ASIA CLASS A-B) ADULTS WITH SPINAL CORD INJURY, 6 WEEKS AFTER DISCHARGE FROM REHABILITATION, DURING REST AND PEAK ARM ERGOMETRY (25)

	HR (bpm)	SBP (mm Hg)	DBP (mm Hg)	$\dot{V}O_2$ (mL/kg/min)	$\dot{V}_E$ (L/min)	RPE (6–20)	PO (W)
Rest							
Tetraplegia	83 ± 16	98 ± 16	66 ± 13	–	–	–	–
High Paraplegia	92 ± 19	104 ± 12	72 ± 11	–	–	–	–
Low Paraplegia	97 ± 14	119 ± 13	79 ± 11	–	–	–	–
Peak Arm Ergometry							
Tetraplegia	117 ± 16	95 ± 22	65 ± 14	8.3 ± 2.9	30 ± 12	17 ± 2	34 ± 11
High Paraplegia	152 ± 29	107 ± 30	67 ± 13	8.9 ± 2.6	36 ± 11	17 ± 2	51 ± 15
Low Paraplegia	161 ± 11	140 ± 19	81 ± 15	13.5 ± 3.7	46 ± 13	17 ± 2	63 ± 16

Mean age = 30 ± 10 yr (range = 16–58): M, male; F, female.
Tetraplegia (C6–C8): n = 24; 20 M, 4 F; mean ± SD body mass ± 71 ± 13 kg
High-lesion Paraplegia (T1–T5): n = 15; 15 M, 13 F; mean ± SD body mass ± 79 ± 10 kg
Low-lesion Paraplegia (T6–L2): n = 55; 42 M, 13 F; mean ± SD body mass ± 71 ± 18 kg

TABLE 5.2B. MEAN ± SD $\dot{V}O_{2peak}$ (mL/kg/min) FOR 72 WOMEN AND MEN WITH LONG-STANDING SCI (26)

	TETRAPLEGIA (C5–C8)	HIGH PARAPLEGIA (T1–T6)	MID PARAPLEGIA (T7–T11)	LOW PARAPLEGIA (T12–L3)	VERY LOW PARAPLEGIA (L4–S2)	INCOMPLETE TETRAPLEGIA (C5–C8)	INCOMPLETE PARAPLEGIA (T1–L3)
Females							
n	0	0	2	2	1	3	1
$\dot{V}O_{2peak}$	–	–	23 ± 1	23 ± 2	40	20 ± 5	12
Males							
n	10	6	14	8	11	10	4
$\dot{V}O_{2peak}$	14 ± 5	17 ± 6	26 ± 8	28 ± 7	24 ± 7	23 ± 11	23 ± 7

who were 6 months after discharge from SCI rehabilitation. Notable differences among groups with different lesion levels are (*a*) blunted tachycardia in subjects with tetraplegia, (*b*) lack of pressor response and very low $\dot{V}O_{2peak}$ in subjects with tetraplegia and high-lesion paraplegia, (*c*) inverse relationship between lesion level and peak power output (PO), and (*d*) substantial variability of most responses. Also in Table 5.2, the data of Hjeltnes and Jansen (27) are from persons with long-standing SCI (i.e., 4–16 years after SCI). Mean $\dot{V}O_{2peak}$ was substantially higher than in the Morrison et al. study (26). Higher $\dot{V}O_{2peak}$ was also strongly associated with higher functional mobility and lower incidence of secondary conditions, such as chronic pain, spasticity, urinary tract infection, and osteoporosis.

Stewart et al. (28) completed a factor analysis of physiologic and functional data on 102 subjects with SCI from the study by Morrison et al. (26). They concluded that the predominant fitness factor was "aerobic fitness and muscle strength/endurance" as indicated by high loadings on several peak physiologic responses, followed by "blood pressure" (maintenance) and "general health."

Raymond et al. (29) compared cardiorespiratory responses during ACE to those during combined ACE and FES-leg cycle ergometry (FEC-LCE) ("hybrid exercise") in seven subjects with T4–T12 paraplegia. FES-LCE involved 18% (35 versus 30 W) higher PO than ACE alone. Compared with ACE alone, submaximal steady-state ACE + FES-LCE elicited 25% higher $\dot{V}O_2$ (1.58 versus 1.26 L/min), 13% lower heart rate (HR) (132 versus 149 bpm), and 42% higher O_2 pulse ($\dot{V}O_2$/HR, 12.2 versus 8.6 L/b), with no differences in $\dot{V}_E$ expired ventilatory rate or respiratory exchange ratio. These results demonstrate that during submaximal or maximal exercise, a greater metabolic stress is elicited during combined arm and leg ergometry compared with arm ergometry. The higher cardiac stroke volume (SV) observed during submaximal combined arm and leg ergometry in the absence of any difference in HR implies reduced venous pooling and higher cardiac volume loading. These results suggest that training incorporating both arm and leg muscles may be more effective in improving aerobic fitness in people with paraplegia than ACE alone.

Haisma et al. (30) critically reviewed the literature on physical capacity in people with SCI who use wheelchairs. Weighted means were calculated for various fitness parameters in subgroups. In tetraplegia the mean $\dot{V}O_{2peak}$ was 0.89 L/min for WERG and 0.87 for ACE or hand-cycling.

The PO_{peak} was 26 W for WERG and 40 W for ACE. In paraplegia the mean $\dot{V}O_{2peak}$ was 2.10 L/min for WERG and 1.51 for ACE, and the PO_{peak} was 74 W for WERG and 85 W for ACE. In paraplegia, muscle strength of the upper body and respiratory function were comparable to that in the general population. In tetraplegia, muscle strength varied greatly and respiratory function was reduced to 55%–59% of predicted values for the general population matched for age, sex, and height. Physical capacity in SCI is clearly reduced and varies greatly by population and methodologic differences. Haisma et al. (30) contend that standardized measurement of physical capacity is needed to further develop comparative values for clinical practice and rehabilitation research.

Paraplegia

In persons with paraplegia, the primary neuromuscular effect is paralysis of the lower body, precluding exercise modes, such as walking, running, and voluntary leg cycling. Therefore, the upper body must be used for all voluntary activities of daily living (ADLs) and exercise: arm cranking, wheelchair propulsion, and ambulation with orthotic devices and crutches. The most common clinical exercise modes for exercise testing of persons with paraplegia are ACE and WERG. ACE is believed to be the more general exercise stressor and less likely to be influenced by the specific wheelchair skill of the user. It is the most available and standardized instrumentation for upper body exercise testing. WERG is specific to wheelchair propulsion, and if the person's own everyday or sports or racing wheelchair can be used for testing, it is also highly specific to the wheelchair task. WERGs are constructed by research laboratories and can take the form of a standardized wheelchair linked with a flywheel or rollers (31–33), or a wheelchair on a wide treadmill (34).

In paraplegia, the proportionally smaller active upper-body muscle mass typically restricts peak values of PO, $\dot{V}O_2$, and CO to approximately one-half of those expected for maximal leg exercise in individuals without SCI (16). Additionally, "circulatory hypokinesis," a reduced CO for any given $\dot{V}O_2$, has been reported by several investigators. Presumably, this condition is caused by a lack of the leg muscle pump to assist venous return during exercise, excessive venous pooling owing to vasomotor paralysis, excessive skin perfusion to aid thermoregulation (35), or subnormal blood volume (36). The effect of this condition would be to impair delivery of O_2 and nutrients to, and removal of, metabolites and CO_2 from working muscles, facilitating muscle fatigue.

The most active people with SCI can achieve high upper body fitness levels. Veeger et al. (37) reported that the average PO_{peak}, HR_{peak}, and $\dot{V}O_{2peak}$ of 17 elite adult wheelchair athletes (basketball and track and field) were 93 W, 184 bpm, and 2.8 L/min (40 mL/kg/min) during maximal wheelchair treadmill exercise.

Tetraplegia

In persons with tetraplegia, the pathologic effects on neuromuscular and autonomic function are more extensive than with paraplegia. The active upper body muscle mass will be partially paralyzed, and the sympathetic nervous system may be completely separated from control by the brain. Upper body PO, $\dot{V}O_2$, and CO are typically reduced to approximately one-half to one-third of those levels seen in individuals with paraplegia (38–40). In the upright sitting posture, peak HR, CO, SV, and arterial blood pressure (BP) are often subnormal for given levels of $\dot{V}O_2$ (41–43). Furthermore, strenuous exercise may not be tolerated because of orthostatic and exercise hypotension, which may produce overt symptoms of dizziness, nausea, and so on (44,45). Peak HRs for persons with tetraplegia typically do not exceed approximately 125 bpm owing to small exercising muscle mass, impaired sympathetic adrenal and cardiac innervation, and vagal cardiac dominance (16).

Posture of subjects with tetraplegia affects peak hemodynamic and metabolic responses to ACE. Figoni et al. (46) compared peak physiologic responses in supine versus upright sitting postures in 11 subjects with tetraplegia. Supine posture produced higher PO by 39%, $\dot{V}O_2$ by 26%, CO by 20%, and SV by 14%, although mean arterial pressure was lower (75 versus 83 mm Hg). Pitetti et al. (34) observed higher peak $\dot{V}O_2$, pulmonary minute ventilation ($\dot{V}_E$), and PO during ACE and higher $\dot{V}O_{2peak}$ during treadmill wheelchair exercise in 10 men with tetraplegia using an anti-G suit to compress the abdomen and legs. Hopman et al. (47) also found 12% higher $\dot{V}O_{2peak}$ during supine ACE in five men with tetraplegia. These support the concept that excessive lower body venous pooling limits maximal arm exercise performance in this population with severe autonomic impairment.

Ready (48) studied acute responses of athletes with tetraplegia during prolonged ACE at 75% $\dot{V}O_{2peak}$ and found no changes in HR or skin or rectal temperatures across 10 exercise stages. They attributed the surprising lack of "cardiovascular drift" to lack of adequate muscle mass to increase body temperature and lack of skin vasodilation to compete with CO, thus maintaining a more stable SV.

Hooker et al. (49) compared acute physiologic responses of eight subjects with tetraplegia performing moderate-intensity voluntary ACE, FES-LCE, and hybrid exercise. Although each mode elicited a $\dot{V}O_2$ of 0.66 L/min separately, the POs used to elicit this metabolic response were very different (arms 19 W versus legs 2 W). This indicates markedly lower efficiency of FES-LCE compared with voluntary ACE. Compared with ACE or FES-LCE, hybrid exercise elicited higher levels of $\dot{V}O_2$ (by 54%), $\dot{V}_E$ (by 33%–53%), HR (by 19%–33%), and CO (by 33%–47%). Total peripheral vascular resistance during hybrid exercise was also lower (by 21%–34%). Compared with ACE, FES-LCE and hybrid exercise produced higher SV by 41%–56%.

Takahashi et al. (50) investigated hemodynamic responses during isometric exercise in 6 men with ASIA A (complete) tetraplegia using a Modelflow method simulating aortic input impedance from arterial blood pressure waveform. CO increased during exercise with no or slight decrease in SV. Mean arterial pressure increased one-third above the control pressor response, but total peripheral vascular resistance did not rise at all during static exercise, indicating that slight pressor response is determined by the increase in CO. They concluded that sympathetic decentralization causes both absent peripheral vasoconstriction and a decreased capacity to increase HR, especially at the onset of exercise, and that the cardiovascular adjustment during voluntary static arm exercise is mainly accomplished by increasing cardiac pump output by means of tachycardia controlled by intact cardiac vagal outflow.

Spina Bifida

Few investigators have reported physiologic responses to exercise in children or adults with SB. Krebs et al. (51) observed the cardiorespiratory and perceptual or cognitive responses to a 6-minute bout of moderate calisthenics in a small group of children 9–12 years of age with SB. Besides normal increases in HR, $\dot{V}_E$, respiratory rate, and tidal volume, they noted acute improvements in peripheral vision, learning, and memory. Agre et al. (52) conducted aerobic and strength testing on 33 children and adolescents, ages 10–15 years, with SB of various functional levels. As shown in Table 5.3, peak $\dot{V}O_2$, HR, and $\dot{V}_E$ during walking or wheeling treadmill exercise varied inversely with functional level. Overall, the data suggest that people with SB respond similarly to people with SCI with comparable functional status.

TRAINING RESPONSES

Spinal Cord Injury

Activities of daily living for (self-care and mobility) those with SCI have been shown to require only 15%–24% of their $HR_{reserve}$. This level of exertion is insufficient for developing physical fitness in people with SCD (53,54). The exception was propulsion of a manual wheelchair up inclines or crutch walking, which elicited 50% $HR_{reserve}$,

the equivalent to moderate exercise intensity. After acute inpatient SCI rehabilitation (mean of 76 days for paraplegia, 96 days for tetraplegia), the mean aerobic fitness ($\dot{V}O_{2peak}$) plateaued and remained stable for at least 8 weeks (27).

Arm exercise training adaptations are believed to be primarily peripheral (muscular) in nature and may include increased muscular strength and endurance of the arm musculature in the exercise modes used. These may result in 10%–60% improvements in peak PO and $\dot{V}O_2$ and an enhanced sense of well-being. Central cardiovascular adaptations to exercise training, such as increased maximal SV or CO, have not yet been documented (55), however, suggesting that increases in $\dot{V}O_{2peak}$ are probably not caused by central cardiovascular limitations, but increases in muscular strength, anaerobic metabolism, and O_2 absorption or utilization by trained muscle tissue. Physiologic effects of exercise training in SCI subjects are well summarized by Devillard et al. (56). Valent et al. (57) attempted a meta-analysis of upper-body exercise on the physical capacity in SCI. In 14 articles of acceptable quality, the mean ± SD increase in peak $\dot{V}O_2$ and PO following training was 17.6 ± 11.2% and 26.1 ± 15.6%, respectively. Representative training studies are discussed below.

Arm Ergometry

Since 1973, several investigators have reported a variety of training effects of ACE or WERG in persons with SCI. Knutsson et al. (58) trained one group of SCI patients during initial rehabilitation with ACE 4–5 days/wk for 6 weeks. A second similar group trained with calisthenics. Both groups increased ACE PO_{peak} by about 40%.

Nilsson et al. (59) trained 12 people with paraplegia for 7 weeks with both ACE and resistance training. Subjects increased their $\dot{V}O_{2peak}$ significantly by 0.20 L/min (10%), muscular strength by 16%, and muscular endurance (bench press) by 80%.

Davis et al. (55) compared training responses of nine men with SCI paraplegia with those of five controls without SCI. After 16 weeks of ACE exercise, HRs of trained individuals were 9 bpm lower during isometric handgrip effort (30% of maximal voluntary contraction for 3 minutes), with a substantial (20%) and decrease of rate-pressure product. Despite a significant increase of $\dot{V}O_{2peak}$ (19% and 31% after 8 and 16 weeks, respectively), left ventricular mass and dimensions and indices of left

TABLE 5.3. MEAN ±SD PEAK PHYSIOLOGIC RESPONSES AND USUAL WALKING SPEED OF CHILDREN WITH SPINA BIFIDA DURING TREADMILL WALKING OR WHEELING (48)

FUNCTIONAL LEVEL	$\dot{V}O_2$ (mL/kg/min)	HR (bpm)	$\dot{V}_E$ (L/min)	USUAL SPEED (km/hr)
L2 and above (n = 6)	17.7 ± 3.8	167 ± 9	32.6 ± 6.7	1.9 (n = 1)
L3–L4 (n = 7)	20.2 ± 3.8	172 ± 9	36.4 ± 6.7	3.5 ± 0.6 (n = 5)
L5–S (n = 17)	29.6 ± 2.2	186 ± 5	49.1 ± 3.8	3.9 ± 0.3 (n = 16)
No motor deficit (n = 3)	41.6 ± 5.3	202 ± 12	63.6 ± 9.4	4.8 ± 0.7 (n = 3)

ventricular performance at rest were unchanged by training. SVs were increased by 12%–16% after training during submaximal and maximal ACE, with a trend toward higher CO_{peak}. A short period of arm training was apparently insufficient to induce cardiac hypertrophy. An increase of SV with a decreased rate-pressure product, but no change in indices of left ventricular performance, implies improved myocardial efficiency. Possible explanations are a greater strength of the trained arms and increased cardiac preload.

Davis and Shephard (60) examined cardiorespiratory responses to four patterns of ACE training (50% or 70% $\dot{V}O_{2peak}$, 20 or 40-min/session, 3 sessions/wk, 24 weeks) in 24 initially inactive subjects with paraplegia. Training was associated with a significant increase of the $\dot{V}O_{2peak}$ during ACE tests, except in control subjects and those combining a low intensity (50% peak) with short-duration training (20 min/session). There were associated increases in SV during submaximal exercise. They suggest that the performance of inactive wheelchair users is limited by a pooling of blood in paralyzed regions, with a reduction of cardiac preloading.

Based on the demonstrated hemodynamic advantages of arm exercise in the supine posture for people with tetraplegia (44), McLean and Skinner (61) conducted a 10-week training study to compare training responses in each posture. Seven subjects with tetraplegia used ACE in the upright sitting posture, whereas another seven subjects used the supine posture. Both posture groups improved comparably: 0.08 L/min increase in $\dot{V}O_{2peak}$, 160% increase in arm exercise endurance, 7-mm decrease in the sum of four skinfolds, 5-bpm increase in resting HR, and nearly significant increase in HR_{peak}.

Lassau-Wray and Ward (62) compared the cardiorespiratory and metabolic responses to ACE in 25 men with cervical and thoracic SCIs and five controls without SCI. $\dot{V}O_{2peak}$ decreased progressively with increasing impairment (i.e., from subjects without SCI to paraplegia to tetraplegia). Great variability in maximal performance levels among groups were noted.

FES Leg Cycle Ergometry (FES-LCE)

Several studies have documented physiologic training effects of FES-LCE. Hooker et al. (63) trained 18 subjects with SCI for 12 weeks with FES-LCE and noted higher posttraining peak PO (+45%), $\dot{V}O_2$ (+23%), $\dot{V}_E$ (+27%), HR (+11%), and CO (+13%) and lower total peripheral resistance (−14%). Nash et al. (64) trained eight subjects with tetraplegia using FES leg cycle ergometry for 6 months and noted reversal of echocardiographically determined myocardial atrophy with the increased volume load during exercise (65). Faghri et al. (66) reported FES-LCE training responses of seven subjects with tetraplegia and six subjects with paraplegia. Twelve weeks of LCE training resulted in a 270% increase in 30-minute training PO (4.6 versus 17.3 W). Resting HR, SBP, and SV increased in subjects with tetraplegia (suggesting more

cardiovascular stability), whereas they decreased in subjects with paraplegia. SBP, DBP, and MAP responses decreased during submaximal exercise in both groups. Janssen et al. (67) have summarized the training effects and clinical efficacy of training with FES-LCE. Although many studies have documented physiologic training effects, no randomized, controlled clinical trials have been conducted to determine efficacy or effectiveness of FES-LCE for improving health or functional status.

Combined Arm and Leg (Hybrid) Ergometry

Two groups have trained SCI subjects using voluntary ACE combined with FES-LCE (hybrid exercise). Figoni et al. (68) trained 14 subjects with tetraplegia for 12 weeks on a hybrid ergometer and observed the following increases in peak responses: PO by 18% (40 versus 47 W), $\dot{V}O_2$ by 18% (1.28 versus 1.51 L/min), and $\dot{V}_E$ by 36% (49 versus 66 L/min). No changes in peak cardiovascular responses (HR, SV, CO, or BP) were observed. Thijssen et al. (69) studied arterial adaptations resulting from 6 weeks of hybrid FES training in 9 subjects with SCI. They found increases in resting and peak blood flow, resting arterial diameter, and flow-mediated diameter in the femoral artery. Six weeks of detraining reversed changes in blood flows, vascular resistance, and femoral diameter (but not flow-mediated diameter) within 1 week.

Resistance Training

Cooney and Walker (70) trained 10 SCI subjects (with tetra- or paraplegia) with hydraulic resistance exercise (3 sessions/wk, 9 weeks, 60–90 HR_{peak}). Mean peak PO and $\dot{V}O_2$ during ACE increased 28% and 37%, respectively. Also, Jacobs et al. (71) tested the effects of circuit resistance training on peak upper-body cardiorespiratory endurance and muscle strength in 10 men with T5–L1 SCI paraplegia. Subjects completed 12 weeks of training, using isoinertial resistance exercises on a multistation gym and high-speed, low-resistance ACE. Peak ACE tests, upper-extremity isoinertial strength testing, and testing of upper-extremity isokinetic strength were all performed before and after training. Subjects increased peak $\dot{V}O_2$ and PO by 30%. Increases in isoinertial muscular strength ranged from 12% to 30%. Increases in isokinetic strength were also observed for shoulder internal rotation, extension, abduction, adduction, and horizontal adduction.

Improper upper-extremity resistance training can induce or aggravate shoulder pain in SCI persons. However, Nash et al. (72) reported both increases in upper-body muscular strength, endurance, and anaerobic power and decreases in shoulder pain resulting from 4 months of circuit resistance training in 7 middle-aged men with thoracic paraplegia. The training involved alternating high-resistance exercises and high-speed, low-resistance arm exercises. Two randomized controlled trials (73,74) have demonstrated the efficacy of therapeutic shoulder exercises for decreasing shoulder pain in adults with SCI and SB. Both programs involved home-based exercises to stretch anterior shoulder musculature and to strengthen posterior shoulder musculature.

Mixed Fitness Training

Hicks et al. (75) conducted a randomized controlled trial of mixed fitness training (aerobic and resistance exercises for 9 months, twice weekly) with a diverse group of 23 men and women (ages 19–65 years, SCI levels C4-L1, ASIA A-D). The training intervention primarily used ACE, pulley and free weights, and accessible Equalizer weight machines. Compared with an educational intervention control group (n = 13), the exercise training group significantly increased submaximal ACE power output by 81%) and 1-RM strength in upper body muscle groups (19%–34%). The training group also reported less pain, stress, and depression after training and scored higher than the control group on indices of satisfaction with physical function, perceived health, and quality of life.

Body Weight Supported Treadmill Training (BWSTT)

Early animal studies examining recovery of hindlimb stepping after complete low thoracic SCI have evolved into human trials. An experimental training method for persons with SCI involves manual positioning of the legs by therapists or robotic devices while subjects perform limb-loaded stepping movements on a treadmill with their body weight partially suspended by a harness, with or without electrical stimulation of paralyzed muscles. Several reports describe subjects with complete and incomplete SCI recovering therapeutic or functional levels of ambulation (76,77). Nash et al. (78) demonstrated in a case report that robotically assisted BWSTT can induce slight acute increases in metabolic rate (by 2.4 metabolic equivalents [METs]) and HR (by 17 bpm). The potential for BWSTT to improve fitness and health in selected SCI individuals is largely undocumented. Dobkin et al. (79) reported a recent clinical trial to compare the functional outcomes of BWSTT with conventional ambulation training and concluded no differences between the interventions in persons with incomplete SCI.

Spina Bifida

Arm Ergometry

Ekblom and Lundberg (80) trained 10 adolescents (7 SB and 3 SCI, mean age 17 years, 6 female and 4 male) with wheelchair exercise (30 min/session, 2–3 sessions/wk, 6 weeks). Although $\dot{V}O_{2peak}$ (1.1 L/min) did not change, PO_{peak} increased by 5.5 W (10%) to 60 W.

Resistance Training

Although no resistance exercise training studies are published that utilized adults with only SB, a few small-scale studies have documented training responses of children or adolescents with SB. Andrade et al. (25) found that a 10-week exercise program significantly increased cardiovascular fitness, isometric muscle strength, and self-concept in eight children with SB compared with control children. Also, O'Connell and Barnhart (81) resistance-trained three children (ages 4, 5, and 16) with thoracic SB. Training consisted of seven upper body exercises using free weights: 30 min/session, 3 sets × 6-repetition maximum (RM), 3 sessions/wk for 9 weeks. All children improved 6-RM muscular strength by 70%–300%, 50-m dash time by 20%, and 12-min wheelchair propulsion distance by 29%. Thus, similar to youth without SCD, resistance training improves strength and general fitness.

PHYSICAL EXAMINATION

To design a program for the participant with SCD adequately, a systematic neurologic examination of the sensory and motor function is required. A well-defined sequence is provided in the International Standards for Neurological and Functional Classification of Spinal Cord Injury (6). Beyond motor and sensory evaluation, attention must be paid to joint range of motion (ROM), spasticity status, and skin integrity. Programs will need to be tailored depending on contracture status, severe spasticity or flaccidity, and the presence of open pressure sores in weight-bearing areas. Some people with SCI require comprehensive pain management for chronic dysesthetic, spinal, or upper-extremity overuse syndromes. These and other functional tests (82,83) may include joint flexibility or ROM; manual muscle testing to determine muscle imbalance and risk of contracture; testing of reflexes, muscle tone, and spasticity; equipment evaluation (wheelchair and cushion, assistive and orthotic devices); home evaluation for accessibility and modification; and psychological evaluation to promote adjustment or coping and to assess or control depression and substance abuse. Because of susceptibility to pressure sores, people with SCD also need to perform frequent inspections of insensitive weight-bearing skin areas to assess skin integrity.

MEDICAL AND SURGICAL TREATMENTS

Multiple medical, nursing, and allied health professional services are utilized during SCD rehabilitation (84). Shortly after injury, neurosurgery, orthopedic surgery, or both are usually necessary to stabilize spinal fractures and dislocations. Internal fixation devices and fusion (rodding, plating, screws, bone grafts) are often necessary to accomplish this after traumatic SCI. The instrumentation and postsurgical healing must be adequate to withstand exercise demands. External spinal orthoses, such as halo, and other spinal orthoses are common for several weeks after surgery to stabilize the healing spine. Other orthopedic injuries often acquired during traumatic SCI include limb fracture and closed head injury.

Physiatrists usually coordinate the rehabilitation team (84). Typically, physical therapists, occupational therapists, clinical exercise physiologists, or kinesiotherapists mobilize patients as soon as possible after SCI to restore tolerance of upright posture, joint flexibility and RON, muscular strength, and independence in ADLs (bed and mat mobility, transfers, wheelchair propulsion, ambulation, orthotic self-care activities, such as dressing, eating, grooming). They also provide adapted driver education and training, home exercise programs, referral to community fitness programs, and prescribed self-care equipment and assistive technology, including a wheelchair with cushion. Nursing coordinates inpatient personal care, education, and followup, especially bowel, bladder, and hygienic concerns. Therapeutic recreation contributes to community reintegration through leisure counseling, social activities, and sports. Other rehabilitation team members include (*a*) the dietician for nutrition assessment and education and (*b*) the social worker for planning about financial, discharge, placement, and family and social support issues. A vocational rehabilitation specialist will deal with reemployment training and education. A urologist will treat bladder dysfunction with medications or surgery to improve bladder filling and emptying and urinary drainage (85). Further, a careful history of adequate bowel and bladder management should be obtained. These programs should be well managed before initiation of exercise therapy. A detailed history of the patient's autonomic dysreflexia status should be investigated, including identification of known stimuli to prevent exacerbating the condition with exercise. Also, any implanted device, including cardiac pacemakers, intrathecal pumps, and FES devices, should be checked for adequate functional status and to be sure that the system or device does not preclude exercise interventions.

PHARMACOLOGY

Table 5.4 summarizes medications commonly used by people with SCD (86). These fall into three classes: spasmolytics (antispasticity, e.g., baclofen and Valium) and

TABLE 5.4. COMMON MEDICATIONS IN PEOPLE WITH SCD (72)

BRAND NAME	GENERIC NAME	DAILY DOSAGE	ACTION	THERAPEUTIC PURPOSE	EXERCISE SIDE EFFECTS
Spasmolytics					
Dibenzyline	Phenoxybenzamine	20–40 mg, BID/TID	Long-acting adrenergic alpha-receptor blocking agent	Relax bladder smooth muscle, prevent autonomic dysreflexia	Tachycardia, hypotension, palpitations
Ditropan	Oxybutynin hydrochloride	5–15 mg	Direct spasmolytic and antimuscarinic (atropinelike) effect on bladder smooth muscle	Facilitate bladder filling and emptying	Tachycardia, hypotension
Lioresal	Baclofen	20–80 mg	Centrally acting GABA agonist	Decrease spasticity	CNS depression, hypotension
Valium	Diazepam	15–30 mg	Centrally acting, facilitates postsynaptic effects of GABA	Decrease spasticity	Transient CV depression, sedation, dizziness, incoordination
Dantrium	Dantrolene sodium	50–400 mg	Decrease calcium release from sarcoplasmic reticulum at neuromuscular junction in spinal cord	Decrease spasticity	Sedation, dizziness, weakness
Catapres	Clonidine hydrochloride	1–2 mg	Centrally acting alpha-2 adrenergic antagonist	Decrease spasticity	Hypotension, bradycardia
Zanaflex	Tizanidine hydrochloride	8 mg/8 hr	Alpha-2 adrenergic antagonist	Decrease spasticity	Mild sedation
Antithrombotic/Coagulants					
Coumadin	Warfarin	—	Blood anticoagulation	Prevent/treat blood clots	Hemorrhage, bruisability
Heparin	Heparin sodium	100 units/kg/ 4 hr via IV	Blood anticoagulation	Prevent/treat blood clots	Hemorrhage, bruisability
Antibiotics					
Bactrim	Cotrioxazole (sulfamethoxazole-trimethoprim)	800 mg tablet PO q 12 hr × 14 days	Inhibits formation of dihydrofolic acid from PABA bacteriocidal	Prevent/treat urinary tract infections	None

BID, twice daily; CNS, central nervous system; CV, cardiovascular; GABA, γ-aminobutyric acid; PABA, para-aminobutyric acid; PO, orally; TID, three times daily.

antithrombics (anticoagulation, e.g., warfarin), and antibiotics (e.g., Bactrim). Neurogenic bladder treatment may require alpha-blocking agents that induce hypotension, especially in persons with tetraplegia (86). Persons with a history of deep venous thrombosis may be taking warfarin, which leads to easy bruisability. Aging persons with SCD are at risk for cardiovascular and metabolic disease and may take medications for hypertension, diabetes, dyslipidemia, dysrhythmia, and congestive heart failure.

DIAGNOSTIC PROCEDURES

The physician will judge the necessity and extent of initial diagnostic procedures that will depend on the prospective participant's documented medical history and physical examination. If FES-LCE exercise will be utilized in exercise programming, the participant's file should include baseline radiographs (including plain x-rays, scans for osseous tissue, and magnetic resonance imaging [MRI] for soft tissues) showing adequacy of spinal alignment and integrity of internal stabilization. Baseline pulmonary function tests are desirable for those with tetraplegia or tetraparesis. The nature and extent of the changes in ventilatory function and cough depend to a great extent on level of neurological injury or dysfunction. If the client is middle-aged or older or if sufficient coronary risk factors exist, electrocardiograms (ECG) and myocardial perfusion tests should be obtained as baseline evaluations of the participant's cardiac status. Also, laboratory analysis of baseline hematologic and metabolic status would be useful, including a complete blood count, electrolytes, renal indices, thyroid and liver function, lipid panel, fasting blood sugar, and glucose tolerance. Urodynamic evaluation is necessary to assess bladder responses to filling and emptying (e.g., voiding cystourethrogram). Finally, because osteoporosis is common below the level of injury in SCD and, with immobilization in other conditions, consider evaluation of bone mineral status (bone densitometry) as part of the initial workup.

EXERCISE/FITNESS/FUNCTIONAL TESTING

GUIDELINES

During rehabilitation of persons with SCD, functional testing takes priority over physiologic testing to promote functional independence at the fastest rate possible. For example, rehabilitation goals usually include independent mobility via weight-bearing or wheelchair ambulation, transfers, and self-care with or without assistive devices. The fitness requirements of these tasks are specific to the functional tasks themselves. The cardiovascular and metabolic demands of walking and wheelchair ambulation are the greatest of all functional tasks, hence, the importance of exercise tolerance and capacity during rehabilitation. Aerobic fitness is necessary for long-distance mobility, some recreational activities, competitive sports, and long-term cardiovascular health. Neuromuscular coordination and skill, balance and stability, and muscular strength and endurance are necessary to various degrees for safe standing, ambulation, transfers, driving, and other self-care activities.

Table 5.5 lists relative and absolute contraindications for cardiovascular exercise testing of persons with SCD. These are the same as for people without disabilities and include several disability-specific conditions.

Advice from the person with SCD concerning exercise modes and proper positioning or strapping is often useful. Adapt the exercise equipment, as needed, and provide for the following special needs (87):

TABLE 5.5. DISABILITY-SPECIFIC RELATIVE AND ABSOLUTE CONTRAINDICATIONS FOR EXERCISE TESTING OF PERSONS WITH SPINAL CORD INJURY (SCI) AND SPINA BIFIDA (SB)

	SCI		
RELATIVE	Tetraplegia	Paraplegia	SB
Asymptomatic hypotension	X		
Muscle and joint discomfort	X	X	X
ABSOLUTE			
Autonomic dysreflexia	X		
Severe or infected skin pressure sore on weight-bearing skin areas	X	X	X
Symptomatic hypotension (dizziness, nausea, palor, extreme fatigue, visual disturbance, confusion)	X		
Illness caused by acute urinary tract infection	X	X	X
Uncontrolled spasticity or pain	X	X	X
Unstable fracture	X	X	X
Uncontrolled hot humid environments	X		
Inability to safely seat and stabilize the person on well-cushioned or padded ergometers or equipment	X	X	X
Insufficient range of motion to perform exercise task	X	X	

X, special relevance to SCI or SB.

1. Trunk stabilization (straps)
2. Securing hands on crank handles (holding gloves)
3. Skin protection (seat cushion and padding)
4. Prevention of bladder overdistension (i.e., empty bladder or urinary collection device immediately before test)
5. Vascular support to help maintain BP and improve exercise tolerance (elastic stockings and abdominal binder)
6. Use an environmentally controlled thermoneutral or cool laboratory or clinic to compensate for impaired sweating and thermoregulation. If necessary, use fans and water for compresses, misting, and hydration.
7. Design a discontinuous incremental testing protocol that allows monitoring of both HR, BP, rating of perceived exertion (RPE), and exercise tolerance at each stage. PO increments may range from 1 to 20 W, depending on exercise mode, level and completeness of injury, and training status.
8. Expect PO_{peak} for persons with tetraplegia to range from 0 to 50 W and 50 to 150 W for persons with paraplegia. The workloads are dependent on the mode used (e.g., ACE versus WERG versus FES-LCE)
9. Treat postexercise hypotension and exhaustion with rest, recumbency, leg elevation, and fluid ingestion.

AEROBIC EXERCISE TEST PROTOCOLS

A. Field Tests

1. University of Toronto Arm Crank Protocol (15,88): This field test is a discontinuous submaximal protocol to predict $\dot{V}O_{2peak}$ from submaximal HR responses to arm-crank ergometry. Subjects performed three 5-minute exercise stages at approximately 40%, 60%, and 80% of age-predicted HR_{peak} with 2-minute rest periods between stages. HR was monitored continuously and recorded during the last 10 seconds of each stage. Based on laboratory assessment of $\dot{V}O_{2peak}$ in 49 subjects with lower-limb disabilities, including tetraplegia and paraplegia, the following regression equations were developed to predict $\dot{V}O_{2peak}$ in L/min; for males: $\dot{V}O_{2peak} = 0.018 \times$ (ACE PO in watts) $+ 0.40$ ($r = 0.88$, SEE = 0.20 L/min); for females: $\dot{V}O_{2peak} = 0.017 \times$ (ACE PO in watts) $+ 0.37$ ($r = 0.85$, SEE = 0.15 L/min). The coefficient of variation of individual differences between direct and predicted values was 12.5% for males and 14.5% for females.
2. Franklin et al. (89) developed a wheelchair field test to estimate $\dot{V}O_{2peak}$. Thirty male adult wheelchair users (mean age 34 years) performed an arm-crank $\dot{V}O_{2peak}$ test in a laboratory and a 12-minute maximal wheelchair propulsion test for distance using a standardized lightweight wheelchair (Quickie II) on a 0.1-mile indoor synthetic track. The mean peak PO, $\dot{V}O_2$ and wheelchair propulsion distance were 89 W, 22 mL/kg/min, and 1.11 mile, respectively. The following regression equation was developed to predict $\dot{V}O_{2peak}$ in mL/kg/min: $\dot{V}O_{2peak} =$ (distance in miles $- 0.37$) $\div 0.0337$; $r = 0.84$.

3. Pare et al. (90) developed a regression equation to predict $\dot{V}O_{2peak}$ from submaximal wheelchair ergometry PO in 35 adults with SCI paraplegia: $\dot{V}O_{2peak}$ in L/min = (0.02 $\times$ PO_{peak} in watts) + 0.79; $r = 0.80$, SEE = 0.22 L/min). Prediction improved slightly when predicted $\dot{V}O_{2peak}$, %HR_{peak}, and body mass were included in the equation, but they admitted great variability among subjects.

B. Laboratory Tests

Generally, graded exercise testing for people with SCD involves discontinuous arm-crank ergometry protocols with five to six stages/test, 2–4 min/stage, and an initial stage of 0–20 W (warm-up). PO increments must be appropriate for the individual, depending on his or her functional level of SCI, muscular strength, and conditioning level. Most persons with tetraplegia require very small PO increments (5–10 W/stage). People with paraplegia may require PO increments of 10–20 W/stage. If deconditioned, PO increments may be lower. Allow 2- to 3-minute rest periods between stages to prevent premature fatigue and to allow monitoring of HR, ECG, BP, RPE, and symptoms. After the test, allow several minutes for cool-down and recovery, especially if the subject experienced symptoms of hypotension or severe exhaustion (87). Similar protocols have been utilized by Glaser et al. (91,92), Kofsky et al. (88), Franklin et al. (89), and Morrison et al. (26).

FITNESS TESTING

Winnick and Short (24) have published detailed physical fitness assessment protocols and standards for youths with SCD, ages 10–17 years. The recommended test items include the "Target aerobic movement test" (93); triceps skinfold or triceps + subscapular skinfolds for body composition; reverse curl, seated push-up, and dominant handgrip; modified Apley and Thomas tests; and target stretch tests adapted for specific joint motions for musculoskeletal functioning. No such standardized tests exist for adults with SCD, but the above items could be adapted for adults. The field tests of Kofsky et al. (88) and Franklin et al. (89) can also be useful for estimating $\dot{V}O_{2peak}$ from arm-crank ergometry or wheelchair propulsion performance.

FUNCTIONAL TESTING

During rehabilitation, the Functional Independence Measure (8,94) is used most often to assess functional independence. Different versions exist for adults and children with SCD. A variety of other functional outcome measures in SCI rehabilitation are discussed by Cole et al. (95). HR responses and timed performances of various daily living functional tasks such as mobility and transfers are also used to reflect functional status (26,51,52).

EXERCISE PRESCRIPTION AND PROGRAMMING

GENERAL GUIDELINES

Rimaud et al. (96) reviewed 25 cardiorespiratory training studies involving SCI subjects that varied greatly in program parameters and outcomes. As a starting point and on the basis of proven efficacy and specificity to daily activity patterns, they recommended interval WERG training at $\geq 70\%$ HR_{peak} for 30 minutes per session, three sessions per week for 8 weeks. The following general guidelines can contribute to the development of safe, effective, and standardized methods for rehabilitative exercise evaluation and treatment and long-term fitness services and sports programming for people with SCD:

1. *Exercise modes:* Aerobic cardiopulmonary training modes may include ACE, WERG, wheelchair propulsion on extra-wide treadmill or rollers; free wheeling over ground; swimming and other aquatic exercises; vigorous sports, such as wheelchair basketball, quad rugby, and wheelchair racing; arm-powered cycling; seated aerobic exercises; FES-LCE with or without combination with voluntary ACE; and vigorous ADLs, such as ambulation with assistive devices.

2. *Regulation of exercise:* In general, using HR to gauge exercise intensity for the SCD population is problematic because of the poor relationships between HR, $\dot{V}O_2$, and symptoms (98,99). Discrepancies are attributable to varying amounts of active muscle mass, completeness of spinal cord lesion, levels of spinal neurologic function, and autonomic control of HR and hemodynamics. However, within individuals, the relationship between HR and $\dot{V}O_2$ is likely to be more predictable and may be useful to guide exercise training intensity. Janssen et al. (53) and Dallmeijer et al. (54) have used percentage of $HR_{reserve}$ successfully to gauge the relative exercise intensity (physical strain) of various daily activities and exercise performance relative to individually determined HR_{peak} values. With continuous HR monitoring, $\%HR_{reserve}$ can be calculated as follows: $\%$ $HR_{reserve} = (HR_{peak} - HR_{observed}) \div (HR_{peak} - HR_{rest}) \times 100$. Hayes et al. (100) used HR from a maximal ACE test to predict energy expenditure (EE) during five ADLs in a diverse group of 13 nonambulatory SCI persons (ages 35–72, levels C5-L5, ASIA A-D, HR_{peak} 96–216 bpm). The ADLs included desk work, washing dishes, transfer between wheelchair and beds, wheeling on tile, and laundry tasks. In general, HRs derived from individualized regression equations explained 55% of the variance in measured EE. However, EE from calibrated HR consistently overestimated the actual EE by about 25%. Therefore, HR can be used only as a gross estimate of EE during higher-intensity ADLs.

   If accurate HR monitoring is not possible, the Borg CR-11 RPE scale (101) can be used to obtain a reliable estimate of relative exercise intensity. Therefore, "moderate"-intensity exercise would be perceived as RPE = 3, "strong" as RPE = 5, "very strong" as RPE = 7, "extremely strong" as RPE = 10, and "absolute maximum" as RPE = 11. As exercise tolerance and fitness improves through training, the exerciser performs at higher POs while reporting the same RPE values.

3. *Environment:* For training, use an environmentally controlled, thermoneutral or cool gym, laboratory, or clinic for persons with tetraplegia. Individuals with impaired thermoregulation can exercise outdoors if provisions are made for extreme conditions. If necessary, drink fluids before, during, and after exercise. Exercise only in thermally neutral environments such as in a laboratory or clinic with air-conditioning to control temperature and humidity, especially for persons with tetraplegia.

4. *Safety:*
   - Always supervise persons with SCD, especially those with SCI tetraplegia.
   - If they are not exercising in their wheelchairs, two people may be necessary for manual transfer of large individuals to and from exercise equipment.
   - A person with tetraplegia may need assistance to perform an exercise, to adjust machines and selected weights, and to perform flexibility exercises.
   - Follow all disability-specific precautions concerning skin, bones, stabilization, handgrip, bladder, bowels, illness, hypo- or hypertension, pain, orthopedic complications, and medications. For individuals with tetraplegia who are susceptible to orthostatic and exercise hypotension, monitor BP and symptoms regularly. Be prepared to reposition a symptomatic hypotensive person with tetraplegia to a more recumbent posture, and apply support stockings and abdominal binder to help maintain BP. The latter may influence exercise options.
   - To prevent and treat upper-extremity overuse syndromes, vary exercise modes from week to week, strengthen muscles of the upper back and posterior shoulder (especially shoulder external rotators), and stretch muscles of anterior shoulder and chest.
   - Emptying the bladder or urinary collection device immediately beforehand may prevent dysreflexic symptoms during exercise. People with tetraplegia should *not* "boost" (i.e., self-induce "controlled" autonomic dysreflexia) during exercise to improve exercise tolerance (i.e., prevent hypotension) because of the danger of stroke and renal infection or damage.

5. *Follow-up:* Consult a physician and appropriate nursing or allied health personnel to answer specific questions concerning medical complications to which the persons with SCD may be susceptible.

6. *Training principles:* Following the universal training principles is necessary for achieving training outcomes.
   - Specificity: Focus exercise training activities on functional tasks to improve mobility and increase

general lifestyle physical activity for health. Include all components of fitness: flexibility, muscular strength and endurance, aerobic fitness, and coordination for high-skill functional or recreational tasks. For aerobic training, the greater the exercising muscle mass, the greater the expected improvements in all physiologic and performance parameters. Arm training may prevent profound deconditioning, but will probably only induce peripheral training effects in the arm muscles. Combined arm and leg ergometry or exercise may induce both muscular and central cardiopulmonary training effects.

- Overload: Perform exercise at a higher intensity, duration, or frequency than that to which the person is accustomed. Fine-tune these according to feedback from the exerciser's subsequent soreness, and so forth.
- Progression: Expect small absolute (peak PO or $\dot{V}O_2$) improvements. Health maintenance and prevention of secondary conditions are essential for progressing to high levels of fitness for sports and optimal functional performance. Increases in exercise duration are more likely to be seen in persons with SCD before absolute improvements in peak PO or $\dot{V}O_2$.
- Regularity: Exercise every week for at least three sessions per week as per American College of Sports Medicine/American Heart Association (ACSM-AHA) recommendations (102). Plan to continue the exercise training program indefinitely. Fulfill the recommendation of at least 30 minutes of daily, moderate, and varied physical activities.

EXERCISE PRESCRIPTION

Useful exercise prescriptions specify the modes, frequency, intensity, and duration of exercises for an individual with known abilities and needs. Because of the diverse functional presentations of SCD and varying fitness goals, it is impossible to specify these parameters. However, approximations for beginners and advanced exercisers with SCD are listed in Table 5.6.

TABLE 5.6. COMPONENTS OF THE BEGINNING AND ADVANCED EXERCISE PRESCRIPTION FOR PERSONS WITH SPINAL CORD DYSFUNCTION

COMPONENT	BEGINNING (MINIMUM)	ADVANCED (MAXIMUM)
Flexibility		
Modes	Static or dynamic stretching, standing frame, Partner stretching, PNF stretching (contract-relax, and so forth), standing frame	Joint motions Scapular adduction, shoulder horizontal abduction and extension, elbow extension, hip extension, knee extension, ankle dorsiflexion
Frequency	Daily	Twice daily
Intensity	Moderate	Moderate
Duration	30 s/stretch, 10 min/session	30 s/stretch, 30 min/session
Muscular Strength		
Modes	Active assistive, dumbbells, wrist weight, body weight resistance, elastic bands or tubing	Resistance machines, barbells, Smith machine, medicine ball, high-speed isokinetics, plyometrics
Muscle groups	Scapular depressors, elbow extensors, latissimus dorsi, and so on. (all innervated muscle groups in balance, if possible)	
Frequency	2 ×/wk	Daily
Intensity	15-RM	1–10-RM
Duration	1 set × 15 repetitions/exercise × 5 exercises	2–3 sets × 1–10 repetitions/exercise × 15 exercises
Muscular Endurance		
Modes	Same as above for muscular strength, aquatics	Same as above for muscular strength, circuit training, medicine ball
Muscle groups	Same as for muscular strength	Same as above for muscular strength
Frequency	2 ×/wk	Daily
Intensity	Moderate (RPE = 4/11)	Maximal (RPE = 10/11)
Duration	1 set × 1 min/exercise	2–3 sets × 2–5 min/exercise
Aerobic/Cardiopulmonary Fitness		
Modes	Walking, wheeling, seated or standing aerobics, sports, interval training, fartlek	Fast walking, jogging, wheeling, arm or leg cycling, swimming, racing, rowing, arm or leg cycling
Frequency	2–3 × /wk	1–2 daily
Intensity	Moderate (RPE = 3/11)	Moderate-extremely strong (RPE = 3–10)
Duration	5 min/session	60+ min/session
Coordination/Skill		
Modes	Skill-specific	Skill-specific
Frequency	Daily	Twice daily
Intensity	Low (avoid fatigue)	Low (avoid fatigue)
Duration	20 min/session	60+ min/session

PNF, proprioceptive neuromuscular facilitation; RM, repetition maximum; RPE, rating of perceived exertion.

EDUCATION AND COUNSELING

Coyle and Kinney (103) indicated that leisure satisfaction was the most important and significant predictor of life satisfaction among adults with disability. Edwards (104) noted that the leading two services desired but not received by individuals following SCI were planning an exercise program (43%) and providing a referral to a fitness center (26%). Moreover, the ability to meet the physical and psychosocial needs of the person affected by SCD is critical to the pursuit of independent productivity (105). Figoni et al. (106) identified multiple physical barriers and inaccessibility of fitness facilities and services. Scelza et al. (107) surveyed 72 people with SCI about perceived barriers to exercise. The most frequently cited concerns fell into three areas: (a) intrapersonal or intrinsic (e.g., lack of motivation, lack of energy, lack of interest), (b) resources (e.g., cost of an exercise program, not knowing where to exercise), and (c) structural or architectural (e.g., accessibility of facilities and knowledgeable instructors). More individuals with tetraplegia reported concerns over exercise being too difficult and that health concerns kept them from exercising. Greater number of concerns were significantly related to higher levels of perceived stress. These findings underscore the need for rehabilitation and exercise providers to promote lifelong fitness, to provide instruction and guidelines, and to refer to accessible fitness centers to assist in meeting the identified needs of this population.

With the decline in the duration and reimbursement of (re)habilitation services (108) and the scarcity of frequent adapted physical education in schools, more and more people with SCD are seeking community-based exercise and fitness opportunities (109). Because many people with SCD are marginally independent, deconditioning and activity-related secondary conditions will make independence more difficult or impossible. Along with physical education and fitness education that all students should receive, people with SCD need physical activity and exercise counseling to learn about benefits of activity, to identify and remove barriers to exercise, and to solve problems related to accessibility or availability of adapted fitness services (110). In particular, the many barriers to physical activity and exercise for people with SCD may not be readily apparent to professionals.

Adherence to physical activity and exercise programs is as important as the programs themselves. People without SCD report that their main barriers (111) are lack of social support, unavailability of facilities, time constraints, and cost. Persons with SCD may face additional barriers, such as muscle paralysis, secondary medical conditions and symptoms, need for physical assistance, inaccessibility of facilities, and inappropriateness of equipment and services (106,111). Table 5.7 summarizes many of these barriers and some potential solutions. One recent publication makes many suggestions for accessibility or universal design of fitness facilities and adaptation of exercise programs and equipment for people with SCD (112).

TABLE 5.7. FACILITATING FACTORS AND INTRINSIC/EXTRINSIC ALTERABLE/UNALTERABLE INHIBITING FACTORS AFFECTING ADHERENCE OF PERSONS WITH SPINAL CORD DYSFUNCTION TO EXERCISE PROGRAMS

FACILITATORS

Dedication to specific goals, intention to exercise	Not currently ill
Belief that benefits will outweigh costs/risks (improved function, health, and so on)	Access to lots of exercise equipment at home or facility
Reliable transportation to facility	Free accessible parking available
Good weather/driving conditions	Accessible facility entrances and halls
Bowels/bladder managed OK today	Accessible scale
Clean exercise clothes	Appropriate accessible equipment
Enjoy fun physical activity/exercise	Appropriate adaptations to equipment
Comfortable with (accepted by) other people at facility	Assistance available
Attendance has priority over other competing activities	Expert staff
Expectation of staff and peers to attend	Social activity (meet friends at facility)
Clean, safe, air-conditioned facility	Service charges covered by project (affordable)
Can participate year-round indoors	Culturally sensitive environment
Competition, adherence	Child care available

INHIBITORS OR BARRIERS	**STRATEGY TO REMOVE BARRIER**

INTRINSIC (DISABILITY, PERSONALITY, BELIEFS, ATTITUDES, PREFERENCES, INTERESTS)

Alterable

Exercise is boring	Listen to music, keep mind occupied, wheel/bike outdoors
Muscle or joint soreness	Initial soreness will go away in a few days, build up gradually, stretch after activity, analgesics
Fear of injury	See staff/healthcare provider, education
Frequent temporary illness (cold, flu, allergy, UTI, sores)	See healthcare provider, education
Lack of goal orientation	See staff/healthcare provider, education
Belief that costs/risks will outweigh benefits	See staff/healthcare provider, education
Cannot stick with it (low self-efficacy/will-power)	Try it, improve confidence/success/discipline, social support, rewards, benefits, record-keeping, adherence

(continued)

TABLE 5.7. FACILITATING FACTORS AND INTRINSIC/EXTRINSIC ALTERABLE/UNALTERABLE INHIBITING FACTORS AFFECTING ADHERENCE OF PERSONS WITH SPINAL CORD DYSFUNCTION TO EXERCISE PROGRAMS (*Continued*)

INHIBITORS OR BARRIERS	STRATEGY TO REMOVE BARRIER
INTRINSIC (DISABILITY, PERSONALITY, BELIEFS, ATTITUDES, PREFERENCES, INTERESTS)	
Alterable	
Prefer outdoors to indoors	Do outdoor activities
Cultural insensitivity of staff/participants	Staff training
Bowel/bladder accident before attendance	See healthcare provider
No previous experience or sport history	Start hobby or enjoyable activity that gets you moving
Does not enjoy exercise	Do not "exercise," try different activities, Do not focus on discomfort
Uncomfortable with (not accepted by) other people	See healthcare provider (psychology)
Dislike staff or participants	Be tolerant of diversity (race, gender, level of SCI, athletes), change location of exercise
Persistent hypotensive symptoms (dizzy, sick, weak), poor orthostatic tolerance	Supine posture, aquatics, support hose, binder, orthostatic training (tilt tolerance table, standing), see healthcare provider, meds
Too tired, not enough energy, too much effort	Regular activity improves your energy level
Poor balance	Use straps or partner/staff to stabilize
Poor hand grip	Use holding gloves, wraps, or wrist cuffs
Cannot use equipment (transfer, change weight, grasp)	Use adapted exercise equipment
Severe arthritis or joint pain	See healthcare provider
Embarrassment (poor body image)	See healthcare provider, psychology
Substance abuse	See healthcare provider
Does not like to ask for help	Assertiveness and social skills training
Likes to be alone	Social skills training, use social support
Family does not encourage me to exercise	Convince family of benefits of exercise
Exercise has low priority	See staff/healthcare provider, prioritize and plan
Never see anyone else exercising	Attend a fitness facility or our program
No friends or family who exercise	Find a partner who will exercise, meet other participants
Do not know how to exercise or what to do	See healthcare provider, education
Too old to exercise	See healthcare provider, education
Healthcare provider said not to exercise	See healthcare provider, education
Never had P.E., sport, or activities when I was younger	Never too late to learn and benefit
Unalterable	
Paralysis	Exercise innervated muscles, FES for paralyzed muscles
Incoordination, spasticity	Use simpler/slower exercises, practice skills
Low pain threshold	Build up gradually, analgesics
Occasional illness	Be patient
Cognitive impairment, ADD, mental illness	See healthcare provider
Alterable	
Medications make me drowsy	See healthcare provider
No clean exercise clothes	Do laundry more often; plan ahead
Neighborhood safety	Bring friend, move
Child care unavailable	Plan ahead, have alternatives, bring child
Family demands	Plan ahead, bring family
No role models present	Find one, Big Brothers, Big Sisters
Unreliable transportation to facility, can't drive	Plan ahead, learn to drive, hand controls, repair car, public transport, alternative means of transport
Bad weather/driving conditions	Exercise at home, have alternate plans
Lack of time, takes time from family/job responsibilities	Time management, shorter exercise sessions, watch less TV, make exercise a high priority, exercise improves function and job performance
Inconvenient facility times	Expand facility hours, change facilities
Exercise is hard work and takes too much energy	Build up gradually
Chronic pain	See healthcare provider (education)
Exacerbates an existing medical condition	See healthcare provider (education)
Hours conflict with work/school	Plan accordingly
Music is too loud	Lower the volume, change facilities
Facility is too far away	Make time for commute, find closer facility
Exercise costs too much	Benefits outweigh costs, find less expensive facility, exercise at home
Heavy work schedule	Plan accordingly
Unalterable	
Emergency, death in family, disaster (tornado, flood, fire)	None
Facility closes down, research project ends	Change facilities, have alternate facility and long-term plan

ADD, attention-deficit disorder; FES, functional electrical stimulation; P.E., physical education; SCI, spinal cord injury; UTI, urinary tract infection.

Less motivated people with or without SCD need structured exercise plans that include behavioral supports to promote adherence. Frequently used supports include self-monitoring (daily activity or exercise log to which they are held accountable), frequent reassessment and tracking of progress with reinforcement, social support (from staff, exercise partner, or fellow members of an exercise group or wheelchair sports team), and provisions for relapse prevention.

All exercise professionals need to be psychologically supportive of efforts made by people with SCD to exercise and remain physically active. They can help them assess their need for specific exercises and activities, set realistic goals, and use effective training methods. Improvements in health, fitness, and function may have profound effects on the lives of people with SCD that professionals may not see in the clinical or fitness setting. If the person with SCD does not seem to be coping with his or her disability, the exercise professional should refer that person to a clinical psychologist for evaluation. Anxiety, depression, and chronic pain are common in the SCD population (113).

Recommended are several excellent practical guidelines on fitness and exercise education and training of people with SCD (96,97,109–122). Additionally, exercise professionals should be aware that competitive wheelchair sports opportunities are available for potential athletes with SCD. They would fit best in events organized by Wheelchair Sports USA with a classification system based on neurologic level of spinal nerve function (123).

CASE STUDY

John sustained a complete spinal cord injury at C8 from a gun shot wound 5 years ago at age 17. His trunk and leg musculature are paralyzed, with marked spasticity in the hip and knee flexors and ankle plantarflexors. The muscle strength of his upper extremities is normal, but his finger extensors and intrinsics, wrist flexors, pectorals, and latissimus dorsi muscles are weak. John is 180 cm tall and weighs 110 kg (BMI = 34 kg/m^2), with a triceps skinfold of 25 mm. He has gained 50 pounds over the past 5 years since his discharge from rehabilitation. He uses a manual wheelchair and lives independently in the community and drives an adapted van.

Subjective Data: John complains of arm muscle fatigue, shoulder pain, dizziness, and shortness of breath when propelling his manual lightweight everyday wheelchair and especially up inclines. He considers himself overweight and out of shape. His posture appears kyphotic with rounded shoulders, forward head, and protruding abdomen.

Objective Data: John's resting HR and BP were 65 bpm and 90/60 mm Hg, respectively. During a graded arm-crank exercise test, his PO$_{peak}$ was 45 W. He became progressively more light-headed during the test as his systolic blood pressure (SBPO decreased to 70 mm Hg and his diastolic blood pressure (DBP) was inaudible. His HR peaked at 125 bpm just before extreme arm muscle fatigue or exhaustion (RPE = 8 on the Borg CR-11 scale). John takes 20 seconds to push his chair up a standard (12:1) 4-meter ramp. During a 6-minute wheeling test, he traveled a distance of 600 meter on a flat, smooth indoor surface. In addition to his daily activities, the only formal exercise that John performs on his own is daily stretching.

Assessment: John is physically deconditioned. He needs improved physical fitness to accomplish his daily activities without exhaustion or pain. Specifically, he needs decreased body fat weight, increased triceps and shoulder depressor strength and endurance, and balanced shoulder muscle strength and flexibility. John needs lifestyle modification education, including exercise and nutrition behavior change to manage his body weight over time. John needs medical evaluation to remediate his symptomatic hypotension.

He has substantial upper body muscle mass and strength, but profoundly impaired autonomic vasomotor and autonomic control over his cardiovascular system.

Plan: John will consult a registered dietician to implement an appropriate diet to lose 20 kg of unnecessary fat weight. John will consult his physician to rule out heart disease and a physical therapist concerning his shoulder pain. He will try using an elastic abdominal binder, support stockings, leg elevation, or supine posture to maintain his BP during exercise. John will continue all normal daily activities with his manual wheelchair. When tolerable, John will increase his general physical activities to help with weight management. John will exercise under the guidance of a Clinical Exercise Physiologist at an accessible fitness facility at least three sessions per week. Assistance will be necessary for postural stability.

John's beginning exercise prescription is as follows.

1. Warm-up (general upper body calisthenics and seated aerobics, dynamic flexibility exercises for upper extremities)
2. Shoulder Balance:
   a. Therapeutic exercises to strengthen the external shoulder rotators and scapular retractors, and stretch the anterior chest and shoulder muscles
3. General Arm Strength, Endurance, and Anaerobic Power Training:
   a. Rickshaw exercise (similar to dips, but on a wheelchair-accessible machine). Two exercises:
      1) With bent elbows (for triceps)
      2) With straight elbows (for shoulder depressors)

b. Lateral pull-downs (pulleys)

c. Rowing (pulleys)

d. Incline press (against light machine weights)

e. Bench press (weight machine)

Day 1: Assessments: Determine 10-RM for each exercise, and perform Wingate anaerobic power test (maximal work performed during maximal-effort, high-intensity arm-cranking for 30 seconds).

Day 2: Training: 2 sets × 10 repetitions at 90% 10-RM

Progress according to principles of progressive resistive exercise and principles of overload, progression, specificity, regularity, and so forth.

4. Aerobic Exercise: Choose two to three acceptable accessible available modes (e.g., arm-crank ergometry):

a. Find workload (≈20–30 W) that elicits RPE = 4/11 for at least 5 minutes or until arm muscle fatigue or dizziness.

b. Perform at least two assessments on different days to establish training baselines. Example:

1) Maximal work performed during 6-minute period

2) ACE field test

c. Progress over time to 30–60 minutes per workout.

d. Vary direction of cranking (forward versus backward).

e. Vary intensities and durations of workouts (i.e., shorter durations with higher intensity [intervals] versus long, slow distance).

f. Watch videos or find partner to combat boredom of arm ergometry.

g. Repeat assessments every 2 weeks.

REFERENCES

1. Nelson MR, Rott EJ. Spina bifida. In: Grabois M, Garrison SJ, Hart KA, et al., eds. *Physical Medicine and Rehabilitation: The Complete Approach.* Malden, MA: Blackwell Science; 2000:1414–1432.
2. Cardenas DD, Burns SP, Chan L. Rehabilitation of spinal cord injury. In: Grabois M, Garrison SJ, Hart KA, et al, eds. *Physical Medicine and Rehabilitation: The Complete Approach.* Malden, MA: Blackwell Science; 2000:1305–1324.
3. Yarkony GM, Chen D. Rehabilitation of patients with spinal cord injuries. In: Braddom RJ, ed. *Physical Medicine and Rehabilitation.* Philadelphia: W.B. Saunders; 1996:1149–1179.
4. Mallory B. Autonomic dysfunction in spinal cord disease. In: Lin VW, ed. *Spinal Cord Medicine: Principles and Practice.* New York: Demos; 2003:477–500.
5. Goshgarian HG. Anatomy and function of the spinal cord. In: Lin VW, ed. *Spinal Cord Medicine: Principles and Practice.* New York: Demos; 2003:15–34.
6. ASIA. International Standards for Neurological Classification of SCI. Atlanta: American Spinal Injury Association; 2002.
7. ASIA. Standard neurological classification of spinal cord injury. Atlanta: American Spinal Injury Association; 2006. (accessed online, 2-17-08: http://www.asia-spinalinjury.org/publications/2006_Classif_worksheet.pdf)
8. Consortium for Spinal Cord Medicine. Outcomes following traumatic spinal cord injury: Clinical practice guidelines for healthcare professions. Washington, DC: Paralyzed Veterans of America; 1999.
9. Furhrer MJ. Rehabilitation and research training center in community-oriented services for persons with spinal cord injury: A progress report. Houston, TX: The Baylor College of Medicine and The Institute for Rehabilitation Research; 1991.
10. Whiteneck GG. Learning from recent empirical investigations. In: Whiteneck GG, Charlifue SW, Gerhart KS, et al., eds. *Aging with Spinal Cord Injury.* New York: Demos Publications; 1993.
11. Anson CA, Shepherd C. Incidence of secondary complications in spinal cord injury. *Int J Rehabil Res* 1996;19:55–66.
12. Johnson RL, Gerhart KA, McCray J, et al. Secondary conditions following spinal cord injury in a population-based sample. *Spinal Cord* 1998;36:45–50.
13. Bauman WA, Spungen AM. Metabolic changes in persons after spinal cord injury. *Phys Med Rehabil Clin N Am* 2000;11:109–140.
14. Washburn RA, Figoni SF. Physical activity and chronic cardiovascular disease prevention: A comprehensive literature review. *Top Spinal Cord Injury Rehabil* 1998;3:16–32.
15. Davis GM. Exercise capacity of individuals with paraplegia. *Med Sci Sports Exerc* 1993;25:423–432.
16. Figoni SF. Exercise responses and quadriplegia. *Med Sci Sports Exerc* 1993;25:433–441.
17. Price MJ. Thermoregulation during exercise in individuals with spinal cord injuries. *Sports Med* 2006;36:863–879.
18. Hopman MTE, Nommensen E, van Asten WNJC, et al. Properties of the venous vascular system in the lower extremities on individuals with paraplegia. *Paraplegia* 1994;32:810–816.
19. Bauman WA. Endocrinology and metabolism after spinal cord injury. In: Kirshblum S, Campagnolo DI, DeLisa JA, eds. *Spinal Cord Medicine.* Philadelphia, PA: Lippincott Williams & Wilkins; 2002:164–180.
20. Kelly LE. Spinal cord disabilities. In: Winnick JP, ed. *Adapted Physical Education and Sport.* 4th ed. Champaign, IL: Human Kinetics; 2005:275–306.
21. Hart AL, Malone TR, English T. Shoulder function and rehabilitation implications for the wheelchair athlete. *Top Spinal Cord Injury Rehabil* 1998;3:50–65.
22. Winnick JP, Short FX. The physical fitness of youngsters with spinal neuromuscular conditions. *Adapted Phys Activ Q* 1984;1:37–51.
23. Shephard RJ. *Fitness in Special Populations.* Champaign, IL: Human Kinetics, 1990.
24. Winnick JP, Short FX. The *Brockport Physical Fitness Test Manual.* Champaign, IL: Human Kinetics; 1999.
25. Andrade CK, Kramer J, Garber M, et al. Changes in self-concept, cardiovascular endurance and muscular strength of children with spina bifida aged 8 to 13 years in response to a 10-week physical-activity programme: A pilot study. *Child Care Health Dev* 1991;17:183–196.
26. Morrison SA, Melton-Rogers SL, Hooker SP. Changes in physical capacity and physical strain in persons with acute spinal cord injury. *Top Spinal Cord Injury Rehabil* 1997;3:1–15.
27. Hjeltnes N, Jansen T. Physical endurance capacity, functional status and medical complications in spinal cord injured subjects with long-standing lesions. *Paraplegia* 1990;428–432.
28. Stewart MW, Melton-Rogers SL, Morrison S, et al. The measurement properties of fitness measures and health status for persons with spinal cord injuries. *Arch Phys Med Rehabil* 2000;81:394–400.
29. Raymond J, Davis GM, Fahey A, et al. Oxygen uptake and heart rate responses during arm vs combined arm/electrically stimulated leg exercise in people with paraplegia. *Spinal Cord* 1997;35:680–685.
30. Haisma JA, van der Woude LH, Stam HJ, Bergen MP, Sluis TA, Bussmann JB. Physical capacity in wheelchair-dependent persons with a spinal cord injury: A critical review of the literature. *Spinal Cord* 2006;44(11):642–652.
31. Glaser RM. Exercise and locomotion for the spinal cord injured. *Exerc Sports Sci Rev* 1985;13:263–303.

32. Dreisinger TE, Londeree BR. Wheelchair exercise: A review. *Paraplegia* 1982;20:20–34.

33. Fuhr L, Langbein E, Edwards LC, et al. Diagnostic wheelchair exercise testing. *Top Spinal Cord Injury Rehabil* 1997;3:34–48.

34. Pitetti KH, Barrett PJ, Campbell KD, et al. The effect of lower body positive pressure on the exercise capacity of individuals with spinal cord injury. *Med Sci Sports Exerc* 1994;26:463–468.

35. Sawka MN, Latzka WA, Pandolf KB. Temperature regulation during upper body exercise: Able-bodied and spinal cord injured. *Med Sci Sports Exerc* 1989;21:S132–S140.

36. Houtman S, Oeseburg B, Hopman MTE. Blood volume and hemoglobin after spinal cord injury. *Am J Phys Med Rehabil* 2000;79: 260–265.

37. Veeger HEJ, Hajd Yahmed M, van der Woude LHV, et al. Peak oxygen uptake and maximal power output of Olympic wheelchair-dependent athletes. *Med Sci Sports Exerc* 1991;1201–1209.

38. Coutts KD, Rhodes EC, McKenzie DC. Maximal exercise responses of tetraplegics and paraplegics. *J Appl Physiol* 1971;55:479–482.

39. Gass GC, Camp EM. Physiological characteristics of training Australian paraplegic and tetraplegic subjects. *Med Sci Sports Exerc* 1979;11:256–265.

40. Van Loan MD, McCluer S, Loftin JM, et al. Comparison of physiological responses to maximal arm exercise among able-bodied, paraplegics, and quadriplegics. *Paraplegia* 1987;25:397–405.

41. Figoni SF, Boileau RA, Massey BH, et al. Physiological responses of quadriplegic and able-bodied men during exercise at the same $\dot{V}O_2$. *Adapted Phys Activ Q* 1988;5:130–139.

42. Hjeltnes N. Capacity for physical work and training after spinal injuries and strokes. *Scand J Rehabil Med* 1982;29:245–251.

43. Hjeltnes N. Control of medical rehabilitation of para- and tetraplegics by repeated evaluation of endurance capacity. *Int J Sports Med* 1984;5:171–174.

44. Figoni SF, Glaser RM. Arm and leg exercise stress testing in a person with quadriparesis. *Clin Kinesiol* 1993;47:25–36.

45. Claydon VE, Hol AT, Eng JJ, Krassioukov AV. Cardiovascular responses and postexercise hypotension after arm cycling exercise in subjects with spinal cord injury. *Arch Phys Med Rehabil* 2006; 87(8):1106–1114.

46. Figoni SF, Gupta SC, Glaser RM. Effects of posture on arm exercise performance of adults with tetrapelgia. *Clin Exerc Physiol* 1999;1: 74–85.

47. Hopman MTE, Dueck C, Monroe M, et al. Limits of maximal performance in individuals with spinal cord injury. *Int J Sports Med* 1998;19:98–103.

48. Ready AE. Responses of quadriplegic athletes to maximal and submaximal exercise. *Physiother Can* 1984;36:124–128.

49. Hooker SP, Figoni SF, Rodgers MM, et al. Metabolic and hemodynamic responses to concurrent voluntary arm crank and electrical stimulation leg cycle exercise in quadriplegics. *J Rehabil Res Dev* 1992;29:1–11.

50. Takahashi M, Sakaguchi A, Matsukawa K, Komine H, Kawaguchi K, Onari K. Cardiovascular control during voluntary static exercise in humans with tetraplegia. *J Appl Physiol* 2004;97:2077-82.

51. Krebs P, Eickelberg W, Krobath H, et al. Effects of physical exercise on peripheral vision and learning in children with spina bifida manifestation. *Perceptual and Motor Skills* 1989;68:167–174.

52. Agre JC, Findley TW, McNally MC, et al. Physical activity capacity in children with myelomeningocele. *Arch Phys Med Rehabil* 1987;68:372–377.

53. Janssen TWJ, van Oers CAJM, van der Woude LHV, et al. Physical strain in daily life of wheelchair users with spinal cord injuries. *Med Sci Sports Exerc* 1994;26:661–670.

54. Dallmeijer AJ, Hopman MTE, van As HHJ, et al. Physical capacity and physical strain in persons with tetraplegia: The role of sport activity. *Spinal Cord* 1996; 34:729–735.

55. Davis GM, Shephard RJ, Leenen FH. Cardiac effects of short term arm crank training in paraplegics: Echocardiographic evidence. *Eur J Appl Physiol Occup Physiol* 1987;56:90–96.

56. Devillard X, Rimaud D, Roche F, Calmels P. Effects of training programs for spinal cord injury. *Ann Readapt Med Phys* 2007;50(6): 490–498.

57. Valent L, Dallmeijer A, Houdijk H, Talsma E, van der Woude L. The effects of upper body exercise on the physical capacity of people with a spinal cord injury: A systematic review. *Clin Rehabil* 2007 Apr;21(4):315–330.

58. Knutsson E, Lewenhaupt-Olsson E, Thorsen M. Physical work capacity and physical conditioning in paraplegic patients. *Paraplegia* 1973;11:205–216.

59. Nilsson S, Staff PH, Pruett ED. Physical work capacity and the effect of training on subjects with long-standing paraplegia. *Scand J Rehabil Med* 1975;7:51–56.

60. Davis GM, Shephard RJ. Strength training for wheelchair users. *Br J Sports Med* 1990;24:25–30.

61. McLean KP, Skinner JS. Effect of body training position on outcomes of an aerobic training study on individuals with quadriplegia. *Arch Phys Med Rehabil* 1995;76:139–150.

62. Lassau-Wray ER, Ward GR. Varying physiological response to arm-crank exercise in specific spinal injuries. *J Physiol Anthropol Appl Human Sci* 2000;19:5–12.

63. Hooker SP, Figoni SF, Rodgers MM, et al. Physiologic effects of electrical stimulation leg cycle exercise training in spinal cord injured persons. *Arch Phys Med Rehabil* 1992;73:470–476.

64. Nash MS, Bilsker S, Marcillo AE, et al. Reversal of adaptive left ventricular atrophy following electrically stimulated exercise training in human tetraplegia. *Paraplegia* 1992;29:590–599.

65. Nash MS. Exercise reconditioning of the heart and peripheral circulation after spinal cord injury. *Top Spinal Cord Injury Rehabil* 1998;4:1–15.

66. Faghri PD, Glaser RM, Figoni SF. Functional electrical stimulation leg cycle ergometer exercise: Training effect on cardiorespiratory responses of spinal cord injured subjects at rest and during submaximal exercise. *Arch Phys Med Rehabil* 1992;73:1085–1093.

67. Janssen TWJ, Glaser RM, Shuster DB. Clinical efficacy of electrical stimulation exercise training: Effects on health, fitness, and function. *Top Spinal Cord Injury Rehabil* 1998;3:33–49.

68. Figoni SF, Glaser RM, Collins SR. Training effects of hybrid exercise on peak physiologic responses in quadriplegics. Proceedings of the 12th International Congress of World Confederation for Physical Therapy. Alexandria, VA: American Physical Therapy Association, 1995, Paper no. PO-SI-0028T on CD-ROM.

69. Thijssen DH, Ellenkamp R, Smits P, Hopman MT. Rapid vascular adaptations to training and detraining in persons with spinal cord injury. *Arch Phys Med Rehabil* 2006;87(4):474–481.

70. Cooney MM, Walker JB. Hydraulic resistance exercise benefits cardiovascular fitness of spinal cord injured. *Med Sci Sports Exerc* 1986;18:522–525.

71. Jacobs PL, Nash MS, Rusinkowski JW Jr. Circuit training provides cardiorespiratory and strength benefits in persons with paraplegia. *Med Sci Sports Exerc* 2001;33:711–717.

72. Nash MS, van de Ven I, van Elk N, Johnson BM. Effects of circuit resistance training on fitness attributes and upper-extremity pain in middle-aged men with paraplegia. *Arch Phys Med Rehabil* 2007;88(1):70–75.

73. Curtis KA, Tyner TM, Zachary L, et al. Effect of a standard exercise protocol on shoulder pain in long-term wheelchair users. *Spinal Cord* 1999;37(6):421–429.

74. Nawoczenski DA, Ritter-Soronen JM, Wilson CM, Howe BA, Ludewig PM. Clinical trial of exercise for shoulder pain in chronic spinal injury. *Phys Ther* 2006;86(12):1604–1618.

75. Hicks AL, Martin KA, Ditor DS, Latimer AE, Craven C, Bugaresti J, McCartney N. Long-term exercise training in persons with spinal cord injury: Effects on strength, arm ergometry performance and psychological well-being. *Spinal Cord* 2003;41(1):34–43.

76. Barbeau H, Nadeau S, Garneau C. Physical determinants, emerging concepts, and training approaches in gait of individuals with spinal cord injury. *J Neurotrauma* 2006;23(3–4):571–585.

77. Field-Fote EC, Lindley SD, Sherman AL. Locomotor training approaches for individuals with spinal cord injury: A preliminary report of walking-related outcomes. *J Neurol Phys Ther* 2005;29(3):127–137.

78. Nash MS, Jacobs PL, Johnson BM, Field-Fote' E. Metabolic and cardiac responses to robotic-assisted locomotion in motor-complete tetraplegia: A case report. *J Spinal Cord Med* 2004;27(1):78–82.

79. Dobkin B, Barbeau H, Deforge D, et al; Spinal Cord Injury Locomotor Trial Group. The evolution of walking-related outcomes over the first 12 wk of rehabilitation for incomplete traumatic spinal cord injury: The multicenter randomized Spinal Cord Injury Locomotor Trial. *Neurorehabil Neural Repair* 2007;21(1):25–35.

80. Ekblom B, Lundberg A. Effect of physical training on adolescents with severe motor handicaps. *Acta Paediatr Scand* 1968;57:17–23.

81. O'Connell DG, Barnhart R. Improvement in wheelchair propulsion in pediatric wheelchair users through resistance training: A pilot study. *Arch Phys Med Rehabil* 1995;76:368–372.

82. Yarkony GM, ed. *Spinal Cord Injury: Medical Management and Rehabilitation.* Gaithersberg, MD: Aspen Publishers; 1994.

83. Nesathurai S. *The Rehabilitation of People with Spinal Cord Iinjury*, 2nd ed. Williston, VT: Blackwell Science; 2000.

84. Stass W, et al. Rehabilitation of the spinal cord injured patient. In: Delisa JA, Gans BM, Bockenek WL, eds. *Rehabilitation Medicine: Principles and Practice.* Baltimore: Lippincott William & Wilkins, 1993:891.

85. Bodner DR, Perkash I. Urological management in spinal cord injury. In: Lin VW, ed. *Spinal Cord Medicine: Principles and Practice.* New York: Demos; 2003:299–306.

86. *Physicians' Desk Reference* (PDR). (accessed online, 2-17-08, http://www.pdr.net)

87. Figoni SF. Spinal cord injury. In: Durstine JL, ed. *ACSM's Exercise Management for Persons with Chronic Diseases and Disabilities.* Champaign, IL: Human Kinetics; 1997:175–179.

88. Kofsky PR, Davis GM, Jackson RW, et al. Field testing—Assessment of physical fitness of disabled adults. *Eur J Appl Physiol* 1983;51:109–120.

89. Franklin BA, Swantek KI, Grais SL, et al. Field test estimation of maximal oxygen consumption in wheelchair users. *Arch Phys Med Rehabil* 1990;71:574–578.

90. Pare G, Noreau L, Simard C. Prediction of maximal aerobic power from a submaximal exercise test performed by paraplegics on a wheelchair ergometer. *Paraplegia* 1993;31:584–592.

91. Glaser RM, Sawka MN, Brune MF, et al. Physiological responses to maximal effort wheelchair and arm crank ergometry. *J Appl Physiol* 1980;48:1060–1064.

92. Glaser RM. Arm exercise training for wheelchair users. *Med Sci Sports Exerc* 1989;21(Suppl 5):S149–S157.

93. Rimmer JH, Connor-Kuntz F, Winnick JP, et al. Feasibility of the target aerobic movement test in children and adolescents with spina bifida. *Adapted Phys Activ Q* 1997;14:147–155.

94. UDS: *Uniform Data System for Medical Rehabilitation.* Accessed 2-17-08 at http://www.fimsystem.com

95. Cole B, Finch, Gowland C, et al. *Physical Rehabilitation Outcome Measures.* Baltimore: Williams & Wilkins; 1995.

96. Rimaud D, Calmels P, Devillard X. Training programs in spinal cord injury. *Ann Readapt Med Phys* 2005;48(5):259–269.

97. Jacobs PL, Nash MS. Exercise recommendations for individuals with spinal cord injury. *Sports Med* 2004;34:727–751.

98. Hooker SP, Greenwood JD, Hatae DT, et al. Oxygen uptake and heart rate relationship in persons with spinal cord injury. *Med Sci Sport Exerc.*1993;25:1115–1119.

99. Irizawa M, Yamasaki M, Muraki S, et al. Relationship between heart rate and oxygen uptake during submaximal arm cranking in paraplegics and quadriplegics. *Ann Physiol Anthrop* 1994;13(5):275–280.

100. Hayes AM, Myers JN, Ho M, Lee MY, Perkash I, Kiratli BJ. Heart rate as a predictor of energy expenditure in people with spinal cord injury. *J Rehabil Res Dev* 2005;42(5):617–624.

101. Borg G. *Borg's Perceived Exertion and Pain Scales.* Champaign, IL: Human Kinetics; 1998.

102. Haskell WL, Lee I-M, Pate RR, et al. Physical activity and public health: Updated recommendation for adults from the American College of Sports Medicine and the American Heart Association. *Med Sci Sports Exerc* 2007;39(8):1423–1434.

103. Coyle CP, Santiago MC. Aerobic exercise training and depressive symptomatology in adults with physical disabilities. *Arch Phys Med* 1995;76:647–652.

104. Edwards PA. Health promotion through fitness for adolescents and young adults following spinal cord injury. *SCI Nurs* 1996;13:69–73.

105. Nichols S, Brasile FM. The role of recreational therapy in physical medicine. *Top Spinal Cord Injury Rehabil* 1998;3:89–98.

106. Figoni SF, McClain L, Bell AA, et al. Accessibility of physical fitness facilities in the Kansas City metropolitan area. *Top Spinal Cord Injury Rehabil* 1998;3:66–78.

107. Scelza WM, Kalpakjian CZ, Zemper ED, Tate DG. Perceived barriers to exercise in people with spinal cord injury. *Am J Phys Med Rehabil.* 2005 Aug;84(8):576–583.

108. Morrison SA, Stanwyck DJ. The effect of shorter lengths of stay on functional outcomes of spinal cord injury rehabilitation. *Top Spinal Cord Injury Rehabil* 1999;4:44–55.

109. Johnson KA, Klaas SJ. Recreation issues and trends in pediatric spinal cord injury. *Top Spinal Cord Injury Rehabil* 1997;3:79–84.

110. Steadward R. Musculoskeletal and neurological disabilities: Implications for fitness appraisal, programming, and counseling. *Can J Appl Physiol* 1998;23:131–165.

111. Sallis JF, Hovell MF, Hofstetter CR. Predictors of adoption and maintenance of vigorous physical activity in men and women. *Prev Med* 1992;21:237–251.

112. North Carolina Office on Disability and Health. *Removing Barriers to Health Clubs and Fitness Facilities.* Chapel Hill, NC: Frank Porter Graham Child Development Center, 2001. (accessed online, 2-17-08, http://www.fpg.unc.edu/~ncodh/)

113. Elliott TR, Rank RG. Depression following spinal cord injury. *Arch Phys Med Rehabil* 1996;77:816–823.

114. Lowe C. Basic training (fitness, exercise, and sports). In: Lutkenhoff M, Oppenheimer SG, eds. *Spinabilities: A Young Person's Guide to Spina Bifida.* Bethesda, MD: Woodbine House; 1997:123–131.

115. Lockette KF, Keyes AM. *Conditioning with Physical Disabilities.* Champaign, IL: Human Kinetics; 1994.

116. Miller P, ed. *Fitness Programming and Physical Disability.* Champaign, IL: Human Kinetics, 1994.

117. Apple DF, ed. *Physical Fitness: A Guide for Individuals with Spinal Cord Injury.* Washington, DC: VA Rehabilitation Research and Development Service; 1996.

118. Youngbauer J, ed. *Deconditioning and Eeight Gain. Secondary Conditions Prevention & Treatment.* B Series, No. 3. Lawrence, KS: Research and Training Center on Independent Living, University of Kansas; 1996.

119. Chase TM. Physical fitness strategies. In: Lanig IS, ed. *A Practical Guide to Health Promotion After Spinal Cord Injury.* Gaithersberg, MD: Aspen Publishers; 1996.

120. Laskin JJ, James SA, Cantwell BM. A fitness and wellness program for people with spinal cord injury. *Top Spinal Cord Injury Rehabil* 1997;3:16–33.

121. Virgilio SJ. Fitness education for children with disabilities. In: Virgilio SJ. *Fitness Education for Children.* Champaign, IL: Human Kinetics; 1997:47–58.

122. Rimmer JH. Fitness and Rehabilitation Programs for Special Populations. Madison, WI: Wm. C. Brown; 1994.

123. Wheelchair Sports USA website. (accessed online, 2-17-08, http://www.wsusa.org)

Postpolio and Guillain-Barré Syndrome

EPIDEMIOLOGY AND PATHOPHYSIOLOGY

POSTPOLIO SYNDROME

Poliomyelitis is an acute viral disease that attacks the anterior horn cells of the lower motor neurons. This disease reached a peak epidemic period in the United States during the 1950s. Poliomyelitis results in flaccid paresis, paralysis, and atrophy in affected muscle groups with accompanying symptoms of fatigue, weakness, and pain. The acute 2-month phase of the disease is followed by a functional recovery period. A greater degree of functional recovery is expected when the percentage of motor neurons damaged, either partially or completely, does not exceed 50% (1). The functional period phase is usually stable for 15 years or more after initial diagnosis. During the stable recovery period, skeletal muscle fibers are reinnervated from the lower motor neurons spared by the polio virus. At some point, however, the remaining motor neurons are unable to generate new sprouts, and denervation exceeds reinnervation (Figure 6.1). Unable to keep up with reinnervation, symptoms such as fatigue, weakness, pain, muscle atrophy, cold intolerance, muscle spasms, and cramps and the difficulty of completing activities of daily living (ADLs) can appear. These symptoms are similar to the original ones and, therefore, this condition is termed postpolio syndrome (PPS) (2).

Postpolio syndrome affects a varyingly large percentage of the almost 1.8 million polio survivors (3–5). Approximately 40% of these survivors have indicated that fatigue, associated with PPS, significantly interferes with occupational performance, and at least 25% of these survivors reported that PPS-related symptoms also interfered with performance of ADLs (4). Conservatively, PPS affects up to one-half million polio survivors, 15–40 years after the original diagnosis, with a peak incidence at 30–34 years.

Two subtypes of PPS are recognized: postpolio progressive muscular atrophy (PPMA) and musculoskeletal postpoliomyelitis symptoms (MPPS). PPMA is equated to neurologic symptoms (i.e., loss of residual motor units) and, therefore, is regarded as PPS. MPPS, on the other hand, is secondary to "wear and tear" on joints and not caused by adverse neurologic changes, and its inclusion may be why PPS has a varyingly large incidence.

Postpolio syndrome is more prevalent and more intense in the muscles of the legs (5). It is also prevelant in the back and arms, but to a lesser degree than the legs (6). The increased stress on progressively weakening and wasting muscles heightens joint instability. PPS is hastened when original paralysis affected all four limbs, a ventilator was required, hospitalization was necessary during acute stages, or the polio virus was contracted after the age of 10 (7).

In addition to physical fatigue and weakness, difficulty in concentration, memory, and attention span have been reported (4). The brain fatigue generator (BFG) model has been used to explain the cognitive and motor activity problems. The BFG model suggests that viral damage to the reticular formation, hypothalamus, thalamic nuclei, and dopaminergic neurons diminishes cortical activity, thereby reducing information processing as well as inhibiting motor processing. Lower levels of dopamine have been found in individuals with PPS, suggesting that depleted dopamine can contribute to cognitive and motor activity problems in PPS. Credibility for this finding was gained when fatigue, attention span, and memory were improved in PPS patients when treated with dopamine receptor agonist medication.

GUILLAIN-BARRÉ SYNDROME

Guillain-Barré syndrome (GBS) is an autoimmune-mediated process that can result in a self-limiting period (8–16 months) of motor, sensory, or autonomic dysfunction. GBS is usually described as an acute inflammatory demyelinating polyneuropathy characterized by progressive symmetric ascending muscle weakness, paralysis, and hyporeflexia, with or without sensory or autonomic symptoms (8). Peripheral nerves and spinal roots are the major sites of demyelination, but cranial nerves also may be involved. GBS is believed to result from an autoimmune response, both humoral and cell mediated, to antecedent infections (bacterial, viral) or immune challenges (rabies, flu, tetanous vaccinations). The identification of various antiganglioside antibodies that crossreact with the ganglioside surface molecules on the myelin sheath of peripheral nerves suggest that molecular mimicry may serve as a possible mechanism for the disease. Recovery is usually associated with remyelination.

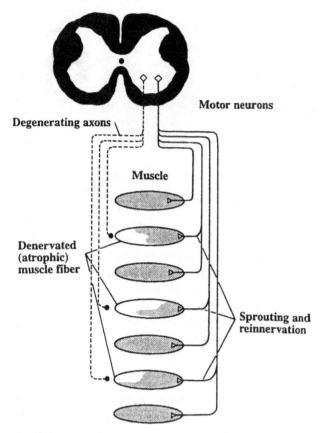

FIGURE 6.1. Denervation and reinnervation of muscle fibers.

Several pathologic and etiologic subtypes exist:

- Acute inflammatory demyelinating polyneuropathy (AIDP)
- Acute motor axonal neuropathy (AMAN)
- Miller-Fisher syndrome (MFS)
- Acute panautonomic neuropathy

Acute inflammatory demyelinating polyneuropathy subtype of GBS is the most common form in the United States. It is generally preceded by an antecedent bacterial (40% of patients are seropositive for *Campylobacter jejuni*) or viral infection (e.g., acute cytomegalovirus mononucleosis syndrome, herpes simplex). Sensory symptoms often precede motor weakness. About 20% of patients develop respiratory failure. The hallmark of classic AIDP is progressive weakness that usually begins in the feet before involving all four limbs. At presentation, 60% of patients have weakness in all four limbs. Weakness plateaus at 2 weeks after onset in 50% of patients and by 4 weeks in more than 90%. Improvement in strength usually begins 1–4 weeks after the plateau. Mortality rate ranges from 2%–6% with death usually caused by complications of ventilation. More than 75% of patients have complete or near-complete recovery with no deficit or only mild residual fatigue and distal weakness. Almost all patients with GBS who required ventilation

report severe dysesthesias (unpleasant, abnormal sensations) or moderately severe distal weakness as residual symptoms and about 15% of these patients end up with significant neurological residuals. Treatment for AIDP, as well as the other subtypes, includes intravenous immunoglobulin or plasma exchange treatment.

Whereas most forms of GBS are AIDP in western countries, an axonal form of GBS, termed acute motor axonal neuropathy (AMAN), has been recognized in northern China and in other Asian countries. It is suggested that AMAN is associated with pure motor axonal involvement.

Miller Fisher syndrome (MFS) is a variant of Guillain-Barré syndrome characterized by the triad of ophthalmoplegia, ataxia and areflexia without significant motor or sensory deficit in the limbs. MFS usually results in complete recovery without specific treatment. Unlike GBS, MFS involves descending paralysis (i.e., paralysis that begins in the upper body and gradually spreads downward). Specifically, in MFS, paralysis starts in the head, affecting eye muscles and balance and slowly descends to the neck, arms, and so on. MFS does not generally have the life-threatening aspects of GBS, but can be very difficult to live through with double vision, nausea, and weakness.

Acute panautonomic neuropathy is among the rarest of all variants and involves both the sympathetic and parasympathetic nervous systems. Cardiovascular involvement is common, and dysrhythmias are a significant source of mortality in this form of the disease. Recovery is gradual and often incomplete. Cardiovascular signs may include tachycardia, bradycardia, wide fluctuations in blood pressure and postural hypotension.

CLINICAL EXERCISE PHYSIOLOGY

POSTPOLIO SYNDROME

Studies using a stationary bicycle protocol have reported that aerobic capacity ($\dot{V}O_{2peak}$) was significantly related to muscle strength in the lower extremities (LEs) for persons with "late effects" of polio (9) or "late sequelae" of PPS (10). This strongly suggests that poor exercise performance on the stationary bicycle was limited by weak muscle function and, therefore, low $\dot{V}O_{2peak}$ was secondary to poor leg strength. In addition, a similar but weaker relationship of leg muscle strength and maximal walking speed has been reported (9). Consequently, the American College of Sports Medicine (11) advocates the use of an ergometer that involves both upper and lower extremities (e.g., Schwinn Air-Dyne ergometer) when evaluating the aerobic capacity of persons with PPS rather than a stationary bicycle or treadmill protocol. For persons with PPS whose condition prevents the use of their legs, armcrank ergometry is recommended to evaluate exercise capacity (11).

Aerobic capacity for persons with PPS was found to be lower than their able-bodied peers or their peers with polio but without PPS (12). Significant increases in $\dot{V}O_{2peak}$ have been observed following exercise programs of stationary bicycling, walking, and arm cranking (6). These increases occurred in aerobic exercise training programs that ranged from 8 to 22 weeks. No adverse effects were reported from participation in these training programs. A recent study found that walking in daily life was more demanding than being tested under standarized conditions and heart rate was 11 bpm less at self-selected testing speed than compared with daily activities (5). Thus, those with PPS tend to have greater cardiovascular stress with everyday walking, do physically less than healthy adults and only somewhat more than those with congestive heart failure.

Concern exists that resistance training of the LEs for persons with PPS could result in loss of strength owing to overtaxed motor neurons. Studies that involved persons with PPS in resistance training regimens of the LEs for a period of 6–12 weeks, however, showed significant increases in LE strength and some participants became less asymptomatic (13–15). Neither muscle nor joint pain was increased, and evidence of weakness was not seen although exercise intensity was classified as "moderate to hard." Considering the results of these studies (13–15), it is recommended that when initiating LE resistance training programs for persons with unstable PPS, a conservative approach should be taken. That is, the person with PPS should begin at a low intensity and gradually (i.e., over 4–6 weeks) increase to a moderate intensity. It is not recommended that high-intensity LE resistance training be performed by persons with PPS (12).

Recent research has also identified impairments of upper extremities secondary to PPS (16,17). In a study by Allen et al. (16), 172 of 177 polio patients reported new generalized PPS symptoms and 16 (9%) and 52 (30%) of the 172 demonstrated reduced elbow fexor strength and function, respectively. Whether these impairments in upper extremity strenght can be improved was the focus of a study by Chan et al. (17). This study (17) introduced a moderate intensity isometric exercise program with PPS patients who demonstrated reduced hand strength. Outcomes were consistent with findings of LE studies in that hand strength was improved with no adverse affect to the remaining motor units. An important secondary finding of this study (17) was that the strength increases were primarily attributed to voluntary motor drive (central), suggesting that PPS may involve central motor drive as well as motor unit transmission defects (peripheral).

GUILLAIN-BARRÉ SYNDROME

Guillain-Barré syndrome is a significant cause of long-term disability for at least 1,000 persons per year in the United States. The age-specific incidence of GBS increased with age from 1.5/100,000 in persons <15 years of age to 8.6/100,000 in persons 70–79 years of age (18). Given the young age at which GBS can occur and the relatively long life expectancies following GBS, it is likely that from 25,000 to 50,000 persons in the United States are experiencing some residual effects of GBS. Approximately 40% of patients who are hospitalized with GBS will require inpatient rehabilitation. Issues that affect rehabilitation are dysautonomia (i.e., orthostatic hypotension, unstable blood pressure, abnormal heart rate, bowel and bladder dysfunction), deafferent pain syndrome (pain originating peripherally, not centrally), and multiple medical complications related to length of immobilization, which include deep venous thrombosis, joint contracture, hypercalcemia owing to bone demineralization, anemia, and decubitus ulcers.

Rehabilitation strategies are similar to those for other neuromuscular illnesses and diseases. (See ref. 19 for a summary of clinical treatment and inpatient rehabilitation therapy for GBS.) Patients with GBS can display such diverse findings as significant involvement with tetraparesis, or isolated weakness of the arm, leg, facial muscles, or oropharynx. Extreme care should be taken not to overfatigue the affected motor units during therapy. In fact, overworked muscle groups in patients with GBS have been clinically associated with paradoxical weakening.

Motor weakness in GBS has been associated with muscle shortening and resultant joint contractures and can be prevented with daily range-of-motion exercises. Depending on the degree of weakness, exercise can be passive, active-assistive, or active. Initial exercise should include a program of low-intensity strengthening that involves isometric, isotonic, isokinetic, manual-resistive, and progressive-resistive exercises carefully tailored to the severity of the condition. Orthotics should be incorporated to properly position the limbs during exercise and optimize residual function.

Proprioceptive losses (i.e., vibratory sensation and joint position) expressed by patients with GBS can cause ataxia (i.e, loss of ability to coordinate muscular movements) and incoordination. Repetitive exercises that involve whole body movements (i.e., picking up an object on a table and placing it onto a shelf) will help improve coordination.

Patients with GBS who enter inpatient rehabilitation are not usually threatened by cardiac arrhythmias; however, 19%–50% will have evidence of postural hypotension. Prevention of hypotensive episodes involves physical modalities, such as compression hose, abdominal binders, and proper hydration. Patients who experience long periods of immobilization will find progressive mobilization on a tilt table to be a useful therapeutic tool for treating orthostatic hypotension.

A patient with GBS is still in the recovery phase during inpatient rehabilitation. Changes in the patient's condition should be monitored by nerve conduction velocity and muscle strength testing.

PHARMACOLOGY

POSTPOLIO SYNDROME

Medications, such as nonsteroidal anti-inflammatory drugs (NSAIDs) and muscle relaxants, are prescribed for persons with PPS to reduce symptoms and do not usually restrict acute or chronic exercise performance. Medications prescribed for reduction of pain and fatigue include tricyclic antidepressants and serotonin blockers. These medications are not only used to reduce pain but to facilitate anxiety reduction, thus enhancing overall relaxation and restful sleep. Selective serotonin reuptake inhibitors (serotonin blockers) have little overall effect on exercise performance, but tricyclic antidepressants have been shown to increase heart rate and decrease blood pressure during rest and exercise. Tricyclic antidepressants can cause ECG abnormalities, resulting in either false-positive or false-negative exercise test results, T-wave changes, and dysrhythmias, particularly in persons with a cardiac history.

Medications such as prednisone, amantadine, pyridostigmine, and bromocriptine mesylate have also been used to diminish fatigue and weakness and enhance physical performance. Prednisone, a corticosteroid, has not significantly increased muscle strength in PPS, and amantadine has not significantly decreased muscle fatigue (20). Pyridostigmine, an anticholinesterase inhibitor that prolongs the effectiveness of acetycholine on neuromuscular signal tranmission, has been investigated and showed muscle fatigue was not significantly diminished in those with PPS (21,22). However, there may be a limited but beneficial effect on walking distance (22). That is, quadriceps strength, walking duration and maximum voluntary activation improved significantly after a dose of 60 mg of pyridostigmine, four times/day for 14 weeks. However the benefits were only found in normal-sized motor units with transmission defects (i.e., subjects who did not show "new weakness" symptoms). In those subjects (n = 23) who did display PPS symptoms (confirmed motor unit abnormalities/changes), pyridostigmine showed no benefit to physical performance. Bromocriptine mesylate, a postsynaptic dopamine receptor agonist, did not show effects on diminishing fatigue, but was found to enhance attention, cognition, and memory (5).

These four drugs (prednisone, amantadine, pyridostigmine, and bromocriptine mesylate) should not negatively affect exercise performance. However, chronic use of prednisone can weaken muscle tissue and cause deposition of fat in the muscle cells, and lead to edema.

GUILLAIN-BARRÉ SYNDROME

Topical analgesics and/or nonsteroidal anti-inflammatory drugs has not been shown to afford sufficient pain relief. During the critical phase (i.e., intensive care) of GBS, gabapentin (seizure medication) and carbamazepine (anticonvulsant and mood stabilizer) are used for acute treatment of pain and along with tramadol and mexiletine may assist in the long-term management of neuropathic pain. Side effects for gabapentin and carbamazepine include dizziness, drowsiness, and motor coordination impairment (23).

PHYSICAL EXAMINATION

POSTPOLIO SYNDROME

An initial physical exam should include medical history of the person with PPS and a description of both central and peripheral complaints and symptoms, particularly new and/or increased overall fatigue and specific muscle(s) weakness or pain. It is important to understand initial polio problems and to determine whether the new and/or increased fatigue, weakness, and pain are associated with areas of the body affected by the initial polio. Symptoms should be analyzed with reference to type, intensity, duration, and frequency of all physical activities (leisure or recreational), including occupational tasks. Daily body postures and positions should also be analyzed, with specific attention to spinal, pelvic, knee, and ankle areas, to determine any abnormal joint mechanics. Since atrophy will likely be presented as an end stage of new neuromuscular deterioration, girth measurements with a tape measure are suggested to determine the extent of tissue lose. Ideally, sequential or at least a baseline girth measurement of a limb can be used for comparison.

The amount of rehabilitation after the initial polio onset and whether assistive devices were used or are still being used for balance and ambulation is important information to more accurately determine the extent of muscle fatigue and weakness. Also, the length of the functional stability period (see Epidemiology and Pathophysiology section), the highest level of physical function achieved during the stability period, and any psychosocial exacerbating factors are important to note.

An extensive neuromuscular exam should begin with a structural/postural evaluation to determine any adverse structural relationships caused by increased fatigue and weakness. The exam should also evaluate muscle size to indicate atrophy in symptomatic areas and test for light touch, sharp/dull touch, vibration, and temperature. Sensory testing of the symptomatic regions will facilitate determination of possible peripheral nerve dysfunction. Reflex testing should also be included in order to differentiate the extent of lower motor neuron involvement, since decreased responses are indicative of increased flaccidity. However, a hyperactive reflex suggests muscle spasm associated with early poliomyelitis.

The motor portion of the exam should include observation of gait and balance testing, including both static and dynamic challenges. Rapid or alternate movement of symptomatic and asymptomatic limbs should be tested for coordination and timing with the evaluator looking for tremors and/or unsteady movements and visual signs. A goniometer is suggested to assess range of motion (ROM) for all symptomatic limbs and joints, including both active range of motion (AROM) and passive range of motion (PROM). Strength can be measured subjectively by manual muscle testing (MMT) to detect gross motor weakness (24). MMT is isometric exercise with the subject required to exert fully to generate sufficient opposing force and activation of muscle fibers to maintain no movement. Isometric exercise more recently has been more widely used for assessing muscle strength in PPS since differentiation of new, weak joint angles are more accurately determined (25). MMT has five grades corresponding from 0, with no contraction, to 5, which is normal strength. MMT should not be used to differentiate nonfunctional contractions, since this musculature has most likely lost a critical number of motor neurons and will not be involved in exercise programs. The MMT should include either several repetitions and/or single repetitions held for a longer period of time because single-effort maximal contraction will not typically show any strength loss, but repetitive contractions will show additional weakness. Consequently, MMT should involve at least 3, and up to 10, repetitions of near-maximal effort at midrange for the symptomatic musculature. Residual fatigue of the tested muscles should be checked within 30 minutes of the initial test and up to 48 hours posttest. This subjective question assessment provides clinical data relevant to the assessment of PPS for the symptomatic musculature. These physical portions of the exam for symptomatic areas should be performed after the less fatiguing portions of the overall exam to avoid possible confounding effects of exertion.

GUILLAIN-BARRÉ SYNDROME

During inpatient rehabilitation, GBS patients can have a relapse of the disease (~10%), so close supervision during inpatient rehabilitation is warranted. Detailed daily physical exams should occur involving motor (i.e., strength), sensory, and autonomic tests to identify relapses and/or complications.

MEDICAL AND SURGICAL TREATMENTS

POSTPOLIO SYNDROME

Medications, as described under Pharmacology. have not been shown to significantly reduce fatigue or weakness associated with PPS; therefore, management of PPS is based largely on treating symptoms. Soft tissue, joint pain, and fatigue have been treated with various local medications and systemic medications such as selective serotonin reuptake inhibitors and tricyclic antidepressants. Success of these medications to modify pain and fatigue has varied.

Intravenous immunoglobulin (IvIg) has recently been studied as a method to reduce inflammation in the spinal cord, in a pilot study of 20 people with PPS (26). Tumor necrosis factor-α (TNF-α) was increased in the cerebral spinal fluid of the subjects with PPS. TNF-α is a potent pro-inflammatory cytokine. The level of TNF-α is influenced by the inflammation. TNF-α was significantly reduced as was pain after the 3 months of treatment, but whether IvIg was directly responsible for the TNF-α reduction was difficult to ascertain due to differing baseline values. Two other key outcomes, muscle strength and fatigue, were not changed. It could be argued that since muscle strength didn't further diminish during the study that there was a therapeutic effect from the IvIg especially on weight-bearing musculature. But, these results although provocative, can't be termed conclusive secondary to the small number of subjects in this pilot study.

Orthotic devices have been successfully used to decrease abnormal, excessive force and motion on LE joints. Certain neuromuscular and orthopedic deficiencies, such as dorsiflexor muscle weakness (i.e., dropfoot), genu valgum (i.e., knock-knee), and genu recurvatum (i.e., hyper-extended knee) impose movements that overstress both noncontractile and contractile tissue. For example, ankle-foot orthoses (AFOs) have been fitted to reduce drop-foot and avoid loss of balance and inefficient walking. Gait can be improved with simple heel lifts or shoe inserts, which decrease the amount of dorsiflexion. Knee orthoses, knee-ankle-foot orthoses (KAFOs), and bracing can facilitate balanced compressive forces on the tibia while walking with genu valgum and recurvatum conditions. Abnormal chronic forces on the knee secondary to chronic drop-foot can result in overstretched connective tissue and cartilage shearing. These abnormal changes result in decreased mobility and increased joint-related pain. A KAFO can also spare the other leg from becoming prematurely fatigued and overworked. Orthosis should be made of carbon fiber which are lightweight. The lightweight carbon fiber orthoses should increase walking ability (27). There are also lightweight nylon knee braces can be a benefit and less conspicuous. Orthotic devices use and compliance for persons with PPS need a strong rationale due to early unpleasant memories associated with braces during the acute polio stage.

GUILLAIN-BARRÉ SYNDROME

In terms of the progression of GBS, only plasma exchange therapy (i.e., plasmapheresis) and intravenous immune serum globulin (IVIG) has proven effective. Oral corticosteroids (e.g., methylprednisolone) alone do not produce significant benefit or harm (23). Side effects caused by plasma exchange therapy include vagus nerve syndrome (low or high blood pressure) and impaired hemostasis (i.e., hypocoaguable state). With IVIG, incidence of generalized reactions occur during and/or immediately after (30–60 minutes) administration are mild and self limiting and include: 1) pyrogenic reaction; 2) minor systemic reactions such as headache, myalgia, chills, nausea and/or vomiting; and 3) vasomotor and cardiovascular manifestations are marked by changes in blood pressure and tachycardia.

DIAGNOSTIC TECHNIQUES

POSTPOLIO SYNDROME

PPS is diagnosed by exclusion of multiple sclerosis, amyotrophic lateral sclerosis, myasthenia gravis, chronic infection, hypothyroidism, collagen disorders, neuropathies, and depression. Exclusion or differential diagnosis of painful conditions such as bursitis, tendinitis, myalgias, osteoarthritis, and poliomyositis must also be made because many of these conditions can occur at the same age as late symptoms of polio. Therefore, aging and its effects on the body must also be ruled out when diagnosing PPS. Significant muscle atrophy is a discerning factor since it is not common in aging and is most suggestive of PPS (1).

There are no laboratory procedures that significantly identify PPS, but procedures can rule out other medical conditions. Viral assays can identify the continuance of the polio virus and have been positive in more than 50% of individuals with PPS, but whether the long-term existence of the virus is linked to a progressive onset of PPS is not clear (28). Further evidence has suggested that if the virus remains active, it may not affect the cerebral cortex, and this suggests that fatigue is not of central origin (29).

Electromyography (EMG) and nerve conduction velocity (NVC) assessments have been used to rule out neuropathies and myasthenia gravis and to identify different phases of PPS. EMGs can identify late changes, such as fasciculations, fibrillations, and increased motor unit amplitude and duration (Fig. 6.2) (1). Although nonspecific, these motor unit alterations indicate overall damage to the motor unit. EMG has differentiated new and more severe pathology in PPS and subsequent compensation of the motor unit (30). Even surface EMG has shown good correlation with invasive EMG in identifying enlarged, overburdened motor units (23). While EMG may differentiate new motor unit pathology, it appears to be a poor predictor of muscle strength loss and impaired muscle endurance (31).

Maximal voluntary activation, another type of EMG being used more recently, has been assessed by the twitch interpolation technique, which is to have the limb (often the arm) attached to a myograph at the wrist, and performing three maximal isometric voluntary contractions of 2–3 secs. duration (32). During each maximal effort, a supramaximal electrical stimulus is delivered through surface electrodes over the muscle which is the primary mover of the joint, such as the biceps brachii of the elbow, and the distal tendon. Increments of torque evoked by the stimuli are measured by an amplifier and computerized software.

Biochemical markers showing muscle function decline have gained some attention in diagnosing PPS. Levels of somatomedin C (IGF-1) and serum creatine kinase have been utilized to determine muscle force and muscle strength and endurance, respectively (33) Although decreased levels of IGF-1 may be consistent with a central deficit which could reduce muscle force in PPS, two studies have found no correlation between muscle force and IGF-1 (33). Creative kinase was related to declining elbow flexor muscle endurance after 45 minutes of submaximal exercise, and positively correlated with elbow flexor strength (33). Yet neither IGF-1 or creatine kinase markers were related to current symptoms, which were negative. Increase use of IGF-1 and serum creatine kinase with greater numbers of people with PPS, appears warranted before either marker can be used as an adjunct in the workup of diagnosing PPS.

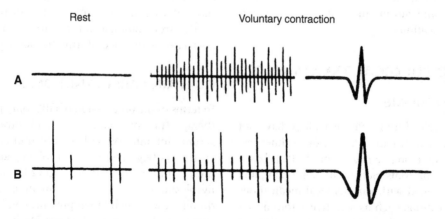

FIGURE 6.2. EMG responses of: A, normal muscle fiber; B, motor neuron disease (PPS) muscle fiber with chronic denervation.

Subjective complaints of pain, particularly in the hip, are the best correlation to new muscle fatigue and dysfunction (34). Since the hip and pelvis are major weight-supporting structures, it follows that pain in this region could present greater estimation of dysfunction than any other area. Diagnostic techniques such as an EMG can be helpful in diagnosis of PPS, but diagnosis is dependent, at least partially, on a good patient interview.

GUILLAIN-BARRÉ SYNDROME

Typical clinical findings such as rapidly evolving flaccid paralysis, areflexia, absence of fever, and a likely inciting event (e.g., bacterial or viral infection, vaccination) are usually followed up by the following laboratory studies. The following laboratory studies are useful in ruling out other diagnoses and to better assess functional status and prognosis. However, because of the acute nature of the disease, they may not become abnormal until 1–2 weeks after onset of weakness.

Typical findings for lumbar puncture and cerebral spinal fluid (CSF) analysis include an elevated protein level (>400 mg/dl) without accompanying pleocytosis (increased cell count). An elevation in CSR cell count may indicate an alternative diagnosis such as infection.

Electromyography (EMG) and nerve conduction study (NCS) may show prolonged distal latencies, conduction slowing, conduction block, and temporal dispersion of compound action potential in demyelinating cases. In primary axonal damage, the findings included reduced amplitude of the action potential without conduction slowing. Rarely EMG and NCS are normal in patients with GBS. This is thought to be due to the location of demyelinating lesions in proximal sites not easily accessible.

Forced vital capacity (FVC), measured by spirometry, is useful in guiding therapy. Patients with an FVC less than 15–20 mL/kg, maximum inspiratory pressure less than 30 cm H_2O, or a maximum expiratory pressure less than 40 cm H_2O generally progress to require prophylactic intubation and mechanical ventilation (35).

EXERCISE/FITNESS/ FUNCTIONAL TESTING

The basic principles for exercise testing stated in *ACSM's Guidelines for Exercise Testing and Prescription* (36) provide the foundation for this section and the next section, "Exercise Prescription and Programming." When not otherwise stated, these basic principles will apply. In addition, the basic principles for exercise testing and exercise management outlined for polio and postpolio syndrome in *ACSM's Exercise Management for Persons with Chronic Diseases and Disabilities* (11) also provide a foundation for this section and the next section. Special situa-

tions created by PPS and GBS will be addressed in these sections.

POSTPOLIO SYNDROME

Evaluation of aerobic capacity for persons with PPS should be performed with an ergometer that involves both upper and lower extremities (e.g., Schwinn Air-Dyne ergometer) (11). A discontinuous protocol should be performed, with initial workloads of 10–25 W and incremental increases of 10–25 W every 2 minutes. Rest periods of 2–4 minutes are recommended between each stage. Persons with PPS whose condition prevents the use of their legs should use an arm-crank ergometer, with an initial workload of 5–10 W, incremental increases of 5–10 W every 2 minutes, and rest periods of 2–4 minutes between each stage. Validity and reliability of a functional ability assessment of PPS, using an effort-limited treadmill walk test, has recently been established (37). Subjects walked at their determined speed, on a treadmill, for as long as it took until an rate of perceived exertion (RPE) of "15" or "hard" or pain level of 7/10, was expressed. The distance achieved was a reproducible measure over the 3 trials on the treadmill and was significantly associated with the timed "get up and go" test. There was also a good correlation between distance walked on the treadmill and pain with activities of daily living (ADL's). That is, the greater the pain the less the distance walked and ADL's performed.

The guidelines established for GBS (see below) are applicable to persons with PPS for muscle strength, endurance, and range-of-motion evaluations. Additionally, and as mentioned earlier, isometric exercise whether for evaluation or training has gained popularity (17). Isometric exercise while taking longer to perform has advantages in that it facilitates greater control of intensity, duration, rest periods and angle of work. These advantages reduce the likelihood of overtraining, possibly sparing some over extended neuromuscular units, but still facilitating training effects for the remainder of the muscle groups.

Muscle strength measurements are used to assess muscle dysfunction, but muscle strength has not been shown to have a good correlation with functional performance (i.e., ADL tasks) (19,27–29). Consequently, recommendations for evaluating functional performance of such ADL activities as walking, rising from a chair, and rising from supine to standing include: (1) walking capacity—timing a distance of 300 feet with at least three changes in direction and two different grades; (2) stepping capacity—timing the ascent and descent on a flight of 10 steps, twice, using conventional 7–8 inch household steps; and (3) orthostatic capacity—timing 10 repetitions of sit-to-stand from a conventional chair (i.e., 52 cm in height).

These functional tests can be difficult for persons with PPS who have MMT scores of less than 3/5 for knee extension and/or hip abduction for one leg, and extremely difficult for individuals with MMT scores of less than 3/5 for both legs. When persons with PPS are using orthosis or assistive devices, these devices should be worn during functional evaluation.

GUILLAIN-BARRÉ SYNDROME

It is important to recognize two distinct phases of rehabilitation for persons with GBS. Testing procedures for inpatient rehabilitation are covered in the sections on clinical exercise physiology and diagnostic techniques. This section and the next section, "Exercise Prescription and Programming," address the "outpatient" phase of rehabilitation and recovery. The outpatient phase is when the patient has been released from a rehabilitation center and is no longer under direct medical care.

The study by Pitetti and colleagues (38) reported methodologies for cardiovascular and strength testing of a GBS patient. Pitetti et al. (38) evaluated the cardiovascular fitness and muscle strength of a 58-year-old male GBS patient, 3.5 years after being released from the hospital. At the time of his discharge from the hospital, this patient had severe muscle atrophy and was unable to ambulate without crutches and ankle orthoses. He also had significant weakness, bilateral foot drop, and some sensory loss in the hands. Three and one-half years later, at the time of exercise evaluation, this patient was able to ambulate with the assistance of one crutch and experienced minimal weakness in the hands and feet.

This patient's peak exercise capacity was evaluated using three different modes of exercise: a Schwinn Air-Dyne ergometer (SAE), an electrically braked bicycle ergometer (BE), and an arm-crank ergometer (ACE). The testing protocol for the SAE and BE was similar, with each exercise starting at an initial workload of 25 W for 2 minutes and increasing workload 25 W every 2 minutes until volitional exhaustion. The protocol for the ACE started the participant with arm cranking at 10 W (50 rpm) for 2 minutes, increasing workload by 10 W every 2 minutes until volitional exhaustion. The peak physiological parameters measured were peak oxygen consumption ($V \cdot O_{2peak}$, mL $\cdot$ min^{-1} and mL $\cdot$ kg^{-1} $\cdot$ min^{-1}), heart rate (HR, bpm), ventilation ($V \cdot_E$, l $\cdot$ min^{-1}), and respiratory exchange ratio (RER, $V \cdot CO_2/V \cdot O_2$). Peak work capacity (in watts) and length of test time were also measured on the BE. The highest peak physiological parameters were seen using the SAE followed by the BE. The highest work level reached (175 W) was also achieved on the SAE followed by the BE (100 W). Arm-crank ergometry produced the lowest work level (75 W) of all parameters measured. Blood pressure responses (taken 2 min before, 2 min after exercise, and the last minute of each work level) throughout all three tests were normal.

Knee extension and flexion were evaluated using the Cybex 340 dynamometer. It was the opinion of these authors (30) that, given the physical capacities of this GBS participant, he was capable of performing most any test of flexibility, muscle strength and endurance, or cardiovascular fitness that could be performed by able-bodied individuals, with the exception of a treadmill protocol.

Upper body measurement techniques used to assess range of motion, as well as upper body strength and endurance test protocols used to evaluate able-bodied individuals, should be applicable to most GBS patients. Variations for lower-extremity testing protocols depend on the residual weakness of the lower limbs. Knee flexion and extension and hip measurements (e.g., flexion, extension, adduction, abduction) used to evaluate able-bodied individuals are applicable to GBS patients. As with upper body measurements, GBS patients should be sitting (as with knee or hip flexion and extension measurements) or prone (as in leg press) in order to maintain balance. Standing test measurements, like a squat, should be performed with caution and in the presence of an assistant.

EXERCISE PRESCRIPTION AND PROGRAMMING

POSTPOLIO SYNDROME

Five classifications of PPS have been developed to facilitate safer and more effective exercise programs (39). If a person is not correctly classified, the exercise program could injure unstable motor units.

Classification I (no clinical polio) is the highest functional and least symptomatic. Individuals with this classification have no history of recent muscle weakness. Their physical exam shows good to normal strength, sensation, and reflexes and no muscle atrophy. EMG and NCV results are normal. Persons in Classification I should be able to exercise aerobically at intensities of 50%–70% heart rate reserve (HRR), rating of perceived exertion (RPE) of 12–14 (on the 6–20 scale), or MET levels in the 6–9 range; durations of up to 30 minutes; with frequencies of 3–5 days/week. It is recommended that the mode of exercise involve both upper and lower body musculature (i.e., Schwinn Air-Dyne, swimming).

Classification II (subclinical polio) shows no new weakness but a history of weakness with full recovery. EMG and NCV testing should exhibit chronic denervation or large polyphasic motor unit action potentials but no acute denervation. Exercise for this classification includes similar MHRR and RPE intensities as Classification I, but MET levels should be in the 5–8 range. However, exercise duration should include intervals of 5 minutes, with a "rest" period of 1 minute between intervals. Exercise days should alternate with 1 day of rest, and the suggested exercise mode is the same as Classification I.

Classification III (clinically stable polio) shows a history of weakness with variable recovery and no new weakness. Physical exam results include poor to good strength, normal sensation, normal to decreased reflexes, and possible muscle atrophy. EMG and NCV results indicate chronic denervation. Exercise intensity should include an MHRR of 40%–60%, RPE of 11–13, with MET levels in the 4–5 range. Duration should be up to 20 minutes total, with intervals of no more than 3 minutes and recovery time of 1 minute. Frequency and modalities are similar to Classification II.

Classification IV (clinically unstable polio) shows a history of weakness with variable recovery and a recent history of new weakness. The physical exam and EMG/NCV results are similar to Classification III. Exercise activities should include durations of 2–3 minutes followed by a 1–2 minute recovery for a total exercise time of 15 minutes, 3 times per week. Intensity level should be HRR of 40%–50%, RPE of 11–12, and MET levels at 3. Nonfatiguing resistance exercise can be supplemented.

Classification V (severely atrophic polio) is the lowest functional and most symptomatic, with new weakness and little recovery from the acute stage. The physical exam results show poor muscle strength, normal sensation, areflexic and severe limb atrophy. EMG and NCV tests show decreased insertional activity with few to no motor unit action potentials and acute denervation. Exercise is generally contraindicated. ADL should be the extent of exercise programming. Orthotic and bracing devices are indicated, and often a wheelchair is required for mobility.

Significant increases have been shown in muscle strength of elbow and knee extensors in persons with PPS using concentric contraction training, 3 nonconsecutive times/week, with 3 sets of 20, 15, and 10 repetitions (14). Resistance intensity was 75% of 3-RM with 90 seconds' recovery between sets and 3 minutes' rest between exercises. Another study (13) reported strength gains using isotonic training that consisted of 3 sets, 12 repetitions each, twice a week on nonconsecutive days. Initial weight or resistance was at a differentiated RPE of 13–14.

Recent studies have focused on the effects of climate and water on training efficacy. Warm climate has been shown to decrease pain, health related problems and depression (40). However, differences in walking were not reported between the warm and colder climate groups (40). Warm water exercises were found to reduce pain and improve cardiovascular conditioning (41). It should be noted that both studies (40,41) used exercise regimens of moderate intensity and duration.

GUILLAIN-BARRÉ SYNDROME

The course of illness can be more prolonged in adults, particularly older adults, than in children. Improvement can continue for up to 2 years after onset, with rate and variability of neurological recovery related to age, requirement for respiratory support, and rate of progression. The course of illness can also result in chronic-relapsing GBS.

Questions regarding the usefulness of exercise to help maintain health for patients with GBS remains unanswered because of the dearth of research regarding the effects of exercise on GBS. The "Medical News" section of the *Journal of the American Medical Association* (42) reported a paper written by Dr. Bensman, who at that time was an assistant professor at the University of Minnesota Medical School. The paper discussed the clinical course of eight GBS patients who were adversely affected by "excessive physical activity" that was part of their inpatient rehabilitation. The phrase "excessive physical activity" was never defined. Three of the eight patients were placed on a nonfatiguing program including passive range-of-motion exercises, which quickly resulted in an increase in muscle strength and no more periods of functional loss. Another three of the eight patients had already been discharged, but loss of function due to weakness and/or paresis reappeared after "exercising too strenuously." These three GBS patients improved after bedrest and limitation of activity, but relapses continued "to be associated with fatigue." The two remaining patients returned to the hospital because of a recurrence of GBS 1 year after the onset of symptoms.

Steinberg (43) noted that excessive exercise, especially fatiguing activity, often causes abnormal sensations for various periods of time. Steinberg (43) suggested that GBS patients be allowed to engage in physical activity up to the point where muscle ache/fatigue begins. Fatigue declined after their activity was "carefully controlled."

The GBS participant in the study by Pitetti et al. (38) performed 40 exercise sessions during a 16-week period on an SAE following initial cardiovascular and strength testing. The GBS participant exercised for 20–30 minutes per session at 70% of peak heart rate as determined by a pretraining exercise test on the SAE. The GBS participant increased cardiopulmonary capacities, peak work level, total work capacity, and isokinetic leg strength following this supervised exercise regimen without any GBS-related complications.

Karper (44) reported the effects of a low-intensity aerobic exercise regimen on a female (18 yr) with chronic-relapsing GBS. The exercise regimen consisted of a 10-week walking phase followed by a 15-week cycling phase. The GBS patient exercised 3 days a week for 20 to 37 minutes as a walking phase and 15 to 32 minutes as a cycling phase. The GBS patient was not allowed to exercise over 45 percent of her HRR (220 – age) reserve. During cycling, the participant stopped every 5 minutes and rested for 2 minutes. No rest periods were reported for the walking phase. Following both exercise phases, the GBS patient improved in walking distance, speed of walking, and riding time (cycle ergometer) without any GBS relapse or side effects.

Given the above reports, a very conservative approach should be taken for both inpatient and outpatient rehabilitation. Once the disease begins to stabilize, inpatient rehabilitation should begin using short periods of nonfatiguing activities (i.e., passive range of motion and active range of motion). As the patient improves (noted by increase in muscle strength and nerve conduction), light muscle strengthening exercises should be initiated. As the patient continues to improve, more exercises and activities for physical therapy and occupational therapy, as well as training for ADL can be added to the overall rehabilitation plan. During the first 3 to 6 months after onset of the disease, the medical staff should be vigilant to signs of fatigue in their patients, and it is important for the patient to know his/her own limitations and be able to exercise without causing fatigue.

No exercise regimens involving flexibility and muscle strength and endurance exercises, have been reported for GBS patients. However, the GBS patient in the study by Pitetti et al. (38) showed increases in leg strength and the patients in the study by Karper (44) showed improved grip strength following their aerobic exercise regimen. This suggests that an exercise program involving not only aerobic exercise but also resistance training would be beneficial for GBS patients.

In addition to cardiopulmonary improvement, work and strength improvements were seen in the GBS patient in the study by Pitetti et al. (38). The patient also reported subjective improvements in activities of daily living. Housework and yardwork activities had been expanded following the exercise regimen. For instance, the GBS patient was able to mow his yard (self-propelled mower) without rest periods and returned to gardening because weeding, digging up roots, and rototilling were feasible again. He also reported being able to walk up stairs without the use of railings plus an overall reduction in daily fatigue. That is, following the exercise regimen, he seldom took naps, whereas before training, they were daily necessities.

Undoubtedly, a significant number of patients discharged from inpatient rehabilitation who return to their homes could benefit from outpatient rehabilitative services or individualized exercise programs at community health clubs who have someone who is, at the least, certified as a Health Fitness Instructor by the American College of Sports Medicine. A certified Exercise Specialist or Registered Clinical Exercise Physiologist would be preferred for working with these clinical populations.

EDUCATION AND COUNSELING

POSTPOLIO SYNDROME

Persons with PPS experiencing new and/or increased weakness could employ several strategies to slow further debilitating decline. First, education about ADL and physical activities is important to minimize effects of fatigue, including the pace used in task completion. Depending upon new weakness and fatigue, physical work simplification skills and frequent rest periods should be learned and practiced (45). Second, the use of orthoses can reduce stress and possibly decrease pain and fatigue. Accepting the need for orthoses or accepting the need for assistive devices such as wheelchairs or scooters may require counseling. Assistive devices are particularly helpful when long periods of standing or walking are necessary and when recovery from fatigue has been slow.

If breathing becomes more difficult, especially with exertion, respiratory muscle training is recommended (46). These exercises of the upper trunk musculature should facilitate greater chest expansion, tidal volume and exhalations. Also, if pulmonary problems become prevalent, pursed lip and diaphragmatic breathing techniques should be practiced. These techniques will assist more oxygen delivery to the lungs and greater carbon dioxide expiration.

A person with PPS can have many adverse problems that surface after many years of status quo. Abrupt changes affecting ADL mobility and independence usually result in increased stress. Consequently, individuals with PPS can be candidates for anxiety and depression. Counseling may be needed along with adequate family support to overcome the changes brought on by PPS.

GUILLAIN-BARRÉ SYNDROME

Psychological variables such as symptoms of mild depression occurring after initial disease onset are common. Research is needed to determine the severity of psychological and social issues with severely involved GBS patients (i.e., months to years of ventilatory dependence with chronic-relapsing GBS).

Additionally, the extent and duration of the physically disabling sequelae in GBS has not been adequately described. That is, with regard to motor function and the loss of the active number of motor units with aging, poliomyelitis and GBS have similar clinical issues.

Of note to this issue, a study by Burrows (47) reported on the residual subclinical impact of GBS in four military personnel (3 males and 1 female; ages 19, 21, 58, and 27 years, respectively) who were medically pronounced "totally recovered" from the syndrome. Prior to the onset of GBS, all four individuals exceeded requirements to pass the Army Physical Fitness Test (APFT). The APFT includes performing 15 push-ups and 40 sit-ups in 2 minutes and completing a 2-mile run in 21 minutes. All four soldiers were unable to pass the APFT 1 to 3 years following onset of GBS.

Other studies have reported residual long-term disabilities. Melillo and colleagues (48) studied the course of 37 patients following discharge and reported that 13 developed long-term disability. Bernsen et al. (49) reported that 3 to 6 years after onset of Guillain-Barré syndrome, 63% of 122 patients showed one or more changes in their lifestyle, work, or leisure activities due to loss of muscle strength and poor coordination. And Soryal and colleagues (50) reported that residual skeletal problems and complications (i.e., marked joint stiffness and contractures) in GBS patients became major components of disability despite having physiotherapy from the onset and improving neurological status.

Similar residual disabilities were also noted in children and adolescents, which indicates special consideration is needed for children and adolescents recovering from GBS. A report by Berman and Tom (51) indicated that significant and permanent motor loss in extremities was still present 1.5 years following discharge. The authors (51) noted that the late permanent motor paralysis and residual joint deformities secondary to GBS occur in children and adolescents at a higher incidence and severity than in adults. This would suggest that an intensive inpatient and outpatient rehabilitation program is imperative for children and adolescents, including frequent and extended follow-up strength and motor evaluations.

REFERENCES

1. Thornsteinsson G. Management of postpolio syndrome. *Mayo Clin Pros* 1997;72:627–628.
2. Dalakas MC, Hallett M. The Post-Polio Syndrome: In: Plum F, ed. *Advances in contemporary neurology*. Philadelphia: F.A. Davis, 1988; 15–95.
3. Widar M, Ahlstrom G. Pain in persons with post-polio. *Scand J Caring Sci* 1999;13:33–40.
4. Bruno RL, Crenge SJ, Frick NM. Parallels between post-polio fatigue and chronic fatigue syndrome: a common pathophysiology? *Am J Med* 1998;105:665–738.
5. Horemans HL, Johannes BJ, Beelen A, Stam HJ, Nollet F. Walking in postpoliomyelitis syndrome: The relationships between time-scored tests, walking in daily life and perceived mobility problems. *J Rehabil Med* 2005;37:142–146.
6. Aurlien D, Strandjord RE, Hegland O. Postpolio syndrome—a critical comment to the diagnosis. *Acta Neurol Scand* 1999;100:76–80.
7. Birk TJ. Poliomyelitis and the post-polio syndrome: exercise capacities and adaptation-current research, future directions, and widespread applicability. *Med Sci Sports Exerc* 1993;25:466–472.
8. Miller A, Ali OE, Sinert R. Gullian-Barré syndrome. http://www.emedicine.com/EMERG/topic222.htm
9. Willen C, Cider A, Summerhagen KS. Physical performance in individuals with late effects of polio. *Scand J Rehabil Med* 1999;31: 244–249.
10. Stanghelle JK, Festvag L, Aksnes A. Pulmonary function and symptom-limited exercise stress testing in subjects with late sequelae of postpoliomyelitis. *Scand J Rehab Med* 1993;25:125–129.
11. Birk TJ. Polio and post-polio syndrome. In: *ACSM's exercise management for persons with chronic diseases and disabilities*. Champaign, IL: Human Kinetics, 1997.
12. Stanghellod JK, Festvag LV. Postpolio syndrome: a 5 year follow-up. *Spinal Cord* 1997;35:503–508.
13. Agre JC, Rodriquez AA, Franke TM. Strength, endurance, and work capacity after muscle strengthening exercise in postpolio subjects. *Arch Phys Med Rehabil* 1997;78:681–687.
14. Spector SA, Gordon PL, Feuerstein IM, et al. Strength gains without muscle injury after strength training in patients with postpolio muscular atrophy. *Muscle & Nerve* 1996;19:1282–1290.
15. Einarsson G, Grindy G. Strengthening exercise program in postpolio subjects. In: Halstead LS, Wiechers DO, eds. *Research and clinical aspects of late effects of poliomyelitis*. White Plains, NY: March of Dimes Birth Defects Foundation, 1987.
16. Allen GM, Middleton J, Katrak PH, Lord SR, Gandevia SC. Prediction of voluntary activation, strength and endurance of elbow flexors in postpolio patients. *Muscle & Nerve* 2004;30:172–181.
17. Chan KM, Amirjani N, Sumrain M, Clarke A, Strohschein FJ. Randomized controlled trial of strength training in post-polio patients. *Muscle & Nerve* 2003;27:332–338.
18. Prevots DR, Sutter RW. Assessment of Gullian-Barré syndrome mortality aned morbidity in the United Staes: implications for acute flaccid paralysis surveillance. *J Infect Dis* 1997;175:S151–S155.
19. Meythaler JM. Rehabilitation of Gullian-Barré syndrome. *Arch Phys Med Rehabil* 1997;78(8):872–879.
20. Dalakas MC, Bartfeld H, Kurland LT. The pospolio syndrome: advances in the pathogenesis and treatment. *Ann N Y Acad Sci* 1995; 753:1–411.
21. Trojan DA, Collet JP, Shapiro S, et al. A multicenter, randomized, double-blinded trial of pyridostigmine in postpolio syndrome. *Neurology* 1999;53:1225–1233.
22. Horemans HL, Nollet F, Beelen A, Drost G, et al. Pyridostigmine in postpolio syndrome: no decline in fatigue and limited functional performance. *J Neurol Neurosurg Psychiatry* 2003;74:1655–1661.
23. Shahar E: Current therapeutic options in severe Guillain-Barre syndrome. *Neuropharmacol* 2006;29:45–51
24. Nollet F, Beelen A, Prins MH. Disability and functional assessment in former polio patients with and without postpolio syndrome. *Arch Phys Med Rehabil* 1999;80:136–143.
25. Farbu E, Gilhus NE, Barnes MP, et al. EFNS guideline on diagnosis and management of post-polio syndrome. Report of an EFNS task force. *European J Neurol* 2006;13:795–801.
26. Farbu E, Rekand T, Vik-Mo E, Lygren H, Gilhus NE, Aarli JA. Postpolio syndrome patients treated with intravenous immunoglobin: a double-blinded randomized controlled pilot study. *European J Neurol* 2007;14:60–65.
27. Heim M, Yaacobi E, Azaria M. A pilot study to determine the efficiency of lightweight carbon fibre orthoses in the management of patients suffering from post-poliomyelitis syndrome. *Clin Rehab* 1997;11:302–305.
28. Julien J, Leparc-Goffart I, Lina B, et al. Postpolio syndrome: poliovirus persistence is involved in the pathogenesis. *J Neurol* 1999; 246:472–476.
29. Samii A, Lopez-Devine J, Wasserman EM, et al. Normal postexercise facilitation and depression of motor evoked potentials in postpolio patients. *Muscle Nerve* 1998;21:948–950.
30. Cywinska-Wasilewaska G, Ober JJ, Koczocik-Przedpelska J. Power spectrum of the surface EMG in post-polio syndrome. *Electromyogr Clin Neurophysiol* 1998;38:463–466.
31. Roeleveld K, Sandberg A, Stalberg EV, et al. Motor unit size estimation of enlarged motor units with surface electromygraphy. *Muscle Nerve* 1998;21:878–886.
32. Rodriquez AA, Agre JC, Franke TM. Electromyographic and neuromuscular variables in unstable postpolio subjects, stable postpolio subjects, and control subjects. *Arch Phys Med Rehabil* 1997;78: 986–991.
33. Sunnerhagen KS, Bengtsson BA, Lundberg PA, Landin K, Lindstedt G, Grimby G. Normal concentrations of serum insulin-like growth factor-1 in late polio. *Arch Phys Med Rehabil* 1995;76:732–735.
34. Nordgren B, Falck B, Stalberg E, et al. Postpolio muscular dysfunction: relationships between muscle energy metabolism, subjective symptoms, magnetic resonance imaging, electromyography, and muscle strength. *Muscle Nerve* 1997;20:1341–1351.
35. Hughes RA, Wijdicks EF, Benson E. Supportive care for patients with Guillain-Barré syndrome. *Arch Neurol* 2005;62:1194–1198.
36. American College of Sports Medicine. *ACSM's guidelines for exercise testing and prescription*, 7th ed. Baltimore: Lippincott Williams & Wilkins, 2007.
37. Finch LE, Ventruini A, Mayo NE, Trojan DA. Effort-limited treadmill walk test-reliability and validity in subjects with postpolio syndrome. *Am J Phys Med Rehabil* 2004;83:613–623.

38. Pitetti KH, Barrett PJ, Abbas D. Endurance exercise training in Guillain-Barré syndrome. *Arch Phys Med Rehabil* 1993;74:761–765.

39. Halstead L, Gawne AC. NRH proposal for limb classification and exercise prescription. *Disabil Rehabil* 1996;18:311–316.

40. Strumse YAS, Stanghelle JK, Utne L, Ahlvin P, Svendsby EK. Treatment of patients with postpolio syndrome in warm climate. *Disabil Rehabil* 2003;25:77–84.

41. Willen C, Scherman MH, Grimby G. Dynamic water exercise in individuals with late poliomyelitis. *Arch of Phys Med Rehabil* 2001;82:66–72.

42. Staff. Strenuous exercise may impair muscle function in Guillain-Barré patients. *JAMA* 1970;214:468–469.

43. Steinberg JS. *Guillain-Barrè syndrome (acute idiopathic polyneuritis): an overview for the lay person.* Wynnwood, PA: The Guillian-Barrè Syndrome Support Group International, 1987.

44. Karper WB. Effects of low-intensity aerobic exercise on one subject with Chronic Relapsing Guillian-Barrè syndrome. *Rehabil Nurs* 1991;16(2):96–98.

45. Packer TL, Martins I, Krefting L, Brouwer B. Activity and post-polio fatigue. *Orthopedics* 1991;14:1223–1226.

46. Klefbeck B, Lagerstrand L, Mattsson E. Inspiratory muscle training in patients with prior polio who use part-time assisted ventilation. *Arch Phys Med Rehabil* 2000;81:1065–1071.

47. Burrows DS. Residual subclinical impairment in patients who totally recovered from Guillain-Barrè syndrome: impact on military performance. *Mil Med* 1990;155:438–440.

48. Melillo EM, Sethi JM, Mohsenin V. Guillain-Barré syndrome: rehabilitation outcome and recent developments. *Yale J Biol Med* 1998;71(5):383–389.

49. Bernsen RA, de Jager AE, Schmitz PI, et al. Residual physical outcome and daily living 3 to 6 years after Guillain-Barrè syndrome. *Neurology* 1999;53(2):409–410.

50. Soryal I, Sinclair E, Hornby J, et al. Impaired joint mobility in Guillain-Barré syndrome: a primary or a secondary phenomenon? *J Neurol Neurosurg Psychiatry* 1992;22(11):1014–1017.

51. Berman AT, Tom L. The Guillain-Barrè syndrome in children. *Clin Ortho Related Resp* 1976;116:61–65.

Muscular Dystrophy and Other Myopathies

EPIDEMIOLOGY AND PATHOPHYSIOLOGY

Myopathies encompass a wide range of disorders that can be broadly considered as either congenital, inherited, or acquired. The congenital forms include the muscular dystrophies, congenital myopathies, channelopathies, and metabolic myopathies (Table 7.1). The acquired myopathies include endocrine myopathies, inflammatory myopathies, toxic myopathies (including drugs), and primary infectious myopathies (Table 7.2). The incidence and prevalence of muscle disorders varies widely, with myotonic dystrophy and Duchenne dystrophy (DMD) ocurring in about 1 of 3,500 live births (DMD only in men), whereas other disorders, such as MELAS 3271 (mitochondrial myopathy), is present in only about 40 people in the world (10,42).

Most of the genetically based myopathies are caused by mutations in structural or metabolism linked proteins. These can be categorized as autosomal dominant (AD), autosomal recessive (AR), X-linked recessive (XR), maternally inherited (MI, mitochondrial disorders), or sporadic spontaneous mutations. In general, the dystrophies often result from abnormalities in the cytoskeleton (e.g., dystrophin in DMD), whereas the metabolic myopathies are caused by mutations in the energy transduction enzymes (e.g., carnitine palmitoyl transferase deficiency [CPT-2]). Some exceptions to this general rule exist, such as calpain-3 deficiency (a proteolytic enzyme) seen in a form of AR limb girdle dystrophy. The inheritance pattern and gene product of many of the inherited myopathies are presented in Table 7.3.

The acquired myopathies encountered in North America are usually inflammatory, endocrine, or toxic. Acute viral myopathies, which are frequently encountered with a wide spectrum of severity, are most commonly caused by influenza or coxsackie viruses. The most common toxic myopathies are those caused by lipid-lowering agents, primarily the statins (hydroxymethylglutaryl-coenzyme A [HMG-CoA]-reductase inhibitors) (36). Fungal and bacterial myopathies rarely occur in first-world countries, but should be considered in recent immigrants or those with travel histories to developing countries (Table 7.2).

SYMPTOMS AND FUNCTIONAL CONSEQUENCES

Progressive muscle weakness is the most common symptom of structural myopathies, and episodic fatigability is the most common symptom of the metabolic myopathies and channelopathies. Most of the congenital myopathies or dystrophies start with weakness in the proximal muscles that eventually spreads more distally. Notable exceptions are fascioscapulohumeral dystrophy (FSHD), where facial weakness may be a prominent and early sign, myopathies with distal weakness including the "distal myopathies," and myotonic muscular dystrophy. In general, the disorders of fat metabolism and mitochondrial cytopathies present with impairment in endurance-type activities, whereas glycogen storage diseases present with symptoms during higher-intensity muscle contractions.

A common outcome from prolonged weakness is joint contracture and secondary bony abnormalities, including osteoarthritis, osteoporosis, and scoliosis. Contractures are most commonly seen at the shoulders, elbows, ankles, knees, and hips. Several of the myopathies can also affect cardiac muscle with conduction block (e.g., myotonic dystrophy) and cardiomyopathy (dystrophinopathy, Emery-Dreifuss) (Table 7.4).

In general, because most myopathies initially affect proximal limb muscles, early in the course of the disease individuals with these conditions will often experience difficultly arising from a low chair, climbing stairs, or rising from a kneeling position or from the ground (e.g., after a fall). As weakness progresses, gait disturbance and limitations in functional mobility become more problematic. Most children with DMD become wheelchair dependent for mobility by 10 to 12 years of age. The requirement for power mobility is extremely variable in other forms of acquired and inherited myopathy.

PHYSICAL EXAMINATION

As stated above, most people with myopathy will have significant proximal weakness without any sensory signs or symptoms as primary manifestations of their disorder. Mental status is usually unaffected, with the exception of some children with DMD, myotonic muscular dystrophy

TABLE 7.1. OVERVIEW OF THE COMMON INHERITED MYOPATHIES

Muscular Dystrophies
- Congenital muscular dystrophy
- Dystrophinopathies (Becker's and Duchenne)
- Fascioscapulohumeral
- Limb girdle
- Distal dystrophies
- Hereditary inclusion body myositis
- Myotonic
- Emery-Dreifuss
- Oculopharyngeal

Channelopathies
- Myotonia congenita (Thomsen's and Becker's)
- Malignant hyperthermia
- Hyperkalemic periodic paralysis
- Hypokalemic periodic paralysis
- Potassium sensitive myotonia congenita
- Paramyotonia congenita

Congenital Myopathies
- Nemaline rod
- Central core
- Centronuclear
- Minicore/multicore

Metabolic Myopathies
- Glycogen storage disease (GSD)
- Fatty acid oxidation defects (FAOD)
- Fatty acid transport defects
- Mitochondrial myopathies
- Myoadenylate deaminase deficiency

(somnolence is very common and cognitive impairment is seen in more severe forms), and congenital myopathy with central nervous system involvement. Cranial nerve examination findings are usually normal. Facial weakness, however, is manifested in FSHD and some cases of central nuclear myopathy and myotonic dystrophy. Prox-

TABLE 7.2. ACQUIRED MYOPATHIES

Endocrine
- Hypothyroidism
- Hyperthyroidism
- Vitamin D deficiency
- Cushing's syndrome-hypercortisolemia
- Hypocortisolemia (Addison's disease)
- Acromegaly (growth hormone excess)

Inflammatory Myopathies
- Polymyositis
- Dermatomyositis
- Inclusion body myositis
- Myositis with connective disease
- Transient viral myositis
- Bacterial/fungal myositis

Drugs
- Zidovudine (AZT)
- Adriamycin
- Chloriquine
- Corticosteroids
- Statins (HMG-CoA Reductase Inhibitors)

imal muscle bulk is reduced in later stages of myopathies, with the exceptions noted previously. Some of the inherited myopathies have very specific patterns of weakness, for example, high riding scapulae, horizontal clavicles, and accentuated pectoral creases are typical of FSHD. Muscle weakness follows a proximal to distal pattern with the notable exceptions above. As such, the shoulder abductors, shoulder internal and external rotators, abdominals, paraspinals, hip girdle muscles, and knee extensors and flexors are usually affected early in varying degrees. Muscle stretch reflexes are normal in the early stages of disease but are suppressed later as weakness progresses.

Sensory examination is usually normal. Significant sensory abnormalities prompt investigation into possible concurrent acquired causes of neuropathy (e.g., compression or entrapment, monoclonal gammopathy of uncertain significance, diabetes, autoimmune disease, vitamin B_{12} deficiency, thyroid abnormalities, toxin exposure, drugs), as opposed to a myopathic etiology. Orthopedic deformities of the foot and ankle (e.g., equinovarus ankle deformity) can be seen in the congenital myopathies owing to intrauterine weakness. Secondary orthopedic manifestations include knee, ankle, and hip contractures as weakness progresses. Dermatomyositis and Emery-Dreifuss muscular dystrophy are susceptible to elbow joint contractures, and the former may also result in subcutaneous calcifications. Scoliosis is common in many of the congenital myopathies. The gait abnormalities associated with myopathies include a compensated Trendelenberg gait pattern owing to hip abductor weakness whereby the trunk bends laterally over the hip during the stance phase of the gait cycle, hyperlordosis because of abdominal and hip extensor weakness, and knee hyperextension through midstance resulting from quadriceps weakness.

DIAGNOSTIC TECHNIQUES

The approach to a patient with suspected myopathy involves a very careful history, physical examination, and family history. Acute and subacute conditions coming on later in life are often acquired. Some of the metabolic myopathies may, however, initially present rather acutely in midlife (e.g., McArdle's disease). The pattern of weakness, absence of sensory symptoms, presence or absence of muscle cramping, pigmenturia, and onset of symptoms with endurance or high-intensity exercise are all helpful in the evaluation. More often than not, the tentative diagnosis can be made from the history and physical examination. For example, a classic history of distal weakness, frontal balding, cataracts, hypersomnolence, and grip myotonia would prompt genetic testing for the diagnosis of myotonic dystrophy type 1 (DM1), and further testing would not be required to establish the diagnosis. In less

TABLE 7.3. MUSCULAR DYSTROPHIES/CONGENITAL MYOPATHIES/CHANNELOPATHIES

	INHERITANCE PATTERN	GENE PRODUCT	SYMBOL
Duchenne muscular dystrophy	XR	Dystrophin	DYS-DMD
Becker's muscular dystrophy	XR	Dystrophin	DYS-BMD
Limb girdle muscular dystrophy	AR	Dysferlin	LG-MD2B
	AR	α-sarcoglycan	LG-MD2D
	AR	β-sarcoglycan	LG-MD2E
	AR	γ-sarcoglycan	LG-MD2C
	AR	Calpain-3	LG-MD2A
Limb girdle muscular dystrophy (dominant)	AD	Caveolin-3	LG-MD1C
	AD	Laminin A/C	LG-MD1B
Distal Muscular Dystrophy			
• Miyoshi	AR	Dysferlin	MM
• Miscellaneous (Nonaka, Udd, and Bethlem)			
Hereditary inclusion body myopathy IBM2	AR	?	
Oculopharyngeal muscular dystrophy	AD	Poly(A) binding Protein	OPMD
Congenital Myopathy/Dystrophy			
• Myotubular myopathy	XR	Myotubularin	MTMX
• Central core	AD	Ryanodine receptor	CCD
• Nemaline myopathy	AD	α-tropomyosin	NEM1
	AR	Nebulin	NEM2
• Emery-Dreifuss	XR	Emerin	EMD1
	AD	Laminin A/C	EMD2
Fascioscapulohumeral	AD	?	FSHD
Myotonic muscular dystrophy–1	AD	Myotonin	DM
Proximal myotonic myopathy	AD	Zinc finger protein 9	DM2
Congenital muscular dystrophy	AR	α-2 laminin	LAMA2
	AR	Integrin α 7	ITG7
Congenital muscular dystrophy	AR	Fukutin	FCMD
Channelopathies			
Malignant hyperthermia	AD	Ryanodine receptor	MHS1
Myotonia congenita	AD	Chloride channel	CLC-1
	AR	Chloride channel	CLC-1
Hyperkalemic periodic paralysis	AD	Sodium channel α subunit	SCN4A
Hypokalemic periodic paralysis	AD	Dihydropyridine receptor	CACNL1A3

classic cases, further testing is required, including serum chemistries for creatine kinase (CK) activity, electrolytes, and thyroid function as an initial screen. The finding of rash, joint involvement, or other autoimmune features would prompt further investigation for underlying connective tissue disease as part of the initial investigation of a potential inflammatory myopathy. In suspected metabolic myopathy, forearm ischemic testing may be helpful in showing absence of lactate rise with normal ammonia rise (a classic glycogen storage disease pattern), or normal lactate rise with absent ammonia rise (myoadenylate deaminase deficiency). Evaluation of suspected free fatty acid (FFA) oxidation defects, FFA transport abnormalities, and mitochondrial cytopathy requires referral to tertiary and quaternary centers that are skilled in the assessment of these disorders (e.g., Institute for Exercise and Environmental Medicine, Southwestern Medical Center, University of Texas, Dallas, Texas; Neuromuscular and Neurometabolic Clinic, McMaster University Medical Center, Hamilton, Ontario).

Most people with a suspected acquired myopathy should have a number of routine investigations, including a complete blood count, CK, creatinine, liver enzymes, thyroid function (thyroid-stimulating hormone [TSH]), antinuclear antibody (ANA), and an erythrocyte sedimentation rate (ESR). With any suspicion of respiratory involvement, both sitting and supine pulmonary function studies and oximetry are of value. People with suspected cardiac involvement or with possible conduc-

TABLE 7.4. MYOPATHIES ASSOCIATED WITH CARDIAC ABNORMALITIES

MYOPATHY	CARDIAC DEFECT
Dystrophinopathies (Becker's and Duchenne)	Cardiomyopathy
Myotonic dystrophy, types I & II	Cardiac conduction block
Emery-Dreifuss muscular dystrophy	Cardiac conduction block
Nemaline rod myopathy	Cardiomyopathy
Centronuclear myopathy	Cardiomyopathy

tion defects (e.g., DM1 and myotonic dystrophy type 2) require annual screening with electrocardiography (ECG), echocardiography (e.g., DMD, Becker's), or both.

Electrodiagnostic investigation or electromyography (EMG) is often helpful in the initial investigation of a potential myopathic disorder. EMG is perhaps most helpful in cases where the clinical presentation is not clear cut and when atempting to distinguish between disorders affecting the motor neurons or axons versus muscle. The classic findings on needle EMG studies of early recruitment and brief- or low-amplitude polyphasic motor unit action potentials would all point toward a potential myopathy (7). Spontaneous activity (fibrillation potentials and positive sharp waves) are usually indicative of muscle fiber necrosis and functional denervation. These findings are typically present in inflammatory myopathies, but can be seen in inherited forms as well (e.g., DMD). The presence of myotonia on EMG testing can help to confirm the suspicion of DM1 or DM2. It is imporant to note that for many of the inheritied myopathies, especially in milder disease or early presentations, needle EMG findings can be completely normal, even in clnically weak muscles. Abnormalities on nerve conduction testing indicating sensory involvement, presence of demyelinating features on motor nerve conduction testing, and neuropathic motor unit action potentials on needle EMG testing would all point toward a primary neuropathic disorder or, in some cases, an associated focal neuropathy (e.g., ulnar nerve entrapment related to pressure from arm rest and prolonged seating).

The muscle biopsy is an essential part of the workup in many myopathies. We routinely use a modified 5-mm Bergstrom needle with a custom-made apparatus, such that a 60-mL syringe can provide airtight suction via a plastic hose inserted into the end using a pipette tip. We routinely obtain sufficient muscle for histochemistry (~40 mg), electron microscopy (~10 mg), and another piece (~60–100 mg) for enzyme and genetic testing. Light microscopy allows for the assessment of morphometry, accumulation of substrates (i.e., glycogen), fiber type, and immunohistochemistry can be used to assess proteins (Table 7.5). Electron microscopy can be useful in the assessment of ultrastructural details, such as mitochondrial morphology, Z-disc streaming, and inclusions.

We have found cranial magnetic resonance imaging (MRI) to be particularly helpful in assessment of mitochondrial cytopathies and also in the evaluation of the hypotonic (floppy) infant, particularly if there are developmental delays in more than one sphere. ^{31}-phosphorous MR spectroscopy is also helpful, particularly when combined with exercise, and it may show delayed phosphocreatine resynthesis rates with fatty acid oxidation defects and mitochondrial cytopathy (4). Near-infrared spectroscopy can contribute significantly to a diagnosis by showing characteristic patterns in metabolic cytopathies (46).

TABLE 7.5. COMMON MICROSCOPY TECHNIQUES

HISTOCHEMICAL ANALYSES	UTILITY
Adenosine triphosphatase (ATPase)	Fiber typing
Hematoxylin and eosin	Central nuclei, inflammatory cells
Modified gomori trichrome	Mitochondria, nemaline rods
Periodic acid Schiff	Glycogen
Oil red-O	Lipid content
Myoadenylate deaminase	AMPD1 deficiency
Cytochrome oxidase	COX deficiency, ragged red fibers
NADH tetrazolium	Reductase NADH deficiency, ragged red fibers
Succinate dehydrogenase	CMPLX II deficiency, ragged red fibers
Elastic Van Giesson	Connective tissue

Aerobic exercise testing can be helpful in determining physical fitness of individuals for exercise prescription and is also very useful in the evaluation of peoplewith suspected metabolic disorders. A low $\dot{V}O_2$ peak is seen in patients with mitochondrial cytopathies. For example, in our recent study with predominantly MELAS participants, the mean $\dot{V}O_2$ peak was approximately 10 mL/kg/min (39). The respiratory exchange ratio also increases rapidly and to a very high level in participants with mitochondrial cytopathies (39). A recent review of exercise testing for the mitochondrial cytopathies is found in reference (40).

EXERCISE, FITNESS, AND FUNCTIONAL TESTING

Most physicians and physiotherapists use the Medical Research Council scale to semiquantitatively categorize muscle strength during manual muscle testing (Table 7.6). Manual muscle testing is relatively quickly and easily carried out in the clinic by a trained examiner and is sensitive to major changes in strength (e.g., reduction from the ability to apply resistance to the examiner, grade 4, to antigravity strength, grade 3). Although useful clinically, this testing is often not helpful in evaluating an experimental therapeutic substance in a clinical trial (i.e., deflazacort or creatine monohydrate) owing to insensivity of the categorical scale and the wide range of strength that accompanies grade 4.

More objective strength outcome measures include isokinetic and isometric dynamometry (i.e., Cybex, Biodex,) as well as hand-held dynamometry. In our experience, we have found these to be very helpful in making treatment decisions, such as tapering corticosteroids in inflammatory myopathies, and in following individuals on a prescribed exercise regimen to ensure that they are not overtraining and losing strength.

Forearm ischemic testing is helpful in the evaluation of suspected myoadenylate deaminase deficiency or glycogen

TABLE 7.6. MEDICAL RESEARCH COUNCIL (MRC) SCALE

0 = No contraction
1 = Flicker of contraction
2 = Movement through a full range without gravity
3 = Movement through a full range against gravity
4− = Movement against minimal resistance
4 = Movement against some resistance
4+ = Movement against moderate resistance
5 = Full muscle power

storage disease (GSD). This test requires basal lactate and ammonia determination (both immediately placed on ice and transported to the laboratory). Following this, a sphygmomanometer cuff is inflated to 20 mm Hg beyond the arterial pressure, and the individual performs rhythmic isometric exercise with a 9:1 exercise-to-rest duty cycle. After 60 seconds of exercise, the manometer cuff is released and recovery samples are taken at 1, 3, and 5 minutes postexercise. Most texts suggest a 10- or even 20-minute recovery. However, we have found that this does not add to the sensitivity and specificity of the test. The recovery samples must be taken and placed immediately on ice and analyzed rapidly to avoid false elevations in lactate and ammonia from red blood cell metabolism. It is critically important when performing this test to terminate immediately if the individual develops a painful muscle contracture, and not to proceed with this type of testing if the individual has had definite myoglobinuria with high-intensity exercise in the past. Under these circumstances, semi-ischemic protocols have been developed, although in reality the muscle is highly ischemic because of the isometric nature of the contractions and all precautions regarding a painful contracture and termination of the test must be assessed and followed.

Submaximal aerobic activity on the cycle ergometer (3) can be helpful to determine the efficacy of a given intervention (i.e., frequent glucose meals for carnitine palmitoyl transferase deficiency, type 2).

PHYSICAL INTERVENTIONS

Physical therapeutic interventions for most myopathies consist minimally of moderate exercise, regular static stretching, and range-of-motion exercise. Stretching and range-of-motion exercises may be of benefit in preventing contractures. When contractures are emerging, serial casting, preventive bracing, and more intensive stretching with a physiotherapist are warranted. If this fails, a surgical procedure, such as tendon lengthening, may become necessary. People with myopathies are very sensitive to the immobility associated with surgery or other forced periods of immobility, which can cause a rapid step-wise decline in motor function.

Gait aids, such as canes and walkers, can be of benefit for those with myopathies by improving balance and overall endurance. In many cases, however, it is difficult for those with myopathic gait patterns to utilize these devices, because their use often requires substantial upper body strength and excessive trunk or hip flexion.

Bracing is a challenge for those with proximal weakness because the weight and complexity of these devices (e.g., knee-ankle-foot orthoses) often results in poor compliance. Some patients with weakness in the knee extensors benefit from knee stabilizing ankle-foot orthoses, but in our experience, simple knee orthoses are usually poorly tolerated and not helpful functionally for those with myopathies. Power mobility devices (wheelchairs and scooters) require indivdualized consideration and prescription. When functional mobility limits the individual from taking part in activities of daily living (ADL) or becomes a barrier to full partcicipation in vocational or avocational pursuits, it is very reasonable to prescribe a power mobility device. When possible, this is best done through a specialized seating clinic with experience in neuromuscular disorders or through referral to a community-based occupational therapist with appropriate training and expertise. Regular standing or walking should be encouraged for those still able to do so.

PHARMACOLOGIC INTERVENTIONS

Most children with DMD and Becker's muscular dystrophy will be treated with corticosteroids (prednisone or deflazacort), which have become an accepted mainstay of treatment in patients with dystrophinopathies (32). Side effects of long-term (weeks to months) corticosteroid use are weight gain, elevated blood pressure, insulin resistance and elevated blood glucose, elevated serum lipids, cataract formation, and osteoporosis (1). Despite their negative side effects, studies show that corticosteriods lead to an overall improvement in muscle strength and function in this population (1). Nevertheless, each child must be treated on an individual basis, and we recommend objective and subjective evaluation and follow-up in a tertiary care center familiar with the use of corticosteroids in dystrophinopathy.

Although limited evidence of functional benefit exists, some people with FSHD are prescribed β-2 agonists, which can produce side effects of tachycardia and possibly cardiac dysrhythmia. Many people with myopathies are also taking creatine monohydrate, which probably has a positive effect on exercise capacity (25,43). A recent Cochrane review has also concluded that creatine monohydrate is of some clinical utility in the muscualr dystrophies (25). Another study found that creatine monohydrate supplementation enhanced function in people with polymyositis and dermatomyositis. Alph-lipoic acid and coenzyme Q10, in combination with creatine monohydrate, appear to confer some efficacy on surrogate markers of disease severity, including lower serum lactate and urineary oxidative stress markers. Currently, however, few other pharmacologic treatment options have been show to alter progression of the major manifestations of inherited myopathies (muscle wasting and weakness).

Acetaminophen and nonsteroidal anti-inflammatories are useful for musculoskeletal pain associated with immobilty or secondary degenerative joint disease. Some people with more severe joint pain require the use of narcotic analgesics. Immunosupression is the mainstay of treatment for the inflammatory myopathies (polymyositis, dermatomyositis). For these disorders, treament is usually initiated with high-dose prednisone, which is tapered following initial treatment reponse. Azathioprine and methotrexate are commonly used as steroid-sparing immunosuppresive agents for inflammatory myopathies. Currently, no benefit is demonstrated of immunosupression for inclusion body myositis.

EXERCISE PRESCRIPTION AND PROGRAMMING

The goal of any therapeutic intervention for patients with progressive disorders involving the neuromuscular system is the maintainance of independence and the ability to perform typical ADL, including vocational and avocational pursuits, to as full an extent as possible (23,48). The means of achieving these goals include (a) the maintenance of maximal muscle mass and strength within the limitations imposed by the disease process, and (b) the prevention or slowing of secondary complications, including disuse weakness and atrophy as well as the development of contractures that lead to the premature loss of ambulation and functional independence. The extent to which exercise therapy is able to improve skeletal muscle strength and function will be reviewed in the following sections.

The hallmark of any progressive myopathy is muscle atrophy and associated weakness. In addition to strength losses associated with the underlying disease, most individuals with neuromuscular disorders lead sedentary lifestyles that likely contribute significantly to their degree of impairment and disability (23). The reasons for this are multifactorial and include (a) concern among parents, educators, physicians, and therapists that exercise may be detrimental to children with progressive myopathic disorders; (b) limited opportunities for children and adults with progressive myopathies to take part in activity owing to lack of available, accessible programming in many communities; (c) lack of early development of adequate motor skills in typical sports and games during childhood that limits participation later in life; and (d) minimal positive reinforcement associated with sport and physical activity in these populations. As a result, lack of

physical activity likely contributes significantly to the overall disability in patients with progressive neuromuscular disorders and, specifically, myopathies. Thus, there has been interest in examining the extent to which exercise therapy can reverse or delay some of the maladaptive changes associated with inactivity.

GENERAL ISSUES IN EXERCISE PRESCRIPTION IN MYOPATHIC DISORDERS

Muscular Dystrophy and Congenital/ Inflammatory Myopathies

Individuals should first be screened for evidence of cardiac conduction defects (i.e., myotonic dystrophy) and cardiomyopathy (i.e., DMD). We recommend stress testing and echocardiography in all individuals in whom cardiac pathology is known to exist (Table 7.5). It is very important that individuals stretch and warm up before exercise. With weight training, we encourage a higher number of repetitions and low percentage (40%–50%) of one-repetition maximum (1-RM) for the first few weeks, with individuals gradually increasing their percentage (1-RM) as they adapt to the activity (no more intense than 3 sets of 10 repetitions) (24). It is very important that each person "listen to his or her body" and report any abnormal muscle or joint pain. We recommend that a muscle group be exercised with resistance training no more frequently than every 48 hours. With endurance exercise, most structural myopathies, and well-treated inflammatory and recovering endocrine myopathies, can follow a standard exercise prescription similar to that for individuals without disabilities starting an endurance exercise program.

A special concern for both endurance and strength training is the individual with a recently diagnosed inflammatory myopathy whose condidtion is not yet well controlled with corticosteroids or other therapies, or has just undergone an exacerbation of his or her condition with increased weakness and elevated CK. We usually have these individuals reduce their training or delay the initiation of onset, and perform gentle static stretching until the CK values are returning toward normal, and the individual feels subjective improvements in his or her strength (Table 7.7). All individuals who are taking corticosteroids should be taking vitamin D and calcium and, under some circumstances, bisphosphates.

Channelopathies

Many people with channelopathies, for example the periodic paralyses, are at risk for malignant hyperthermia (MH). Although the main trigger for malignant hyperthermia is exposure to anesthesia with succinyl choline, volatile halogenated anesthetic agents, or both, individuals harboring malignant hyperthermia may also have episodes of potentially fatal hypermetabolic crisis precipitated by prolonged or severe exercise in very hot and humid conditions

TABLE 7.7. GENERAL RESISTANCE EXERCISE PRESCRIPTION GUIDELINES FOR PATIENTS WITH MYOPATHIES

WEAKNESS	MRC GRADE	EXERCISE PRESCRIPTION
None to mild	4, 4+, 5	May perform moderate to high intensity resistance exercise with appropriate monitoring (8–12 repetition maximum sets)
Moderate	3, 4–	May perform moderate intensity exercise with appropriate monitoring (15–20 repetition maximum sets)
Severe	1, 2	Passive and active assisted range-of-motion exercise to maintain range and prevent contractures

(44). People with MH should follow the *ACSM Guidelines* for exercise in the heat, and we would recommend avoidance of prolonged or very high-intensity repeated activities in hot or humid environments. The medication dantrolene sodium has dramatically decreased the mortality from anesthesia-related MH deaths (44) and would certainly be indicated in a rare case of MH crisis precipitated by exercise. All patients with malignant hyperthermia should wear a Medic-Alert bracelet and, if exercise must be performed in hot or humid environments, prophylactic oral dantrolene sodium may be of benefit, but it may reduce strength.

People with myotonia congenita develop extreme muscle hypertrophy. Most of these individuals avoid resistance training because of precipitation of extreme hypertrophy that can be so extensive that it is disfiguring. Rapidly initiating exercise results in myotonia, and slowly warming up helps to prevent the myotonia. These individuals tolerate endurance exercise quite well, which does not result in muscle hypertrophy. In persons with paramyotonia congenita, the main issue with exercise is severe symptomatic exacerbation when exposed to the cold. For this reason, these individuals should not perform winter activities when the potential for hypothermia or a severe cold exposure exists. Under no circumstances should these individuals participate in swimming sports in open water, where cold-induced myotonia could be fatal. In paramyotonia and hyperkalemic periodic paralysis, profound muscle weakness can occur in the minutes to hours following exercise. This is exacerbated with complete inactivity (i.e., driving home in a car after activity). For this reason, we recommend that these individuals try to perform a gentle warm-down and keep their legs moving at low intensities following exercise to avoid the paralysis.

Metabolic Myopathies

It is of primary importance for those with fatty acid oxidation defects to avoid fasting and never exercise during a period of concurrent illness. Most patients should start the consumption of carbohydrates at approximately 1 g/kg/h in the hour before exercise and consume at least 0.25 g/kg at 15-minute intervals during endurance exercise. Persons with CPT-2 deficiency and other fatty acid oxidation defects should adopt a high carbohydrate diet (27). If muscle cramping, shortness of breath, or tachycardia occurs in patients with fatty acid oxidation defects, they should stop their activity, continue to consume fluids with high carbohydrate content, and if symptoms persist, (44) the clinical exercise physiologist should implement the facility's emergency procedures protocol. In our experience, we have found that these exercise and dietary strategies have allowed most of our patients with CPT-2 to perform endurance-type activities, some even at rather surprising intensity or duration.

For the person with GSD, it is imperative to perform a long warm-up period to increase the delivery of blood-borne substrates, such as glucose, FFA, and proteins, to "bypass the defect" and get into the "second wind" (50). Most people with this condition report a very idiosyncratic feeling of "getting their second wind" when the body can aerobically utilize lipids. Studies have shown that persons with McArdle's disease (GSD, type 5) may also benefit from frequent sips of carbohydrate during exercise as the glucose bypasses the metabolic defect (27,28). Carbohydrate intake before and during exercise in patients with GSD type 7 (Tarui's disease) inhibits fatty acid mobilization and utilization, and significantly impairs exercise performance (14). Avoidance of carbohydrates before and during exercise is also prudent for those with other glycogenoses affecting glycolysis (i.e., phosphoglycerate mutase, phosphoglycerate kinase). Several studies have demonstrated the benefits from slowly progressive endurance exercise training programs in people with McArdle's disease (15).

SPECIFIC CONCERNS DURING EXERCISE TRAINING

Overuse Weakness

Overuse or overwork weakness, a concern first identified in those recovering from the effects of poliomyelitis, is a major concern among patients, their parents, clinicians, and therapists. There have been anecdotal case reports of increased weakness following strengthening exercise in people with amyotrophic lateral sclerosis, peripheral nerve lesions, and DMD (6,16,26). Additionally, overuse was suggested in several family members with FSHD based on asymmetric weakness in the upper extremities (21). The affected family members showed greater weakness on the dominant side, with the exception of one individual, a heavy equipment operator, who used his non-dominant left arm to operate the equipment and exhibited greater weakness on that side. This description is obviously anecdotal and uncontrolled. Additionally, it fails to take into account the common observation of significant asymmetry in the pattern of weakness typically found in people with FSHD. In one controlled study, participants with DMD performed submaximal knee extension exercise for 6 months and showed no evidence of overuse weakness in comparison to the nonexercised control leg (19). Thus, no definitive evidence currently exists to support overuse weakness in persons with myopathic disorders (see later). It is most prudent, however, that exercise programs be appropriately adapted to individual needs and that adequate supervision and monitoring is in place.

Resistance Exercise in Rapidly Progressive Myopathies

In DMD, there is rapid and progressive loss of strength and functional capacity. Boys are typically dependent on wheelchairs for mobility between the ages of 8 and 12 years (48). Because of this rapid progression, these boys are limited in the extent to which they can participate with their peers in normal age-appropriate physical activity and play. There is, therefore, considerable risk of isolation and lack of social interaction, as well as the aforementioned additive problems of disuse weakness and atrophy, as well as obesity from inactivity, potentially complicated by corticosteroid use (23). Thus, considerable interest exists in the potential benefits of strengthening exercise to slow the progression of weakness, improve functional capacity, and allow for more natural social development.

In general, resistance exercise in children with DMD has been shown to either maintain strength or result in mild improvement. Little consensus is found among experts, however, to the clinical utility of strength training in this population (13,24,47). The few studies in the literature are limited by (a) frequent use of nonquantitative, insensitive outcome measures; (b) often poorly defined exercise programs; (c) lack of a control group in many cases or use of the opposite limb as a control; (d) heterogeneity in the treatment groups regarding age, specific type of disease, disease progression, functional level, and degree of contracture present; and (e) small sample sizes in the treatment and, when present, control groups. Additionally, any intervention trial directed toward DMD must take into account the rapidly progressive nature of this disease (13,24).

Two pioneering studies that examined resistance exercise in children with DMD were carried out by Abramson and Rogoff (2) and Hoberman (19). Strength was assessed by manual muscle testing in both studies. Abramson and Rogoff (2) reported slight improvement by about one-half to one grade on the Medical Research Council (MRC) scale in half of their subjects, with the other half remaining unchanged in response to a 7-month program consisting of active, active-assisted, and resistance exercise performed three times per week. Although poorly

quantified, mention was also made of improved mobility in 8 of 27 subjects.

Hoberman (19) examined 10 patients over a 4-month daily program of resistance exercise, gait training, and stretching. There were no reported improvements in strength defined as a gain of one full MRC grade. The author noted, however, in some participants for whom there were records, there was less decline in strength during the program than in the previous year.

The lack of positive results in this study and the failure of one-half of the patients to respond in the former study may have been influenced by the high proportion of subjects in each with severe disease progression. Two-thirds of the patients in both studies were using wheelchairs for mobility. It has been suggested that, by the time patients with DMD are wheelchair dependent, they have lost half of their muscle mass (48). Additionally, contractures were present in most subjects, which further reduces the ability of the muscle to respond optimally to resistance exercise training.

Wratney (52) provided a home-based, unsupervised exercise program for 75 people with muscular dystrophy (most with DMD) between the ages of 12 and 16 years. The program consisted of arm and leg exercises against gravity for an unspecified length of time within a 3-year period. No gains in strength were reported; however, it was suggested that a program of this nature may prevent disuse atrophy and maintain range of motion.

Vignos and Watkins (49) attempted to improve on these earlier studies and examined the effects of a 1-year, home-based, higher-intensity resistance-training program in a group of still ambulatory persons with muscular dystrophy (14 DMD, 6 LGMD, 4 FSHD). The DMD participants were compared with a nonexercised control group of age, strength, and functional ability matched people with DMD. As determined by manual muscle testing, measurable increases in strength were reported for all three groups. In all three forms of dystrophy, the strength gains occurred in the first 4 months; however, the gains were maintained during the subsequent 8 months. In general, participants with less severe disease improved more so and greater gains were noted in muscles that were initially stronger. The muscle strength had declined in both the exercised and nonexercised subjects with DMD in the year before the study. The control subjects continued to decline during the second year. The exercised group showed no loss in strength and exhibited a minimal increase, thus suggesting some longer term benefit.

Finally, DeLateur and Giaconi (8) isokinetically (Cybex) trained the quadriceps of one leg in four participants with DMD four to five times per week for 6 months. The nonexercised leg served as a control. All five subjects were ambulatory at the onset of the study and had at least grade 3/5 strength in the knee extensors. One subject, however, with rapidly progressive disease became nonambulatory during the study. Strength was tested on the same device at monthly intervals during the 6-month training period and for the first 6 months after training, and at 18 and 24 months after training. Increases in maximal strength in response to this program were modest, and strength was greater in the exercised leg at only the 5- and 9-month test periods. It should be noted, however, that the maximal strength of the exercised leg was equal to or stronger than the control leg for all months of follow-up except at 2 years. Additionally, one of the subjects appeared to have deteriorated rapidly during the course of the study, which likely biased this small data set. An important additional conclusion of this study was the lack of any evidence for overuse weakness in the trained legs as compared with the control legs.

In summary, it can be concluded that little evidence supports overuse weakness in response to controlled resistance training programs, at least in cases of DMD. For the most part, studies have shown either maintenance of strength and, in some cases, modest improvements. In general, the most significant gains have been noted in people with less disease progression and in their less severely affected muscle groups. These latter points may indicate the need to intervene as early as possible to obtain maximal benefits. Further investigation into the potential benefit of resistance exercise in DMD is required. These studies will require adequate sample sizes, matched controls, carefully designed and monitored programs, and sensitive strength and functional outcome measures. In addition, as noted earlier, most boys with DMD are now treated with either oral prednisone or deflazacort. The additive effect of well-controlled resistance training programs in conjunction with corticosteroids has not yet been assessed.

Resistance Exercise in Slowly Progressive Myopathy

In more slowly progressive myopathies, such as myotonic dystrophy (DM1), LGMD, FSHD, and most of the congenital myopathies, the goal of resistance exercise programs has been to improve strength and function rather than simply slow the pace of disease progression. Most studies in this regard have grouped people with different disorders to achieve adequate sample sizes.

McCartney and coworkers (30) dynamically trained the elbow flexors of one arm and the knee and hip extensors bilaterally in five persons with slowly progressive neuromuscular disorders (three with spinal muscular atrophy, one with LGMD, and one with FSHD) three times per week for 9 weeks. Strength was objectively determined with isometric dynamomoetry before and after training while the extent of motor unit activation was determined with the twitch interpolation technique (5). Force in the trained elbow flexors increased from 19% to 34% and from −14 to +25% in the control arm. Leg strength improved on average by 11%. Three subjects who were unable to activate their muscles completely

pretraining, as determined by twitch interpolation, were able to do so after training, suggesting a significant central neural component to their strength increases.

Milner-Brown and Miller (33) similarly trained a group of people with slowly progressive neuromuscular disorders (six with FSHD, four with DM, one with LGMD, three with spinal muscular atrophy, and one with polyneuropathy). The elbow flexors and knee extensors were trained with a standard progressive-resistance exercise program, and quantitative measures of strength and fatigue were performed with isometric dynamometry. Significant increases in strength and endurance were noted for mildly to moderately weak muscles. Severely weak muscles (<10% normal), however, generally did not improve.

The impact of a moderate-resistance, home-based exercise program for patients with slowly progressive neuromuscular disease was reported by Aitkens et al. (3). Subjects trained their knee extensors and elbow flexors unilaterally with weights 3 days per week for 12 weeks. A healthy control group was studied for comparison. Training loads were designed to be moderate in intensity and ranged from 10%–40% of maximum (except handgrip at 100%). Both the experimental and control groups demonstrated similar modest increases in strength, and there were similar gains for both the exercised and nonexercised limbs. This provides evidence that even a very modest training program can result in improvements in this population. This same group of researchers examined the effects of a higher-resistance, home-based, resistance training program (22). The training load for the knee extensors and elbow flexors was based on a 10-RM load (approximately 80% of maximum). The authors expressed concern that a program of this nature may be harmful to persons with neuromuscular diseases because a number of the isokinetic indices for the elbow flexors failed to show any statistical improvement. It should be noted, however, that the healthy control subjects also failed to show improvement in most of the isokinetic elbow flexion variables, perhaps related to the lack of similarity between the training regimen and testing condition (isotonic versus isokinetic). Therefore, the expressed concern over higher-intensity training by the authors in this study may not be valid. More recently, Tollbäck et al. (45) reported the effects of a supervised high-resistance training program in a small group of persons with mytonic dystrophy type 1 (DM1). Subjects performed supervised unilateral knee extension exercises three sets of 10 repetitions at 80% of 1-RM three times per week for 12 weeks. In the trained leg, the 1-RM load increased significantly by 25%. No significant improvements were noted in isokinetic concentric or eccentric values. Muscle biopsy revealed no change in the degree of histopathology, and a trend noted toward increased type I fiber cross-sectional area. These authors stressed the importance of supervision during programs of this nature to ensure compliance.

Finally, Lindeman and coworkers (29) reported the results of a study that examined the effects of a 24-week strength training program in persons with DM1 and hereditary motor sensory neuropathy. Matched subjects were randomly assigned to either a training or control group. The training group performed knee extension exercise three times per week with loads increasing gradually from 60% to 80%. Maximal isometric and isokinetic strength, functional tasks, ADL questionnaires, and serum myoglobin were measured before and after training. Subjects with DM1 showed no deleterious effects of training, and all subjects progressed with regard to their training loads. None of the less-specific strength or timed functional tasks, however, exhibited any significant improvement. Myoglobin levels were not significantly changed from pretraining levels.

In summary (Table 7.7), although not all studies have shown consistent positive effects, moderate- to high-intensity resistance training generally has been found to maintain or improve strength in people with a variety of myopathic disorders. As with DMD, strength gains tend to be greatest for muscles with mild-to-moderate weakness and are minimal in muscle groups with severe weakness. Strength training programs for these populations should be designed by experienced, trained personnel, and the program must be specifically tailored to the needs and limitations of the participants. Programs should be supervised, at least during their initial stages, and objective monitoring should be in place. High-intensity resistance training has no advantage over moderate-intensity resistance programs and may lead to a greater liklihood of joint pain, injury, and, possibly, overtraining. Training the major muscle groups two to three times per week with intensities allowing 12–15 repetitions maximum is appropriate. The required frequency and intensity for *maintenance* of strength gains have not been adequately addressed in these patient populations.

Future high-quality studies are required to better define minimal and optimal training intensities and volumes (13,24). Ideally, these studies should include randomized control groups, completely supervised training programs, blinded assessors, and homogeneous training groups. The latter may require a multicentered approach. Functional, person-centered outcomes are crucial to examine the potential impact of these interventions on disability, participation, and quality of life.

Resistance Exercise in Inflammatory Myopathy

Exercise therapy in inflammatory myopathies has traditionally been confined to range-of-motion exercises and stretching in an attempt to prevent contractures and restricted joint motion. Traditional teaching has promoted rest and energy conservation in these disorders, because it was felt that exercise would potentially harm inflamed muscles. Although this may still hold true for the initial stages of treatment in inflammatory myopathies, evidence now indicates that a more active approach is safe and of potential benefit in the overall management of these disorders (18).

A single case report was the first indication that resistance exercise could be of potential benefit in the rehabilitation of polymyositis (17). In this case, a 42-year-old man with a stable course of at least 4 months' duration performed isometric resistance exercise (6- × 6-second maximal isometric contractions) for the biceps and quadriceps for 1 month. There was a gradual and significant increase in peak isometric force over the course of the study and, if anything, a slight decrease in the postexercise CK activity. Thus, there was evidence to support potential strength increase and no indication of increased muscle damage.

Escalante et al. (11) similarly reported a small case series of five subjects with stable polymyositis or dermatomyositis who underwent successive 2-week periods of generalized rehabilitation and resistance exercise. Four of the five subjects had significant increases in strength associated with the periods of resistance exercise. A small and likely clinically insignificant 7.7% mean rise in CK was seen postexercise.

Wiesinger et al. (53) reported the results of a randomized, controlled trial of progressive bicycle ergometer and step aerobic exercise in a group of individuals with stable inflammatory myopathy. As with the resistance training programs described above, significant gains were achieved in peak isometric strength, and additionally improvements in an ADL questionnaire and maximal oxygen consumption in the trained group in comparison to controls. No evidence was seen of any deleterious effects with this type of program.

Finally, Spector et al. (37) examined the potential efficacy and safety of resistance training in five people with inclusion body myositis (a chronic inflammatory myopathy that typically affects older adults with quadriceps weakness as initial manifestation). Four men and one woman trained 3 days per week for 12 weeks with a program consisting of concentric exercises for the knee flexors and extensors and the elbow flexors. Following the 12-week program, no significant increase was seen in MRC scores or the Barthel Index. Three subjects, however, reported improved function as a result of the program. Mean 3-RM values were significantly improved for all muscle except the right knee extensors. Strength gains were greatest for the initially stronger muscle groups. Serum CK, B cells, T cells, and natural killer cells (all markers of inflammation) remained unchanged. These results were interpreted as suggesting that resistance exercise was safe and may be functionally beneficial for people with this diagnosis. This is an important finding because, as opposed to polymyositis and dermatomyositis, there is no proved benefit of immunosuppression or other medical therapy at this point for inclusion body myositis.

In summary, reasonable evidence indicates that resistance training and general conditioning are safe and potentially beneficial in people with inflammatory myopathy. As with the dystrophies, need exists for appropriate monitoring and follow-up. Participants should be exposed to active exercise programs only when they have been stable for 3 or more months, and programs should initially be supervised. In general, training should be approached very cautiously in muscle groups with less than antigravity strength. If these muscle groups are trained, it is best done with the supervison of a trained therapist. There is a considerable need for future well-designed studies.

Respiratory Muscle Training in Myopathies

Although limb and trunk muscle weakness is responsible for much of the functional limitation in progressive myopathies, deterioration of respiratory muscle function is primarily responsible for the high mortality rate among these individuals (31). Respiratory insufficiency and associated hypercapnia, loss of lung volume, impaired cough, and pneumonia are leading causes of morbidity and mortality among people with DMD (31). Thus, along with appropriate respiratory therapy and support, there has been interest in the potential benefit of inspiratory muscle training to improve respiratory muscle force and endurance in this population. As with other muscle groups, concern exists over the possibility of overuse weakness with inspiratory muscle training and the extent to which improvement on pulmonary function indices may translate to decreased morbidity.

The results of studies that have assessed the effectiveness of inspiratory muscle training are varied. DiMarco et al. (9) examined the effects of inspiratory muscle resistance training on inspiratory muscle function in 11 patients with muscular dystrophies (DMD, LGMD, FSHD). After 6 weeks of training with inspiratory resistive load, improvements were noted in the maximal inspiratory resistance that could be tolerated for 5 minutes and maximal sustainable ventilation. The degree of improvement with training, as noted previously for limb muscles, was directly related to the person's baseline vital capacity. Wanke et al. (51) studied the effects of a 6-month inspiratory muscle training program on 15 subjects with DMD in comparison to a DMD control group. The authors found that the 10 subjects who completed the training protocol had improvements in force as measured by maximal transdiaphragmatic pressure and maximal esophageal pressures. No changes were reported, however, for vital capacity, forced expiratory volume in 1 second, or maximal voluntary ventilation. Again, persons with the most severely reduced function responded less or not at all.

Gozal and Thiriet (12) examined the effects of a 6-month respiratory muscle training program on respiratory muscle strength and respiratory load perception in 21 children with DMD and spinal muscular atrophy type III. They were compared with 20 matched controls. Subjects were randomized to undergo incremental respiratory muscle training against inspiratory and expiratory loads, or against no load. In controls, no change in maximal static pressures or load perception was found. Respiratory training in the neuromuscular patients, alternatively, was associated with improvements in maximal inspiratory and expiratory pressures. Additionally, respiratory load perception improved in the group that trained against higher inspiratory and expiratory loads. Static pressures returned to baseline values within 3 months, whereas respiratory load perception was still improved after 3 months.

In general, as with the limb muscles, some evidence indicates that respiratory muscle training can improve some measures of maximal respiratory muscle function and may decrease the perceived respiratory effort. Those with high pretraining values tend to improve more so, which as with limb muscle training may support the role for early intervention. No definite evidence at this time suggests that respiratory muscle training is able to decrease incidence of chest infection and associated morbidity.

Aerobic Training in Muscle Disease

Although most exercise studies for myopathies have addressed the cardinal features of weakness and muscle wasting with resistance exercise, a few studies have also addressed the potential benefit of aerobic or endurance exercise (47). Olsen et al. (34) reported improved maximal oxygen uptake and training workloads in a group of people with FSHD in response to a 12-week cycle training program of moderate intensity (heart rate corresponding to 65% of $\dot{V}O_2$max). Similar results were reported for groups with LGMD, DM1, and mitochondrial myopathy (20,35,38). In some cases, the improvements in endurance translated to improvement in performance of ADL and quality of life. Based on these studies, it would appear that endurance or aerobic exercise training is safe and effective for patients with moderately severe myopathies. In general, the relative improvements in aerobic capacity are similar to controls. Whether endurance training is safe and effective for those with severe weakness has not been addressed in the literature.

EDUCATION AND COUNSELING

With careful monitoring and appropriate treatment, many people with myopathies live a normal, or only a minimally reduced, life span. For these reasons, a healthy lifestyle with respect to nutrition and physical education is important, and general guidelines are not much different than for those without disabilities with the caveats described above. Barriers to participation are much higher for those who require assistive devices, ranging from orthoses and canes to scooters and wheelchairs. Many universities and fitness facilities, however, are now wheelchair accessible. Many of these individuals, however, still feel embarrassed or different when going to a public gymnasium, although these barriers are also falling. A major factor we have encountered, particularly in children with DMD and most patients with myotonic dystrophy, is disinterest and poor compliance with exercise programs. Therefore, to improve compliance, it is important to make the activities enjoyable and age-specific.

REFERENCES

1. Angelini C. The role of corticosteroids in muscular dystrophy: A critical appraisal. *Muscle Nerve* 2007;May 31.
2. Abramson AS, Rogoff J. An approach to rehabilitation of children with muscular dystrophy. Proceedings of the First and Second Medical Conferences of the MDAA, Inc. New York, MDAA; 1953. p. 123–124.
3. Aitkens SG, McCrory MA, Kilmer DD, et al. Moderate resistance exercise program: Its effect in slowly progressive neuromuscular disease. *Arch Phys Med Rehabil* 1993;74:711–715.
4. Argov Z, Arnold DL. MR Spectroscopy and imaging in metabolic myopathies. *Neurol Clin* 2000;18:35–52.
5. Belanger AY, McComas AJ. Extent of motor unit activation during effort. *J Appl Physiol* 1981;51:1131–1135.
6. Bonsett CA. Pseudohypertrophic muscular dystrophy: Distribution of degenerative features as revealed by anatomical study. *Neurology* 1963;13:728–738.
7. Buchthal F, Rosenfalck P. Action potential parameters in different human muscles. *Acta Physiol Scand* 1955;30:125–131.
8. DeLateur BJ, Giaconi RM. Effect on maximal strength of submaximal exercise in Duchenne muscular dystrophy. *Am J Phys Med* 1979;58:26–36.
9. DiMarco AF, Kelling J, Sajovic M, et al. Respiratory muscle training in muscular dystrophy. *Clin Res* 1982;30:427A.
10. Dubowitz V. *Muscle Disorders in Childhood.* 2nd ed. Philadelphia: W.B. Saunders; 1995:1–133.
11. Escalante A, Miller L, Beardmore TD. Resistive exercise in the rehabilitation of polymyositis/dermatomyositis. *J Rheumatol* 1993;20: 1340–1344.
12. Gozal D, Thiriet P. Respiratory muscle training in neuromuscular disease: long-term effects on strength and load perception. *Med Sci Sports Exerc* 1999;31:1522–1527.
13. Grange RW, Call JA. Recommendations to define exercise prescription for Duchenne muscular dystrophy. *Exerc Sport Sci Rev* 2007; 35:12–17.
14. Haller RG, Lewis SF. Glucose-induced exertional fatigue in muscle phosphofructokinase deficiency. *N Engl J Med* 1991;324:364–369.
15. Haller RG, Wyrick P, Taivassalo T, Vissing J. Aerobic conditioning: An effective therapy in McArdle's disease. *Ann Neurol* 2006;59(6): 922–928.
16. Hickok RJ. Physical therapy as related to peripheral nerve lesions. *Phys Ther Rev* 1961;41:113–117.
17. Hicks JE, Miller F, Plotz P, et al. Isometric exercise increases strength and does not produce sustained creatinine phosphokinase increases in a patient with polymyositis. *J Rheumatol* 1993;20: 1399–1401.
18. Hicks JE. Role of rehabilitation in the management of myopathies. *Curr Opin Rheumatol* 1998;10:548–555.
19. Hoberman M. Physical medicine and rehabilitation: Its value and limitations in progressive muscular dystrophy. *Am J Phys Med* 1955;34:109–115.
20. Jeppesen TD, Schwartz M, Olsen DB, et al. Aerobic training is safe and improves exercise capacity in patients with mitochondrial myopathy. *Brain* 2006;129:3402–3412.
21. Johnson EW, Braddom R. Over-work weakness in facioscapulohumeral muscular dystrophy. *Arch Phys Med Rehabil* 1971;52: 333–336.
22. Kilmer DD, McCrory MA, Wright NC, et al. The effect of a high resistance exercise program in slowly progressive neuromuscular disease. *Arch Phys Med Rehabil* 1994;75:560–563.
23. Kilmer DD. The role of exercise in neuromuscular disease. *Phys Med Rehabil Clin N Am* 1998;9:115–125.
24. Kilmer DD. Response to resistive strengthening exercise training in humans with neuromuscular disease. *Am J Phys Med Rehabil* 2002; 81(11 Suppl):S121–S126.
25. Kley RA, Vorgerd M, Tarnopolsky MA. Creatine for treating muscle disorders. *Cochrane Database Syst Rev* 2007(1):CD004760.
26. Lenman JA. A clinical and experimental study of the effects of exercise on motor weakness in neurological disease. *J Neurol Neurosurg Psychiatry* 1959;22:182–194.
27. Lewis SF, Haller RG. Skeletal muscle disorders and associated factors that limit exercise performance. *Exerc Sport Sci Rev* 1989;17: 67–113.
28. Lewis SF, Haller RG, Cook JD, et al. Muscle fatigue in McArdle's disease studied by 31P-NMR: Effect of glucose infusion. *J Appl Physiol* 1985;59:1991–1994.
29. Lindeman E, Leffers P, Spaans F, et al. Strength training in patients with myotonic dystrophy and hereditary motor and sensory neuropathy: A randomized clinical trial. *Arch Phys Med Rehabil* 1995; 76:612–620.
30. McCartney N, Moroz D, Garner SH, et al. The effects of strength training in patients with selected neuromuscular disorders. *Med Sci Sports Exerc* 1988;20:362–368.
31. McCool FD, Tzelepis GE. Inspiratory muscle training in the patient with neuromuscular disease. *Phys Ther* 1995;75:1006–1014.
32. Mendell JR, Moxley RT, Griggs RC, et al. Randomized, double-blind six-month trial of prednisone in Duchenne's muscular dystrophy. *N Engl J Med* 1989;320:1592–1597.
33. Milner-Brown HS, Miller RG. Muscle strengthening through high-resistance weight training in patients with neuromuscular disorders. *Arch Phys Med Rehabil* 1988;69:14–19.
34. Olsen DB, Orngreen MC, Vissing J. Aerobic training improves exercise performance in facioscapulohumeral muscular dystrophy. *Neurology* 2005 22;64(6):1064–1066.
35. Orngreen MC, Olsen DB, Vissing J. Aerobic training in patients with myotonic dystrophy type 1. *Ann Neurol* 2005;57(5):754–757.
36. Radcliffe KA, Campbell WW. Statin myopathy. *Curr Neurol Neurosci Rep* 2008;8(1):66–72.
37. Spector SA, Lemmer JT, Koffman BM, et al. Safety and efficacy of strength training in patients with sporadic inclusion body myositis. *Muscle Nerve* 1997;20:1242–1248.
38. Sveen ML, Jeppesen TD, Hauerslev S, Krag TO, Vissing J. Endurance training: An effective and safe treatment for patients with LGMD2I. *Neurology* 2007;68(1):59–61.
39. Tarnopolsky M. Exercise testing as a diagnostic entity in mitochondrial myopathies. *Mitochondrion* 2004;4(5-6):529–542.
40. Tarnopolsky MA, Raha S. Mitochondrial myopathies: Diagnosis, exercise intolerance, and treatment options. *Med Sci Sports Exerc* 2005;37(12):2086–2093.
41. Tarnopolsky MA, Roy BD, MacDonald JR. A randomized, controlled trial of creatine monohydrate in patients with mitochondrial cytopathies. *Muscle Nerve* 1997;20:1502–1509.
42. Tarnopolsky MA, Maguire J, Myint T, et al. Clinical, physiological, and histological features in a kindred with the T3271C melas mutation. *Muscle Nerve* 1998;21:25–33.
43. Tarnopolsky M, Mahoney D, Vajsar J, et al. Creatine monohydrate increases strength and body composition in boys with duchenne muscular dystrophy. *Neurology* 2004;62(10):1771–1777.

44. Tein I. Metabolic myopathies. *Semin Pediatr Neurol* 1996;3:59–98.

45. Tollbäck A, Eriksson S, Wredenberg A, et al. Effects of high resistance training in patients with myotonic dystrophy. *Scand J Rehabil Med* 1999;31:9–16.

46. van Beekvelt MC, van Engelen BG, Wevers RA, et al. Quantitative near-infrared spectroscopy discriminates between mitochondrial myopathies and normal muscle. *Ann Neurol* 1999;46:667–670.

47. van der Kooi EL, Lindeman E, Riphagen I. Strength training and aerobic exercise training for muscle disease. *Cochrane Database Syst Rev* 2005(1):CD003907

48. Vignos PJ Jr. Physical models of rehabilitation in neuromuscular disease. *Muscle Nerve* 1983;6:323–338.

49. Vignos PJ, Watkins MP. The effect of exercise in muscular dystrophy. *JAMA* 1966;197:89–96.

50. Vissing J, Haller RG. The effect of oral sucrose on exercise tolerance in patients with McArdle's disease. *N Engl J Med* 2003;349(26): 2503–2509.

51. Wanke T, Toifl K, Merkle M, et al. Inspiratory muscle training in patients with Duchenne muscular dystrophy. *Chest* 1994;105:475–482.

52. Wratney MJ. Physical therapy for muscular dystrophy children. *Phys Ther Rev* 1958;38:26–32.

53. Wiesinger GF, Quittan M, Aringer M, et al. Improvement of physical fitness and muscle strength in polymyositis/dermatomyositis patients by a training programme. *Br J Rheumatol* 1998;37:196–200.

Peripheral Neuropathy and Neuropathic Pain

PATHOPHYSIOLOGY

Pain is a common experience, and the capacity to sense pain plays a protective role in warning of current or potential tissue damage. Response to tissue injury (as well as painful stimuli) includes adaptive changes that promote healing and avoid further irritation to the injured tissue.

Peripheral neuropathy is defined as deranged function and structure of peripheral motor, sensory, and autonomic neurons (outside the central nervous system [CNS]), involving either the entire neuron or selected levels (1). Pain and other sensory changes can be produced in a variety of ways and, in peripheral nerves, motor or sensory fibers may be preferentially affected, but in most neuropathies both are involved, leading to various patterns of sensorimotor deficit (2). Pain is not always associated with peripheral neuropathy. Painful neuropathies are usually a result of damage to the axon, in contrast to demyelinating neuropathies that tend, with some exceptions, to cause pronounced motor or sensory loss without pain (3).

The two basic mechanisms by which the experience of pain can be evoked are *somatic tissue injury* (nociceptive) or *nerve injury* (4). In the typical process of nociceptive pain, stimulation of tissue nociceptors (found throughout the musculoskeletal system) causes action potentials to be propagated along nociceptive axons that ultimately enter the limbic sectors of the cerebral cortex where the pain is perceived. Nociceptive pain is typically described by patients as deep, tender, dull, aching, and diffuse (4). Pain induced by nociceptive pain mechanisms is the most common variety seen in clinical practice (5).

In contrast to nociceptive pain syndromes that are typically related to musculoskeletal damage or injury, damage to the peripheral or CNS produces a different type of pain. This type of pain is known as *neuropathic pain*. Often neuropathic pain is chronic and persistent, and patients are more likely to use adjectives such as shooting, stabbing, lancinating, burning, and searing to describe it and often complain of pain worsening at night (6). Patients with neuropathic pain may appear to have continuous or paroxysmal pain without any detectable relationship to stimulus (7). The symptoms can be divided into those that are unprovoked and those that are provoked by maneuvers such as skin stimulation, pressure over affected nerves, changes in temperature, or emotional factors (2).

One key diagnostic feature of neuropathic pain is the presence of pain within an area of sensory deficit (8). Allodynia is also a commonly seen hyperpathic state in neuropathic pain, in which a normally innocuous stimulus produces a sensation of pain whose quality is inappropriate for the stimulus. An example of this is the patient who cannot tolerate a blanket resting on an affected extremity. Another feature suggestive of neuropathic pain is summation, which is the progressive worsening of pain evoked by slow, repetitive stimulation with mildly noxious stimuli, for example, pinprick (8).

Neuropathic pain can be classified on the basis of the cause of the insult to the nervous system, the disease or event that precipitated the pain syndrome, or the distribution of pain. Certain medical conditions are associated with neuropathic pain, and these commonly include diabetes, human immunodeficiency virus (HIV) infection or acquired immunodeficiency syndrome (AIDS), multiple sclerosis, cancer chemotherapy, malignancy, spinal surgery, alcoholism, herpes zoster, and amputation (6). Cancer patients can develop neuropathy from tumor invasion and also are at higher risk for neuropathic pain following chemotherapy or radiation therapy.

Diabetes is associated with peripheral neuropathy and radiculopathy (9,10). HIV is associated with a variety of neuropathies and myelopathies. Multiple sclerosis is associated with neuralgia and neuropathy (11). Failed spine surgery is associated with radiculopathy. Amputation is associated with neuroma and phantom limb pain (6).

Trauma can lead to the development of entrapment neuropathies, as well as partial or complete nerve transection, plexopathies, and painful scars. Entrapment neuropathies, such as carpal tunnel syndrome, are usually characterized in the early stages by paresthesia and pain (2).

CLASSIFICATION

A variety of disease processes can cause, or contribute to, peripheral neuropathy and the possible pain associated with it (12). A working knowledge of these is needed to help identify or establish a specific cause or underlying process and develop a prognosis and treatment plan accordingly. Despite a thorough investigation into the cause of peripheral polyneuropathy, the cause often remains unknown in 25%–50% of cases (13). It is then the goal of treatment to lessen the patient's symptoms or dysfunction.

Based on anatomic distribution, there are four main types of peripheral nervous system disease. It is useful to know their clinical patterns for diagnosis and treatment (14):

1. Symmetric polyneuropathy: affects mainly the distal extremities, usually affects the feet with altered sensation. It is the most common chronic type of peripheral polyneuropathy. Diabetes, metabolic causes, or toxin exposures often cause this type of neuropathy.
2. Mononeuropathy: affects a single nerve and is also a common cause of acute or chronic peripheral neuropathy. This type is often from a focal compression of the nerve, but is often found with chronic disease states, such as diabetes, which make the nerve more susceptible.
3. Plexopathy dysfunction in the nerve plexus): is often the result of injury, but can result from an underlying endogenous process, such as might develop after radiation treatment for a tumor. It may affect several peripheral nerves in a nondermatomal pattern with weakness or sensory changes.
4. Radiculopathies: result from involvement or injury to a nerve more proximally (toward the spinal cord) causing nerve root dysfunction, often with weakness, pain, and peripheral sensory deficit in a specific dermatomal pattern (15). Nerve encroachment from spondylitic degenerative changes or disk herniation can commonly cause this.
5. Facial neuralgias: although not classically considered in a discussion of peripheral neuropathies, must also be considered when discussing pain in the peripheral nervous system.

CLINICAL EXERCISE PHYSIOLOGY

Basic information about nociception and pain has not received systematic coverage in either exercise science textbooks or the sports medicine literature (16). The patient with a chronic pain problem typically has a complicated medical and psychological history. An adequate comprehensive treatment of the problem requires a careful and multidisciplinary assessment. The goal of the assessment is to identify nociceptive factors that may be correctable, psychological factors that can be addressed (pharmacologically or behaviorally), the contribution of disuse to the pain problem, and the socioenvironmental context in which the pain problem is maintained (17).

Physical exercise is widely used in the treatment in patients with chronic pain. Patients with chronic pain have demonstrated highly significant improvements in aerobic fitness measures following a short (4-week) course of exercise intervention (18). Outcomes assessed have included $\dot{V}O_2$ max and metabolic equivalents (METs), and lower body power output. Possible mechanisms underlying such dramatic improvement include improved physical fitness, learning, or desensitization to symptoms associated with exertion, and improved effort. Patients with chronic pain related to peripheral neuropathy have displayed lower health-related quality of life, and patients placed on a 6-week home exercise program demonstrated slight improvements in this measure as well as increases in muscle strength (19).

Patients with peripheral neuropathy involving the median nerve at the wrist (carpal tunnel syndrome) have been treated with nerve and tendon-gliding exercises. A significant number of patients reported excellent results and were spared the morbidity of a carpal tunnel release procedure (20). Other studies have shown that various exercise interventions may prevent or decrease the incidence of carpal tunnel syndrome and other painful cumulative trauma disorders (21,22).

Physical activity, including appropriate endurance and resistance training, is a major therapeutic modality for type 2 diabetes. Too often, however, physical activity is an underutilized therapy. Favorable changes in glucose tolerance and insulin sensitivity usually deteriorate within 72 hours of the last exercise session; consequently, regular physical activity is imperative to sustain glucose-lowering effects and improved insulin sensitivity (23). Modifications to exercise type and intensity may be necessary for those who have complications of diabetes. Autonomic neuropathy affects the heart rate response to exercise. As a result, ratings of perceived exertion (RPE) may need to be used instead of heart rate for moderating intensity of physical activity. Patients with diabetic neuropathy causing sensory loss in the lower extremity may have to alter exercises to focus on the use of non–weight-bearing forms of activity (23).

Exercise has been demonstrated to improve several measures of balance in diabetic patients with peripheral neuropathy (24). This study involved a short (3-week) intervention designed to increase lower-extremity strength and balance. Significant improvement was found in unipedal stance time, tandem stance time, and functional reach. Additional studies are needed to determine if this decreases fall frequency in this population.

Pain can be modulated at peripheral sites by opioids, and peripheral blood concentrations of β-endorphins are increased during exercise (16). Therefore, exercise may play a beneficial role in reducing pain in certain cases, but further research is warranted to understand the specific mechanisms. Also, additional research is needed to understand the conditions (e.g., mode, duration, and intensity of exercise, whether or not the exercise itself is painful, and the nature of the noxious stimulus) under which exercise-related analgesia is produced (16).

PHARMACOLOGY

A variety of pharmacologic approaches to the management of neuropathic pain are in use, although no current consensus exists on optimal strategy. Pharmacologic management is based on the response of the patient and careful titration of dosage to achieve positive results while minimizing side effects. Pharmacologic treatments have generally been selected on the basis of evidence for efficacy in randomized, placebo-controlled trials conducted in disease-based groups of patients, notably in postherpetic neuralgia and diabetic polyneuropathy (25). These studies demonstrate efficacy of tricyclic antidepressants, standard and newer anticonvulsants, and opioids. Evidence for efficacy is less for selective serotonin reuptake inhibitors (SSRIs), antiarrhythmics (mexiletine), and capsaicin. Nonopioid analgesics (aspirin, acetaminophen, and other nonsteroidal anti-inflammatory drugs [NSAIDs]) are often used by patients with neuropathic pain, but they are typically more effective for mild to moderate nociceptive pain. Emerging treatments include pharmocologic blockade of specific ion receptors, ligand-gated channels, and nicotinic receptors, and increasing spinal inhibition (26).

Many patients with mild to moderate pain are helped by the use of aspirin, acetaminophen, and NSAIDs. Acetaminophen is often used initially because of its lower incidence of gastrointestinal toxicity when taken chronically. It has no anti-inflammatory effect and is not appropriate as a primary therapy for an inflammatory process.

A wide variety of NSAIDs are in use, and many patients respond better to one over another, although this is unpredictable in advance of starting on the drug. NSAID use is associated with an increased incidence of gastrointestinal toxicity and should be avoided in patients with peptic ulcer disease or bleeding abnormalities (27). NSAIDs should also be avoided in patients older than 70 years of age and as unsupervised long-term treatment (28). Patients with neuropathic pain will typically be engaged in low-level exercise programs, but it is important to acknowledge a recent study that demonstrated that use of NSAIDs was found to be a risk factor in exercise-associated hyponatremia in high-level physical activity (29).

Many patients with neuropathic pain experience relief with the use of antidepressants. Pain relief is often achieved at doses that are subtherapeutic for the treatment of depression. The analgesic effects of these agents may result from their ability to block reuptake at presynaptic nerve endings of neurotransmitters, such as serotonin and norepinephrine, which are involved in pain and depression (30). Tricyclic antidepressants remain the class most commonly used, and their use has been documented in a variety of pain-related conditions, including postherpetic neuralgia, diabetic neuropathy, arthritis, low back pain, myofascial pain, cancer pain, migraine and tension-type headaches, central pain, and psychogenic pain (30). Common side effects include sedation and dry mouth. In light of recent reports of sudden death in children being treated with desipramine (tricyclic antidepressant), three of which were associated with physical exercise, the effects of this drug on exercise were evaluated (31). Desipramine was found to have only minor effects on the cardiovascular response to exercise, and the effects did not appear to be age related (31). The authors stated that desipramine may increase the risk of exercise-associated arrhythmias in some individuals.

When the previously described drugs are not sufficient, the addition of an anticonvulsant drug to the antidepressant may be useful (32). Anticonvulsants are generally considered to be first-line agents for the treatment of neuropathic pain with a predominantly paroxysmal or lancinating quality, such as trigeminal neuralgia (30). The mechanisms by which anticonvulsants relieve pain may be related to stabilizing neuronal membranes (phenytoin), altering sodium channel activity (carbamazepine), and modulating γ-aminobutyric acid activity (clonazepam and valproate) (30). Carbamazepine (anticonvulsant) produced a significant delay in pain increase in patients with peripheral neuropathy that was previously mediated by spinal cord stimulation (33). In this study, the pain-relieving spinal cord stimulation was inactivated before introduction of medication. Anticonvulsant medication demonstrated better delay in return of pain compared with an opioid analgesic.

The role of opioid analgesics is controversial in the management of neuropathic pain. Most patients do not respond to these drugs and should not receive them (32). Many patients need detoxification from opioids, sedative-hypnotics, and muscle relaxants (32). Some evidence indicates that some patients with neuropathic pain do function well while taking low-dose, regularly scheduled opioids (32).

Neuropathic pain with a major cutaneous component may respond well to topical therapy with the substance P depletor, capsaicin, to reduce elevated prostaglandin levels (32). Animal studies are demonstrating a rationale for the selected use of topical capsaicin in the treatment of pain (34).

Chronic pain and depression are often found to coexist. The use of tricyclic antidepressants in higher therapeutic doses is indicated in these cases. SSRIs, such as fluoxetine (Prozac), paroxetine (Paxil), and sertraline (Zoloft), have generally replaced tricyclic antidepressants for the treatment of depression (30). Although they are typically well tolerated with fewer side effects, SSRIs have not shown significant efficacy for treatment of pain. Sometimes, patients with chronic pain and depression are placed on bedtime dosing of tricyclics and concomitant daytime dosing of SSRIs. Caution is required because some SSRIs can significantly increase tricyclic antidepressant serum levels (30).

HISTORY AND PHYSICAL EXAMINATION

The history the patient gives can be a very important guide toward diagnosis. Specific attempts should be made to determine the following:

1. The time course of the patient's symptoms: When did they start (acute, subacute, chronic, or relapsing)? Was there a specific event associated with onset? What age did symptoms first occur? How fast have the symptoms progressed?
2. What type of distribution or pattern are the symptoms: symmetric or asymmetric, proximal or distal, single nerve, multiple nerves, or diffuse?
3. What type of nerve fibers are affected more: motor (weakness), sensory (pain or anesthesia), or autonomic symptoms (blood pressure, pulse rate, and rhythm changes)?
4. What is the quality and quantity associated with pain or sensory change (dull ache, sharp, burning, numb) and its effects on daily functions or activities.
5. Does it seem to start in a given area and then radiate?
6. Is there anything the patient can identify that causes the symptom to be worse, or that helps alleviate it (body positions, use, rest, movement)?
7. Is there a certain time of day or night when it worsens or improves?
8. Family history: Attempt to search for possible genetic patterns or links to other family members.
9. Social history: Illicit drug use, alcohol use, job history (repetitive strain, toxic exposure, heavy lifting or labor), travel history (exposures and subsequent illnesses), diet changes or patterns (with exposure to toxins or illnesses), and vitamin ingestion (deficiency or toxicities).
10. Medical history: illnesses or conditions affecting organ systems (infections, diabetes, thyroid or endocrine disease, tumors, kidney disease, connective tissue diseases, metabolic diseases or defects, prior disease treatments or prior medications).
11. Current medications
12. Allergies

Many other conditions can mimic the pain or dysfunction of neuropathy, such as myopathy, arthritides, musculoskeletal pain, myofascial pain, visceral conditions, infections, neoplasms, psychological causes, and pain or weakness from CNS conditions.

Peripheral neuropathy affects lower motor neurons, and the neurologic physical examination may uncover any of the constellation of findings that typically result from this. Neurologic findings may include weakness, atrophy, loss of sensation, hypersensation, paresthesia, and decreased deep tendon reflexes in the distribution of the affected nerve or nerves (14). In acute neuropathy, there may be nerve tension signs (e.g., a positive straight leg raise in lumbar radiculopathy) and splinting of muscles, or antalgic body postures. There may be changes in gait due to weakness, pain, or loss of distal sensation. Position sense may be impaired in the extremities and muscles may be atrophied in more chronic nerve disease. In suspected peripheral neuropathy, each of the areas of the neurologic physical examination should be evaluated.

It is important, especially with suspected mononeuropathy or radiculopathy, to compare physical examination findings from the affected side of the body with the unaffected side, looking for objective differences or asymmetry in sensation, reflexes, strength, size, and body position.

In peripheral polyneuropathy, usually a more symmetric neurologic involvement is seen in the distal limbs. The physical examination will often show decreased deep tendon reflexes, decreased or increased sensation (in a nondermatomal stocking-type distribution), and possible weakness in the distal extremities (12). The lower extremities are usually most affected in earlier states of involvement, but eventually all extremities may be affected.

Sensory testing for smaller fiber involvement can be performed by pinprick and ice touching. Larger fibers can be tested better with a tuning fork for vibration, two-point discrimination at the fingertips, or by position sense (by lifting a toe or fingertip slightly superiorly or inferiorly with the patient's eyes closed and then asking them to identify what they felt) (35). Strength can be tested manually with resisted joint range of motion (ROM) against the examiner's own resistance, and with maneuvers that test strength in the lower extremities that the patient can perform (e.g., heel-toe walking, squatting, step-ups, or toe raises). Reflexes should be checked with a reflex hammer with the patient's joint in a neutral, relaxed position. To help facilitate a reflex in an areflexic limb, the patient should clasp his or her hands together in front of the torso and attempt to pull them apart while the reflex is retested. Nerve tension or compression signs may be checked by applying traction to the nerve, by applying focal pressure, or by mechanically tapping over the nerve. Examples would be (a) the straight leg raise test to stretch the sciatic nerve and lumbar nerve roots in evaluating for suspected lumbar radiculopathy; (b) Spurling's (maximal foraminal compression) test in the cervical spine to check for nerve encroachment in the intervertebral foramen; or (c) compression or tapping over the median nerve at the wrist to reproduce symptoms of carpal tunnel syndrome (median neuropathy at the wrist).

MEDICAL AND SURGICAL TREATMENTS

Treatment of neuropathy of any etiology should be aimed at treating or correcting any underlying identifiable cause, if possible (12,14,36). Because many etiologies exist for peripheral neuropathies, numerous approaches also exist to their treatment, whether acute or chronic. Immediate goals of therapy are generally to achieve acceptable pain levels, minimize any functional deficits, and protect from risk of ongoing damage or hypoesthesia.

Acute, painful neuropathies (e.g., acute radiculopathy or acute peripheral nerve trauma) are often treated, depending on severity and cause, with analgesic medications (narcotic and nonnarcotic); appropriate limitations of activity, physical therapy and pain-modulating modalities; appropriate assistive or supportive devices (e.g., upper-extremity sling support, cervical or lumbar support, or functional or static limb bracing); anesthetic nerve blocks; or surgical correction (37,38). Conservative treatments should be implemented first when possible before attempting more invasive measures. Examples: First, lancinating sharp pain of trigeminal neuralgia may be treated conservatively with baclofen or anticonvulsant medications (12,39,40) (starting at a low dose to minimize more common side effects of drowsiness, dizziness, or gastrointestinal problems), or by more invasive surgical or regional anesthetic techniques (including trigeminal nerve anesthetic block, glycerol gangliolysis injections, or surgical decompression of the trigeminal ganglion). Second, acute lumbar radiculopathy may often be treated conservatively with relative rest (up to 2–3 days); oral or intramuscular narcotic and nonnarcotic medications (which may include Tylenol, NSAIDs, antispasmodics or muscle relaxants, tramadol, or antidepressants, which may augment other medications effects); intermittent orthotic splinting with a lumbosacral corset; active and passive physical therapy techniques (often with modalities to minimize pain, dysfunction, disuse, spasm, endocrine dysfunction or irritation); transcutaneous electrical stimulation; oral steroids; epidural injections with steroids, opioids, anesthetics, or a combination of these drugs; or surgical decompression of the nerve (in severe cases).

In more chronic causes of neuropathy or neuropathic pain that may not be correctable, some of the same techniques and medications may be used, but there is a shift toward more chronic or long-term treatment approaches to help manage the disorder. With a chronic underlying disease state causing or contributing to the neuropathy, the initial goal is medically manage that condition to the best degree possible, because it may often have a positive effect on the neuropathy process and the patient's symptoms (14). Examples include: (a) improvement in peripheral polyneuropathy with tight control of blood glucose levels in diabetes mellitus, or (b) appropriate therapeutic control of hypothyroidism with replacement hormone. If the chronic neuropathy has no known underlying cause or cannot be improved by medical intervention, the management of the symptoms or dysfunction is the focus. Often, medications for chronic neuropathic pain may be implemented to help control symptoms

(14,39,40). These often include sympatholytics; oral anticonvulsants; tricyclic antidepressants or sometimes selective serotonin reuptake inhibitors; baclofen; topical medications (26,41) (anesthetics, nonsteroidal drugs, capsaicin, or other neuromodulating medications that are often used orally, alone, or in combinations with each other), which are less proven, but may be tried alone or with oral medications to lessen their side effects; corticosteroids; oral or intravenous anesthetics; and, less often, narcotics (usually only used when other methods to control pain have failed).

Anesthetic approaches may be used transiently or more permanently to block sympathetic or somatic nerve transmission. Techniques include infiltration of involved nerves, perineurally, in the epidural space, or intraspinally, with local anesthetics, corticosteroids, sympatholytics, narcotics, or a combination of these drugs, and sometimes neurolytic substances (42,43). They may be given by single injections or by continuous type of infusion by catheter in patients who fail to obtain sufficient pain relief with less-invasive measures. Examples: (a) lumbar epidural steroid injection for radiculopathy, (b) continual morphine intraspinal infusion for failed low back syndrome. Radio-frequency nerve ablation, cryolysis, or neurosurgical interruptive procedures may also be used as neurodestructive procedures of last resort (44).

Neurostimulatory techniques for neural afferent sensory pathway modulation are other approaches to painful neuropathy. Counter-irritation (rubbing) of the painful area, transcutaneous electrical stimulation, spinal cord stimulation (requires electrode implantation), and acupuncture are examples. Many patients may achieve analgesia soon after implementation of these techniques, but often fewer obtain lasting relief (15).

Physical medicine and rehabilitation are often important in patients with significant dysfunctions from neuropathies for their overall outcome and management. Rehabilitation techniques are used in both acute and chronic neuropathies. They help the patient to accommodate or compensate for deficits; improve strength, coordination, and self-confidence; appropriately use assistive devices (if needed); reduce pain; and help maximize overall functional ability (45). A vast array of active and passive therapy modalities and techniques may be implemented, based on the state and severity of the patient's disease, the degree of dysfunction or pain, comorbid conditions, and the goals for rehabilitation. Generally speaking, passive therapies are used early in the course of treatment, moving to greater use of active therapy as treatment continues. Passive therapy may include various cold or heat techniques, electrotherapies and stimulation, traction, massage, mobilization, manipulation or manual therapy, and compression. Active therapy may include implementation and training with specific orthoses, therapeutic exercise, gait training, adaptation or training for activities of daily living, vocational adaptation or conditioning, and ergonomic considerations (37). Multiple disciplines may be needed to fully assess and implement many of these strategies to best serve the patient's needs (depending on the disease process). These may include the physician, physical therapist, chiropractor, occupational therapist, orthotist, clinical exercise physiologist, kinesiotherapist, recreational therapist, social worker, and psychologist.

DIAGNOSTIC TECHNIQUES

Diagnostic imaging studies, such as computed tomography (CT) or magnetic resonance imaging (MRI) may help detect abnormal causes contributing to an entrapment neuropathy, such as bony encroachments, soft-tissue masses, tumors, infections, vascular lesions, or cysts (46–48). MRI is the study of choice for imaging most soft-tissue types of suspected lesions, whereas scanning visualizes many bony processes better (48). These tests provide an anatomic "picture" of the tissues in question and are best used as an extension to a good history and physical examination to provide further information of an already clinically suspected lesion or process. If not used in this manner, their results are less meaningful toward providing accurate diagnostic information and can sometimes mislead the true diagnosis.

Electrodiagnostic studies are physiologic tests performed on the specific nerves and muscle they innervate. They are often very valuable in objectively confirming the diagnosis of neuropathy and documenting the type of nerve pathology involved (49–52). They can help classify whether the neuropathy is focal or diffuse, sensory or motor, or axonal or demyelinating types of processes. This helps guide a more accurate diagnosis and treatment. Electrodiagnostic nerve conduction studies do have some limitations. These studies test the larger-diameter nerve fiber conduction which may be completely normal in patients with painful diffuse peripheral neuropathy involving only the smaller nerve fibers. Electromyographic findings may also be complicated by the process of reinnervation (53).

Laboratory studies are appropriate with undetermined causes of peripheral neuropathy to help further narrow the diagnosis and appropriate treatment (54). Treatment of neuropathies is usually aimed at correcting deficiencies, removing insultive agents, and treating contributing systemic illnesses. Studies of blood, urine, spinal fluid, antibody assays, and sometimes nerve biopsies are needed to help determine a cause (54). Blood, urine, and cerebrospinal fluid (CSF) tests may need to be done to assess for the following conditions: diabetes, liver or thyroid disease, autoimmune processes, collagen-vascular disease, vitamin deficiency or toxicities, toxin exposures or ingestions, prescription and nonprescription or illicit drug use, infections, neoplasms, or hereditary causes.

Anesthetic approaches, such as regional analgesia, may be implemented in neuropathy to help with diagnosis, prognosis, prophylaxis, or for therapeutic measures (42). Neural blockade (anesthetic) injection procedures may be used to block transiently the somatic or sympathetic nerves for diagnostic analysis, or may be used to block these nerves more permanently to abolish the pain (42,43). Diagnostic (temporary) blocks are directed to affect the afferent pathways involved with pain. They may also be used to prognosticate the affect of a more permanent neurolytic or ablative procedure. Nerve blockade may be performed peripherally in direct proximity of the affected nerve as used with the trigeminal or intercostal neuralgia or sympathetic blocks of the lumbar plexus or stellate ganglion. Regional blockade may be performed intraspinally in the epidural space for conditions such as radiculopathy, or may be performed intrathecally. Repeated blocks may be used therapeutically for patients who obtain relief from an initial trial (42,43).

PAIN MEASUREMENT

Pain measurement is important to monitor effects of treatment. Measurement of pain poses some difficulties because of the subjectivity of the experience and variations in cognitive and emotional factors from person to person. One of the most common ways to measure and document pain is the use of the visual analog scale (VAS) (55). The patient marks or points to a mark on a 10-cm line that corresponds to his or her level of pain with one end point corresponding to "no pain" and the other end point corresponding to "worst pain." The distance in centimeters from the low end of the VAS to the patient's report is used as a numerical index of the severity of pain. High reliability and validity have been reported with this commonly used scaling device (55–59).

Another commonly used instrument is the McGill Pain Questionnaire (60). This questionnaire is designed to assess the multidimensional nature of pain experience and has been demonstrated to be a reliable, valid, and consistent measurement tool (60). A short-form McGill Pain Questionnaire is also available when time limitations are present and a need exists to obtain more than just pain intensity. This questionnaire is widely used and is available in many different languages.

Ongoing assessment of outcomes is vital when dealing with a patient with chronic pain, and quantification of pain is an important part of this process. Providers should periodically assess patients relative to the beginning of care, not just on a visit-by-visit basis. In this way, the risk of losing sight of the overall progress goals in lieu of palliative management can be avoided (61).

EXERCISE/FITNESS/FUNCTIONAL TESTING

Before starting on an exercise program, all patients with peripheral neuropathy or neurogenic pain syndromes should undergo a medical evaluation and graded exercise test to determine their general state of health, the presence and degree of long-term complications, and any limitations or contraindications to exercise. The patient with a chronic pain problem typically has a complicated medical and psychological history. An adequate comprehensive treatment of the problem requires a careful and multidisciplinary assessment. The goal of the assessment is to identify nociceptive factors that may be correctable, psychological factors that can be addressed (pharmacologically or behaviorally), the contribution of disuse to the pain problem, and the socioenvironmental context in which the pain problem is maintained (62).

Exercise tolerance testing in patients with neuropathic pain should be performed only after medical clearance is obtained. Increased activity and exercise may aggravate and increase pain in these patients, so it is important to pay attention to patients having exercise testing and evaluation. Documentation of specific aggravating activities or movement is important.

Muscle weakness, joint contractures, and muscle shortening can occur in patients with peripheral neuropathy. Active and passive ROM of the trunk and extremities should be evaluated using goniometer or inclinometer assessment. Strength of the trunk and extremities can be evaluated manually or with the use of isokinetic testing equipment. Documentation of pain provoked by active and passive movement, as well as pain produced with resisted ROM or strength testing, should be noted, including a description of location and character of pain.

EXERCISE PRESCRIPTION AND PROGRAMMING

Therapeutic exercises represent an important part of the treatment program for most patients with pain, keeping in mind that most patients will have varying degrees of deconditioning that can range from mild to severe. Exercises are utilized to increase flexibility, improve strength and endurance, and stabilize weak or lax joints.

Patients with pain often decrease their level of physical activity because of concern that they may exacerbate pain or produce tissue damage. The consequences may include reduced flexibility, decreased muscle strength, muscle wasting, and overall deconditioning (30). Intervention should include exercises specific for the painful area, in addition to general aerobic exercises. The exercises should encourage flexibility and strength improvement while demonstrating to the patient that no harm is being produced.

As discussed above, muscle weakness, joint contractures, and muscle shortening commonly occur in patients with peripheral neuropathy. This should be addressed with ongoing range-of-motion exercises performed both passively and actively. Graded mild resistance training is added as tolerated, keeping in mind that stress on the affected area can produce a hyperpathic pain response or reports of exaggerated pain intensities following exercise or activity.

Exercise guidelines for the patient with chronic pain differ from those of the acutely injured. Often, medical practitioners use pain as a guideline, telling the patient, "If it hurts, don't do it." This may be appropriate with an acute injury, but not with a chronic condition. As a general rule, exercises that induce more peripheral pain should be avoided, and exercises that centralize the pain should be continued (63).

Prescribed exercises will depend on patient interest and motivation and should minimize risk of exacerbating pain. Examples of appropriate exercises include walking, rapid walking, running, aerobic dance, bicycling, swimming, rowing, and crosscountry skiing. The program should be graduated, starting with exercise to tolerance as determined by pain, weakness, or fatigue. Initially, brief daily periods of exercise should be encouraged, with a goal to exercise 15–30 minutes at least three times per week. The following specific walking program has been recommended as appropriate for patients with chronic pain (30).

1. Achieve activity level of walking 2,000 feet (e.g., 10 laps of 200 feet each) without interruption. If necessary, this goal may be attained by increasing the distance walked by 200–400 feet each day.
2. Increase the distance walked to 2,400 feet at previous pace, or decrease time to walk 2,000 feet by 30 seconds.
3. When this quota is reached, increase distance another 400 feet, or decrease time another 30 seconds.
4. Continue reduction in time quotas until upper speed limit is reached, as determined by repeated time quota failures.
5. Increase time quota to level previously achieved, and expand distance walked on successive days.
6. Provide positive reinforcement for achieving these goals by documenting increments in speed and distance on performance graphs.

Patients with chronic neuropathies (either focal or diffuse) or with neurogenic pain syndromes may not respond positively to increased exercise. With this group of patients, it may be beneficial to prescribe physical activities not clearly defined as exercise (64). Increased walking may be a useful goal for these patients. Increase in recreational activities, such as gardening, may also have some beneficial effects in this group of patients. In addition, these patients will often require formal programs to maintain ROM, improve aerobic conditioning, prevent deconditioning, and enhance strength.

REFERENCES

1. Dyck PJ. Causes, classification and treatment of peripheral neuropathy. *N Eng J Med* 1982;307:283–286.
2. Scadding JW. Peripheral neuropathies. In: Wall PD, Melzack R, eds. *Textbook of Pain*. Edinburgh: Churchill Livingstone; 1999: 1815.
3. Vaillancourt PD, Langevin HM. Painful peripheral neuropathies. *Med Clin North Am* 1999;83:627.
4. Perle SM, Schneider MJ, Seaman DR. Chiropractic management of peripheral neuropathy: Pathophysiology, assessment, and treatment. *Top Clin Chiropr* 1999;6:6–19.
5. Seaman DR, Cleveland C. Spinal pain syndromes: Nociceptive, neuropathic, and psychologic mechanisms. *J Manipulative Physiol Ther* 1998;22:458–472.
6. Belgrade MJ. Following the clues to neuropathic pain. *Postgraduate Med* 1999;106:127–140.
7. Bennett GF. Neuropathic pain. In: Wall PD, Melzack R, eds. *Textbook of Pain*. Edinburgh: Churchill Livingstone; 1994:201–224.
8. Fields HL, Baron R, Rowbotham MC. Peripheral neuropathic pain: An approach to management. In: Wall PD, Melzack R, eds. *Textbook of Pain*. Edinburgh: Churchill Livingstone; 1999:1523–1533.
9. Boulton AJ. Diabetic neuropathy: Classification, measurement and treatment. *Curr Opin Endocrinol Diabetes* 2007;14:141–145.
10. Tracy JA, Dyck PJ. The spectrum of diabetic neuropathies. *Phys Med Rehabil Clin N Am* 2008;19:1–26.
11. Pollmann W, Feneberg W. Current management of pain associated with multiple sclerosis. *CNS Drugs* 2008;22:291–324.
12. Loar, C. Peripheral nervous system pain. In: Raj P. *Pain Medicine: A Comprehension Review*. St. Louis: Mosby Year Book; 1996:453–459.
13. Oh SJ, ed. *Clinical Electromyography: Nerve Conduction Studies*. Baltimore: Williams & Wilkins; 1993.
14. Fisher MA. Peripheral neuropathy. In: Weiner WJ, Goetz CG, eds. *Neurology for the Non-neurologist*, 3rd ed. Philadelphia: JB Lippincott; 1994:154–170.
15. Hogan QH. Back pain and radiculopathy. In: Abram S, Haddox J, eds. *The Pain Clinic Manual*, 2nd ed. Philadelphia: Lippincott Williams & Wilkins; 2000:157–166.
16. O'Connor PJ, Cook DB. Exercise and pain: The neurobiology, measurement, and laboratory study of pain in relation to exercise in humans. *Exerc Sports Sci Rev* 1999;27:119–166.
17. Cardenas DD, Egan KJ. Management of chronic pain. In: Kottke FJ, Lehmann JF, eds. *Krusen's Handbook of Physical Medicine and Rehabilitation*. Philadelphia: WB Saunders; 1990:1162–1191.
18. Davis VP, Fillingim RB, Doleys DM, et al. Assessment of aerobic power in chronic pain patients before and after a multidisciplinary treatment program. *Arch Phys Med Rehabil* 1992;73: 726–729.
19. Ruhland JL, Shields RK. The effects of a home exercise program on impairment and health-related quality of life in persons with chronic peripheral neuropathies. *Phys Ther* 1997;77:1026–1039.
20. Rozmaryn LM, Dovelle S, Rothman ER, et al. Nerve and tendon gliding exercises and the conservative management of carpal tunnel syndrome. *J Hand Ther* 1998;11:171–179.
21. Seradge H, Bear C, Bithell D. Preventing carpal tunnel syndrome and cumulative trauma disorder: Effect of carpal tunnel decompression exercises. An Oklahoma experience. *J Okla State Med Assoc* 2000;93:150–153.
22. Lincoln AE, Bernick JS, Ogaitis S, et al. Interventions for the primary prevention of work-related carpal tunnel syndrome. *Am J Prev Med* 2000;18:37–50.
23. Albright A, Franz M, Hornsby G, et al. American College of Sports Medicine Position Stand. Exercise and type 2 diabetes. *Med Sci Sports Exerc* 2000;32:1324–1360.
24. Richardson JK, Sandman D, Vela S. A focused exercise regimen improves clinical measures of balance in patients with peripheral neuropathy. *Arch Phys Med Rehabil* 2001;82:205–209.
25. Attal N. Pharmacologic treatment of neuropathic pain. *Acta Neurol Belg* 2001;101:53–64.
26. Dray A. Neuropathic pain: Emerging treatments. *Br J Anaesth* 2008; 101:48–58.
27. Julien RM. *A Primer of Dug Action. A Concise, Nontechnical Guide to the Actions, Uses, and Side Effects of Psychoactive Drugs*, 8th ed. New York: W. H. Freeman: 1998:181–222.
28. Pariente A, Danan G. Gastrointestinal disorders. In: Benichou C, eds. *Adverse Drug Reactions: A Practical Guide to Diagnosis and Management*. New York: John Wiley & Sons; 1994:77–86.
29. Davis DP, Videen JS, Marino A, et al. Exercise-associated hyponatremia in marathon runners: A two-year experience. *J Emerg Med* 2001;21:47–57.
30. Hamilton ME, Gershwin ME. Treatment of pain. In: Gershwin ME, Hamilton ME, eds. *The Pain Management Handbook*. Totowa, NJ: Humana Press; 1998:283–235.
31. Waslick BD, Walsh BT, Greenhill LL, et al. Cardiovascular effects of desipramine in children and adults during exercise testing. *J Am Acad Child Adolesc Psychiatry* 1999;38:179–186.
32. Lipman AG. Analgesic drugs for neuropathic and sympathetically maintained pain. *Clin Geriatr Med* 1996;12:501–515.
33. Harke H, Gretenkort P, Ladleif HU, et al. The response of neuropathic pain and pain in complex regional pain syndrome I to carbamazepine and sustained-release morphine in patients pretreated with spinal cord stimulation: A double-blinded randomized study. *Anesth Analg* 2001;92:488–495.
34. Minami T, Bakoshi S, Nakano H, et al. The Effects of capsaicin cream on prostaglandin-induced allodynia. *Anesth Analg* 2001;93: 419–423.
35. Ho J, DeLuca KG. Neurologic assessment of the pain patient. In: Benzon H, Raja S, Borsook D, et al., eds. *Essentials of Pain Medicine and Regional Anesthesia*. New York: Churchill Livingstone; 1999: 14–15.
36. Galluzzi KE. Managing neuropathic pain. *J Am Osteopath Assoc* 2007;107:ES39-ES48.
37. Tan JC. Practical *Manual of Physical Medicine and Rehabilitation*. St. Louis: Mosby Yearbook; 1998:133–155, 607–644.
38. Williams V, Pappagallo M. Entrapment neuropathies. In: Benzon H, Raja S, Borsook D, et al., eds. *Essentials of Pain Medicine and Regional Anesthesia*. Philadelphia: Churchill Livingstone; 1999:298.
39. Rathmell J, Katz J. Diabetic and other peripheral neuropathies. In: Benzon H, Raja S, Borsook D, et al., eds. *Essentials of Pain Medicine and Regional Anesthesia*. Philadelphia: Churchill Livingstone; 1999: 288–294.
40. Backonia M. Anticonvulsants for neuropathic pain syndromes. *Clin J Pain* 2000;16:S67–S72.
41. Tan JC. *Practical Manual of Physical Medicine and Rehabilitation*. St. Louis: Mosby Yearbook; 1998:133–155, 607–644.
42. Abram SE. Neural blockade for neuropathic pain. *Clin J Pain* 2000; 16:S56–S61.
43. Raj P. *Neural Blockade in Clinical Anesthesia and Management of Pain*. St. Louis: Mosby Year Book; 1996:899–934.
44. Levy R. Neuroablative procedures for treatment of intractable pain. In: Benzon H, Raja S, Borsook D, et al., eds. *Essentials of Pain Medicine and Regional Anesthesia*. Philadelphia: Churchill Livingstone; 1999:104–110.
45. Carter GT. Rehabilitation management of peripheral neuropathy. *Semin Neurol* 2005;25:229–237.
46. Kemp SS, Rogg JM. In: Latchaw, ed. *MR and Imaging of the Head, Neck, and Spine*. St. Louis: MosbyYear Book; 1991:1109–1157.
47. Deutsch AL, Mink JH. Magnetic resonance imaging of musculoskeletal disorders. *Radiol Clin North Am* 1989;27:983–1002.
48. Daffner RH, Rothfus WB. In: Latchaw, ed. *MR and Imagining of the Head, Neck, and Spine*. St. Louis: Mosby Year Book; 1999:1225–1255.

49. Intracosa JH, Christopherson LA. Radiology of the spine. In: Benzon H, Raja S, Borsook D, et al., eds. *Essentials of Pain Medicine and Regional Anesthesia*. New York: Churchill Livingstone; 1999: 20–26.

50. Nishida T, Miniek M. Role of neurophysiologic testing for pain. In: Benzon H, Raja S, Borsook D, et al., eds. *Essentials of Pain Medicine and Regional Anesthesia*. New York: Churchill Livingstone; 1999:27–33.

51. Kimura J. *Electrodiagnosis in Diseases of Nerve and Muscle: Principles and Practice*, 2nd ed. Philadelphia: FA Davis; 1989.

52. Wilborn AJ. The electrodiagnostic exam of patients with radiculopathies. *Muscle Nerve* 1998;32:1612–1631.

53. Dumitru D. Electrodiagnostic Medicine. Philadelphia: Hanley and Belfus; 1995.

54. Griffin JW, Hiesch ST, McArthur JC, et al. Laboratory testing in peripheral neuropathy. *Neurol Clin* 1996;14:119–133.

55. Huskisson EC. Measurement of pain. *Lancet* 1974;2:1127–1131.

56. Huskisson EC. Measurement of pain. *J Rheumatol* 1982;9:768–769.

57. Dixon JS. Reproducibility along a 10 cm vertical visual analogue scale. *Ann Rheumatol Dis* 1981;40:87–89.

58. Scott J, Huskisson EC. Vertical or horizontal visual analogue scales. *Ann Rheumatol Dis* 1979;38:560.

59. Maxwell C. Sensitivity and accuracy of the visual analogue scale. *Br J Clin Pharmacol* 1978;6:15.

60. Melzack R, Katz J. Pain measurement in persons in pain. In: Wall PD, Melzack R, eds. *Textbook of Pain*. Edinburgh: Churchill Livingstone; 1999:409–426.

61. Skogsbergh DR, Chapman SA. Dealing with the chronic patient. In: Mootz RD, Vernon HT, eds. *Best Practices in Clinical Chiropractic*. Gaithersburg, MD: Aspen; 1999:120–129.

62. Cardenas DD, Egan KJ. Management of chronic pain. In: Kottke FJ, Lehmann JF, eds. *Krusen's Handbook of Physical Medicine and Rehabilitation*. Philadelphia: WB Saunders; 1990:1162–1191.

63. Yeh C, Gonyea M, Lemke J, et al. Physical therapy. In: Aronoff GM, ed. *Evaluation and Treatment of Chronic Pain*. Baltimore: Williams & Wilkins. 1985:251–261.

64. Kilmer DD, Aitkens S. Neuromuscular disease. In: Frontera WR, Dawson DM, Slovic DM, eds. *Exercise in Rehabilitative Medicine*. Champaign, IL: Human Kinetics; 1999:253–266.

Traumatic Brain Injury

EPIDEMIOLOGY

Traumatic brain injury (TBI) refers to the primary and secondary neurologic consequences of an insult to the brain resulting from the application of an external force. These forces can result from various injury scenarios, such as, falls, direct blows to the head, acceleration-deceleration injury, crush injuries, gunshot wounds, explosive blast injuries, or motor vehicle collisions. TBI is a significant public health issue in that it results in death or long-term disability for many people. In the United States, the incidence of TBI is approximately 100–300 per 100,000 people per year. This amounts to a total of 1.5 million people injured yearly (61). Approximately 50,000–75,000 of these will die from their injuries and 80,000 will acquire long-term disability in any or all of the cognitive, behavioral, or physical function domains (15). It is important to realize that the total number of disabled is cumulative and currently up to 2% of the United States population has disability resulting from TBI (9). In adults, TBI typically has two main incidence peaks: those aged 15–24 years and those more than 75 years of age. Most studies report the top three mechanisms of injury as being motor vehicle collisions, falls, and assaults (61). Transportation-related causes account for most of injuries in the 15–24 year-old age group and falls are the primary mechanism of injury in those more than 75 year of age. In the younger group, males account for about 2 of 3 TBI cases, whereas men and women tend to be more equally represented in the older age group. Overall, TBI is the leading cause of death and disability in young adults, despite the primary causes of injury being eminently preventable (38).

During the last decade, the incidence of TBI in military personnel engaged in the war zones has increased considerably owing to explosions, accidents, and other causes (http://www.tbindc.org). Blast injuries as a result of improvised explosive devices and military ordinance, such as artillery, mortar shells, and aerial bombing, are an increasingly significant cause of TBI in both military personnel and civilian populations. Explosions produce three types of injuries. Injuries owing to the blast wave-induced changes in atmospheric pressure primarily affect areas of the body with air-fluid interfaces, such as the lungs, bowels, and middle ear. It is still not clear whether the brain is vulnerable to the blast wave. It is thought, however, that concussion, hemorrhage, edema, axonal injury, and infarctions caused by the formation of gas emboli are possible consequences of exposure to explosions (58). The other two forms of blast injuries, being struck by objects propelled by the blast and being thrown into a stationary object by the shock wave, have similar consequences as penetrating brain injuries, and automobile accidents, or falls, respectively.

PATHOPHYSIOLOGY

Traumatic damage to the brain can be thought of in terms of both primary and secondary injuries. Primary injury refers to the immediate damage to brain tissue caused by the actual application of force. This may be a shearing, tearing, or laceration wound caused by a knife, bullet, or other object entering the brain; or it may refer to shearing along tissue planes of differential density or fiber tracts caused by rotational torque forces within the brain itself. Widespread disruption of axonal fiber tracts and the gray–white matter interface caused by these torque forces is called *diffuse axonal injury* and can result in widespread brain dysfunction. Injury to brain tissue can also result from cavitational or pressure wave phenomena in situations, such as high-velocity gunshot injuries, or blast-type injures, as in an explosion. These initial applications of force can also disrupt blood vessels and result in contusions (bruises), hematomas (large blood collections), or ischemia (oxygen deficiency) to areas supplied by the affected blood vessels. Besides direct trauma, the brain can also be widely affected by reduced perfusion or oxygenation failure resulting from other concurrent injury, such as shock, pneumothorax, and circulatory collapse. This occurs particularly in cases of high-speed motor vehicle collisions, industrial accidents, and other scenarios that result in a high probability of thoracic injury.

After the initial trauma, secondary causes of injury to the brain evolve over the minutes, hours, and days following the injury. These secondary injuries refer to events such as, cerebral edema (brain swelling) or a cascade of neurotoxic events at the cellular level triggered by the initial injury. Edema is particularly worrisome as the brain is encased in a rigid box (the skull) and there is

113

usually equilibrium in pressure among tissue, blood, and cerebrospinal fluid compartments. Should any one of these compartments enlarge, the intracranial pressure will increase and there is a risk of decreasing cerebral blood flow, as well as tissue injury taking place as the swollen brain attempts to squeeze across or through rigid tissues or bony areas (herniation). The disruptive events at the cellular level include the release of excitatory neurotransmitters (so-called "excitotoxins"), free radicals, lipid peroxidases, and a variety of other proinflammatory mediators that can cause widespread, ongoing neuronal death for a period of time after injury. Current acute treatment for TBI is generally based on interventions directed toward limiting these secondary consequences by controlling intracranial pressure, evacuating space-occupying blood collections, or inhibiting the toxic cellular cascade with treatments such as hypothermia (5,10). Despite many promising animal laboratory findings, there are no currently available, clinically effective, drug treatments available to limit the secondary injury cascade.

SEVERITY OF INJURY

Traumatic brain injury severity is typically graded according to the degree of compromise of neurologic function resulting from the injury. This grading can be done in reference to the person's degree of responsiveness and ability to interact with the environment, or the duration of the characteristic period of anterograde amnesia that accompanies TBI. The most common way of grading responsiveness is the Glasgow Coma Scale (GCS). Initially developed to allow accurate and reliable communication of functional state (59), the GCS score ranges from 3 to 15 on three subscales based on eye-opening, best motor response, and best verbal response. A GCS score of 8 or less constitutes coma and represents severe brain injury, a score of 9–12 constitutes moderate brain injury, and a score of 13–15, mild brain injury. Some controversy remains surrounding the accepted definition of mild TBI (52), perhaps because disabilities associated with this condition are often subtle and difficult to diagnose. It is commonly accepted that injury to the brain may occur without loss or significant alteration of consciousness. About 80% of TBI falls into the mild category, with the remaining 20% representing moderate to severe injury. Mild TBI frequently occurs in contact sports, such as ice hockey, football, boxing, and soccer. These injuries have been reported to alter the acute cardiovascular responses (autonomic control) during exercise (5). Research has indicated that even mild TBI can cause premature fatigue, thereby affecting the person's ability to perform routine (43,73) activities of daily living (ADL).

The duration of posttraumatic amnesia (PTA) has also been used to grade injury severity, with mild TBI defined as PTA less than 1 hour and extremely severe TBI defined as PTA lasting longer than 1 month (43). Both the initial GCS score and the PTA duration are correlated (although not perfectly) with functional outcome following brain injury. In general, lower GCS scores and longer durations of PTA are associated with poorer outcome and increased disability. It should be noted that 10%–15% of even mild TBI survivors have persisting symptoms and impairments (52).

DIAGNOSTIC TECHNIQUES AND NEUROIMAGING

A variety of techniques have been developed to assess structure and function of the brain. Perhaps the most widely available and useful neuroimaging technique is computed tomography or CT scanning. CT is relatively inexpensive and, because CT images clearly show bone, acute blood collections, fluid-filled spaces, and brain tissue, it is very useful in initial trauma evaluation and surgical decision-making. Magnetic resonance imaging (MRI) is a nonionizing radiation technique that has great capacity to show structural details, but has two disadvantages that limit its usefulness in the acute situation: it requires longer scan acquisition times and more complex technology. The greater spatial resolution and range of image manipulation available with MRI does mean, however, that it is more effective than CT in situations where structural injury may be more subtle, diffuse, or earlier in evolution. Other techniques, such as CT angiography, conventional angiography, magnetic resonance angiography (MRA), or radionuclide scanning (single photo emission computed tomography [SPECT]) may be used in some cases to evaluate the integrity of blood vessels and cerebral perfusion (16). These imaging techniques are limited, however, to assessing structure and give little information about function of the neural tissue. Functional brain imaging may be done with positron emission tomography (PET) or functional MRI (fMRI), but these remain largely research techniques and are not presently in widespread clinical use (39). The electrical activity of the brain can also be used to assess brain function (71). Recording of the minute electrical signals across the skull (electroencephalography [EEG]), or recording stimulus-locked brain electrical activity (evoked potentials [EP]) for different sensory systems (e.g., auditory evoked responses, visual-evoked responses, soma-to-sensory evoked responses) can provide at least some crude assessment of functional activity and the integrity of sensory pathways. EEG also has a more specific application in the evaluation of brain death.

Other diagnostic and evaluation techniques rely on behavioral responses to assess brain function. Some of these techniques (e.g., the coma recovery scale-revised) (23) or the Wessex head injury matrix (30) can be applied in the case of the very low functioning patient. In the more alert and higher functioning patient, a comprehensive neuropsychological assessment may be used to obtain a profile of perceptuomotor, cognitive, and behavioral strengths and weaknesses (50). Recently, near infrared spectroscopy, a noninvasive optical technique had been demonstrated to be reliable and useful in evaluating neuronal activation during maximal, rhythmic handgrip contractions in individuals with moderate to severe TBI (6).

MEDICAL CONSEQUENCES AND TREATMENT RELATED TO BRAIN INJURY

SEIZURES

Seizure disorders may complicate long-term recovery in up to 50% of penetrating brain injury survivors (53). Risk factors for posttraumatic epilepsy include severe brain injury, intracranial hemorrhage, the presence of hematomas, and injury in which the dura mater is penetrated. Early seizures (within the first week) are considered minor risk factors for the development of later seizures. Most of the later seizures (75%–80%) will occur within the first 2 years after injury and may require long-term treatment with anticonvulsant medications. Current guidelines, however, suggest no role exists for prophylactic anticonvulsant treatment in prevention of epilepsy (60). The primary concern related to anticonvulsant drug treatment of seizure disorders is the potential for side effects associated with the anticonvulsant drugs (40). These may include cognitive impairment, sedation, balance dysfunction, impairment of liver function, and serious hematologic consequences. In general, if seizure medication is needed, attempts should be made to choose the least-impairing medication.

HYPERTONIA AND SPASTICITY

Excessive muscle tone and exaggerated muscle stretch reflexes may accompany injury in the brainstem, cerebellum or midbrain to motor control pathways as part of the upper motor neuron syndrome. This syndrome can result in poor muscle coordination, flexor or extensor motor patterns, co-contraction, spastic dystonia, or even joint contracture (57). Spasticity, defined as a velocity dependent increase in resistance when a joint is passively moved through its available range of motion (ROM) typically is more pronounced in the flexor muscles of the upper extremities and the extensor muscles of the lower extremities. Increases in tone not only affect the muscles of the limbs but also those in the trunk, neck, and face and may be sufficiently severe to interfere with, or prevent, day-to-day motor activities, such as, speech, feeding, ambulation, and dressing. In some instances, the increased muscle tone can be of functional benefit in some ADL; for example, increased extensor tone may assist in learning to perform independent transfers and walk with an adaptive device. However, not all increased motor tone and dyscoordination is spastic in nature. Motor dysfunction may also result from drug side effects, injury to subcortical motor areas, or impairments in motor planning and execution (dyspraxia). Treatment for excessive motor tone is focused on a number of goals: improving specific functions, such as, gait or transfers; relieving painful spasm; facilitating self or assisted care, such as dressing; improving seating; and preventing joint contracture. A variety of treatments have been proposed (26), including drugs, cryotherapy, hydrotherapy, stretching, exercise, casting and splinting, and electrical stimulation. Drugs can be delivered orally, intrathecally, or focally targeted to specific muscle groups (e.g., botulinum toxin or phenol). Concerns exist regarding the effectiveness and potential for side effects of centrally acting drugs, such as baclofen, diazepam, and tizanidine, and because of this some health professionals prefer more peripherally acting agents, such as dantrolene sodium, as first-line drug treatment. Typically, treatment modalities would be combined to enhance effectiveness (54).

HYPOTONIA

Hypotonia is not as common as increased tone in the people with TBI. When it occurs it is typically associated with injury to the cerebellum. Often, when patients are admitted to rehabilitation, they may exhibit low tone in one or more limbs. In extreme cases, the muscles involved may be described as flaccid. Over time, usually tone increases and treatment is required to prevent the problems associated with high tone, such as the development of contractures. As seen with hypertonia, hypotonia can also affect muscles in the trunk, neck, and face. This can impair motor control of the extremities, balance, and gait, which in turn affects functional activities such as ADL.

HETEROTOPIC OSSIFICATION

Heterotopic ossification (HO) refers to the poorly understood phenomenon of ectopic growth of bony tissue in tissue planes around major joints, such as the shoulders, hips, and knees, following major insults, such as, brain injury, spinal cord injury, burns, or joint replacement (62). Not surprisingly, HO can severely limit joint range and, in extreme cases, prevent joint movement, thus making active or passive use of the joint difficult or impossible. In addition, the ectopic bone can compromise neurovascular structure around joints, leading to such problems as peripheral neuropathy, weakness, or paresis. In the early stages, HO can present as a painful or increasingly range limited joint with x-rays showing the ossified tissue only later in the course of the condition. Early detection for treatment requires a reasonable index of suspicion and the use of radionuclide scanning. Treatment is generally with nonsteroidal anti-inflammatory drugs and sodium etidronate. Once ossification has occurred, the only treatment is surgical resection of the bony overgrowth.

BALANCE DISORDERS

Difficulty with balance is very common after TBI (18). This may relate to motor problems, impaired postural control reflexes, or impaired central processing of balance and stability cues, such as, proprioceptive, visual, and kinesthetic feedback. Central or peripheral damage to the vestibular apparatus may also occur and the patient should be carefully evaluated for easily treatable causes of balance dysfunction, such as benign positional vertigo (49).

MUSCULOSKELETAL INJURIES

Events such as motor vehicle accidents, falls, and artillery blasts where the body is subjected to violence can result in significant musculoskeletal injuries in addition to the brain injury. Fractures, dislocations, tissue lacerations, limb loss, and organ contusions are examples of the types of injuries that can occur. Damage can occur to the median, ulnar, and radial nerves as well as the brachial plexus when musculoskeletal damage involves the upper extremities and neck. The sciatic nerve or lumbosacral plexus may also be damaged when injuries occur to the pelvis and lower extremities. Damage to the spine can result in injury to the spinal cord or the nerve roots innervating associated organs and muscles. Damage to the central and peripheral nervous systems can contribute to impairment in both the motor and sensory systems and negatively affect involvement in rehabilitation efforts. Poorly united fractures of the pelvis and bones of the legs can result in leg length discrepancies affecting gait and the sites of fractures may be painful when stressed during activity.

NEUROCOGNITIVE FUNCTION, SENSORY FUNCTION, SPEECH, AND COMMUNICATION

Behavioral psychiatric disturbance is common after TBI (2). For example, some estimates have placed the incidence of depression as high as 60% after brain injury (37) and newly acquired psychiatric diagnoses, such as anxiety and mood disorders, are common (2). Many individuals experience personality changes, particularly those with frontal lobe damage. Behavioral disturbance can also take the form of agitated behavior, aggressive behavior, or socially inappropriate behavior resulting from impairments in judgment, temper control, planning and problem-solving, and self-awareness. Cognitive problems can include deficits or delays in executive functioning, memory, attention, concentration, information processing, and speech (e.g., word retrieval). Speech and communication disturbances can also occur because of damage to the motor areas of the brain that control physical produc-

tion of speech. Sleep disturbances, chronic pain, and headaches are commonly reported after TBI and can negatively impact cognitive functioning. Individuals who become neurocompromised as a result of TBI often experience changes in sensory systems that can range from heightened sensitivity and difficulty filtering sensory input, to sensory losses in vision, hearing, taste, and smell (2). The importance of these behavioral, psychiatric, speech, and sensory consequences cannot be underestimated because they may be the primary reason for failure of successful community reintegration after brain injury (41). In addition, many people with TBI have multiple symptoms, each of which can exacerbate the effects of another. For example, someone with TBI from a bomb blast may have chronic tinnitus, difficulty articulating, poor concentration, depression, and difficulty self-regulating. The individual gets frustrated because he or she knows what to say during a conversation and understands dialog, but his or her rate of speech is slow. As a result, the person becomes frustrated, which causes trouble with self-regulation and increases depression. Also, the chronic tinnitus can lead to sleep problems, which increase fatigue and have a negative impact on the ability to concentrate, which can also increase depression.

Treatment may consist of psychotherapeutic interventions, behavior modification techniques, speech therapy, cognitive therapy, psychotropic pharmacotherapy, assistive devices (e.g. hearing aids), or a combination of methods. The use of psychopharmacologic agents is somewhat controversial because some of the commonly used drugs have been associated with side effects, such as excessive sedation, cognitive impairment, or even the potential for delaying or retarding functional recovery (24).

IATROGENIC AND TREATMENT-RELATED ISSUES

A number of complications of severe TBI are related to non-neurologic consequences. In cases of extended decreased consciousness, some problems can simply be related to the prolonged periods of bedrest and immobility (42). These complications can include significant loss of lean muscle mass (and associated strength loss) and overall body weight, impaired skin integrity, joint contracture, peripheral neuropathy (intensive care unit [ICU] polyneuropathy or focal pressure palsies), marked loss of cardiovascular reflexes, and decreased general aerobic fitness. These consequences may occur regardless of the extent and type of neurologic injury, and may compound the functional impairments resulting from the brain injury itself.

RISK OF SUBSEQUENT BRAIN INJURY AND SECOND IMPACT SYNDROME

One concern with regard to return to activity after brain injury is the risk associated with possible additional brain injury (33). In general, the consequences of a second or subsequent head injury are felt to be cumulative and more severe than for first injuries of equivalent energy transfer. Related to this is the so-called second impact syndrome. Second impact syndrome refers to the potential for catastrophic injury and even death following a second sequential brain trauma. Concern about second impact syndrome is the main driving force behind guidelines for concussion management and return to play criteria in sport (14).

ASSESSING THE FUNCTIONAL CAPACITY IN TRAUMATIC BRAIN INJURY

Individuals with TBI present with a wide range of physical abilities, depending on the nature and location of their injury. Often, a significant gap exists between what the individual can do, and what he or she believes is possible to do or wants and needs to do. One of the aims of rehabilitation services is to reduce this occupational gap, which persists in those with TBI, even several years after injury. The Functional Assessment Measure (FAM) is a tool that is used by rehabilitation therapists to evaluate the ability of individuals with TBI in the following six areas: mobility, transfers, self-care, cognition, psychosocial, and communication (56). The individual is evaluated on specific skills pertaining to each of these areas that are essential to performing routine ADL. Physical therapy, occupational therapy, and other support services are provided on the basis of their performance on the FAM. The individual's progress can be continually monitored during the course of rehabilitation using this instrument. Examples of the utility of the FAM are provided in the case studies presented at the end of this chapter.

FOCUS OF REHABILITATION: IMPORTANCE OF EXERCISE

Although there is an element of spontaneous recovery from even very severe TBI, this can be enhanced with treatment in a coordinated comprehensive rehabilitation program (32). Spontaneous recovery can take any number of forms, ranging from rapid to slow insidious improvements over multiple years. Emerging evidence suggests that rehabilitation activities may take advantage of the inherent plasticity of the human brain to either restore neurologic function, or facilitate the acquisition of compensatory strategies (12). Factors that influence rehabilitation outcomes include type and severity of injury, age at time of injury, time after injury at rehabilitation entry, duration and intensity of rehabilitation, and support systems (e.g. family, quality of care, community resources) (72). Even those with very severe TBI may benefit from rehabilitation, particularly if rehabilitation can be provided over an extended period (28). Human cerebral tissue is highly dependent on aerobic metabolism to maintain ionic balance and membrane stabilization, neuronal activation, and synthesis of numerous structural components. It has been reported that the mitochondrial oxidative capacity in patients with TBI in the acute stages of recovery is suppressed (64). Whether this is evident in the chronic stage of rehabilitation is not known. Increasing cerebral blood flow as a result of dynamic exercise may be one way of restoring mitochondrial function in cerebral tissue. Furthermore (63), regular exercise can positively influence some aspects of recovery from TBI by elevating the brain-derived neurotrophic factor, which is known to stimulate the proliferation of cells in the central nervous system.

In one retrospective study (25), it was found that individuals with TBI who exercised regularly experienced less depression than nonexercising individuals with TBI. No differences were noted between the two groups of individuals with TBI on measures of disability. In patients with severe head trauma who were in the chronic stages of rehabilitation, it has been demonstrated (55) that a comprehensive rehabilitation program that includes cognitive and perceptual remediation, problem-solving learning, personal counseling, physical exercise and relaxation, social skills, and prevocational training over a 30 week period induces significant improvements in the psychomotor tests of attention, visual information processing, memory, and complex reasoning. Changes in manual dexterity, verbal IQ, and basic academic skills were not, however, evident subsequent to the rehabilitation program. Participants with damage to the motor system gained cognitively as much as those whose motor system was intact. More importantly, these improvements were sustained 3–12 months after rehabilitation. A randomized, controlled trial (3) that examined the effects of 12 weeks of aerobic training in patients with recent TBI demonstrated significant improvements in exercise capacity in the training compared with the control group. These changes, however, were not matched by greater improvements in functional independence, mobility, or psychological function, at either 12 weeks or follow-up.

Participation in group exercise programs and sports or leisure activities also offers the added advantage of social interaction with other participants, which could enhance their chances of successful reintegration into society. Although the importance of regular exercise cannot be overemphasized in this population, it should be recognized that individuals with disabilities face numerous barriers for participation. In one survey conducted in the United States (48), lack of transportation, financial circumstances, lack of energy, poor motivation, uncertainty about suitable fitness facilities for individuals with disabilities, what exercises to perform, fear of leaving home and going into a new environment, and engaging with strangers were reported as barriers to participation.

MEASUREMENT OF PHYSICAL FITNESS IN TRAUMATIC BRAIN INJURY

AEROBIC POWER AND CAPACITY

Selecting the Exercise Mode

The primary physical consideration for implementing an exercise testing and training program for those with TBI is establishing the functional capacity of the participant. Individuals with TBI present with a wide range of functional abilities, depending on the location, nature, and magnitude of the injury. Preliminary screening using the FAM with specific reference to the ambulatory score is a useful starting point. Typically, the exercise mode for measurement of aerobic fitness should incorporate as large a muscle mass as possible so that the cardiorespiratory system can be maximally stressed. This, however, is usually not possible in those with TBI because most of these individuals experience premature fatigue well before their cardiorespiratory system is fully stressed (4,7,31). Individuals with TBI can be tested for aerobic fitness using the following exercise modes: treadmill walking or running (31), upright and recumbent cycle ergometry (4,7,31), arm-cranking (7), wheelchair ergometry, a combination of arm and leg ergometry, and stair climbing (31). Although treadmill walking or running is the most logical choice for testing because it utilizes the largest muscle mass and has the potential for transfer to ambulation and other ADL, this mode may not be feasible and safe for all individuals with TBI. For example, although a participant with TBI may be able to walk independently, he or she may experience balance problems while exercising on the treadmill, which could compromise safety. In such cases, cycle ergometry may be a more appropriate mode for testing and training the individual. Participants who are nonambulatory and are wheelchair dependent can be tested on an arm-crank ergometer or a specially designed wheelchair ergometer. Both these types of ergometers can quantify the power output generated and can be used to monitor the progress of the participant. Wheelchair ergometry is a more valid method of evaluation, however, because it is specific to their mode of ambulation.

Modifications to Exercise Testing Equipment

Many individuals with TBI have sensorimotor impairments and experience a high degree of spasticity, which could affect their ability to exercise on the different devices. In such instances, it may be necessary to make some modifications so that the participant can safely complete the exercise (13). For example, a person who is unable to apply consistent force with the hands or feet on the pedals of the arm-cranking and cycle ergometers, respectively, can be assisted by using Velcro straps to secure the limbs to the pedals. Differences in muscle function between the two limbs should also be considered when selecting the suitability of exercise machines for enhancing muscle strength and endurance.

Modifications to Exercise Testing Protocols

Although the testing protocols for assessment of various fitness parameters have been standardized for able-bodied individuals, this not the case for individuals with disabilities, including those with TBI (13). Therefore, it is recommended that existing protocols for the able-bodied population be modified when evaluating participants with TBI. For example, if the goal of the test is to determine the peak oxygen uptake (peak $\dot{V}O_2$) during cycling, then an incremental protocol with low power output increments should be used when assessing the participant. Most of the cycling protocols for able-bodied individuals utilize power output (PO) increments of 25–30 Watts each minute at a pedaling cadence of 60 revolutions/minute. This may not be suitable for participants with TBI because of their low cardiorespiratory fitness and reduced muscular strength and endurance. Designing a protocol with lower PO increments and pedaling cadence will delay premature fatigue and increase the chances of obtaining a more valid measure of the aerobic fitness of the individual. The same principle can be applied to arm-cranking or treadmill tests that are designed to measure the peak $\dot{V}O_2$ of the participant.

MUSCLE STRENGTH AND ENDURANCE

Likely, the extended periods of bedrest, sedentary lifestyles, and other barriers to physical activity in those with TBI will result in muscle atrophy, thereby reducing muscle strength and endurance (17). As well, muscle weakness, hypertonicity, or the loss of ability to perform isolated movement can occur as a result of the TBI. In the able-bodied population, computerized dynamometers, such as the Cybex and Biodex, have been used to quantify the peak torque, total work done, and fatigue index of various muscle groups under isokinetic, isotonic, and isometric conditions at various limb velocities. Although no compelling neurologic reason exists to why this method of testing cannot be used on people with TBI, some important factors should be considered when using such instrumentation. The participant should: (a) have sufficient cognition to fully understand the test requirements; (b) be completely familiarized with the exercise mode, especially if isokinetic measurements are required because this is not a natural movement; and (c) be tested at the slow to moderate speeds to minimize the risk of injury.

Resistance training machines, free weights, and hand grip dynamaometers can also be used to evaluate the muscle strength and endurance of people with TBI. Caution should be used when using free weights because TBI can often result in an imbalance in strength and ROM between the left and right sides of the body. Evidence from studies that have used circuit training (7,31,36) indicates that individuals with TBI can safely participate in such activities. Resistance training does not increase the muscle tone in people with TBI and hypertonia. Therefore, this method of training should be used to restore the deficits in muscle strength and endurance that occur in this population. Velcro straps should be used to secure the limbs to the machines as required. Seat belts should also be used to stabilize the torso, if necessary. When using the hand grip dynamometer, a record should be kept of the hand position and joint angle at which the measurements are taken. Abdominal muscle strength and endurance can be measured using the modified curl-up test to the point of fatigue or over a fixed duration (22,36). The latter study (36) reported that TBI participants scored in the eighth percentile on this particular test. Because motivation plays a very important role in strength measurement, it is important that the participant is motivated to a similar degree when these assessments are taken.

FLEXIBILITY

Flexibility is necessary to perform many of the ADL without undue stress. Individuals with TBI could have limited joint flexibility because of a variety of reasons including: (a) trauma to one or more joints which could restrict the range of motion, (b) muscle weakness, (c) hypertonia, (d) heterotopic ossification in the joints, and (e) increased incidence of arthritis. The ROM of various joints can be reliably measured using a hand-held goniometer. The sit-and-reach test can also be used to assess the flexibility of the hamstrings and lower back in this population (44). When assessing flexibility, the movement should be performed in a slow and sustained manner to minimize the effects of increasing muscle tone, which could influence the measurement.

BODY COMPOSITION

Individuals with TBI who have been hospitalized for extended periods undergo profound changes in body composition owing to extended periods of bedrest. As well, most of these individuals lead sedentary lifestyles because they may be in-patients in a rehabilitation center where the opportunities for physical activity, unless specifically undertaken as part of their therapy, are often limited by the time demands of therapies addressing other deficits. Those living in the community also face several barriers to participation in physical activity programs. It is likely, therefore, that these individuals will demonstrate an increased proportion of body fat with lower levels of lean body mass. In addition, some people with TBI who have damage to the hypothalamus may have problems in regulating food intake. This could result in ingestion of excessive number of calories and significantly increase the proportion of body fat. One study (29) demonstrated that people with TBI who were in the chronic state of recovery tended to eat larger meals and consume significantly more calories per day than their able-bodied counterparts. The presence of other individuals during the meal influenced the meal size of patients with TBI, but not that of the controls. Whether this is due to alterations in hypothalamic control of food intake in this population is currently unclear. It is well documented that a sedentary lifestyle and excessive amount of body fat can increase the overall risk of cardiovascular disease. It is important, therefore, that the body composition of individuals with TBI be monitored at regular intervals during the rehabilitation program.

The body composition of individuals with TBI has been assessed using simple measurements, such as body weight and the body mass index (BMI). The BMI values calculated can be compared with expected values for nondisabled adults so that an overall index of their health risk is obtained. Conventional methods of measuring body fat, such as densitometry and skinfold thickness, have not been validated for the TBI population. The latter can be influenced by both hypertonia and hypotonia over the measurement sites in this population. Nevertheless, despite these limitations, some researchers (22) have used the sum of skinfolds at selected sites to examine the changes in body composition as a result of exercise training programs in individuals with TBI. The reliability of the bioelectrical impedance technique to measure total body water and estimate body fat in the TBI population has been documented (51). Another study (7) has utilized this technique to examine the changes as a result of a circuit training program in participants with moderate to severe TBI.

VALIDITY OF INCREMENTAL EXERCISE RESPONSES

Participants with TBI usually demonstrate the normal cardiovascular and respiratory responses to exercise, unless specific damage has occurred to the medulla oblongata, which alters their autonomic control. As observed in the able-bodied population, the oxygen uptake ($\dot{V}O_2$) and heart rate (HR) increase linearly during dynamic incremental exercise until the point of fatigue on the treadmill or cycle ergometer (8,19). Alterations in blood pressure during exercise have not been systematically examined in this population. Because of their low levels of aerobic fitness, participants with TBI usually do not meet the American College of Sports Medicine (1) criteria for attaining the maximal aerobic power ($\dot{V}O_2$max). In other words, these participants demonstrate a peak $\dot{V}O_2$ and not a true $\dot{V}O_2$max. No published research exists pertaining to the lactate (ventilatory) threshold in those with TBI. Testing conducted by the authors indicate that TBI participants with sufficient exercise capacity demonstrate the exponential changes in the ventilation rate (V_E), carbon dioxide (VCO_2) production and respiratory exchange ratio (RER) that occur at this intensity during incremental cycling, similar to that observed in able-bodied subjects.

RELIABILITY OF PEAK CARDIORESPIRATORY RESPONSES

Laboratory Tests

Research (8) has demonstrated that the PO and the associated physiologic responses during incremental cycling to voluntary fatigue can be reliably determined in participants with moderate to severe TBI. Significant test–retest reliability coefficients of 0.96, 0.98, 0.97, 0.82, 0.96, and 0.81 were reported for the peak values of the PO, absolute $\dot{V}O_2$, relative $\dot{V}O_2$, HR, V_E and oxygen pulse (O_2 pulse) respectively, during repeated tests conducted within a 1-week period. The reliability of the submaximal and maximal responses of HR, $\dot{V}O_2$, V_E, and RER in participants with TBI has also been demonstrated during treadmill walking (47). The intraclass correlations for the submaximal responses ranged between 0.80 and 93, whereas those for the peak responses were between 0.77 and 0.92. The authors reported strongest correlations between the third and seventh minutes of exercise, with the values during the early and later stages of the exercise test being less than optimal for HR and V_E. These observations have important implications for evaluating the training responses of participants with TBI.

Field Tests

Direct measurement of $\dot{V}O_2$ requires specialized equipment and technical expertise that may not be available at all rehabilitation centers. Several researchers have therefore designed field tests to evaluate the $\dot{V}O_2$ of participants with TBI. One study (45) reported high test–retest reliability of a 6-minute walking test in male and female participants who were assessed 7–38 months after injury. The participants, who were clients in a postacute rehabilitation facility, completed two 6-minute walks on a rectangular track within a 10-day period. Significant intraclass correlations of 0.94, 0.65, and 0.89 were reported for the distance traveled, HR, and the physiologic cost index (ratio between HR and distance traveled). Another investigation (65) demonstrated the reliability of a 20-m shuttle walk or run test in adults with TBI. The participants performed a progressive walking or running shuttle course until the point of fatigue twice within a 1-week period. The intraclass correlations for the number of levels completed, total walk or run test time, and the

maximal HR were 0.97, 0.98, and 0.96, respectively. These observations indicated that simple field tests can be used with confidence to evaluate aerobic capacity in those with TBI.

AEROBIC FITNESS AND ENERGY EXPENDITURE IN TRAUMATIC BRAIN INJURY

Several studies have indicated that the aerobic capacity of participants with TBI is well below that of their age- and gender-matched counterparts. According to the published literature (4,7,31,35) the peak $\dot{V}O_2$ of individuals with TBI before participation in a conditioning program ranged from 67% to 74% of the value predicted for their able-bodied counterparts. It has been reported that the peak PO during incremental cycling is associated with quadriceps muscle strength in participants with moderate to severe TBI (20). This suggests that besides aerobic capacity, the premature fatigue observed during cycling in those with TBI may also be limited by localized muscle strength of the quadriceps muscles. The low levels of aerobic fitness in persons with TBI are also evident during submaximal exercise. In participants recovering from TBI, the O_2 pulse was significantly lower and the $V_E/\dot{V}O_2$ ratio was significantly higher in the TBI participants when compared with a convenience sample of age- and gender-matched controls (46). The lower O_2 pulse suggests that cardiac stroke volume was also reduced in the TBI subjects while the higher $V_E/\dot{V}O_2$ ratio implies that they had a greater energy cost of ventilation. Because most of the ADL performed by these individuals are usually submaximal in nature, these observations have important implications for the rehabilitation of this segment of the population.

The energy expenditure during walking, measured by the amount of oxygen consumed, is significantly higher in people with TBI when compared with that of their able-bodied counterparts (31). Factors such as (altered) muscle tone, spasticity, lack of coordination, reduced ROM, and poor postural control can account for this increase. As well, patients with TBI who ambulate in a wheelchair perform this task with a considerably smaller muscle mass when compared with normal walking. Methods of propulsion include (a) use of both arms or both legs, (b) one arm and one leg typically on the same side of the body, (c) one leg or the use of specialized wheelchairs that enable the use of one arm where the drive wheel on the individual's affected side is mounted inside of the handrim of the unaffected side, or (d) a lever drive mechanism. Where funding is available (sources may include insurance, litigation or private), power wheelchairs can be used and, although these machines significantly improve mobility and community access, users do not obtain the cardiorespiratory benefits that self-propelling in a manual wheelchair provides. These factors, along with their low aerobic fitness levels, impose a substantially greater stress on the cardiorespiratory and metabolic systems in individuals with TBI. Therefore, it is not surprising that fatigue is one of the most commonly reported symptoms in this population (73). Individuals with TBI have a low tolerance for physical activity, which can influence their ability to perform routine ADL. Furthermore, the onset of fatigue could deteriorate the posture and biomechanical aspects of simple tasks, thereby exacerbating this symptom. From a vocational standpoint, it has been reported that the ability to work continuously for 3 hours a day is an important criterion that determines whether a person with a TBI can obtain and keep a job (68). As such, addressing fatigue by increasing physical fitness and stamina is important to helping this population reintegrate into a work setting.

SCREENING FOR HEALTH RISK FACTORS BEFORE INITIATING A PROGRAM

Before initiating an exercise rehabilitation program for an individual with TBI, the person should be screened for pertinent medical and psychological factors to determine suitability for participation. With respect to the medical factors, the attending physician should complete the PARmedX (13) questionnaire to screen the individual for possible medical conditions that could place the individual "at risk" for an active exercise program. Although this is a generic questionnaire that is used for individuals who respond positively to the Physical Activity Readiness Questionnaire (PAR-Q) (13), it is routinely used to screen individuals with a variety of disabilities for exercise and physical activity programs. Besides this preliminary screening, the physician should specifically screen for the following health risk factors that have been identified (67) as extremely important for individuals with TBI: (a) angina pectoris, (b) aortic stenosis, (c) exertional syncope, (d) musculoskeletal sequelae that are exacerbated by exercise, (e) pulmonary embolism, (f) uncontrolled epilepsy (seizures), and (g) ventricular arrhythmias. The participant should be carefully evaluated for sensory deficits (e.g., hearing or vision loss) that may require modification for participation in an exercise program. As well, psychological factors such as cognition, judgment, motivation, outward aggression, and impulsiveness should be evaluated before initiating the training program. This information should be communicated with the members of the rehabilitation team responsible for supervising the participant's physical activity program and should be placed in the participant's file for follow-up if necessary.

EXERCISE TRAINING IN PARTICIPANTS WITH TRAUMATIC BRAIN INJURY

AEROBIC TRAINING

Research (34) has indicated that individuals who have recently acquired a brain injury can participate in an exercise training program during early in-patient rehabilitation. Some of them, however, may take longer to attain the prescribed training intensity corresponding to a HR >60% of the age predicted maximum and a duration of 30 minutes per session that is required to induce aerobic fitness improvements. In participants who have recently acquired a severe TBI (4), 24 sessions of cycle ergometer training for 30 minutes per session at 60%–80% of the age-predicted maximal HR has been reported to induce a significant increase in the peak PO (34%) with a slight decline in the peak HR (4.2%). Moreover, only a slight decline occurred in the peak PO when the participants were reevaluated 12 weeks after the cessation of training. This study did not report the changes in the cardiorespiratory responses of the participants. Another investigation (70) examining the effects of 12 weeks of cycle ergometer training at 60%–80% of the maximal HR for 30 minutes per session in participants with chronic TBI demonstrated significant increases in exercise time to fatigue (59.6%), peak PO (82.7%), and V_E (12.3%). The large increases were most likely due to the low levels of initial fitness of the participants.

CIRCUIT TRAINING

Circuit training is a method of conditioning in which participants exercise at various stations during the session. This type of training is designed to improve the main fitness parameters, such as aerobic capacity, anaerobic capacity, muscle strength and endurance, flexibility, and body composition. In one investigation (35), 16 weeks of circuit training during which the chronic TBI participants completed three 2-hour training sessions per week induced 15.4% increase in the peak $\dot{V}O_2$. The aerobic training component was performed at 70% of the age-predicted maximal HR. These findings were corroborated in another study (31) that demonstrated significant increases of 21.2% and 14.1%, respectively, in the peak PO and peak $\dot{V}O_2$ subsequent to a 12-week circuit training program during which the participants trained five times per week for 50 minutes per session. These investigators also reported that the HR after 4 minutes of exercise was significantly reduced subsequent to training, which is similar to the bradycardia observed in able-bodied subjects. A more recent study (7) examining the effects of circuit training on patients with moderate to severe TBI reported significant increases in the peak values of the PO (41.3%), absolute peak $\dot{V}O_2$ (33.3%), relative peak $\dot{V}O_2$

(22.5%), and O_2 pulse (26.3%). Concomitant declines were observed in the peak values of the V_E and the $V_E/\dot{V}O_2$ ratio. The improvement in the O_2 pulse suggests that cardiac stroke volume was significantly enhanced, whereas the decline in the $V_E/\dot{V}O_2$ ratio indicates an overall improvement in the efficiency of ventilation. The delta values of blood lactate were also significantly reduced as a result of the training program, suggesting less dependency on anaerobic metabolism. The significant improvements in peak physical fitness resulting from exercise training in patients with TBI have been attributed to improvements in localized muscular strength, cardiorespiratory fitness, and mechanical efficiency. The relative contribution of each of these components, however, is difficult to establish because none of these studies measured all these components. Overall, these observations provide sufficient evidence that circuit training can significantly enhance the aerobic fitness of participants with chronic TBI.

CHANGES IN MUSCLE STRENGTH AND ENDURANCE

The effects of regular exercise on the muscle strength and endurance of the major muscle groups in TBI participants have not been systematically researched. One study (35) reported a 92% increase in the number of sit-ups (curls) that TBI participants were able to perform in 1 minute following a 16-week circuit training program. These participants were at least 1 year after injury and performed a variety of aerobic (stationary cycling, jogging, skipping, and stair climbing) and neuromuscular rehabilitation (weight training, shooting, baskets, ring toss, three pin bowling, calisthenics, and dribbling) activities.

CHANGES IN BODY COMPOSITION

A limited number of studies have examined the effects of exercise training on the alterations in body composition in TBI participants. One investigation (4) reported a significant increase in the BMI of participants with recently acquired TBI following 12 weeks of cycle ergometer training. Another study (35) reported no significant changes in body mass and percent body fat (%BF) estimated from skinfold thickness before and following 16 weeks of circuit training in 14 chronic TBI participants. Examination of the individual data indicated that participants increased their body weight between 1.5 and 4.5 kg during this time interval with two of them showing increases in %BF of 3.9% and 3.6%. These observations were supported by a subsequent study (7) that reported no significant changes in the body mass, BMI and %BF measured by bioelectrical impedance in individuals with moderate to severe TBI subsequent to 12 weeks of circuit training. A tendency was noted for each of these variables to increase during this period, however, despite the increase in energy expenditure resulting from the training program. Closer examination of their individual data revealed that 9 of the 14 participants showed increases in all these variables. Two male and one female participant gained considerable body mass (21.5 kg, 11.3 kg, and 11.3 kg, respectively) with concomitant increases in %BF (8.1%, 6.3%, and 6.7%, respectively). This was a very large increase for the relatively short duration of the study. Thus, the overall evidence suggests that (a) regular exercise training performed three times a week for 12–16 weeks is ineffective in reducing the body weight and %BF in patients with TBI, and (b) some patients can increase their body mass, BMI, and %BF during this training period if the caloric intake is not controlled.

AMBULATION TRAINING WITH PARTIAL WEIGHT BEARING

A relatively new method of testing and training individuals with TBI is the use of a weight-supported harness system for treadmill walking. Depending on the participant's functional capacity, a percentage of their body weight is supported by the harness while they are walking on the treadmill. As the functional capacity of the participant improves with time, the amount of weight that is supported by the harness is decreased so that the participant ambulates more independently.

Although research has demonstrated that this method of training can enhance ambulatory parameters, such as gait velocity, step width, and step length of participants with TBI, some evidence indicates that it offers no added advantage when compared with conventional physical therapy that focuses on gait training (11,69).

GUIDELINES FOR IMPLEMENTING AN EXERCISE PROGRAM

EXERCISE PRESCRIPTION

On initial consultation, the exercise specialist must understand the many obvious and subtle global impairments that are consequent to TBI. It is important to gather as much information about the participant beforehand to better address medical, mobility, communication, behavioral, and cognitive needs. Speech and communication difficulties are common in this population, so the exercise specialist will need to be patient in allowing time for delayed responses to inquiries (e.g., slowed information processing), difficulties in speech production (e.g., slurred words, poor pronunciation), and difficulty with expression (e.g., poor word retrieval). Sensory impairments, such as hearing or vision loss, can also have an impact on communication. Alternate methods of communication using written materials and demonstrations may be necessary to augment interaction and understanding. In addition, speech and communication difficulties should not be automatically associated with a cognitive deficit. In many cases, the motor ability to produce speech is impaired, not cognition.

Many individuals with TBI have impaired neurocognitive function that could result in difficulty in understanding simple instructions pertaining to exercise testing and training. Before initiating any exercise program in these individuals, it is imperative that the participants understand what the expectations are. The TBI participant should be oriented to the training facility and be familiarized with the different exercise stations. The exercise specialist or therapist should demonstrate each exercise to the participant or provide other visual cues to ensure that they understand what the requirements are. Techniques, such as maintaining a simple visual tracking system using bar graphs to show progress and set future goals, displaying personal best scores for variables such as HR and exercise time, should also be employed to increase the attention and motivation of the participants during these activities. The risks and potential benefits associated with participation in an exercise program should also be reviewed with the participant and, if present, any legally appointed surrogate decision maker.

The team member supervising the exercise program may choose to provide more individualized training to the participant who lacks sufficient cognition and judgment. On the other hand, a participant who is not motivated to participate in an individual exercise program may be more encouraged to participate in a group setting. Participants who are easily distracted, outwardly aggressive, and overly impulsive could be scheduled to exercise in the facility during nonpeak hours or in areas where the chances of interacting with other clients is minimized.

When conducting exercise rehabilitation programs for individuals with TBI, it is important that each training session be supervised by a qualified person. Because many participants with TBI have special needs, the person supervising the training program should have the expertise in working with individuals with disabilities. As well, experience in adapting equipment and modifying testing and training protocols to suit the individual needs of the participant is an asset.

The use of simple tools such as wrist straps or Velcro fasteners to secure the limbs to weight machines, cycle ergometer pedals, and so on can facilitate exercise performance in these individuals. Care should be taken, however, when using such tools in areas with increased sensation as they can cause discomfort during participation. Similarly, areas of decreased sensation may be subject to injuries, such as blisters or scrapes. During the first few sessions, the participants should be closely monitored to ensure that they can perform the exercises safely (13).

The primary variables that should be considered in implementing an exercise program are the frequency, intensity, and duration of the training sessions, as well as the overall length of the training program. Each training session must be structured to include the following three phases: warm-up, training, and cool-down. The following recommendations for aerobic training are made on the basis of the available evidence (4,7,31,35) on patients with TBI: frequency, three times/week; intensity, 60%–90% of the maximal HR or 60% of the HR reserve; duration, minimum of 30 minutes per session. The overall length of the training program should be at least 12–14 weeks. One study (7) reported that, although some improvement was seen in the peak PO and peak $\dot{V}O_2$ during incremental cycling after 18 training sessions, the values were statistically significant only after the participants had completed 32 sessions. If the individuals with TBI are participating in a circuit training program, then the length of the training session can be increased so that all the stations can be completed. The circuit training stations should include resistance exercise to enhance muscular strength and endurance of the major muscle groups, flexibility training, and balance training, if necessary. A shorter duration of 20 minutes at the aerobic station may be used to avoid undue fatigue and increase compliance. Studies have demonstrated that circuit training sessions for TBI participants can last from 50 minutes (31) to 2 hours (35). The flexibility and balance training can be completed during the warm-up or cool-down phases of the training session. The neurologic and physical effects of TBI often cause the individual to fatigue quickly, and it is likely that some participants, particularly those who are in the early stages of rehabilitation, may not be able to attain the prescribed training intensity for enhancing aerobic fitness (34). These participants should be allowed to rest when necessary and encouraged to resume training after adequate recovery. In addition, at certain times of day the individual may be more alert and function better, depending on sleep patterns, medication administration, and so forth. Attempts should be made to schedule sessions during these periods of optimal arousal. During the aerobic training session, it is important that the HR be monitored at regular intervals so that a record of the training intensity is obtained. However, it has been reported (66) that some individuals with TBI may have difficulty in monitoring their pulse rate during exercise and tend to underestimate it. In such cases, it is advisable that a wireless HR monitor be used to record the training intensity.

It is imperative that the principle of progressive overload be incorporated in the training program for continual adaptation to occur. Usually, changes to the training load are made on the basis of alterations in the training HR and the subjective rating of perceived exertion (RPE). It should be noted, however, that participants with TBI may not be able to provide an accurate estimate of the RPE during exercise (21). Hence, the judgment should be based primarily on the objective HR measurements. The participants should be closely supervised when changes are made to the training loads to ensure that they can perform these exercises safely and are able to cope without premature fatigue. The supervisor should record any mishaps that may occur during training and take the necessary remedial measures. If the TBI participants are involved in a group exercise program, then they should be encouraged to interact with each other after the training session. This could have a positive influence on the mood, psychological well-being and social skills of the participant. It should be recognized that if music is used in a group exercise situation, this could be annoying and distracting to some participants with TBI.

CASE STUDIES

The following two case studies are actual examples of individuals who incurred a moderate to severe TBI. They were admitted into a long-term brain injury rehabilitation program (BIRP) in Alberta, Canada. This in-patient program offers rehabilitation services, including physical therapy, occupational therapy, speech language, recreation therapy, psychological counseling, nutrition counseling, and other support services as required (27,28). These two individuals participated in a research study conducted by the authors (7). Typically, participants in this BIRP arise at approximately 7 AM and complete their morning hygiene, often with nursing assistance, before having breakfast, which is scheduled at 8 AM. Most scheduled therapies begin at 9 AM, although occupational therapy sometimes schedules bathing and dressing training as early as 8:15 AM. The therapy services listed above vary on a daily basis, but are usually offered between 9 AM and 4 PM.

CASE 1

Demographics and Etiology

C, a 23-year-old man, experienced two major accidents. At age 16 he was involved in an accident between a snowmobile and a car. It was reported that he experienced a short bout of unconsciousness. His medical history also suggested that he may have had other concussions as a result of sports, including hockey and boxing. He led an active social life which included weekend parties and reported use of alcohol, marijuana, and other recreational drugs. Seven years later, C incurred a severe TBI as a result of a collision between an all-terrain vehicle, which he was operating, and an automobile. He was assigned a GCS rating of 5/15 at the scene and was airlifted to a major trauma center. The duration of coma was approximately 5 days. CT scans revealed intracerebral hemorrhages to the right cerebral peduncle and in the left parietal lobe, and bilateral frontal lobe subdural and intracerebral hematomas. Blood was seen in both the lateral and fourth ventricles. Musculoskeletal injuries included fractures of the right fibula and right sacrum as well as small diastosis of the left sacroiliac joint. At the time of this second injury, C was unemployed and receiving government social assistance for persons with severe handicaps. He was living with his parents but was independent with respect to all areas of his personal care.

Physical Limitations

On admission to the BIRP, C was independently able to self-propel to and from his therapy programs and to attend recreational and social activities in a manual wheelchair. His admission score on the FAM for mobility was 6 for wheelchair ambulation, indicating that he was able to self-propel independently in his wheelchair distances greater than 50 m and negotiate turns and ramps. He experienced difficulty with high level balance tasks. At the time of admission, he could walk with aids (walker, cane), with one-person assistance and negotiate stairs with two-person assistance.

Cognitive Limitations

Neuropsychological testing completed over the first month of his admission revealed low borderline performance in organization, information processing speed, memory, behavioral control and awareness of his deficits.

Time Course of Rehabilitation

C was admitted 5.5 months after injury into the BIRP where he received treatment for 6 months. The details of the program have been previously reported (27,28). During this period, he participated in a circuit training program conducted by the authors. This program was in addition to the regular physical therapy, occupational therapy, and other treatments that he received as an inpatient. The specific goals of the circuit training program were to (a) increase aerobic capacity to avoid undue fatigue, (b) improve muscular strength and endurance of major muscle groups, (c) minimize weight gain during the rehabilitation program, and (d) be able to walk 50 m independently.

C completed 33 circuit training sessions over a 14-week training period. During each training session, he wore a wireless heart rate monitor to record his training intensity. Each session lasted 1 hour and was divided into three phases: 10 minutes of warm-up, 45 minutes of training, and 5 minutes of cool-down. The supervising therapist demonstrated each exercise to him so that he could perform them safely without assistance. During the warm-up, C completed several stretching exercises of the major muscle groups of the upper and lower body. These exercises were designed to improve his flexibility. During the training phase, C completed 20 minutes of aerobic training on the cycle ergometer, treadmill, or both. He trained at a HR equivalent to 60% of his HR reserve. This was calculated on the basis of the initial cycle ergometer test that was designed to measure his peak $\dot{V}O_2$. C had no difficulty in attaining his prescribed training HR of 138 bpm during the training sessions. During the first few sessions, he could not complete the entire 20 minutes without a break.

He was allowed to rest as required (usually 1–2 minutes) and then complete the required 20 minutes of aerobic training. C then completed the rest of the exercise stations, which were primarily designed to increase his muscle strength and endurance. These exercises were performed on the Total Gym and Hydrafitness equipment. Each exercise was demonstrated to him and he was encouraged to perform them to the best of his ability. Initially C required some assistance because of muscle weakness due to his TBI and sedentary lifestyle. However, he seemed to enjoy these exercises and showed considerable improvement as the training progressed. After completing these circuits, C completed a cooldown phase, which included stretching of the muscle groups that were previously exercised. The supervisor recorded the HR during the various phases of the training session.

The changes in peak exercise capacity and body composition that C demonstrated as a result of the circuit training program are summarized in Table 9.1 and Table 9.2, respectively. He demonstrated increases in all the peak cardiorespiratory responses that were characteristic of an untrained able-bodied subject: PO, 50%;

TABLE 9.1. CHANGES IN PEAK AEROBIC FITNESS FOLLOWING THE CIRCUIT TRAINING PROGRAM

VARIABLE	CASE NO.	PRE-TRAINING	POST-TRAINING	CHANGE (%)
Power	1	60	90	50
watts	2	45	60	33
Oxygen uptake	1	1.43	1.76	23.1
L/min	2	0.95	1.03	7.3
Oxygen uptake	1	16.6	19.3	16.2
mL/kg/min	2	15.7	14.2	9.5
Heart rate	1	183	193	9.8
beats/min	2	135	112	16.1
Ventilation rate	1	54.0	70.6	37.4
L/min	2	23.3	23.1	−0.9
Oxygen pulse	1	7.8	9.1	16.7
mL/beat	2	7.1	9.2	29.6
Ventilatory	1	37.8	40.2	6.3
equivalent	2	24.4	22.5	7.8

TABLE 9.2. CHANGES IN BODY COMPOSITION RESULTING FROM A CIRCUIT TRAINING PROGRAM

VARIABLE	CASE NO.	PRE-TRAINING	POST-TRAINING	CHANGE (%)
Body mass (kg)	1	81.8	89.1	8.9
	2	62.6	64.5	3.0
Body mass index	1	25.9	28.2	8.9
	2	22.5	23.0	2.2
Body fat percent	1	14.8	18.0	21.6
	2	18.6	20.1	8.1
Lean body mass percent	1	85.2	82.0	−3.8
	2	81.4	79.9	−1.8
Body fat (kg)	1	12.1	16.0	32.2
	2	11.5	12.9	12.2
Lean body mass (kg)	1	69.7	73.1	4.9
	2	51.1	51.6	1.0

absolute peak $\dot{V}O_2$, 23.1%; relative peak $\dot{V}O_2$, 16.2%; HR, 9.8%; VE, 37.4%; O_2, 16.7%; $V_E/\dot{V}O_2$ ratio, 12%. The increase in O_2 pulse suggests that C also experienced an increase in cardiac stroke volume during exercise. These results indicate that C was able to tax a greater proportion of his cardiovascular reserve subsequent to the circuit training program. Despite the increase in energy expended as a result of the circuit training program, C gained 7.3 kg in body mass. His %BF increased from 14.0% to 18.0% during this 14-week period, and this was not a healthy development in his program. This increase in body mass would increase the energy cost of weight-bearing activities, such as walking, and cause premature fatigue. This was an activity that he was having considerable difficulty with as a result of the TBI.

Discharge from Rehabilitation Hospital

C was discharged from the hospital 6 months after his admission. The FAM scores assigned 2 weeks after his admission to the rehabilitation program and at discharge are summarized in Table 9.3. These results indicate that, despite his increased body mass, his walking steadily improved and, at discharge, he was able to walk 50 m in 2 minutes independently using a cane. C was assigned a FAM score of walking −6 for locomotion. His FAM score for stairs improved from a 2 to a 5, indicating that at discharge it was recommended that he be supervised but not assisted on stairs. His Berg balance score improved from 31/56 on admission to 41/56 at discharge. Throughout his stay in the rehabilitation program he experienced increased tone in his right side affecting both his upper and lower limb. A right elbow contracture limited extension by 15–20 degrees. At discharge, FAM scores for adjustment to limitations and safety judgment had improved from a 2 to a 4 and from a 3 to a 5, respectively. This represents very limited self-awareness of the significant cognitive deficits he was

TABLE 9.3. CASE STUDIES: FUNCTIONAL ASSESSMENT MEASUREMENT SCORES

FUNCTION	ACTIVITY/PROCESS	CASE STUDY 1		CASE STUDY 2	
		ADMISSION	DISCHARGE	ADMISSION	DISCHARGE
Mobility	Walking	Walking, 6	Walking, 6	W/c, 5	Walking, 5
Transfers	Bed, chair, wheelchair	2	5	4	6
	Toilet	6	6	4	6
	Tub or shower	6	6	4	5
Self-care	Dressing upper body	6	5	5	5
	Dressing lower body	5	6	5	5
	Bathing	5	6	2	5
Cognitive	Problem-solving	5	5	2	2
	Memory	2	3	2	3
	Orientation	2	5	3	4
	Attention	3	7	2	3
	Safety judgment	5	5	2	2
Psychosocial	Adjustment to limitations	3	5	2	2
	Employability	2	4	3	3
Communication	Comprehension	2	3	4	4
	Expression	5	6	4	4
	Reading	4	6	2	5
	Writing	5	6	3	5
	Speech intelligibility	4	4	6	6

W/c, wheelchair dependent.

experiencing and their impact on his ability to live independently. At discharge, C returned to live with his parents. Referrals were made to the appropriate community services to provide on-going support to C and his family. This included recommendations for participation in active living programs so that he could improve or maintain his existing fitness levels.

CASE 2

Demographics and Etiology

M, a 34-year-old woman, incurred a TBI as a result of a motor vehicle accident. At the time of her injury, she was married to a farmer and had two school-aged children. For the previous 9 years she worked primarily as a homemaker and mother and assisted with farming activities. Before that, she was employed as a designer for a monogram company. Her GCS rating was 3/15 at the scene, implying a very severe brain injury. Her GCS was between 5 and 7/15 in the emergency department and subsequently dropped to 3 again. A CT scan the day after her accident revealed petechial hemorrhages in the frontal lobes bilaterally and in the left parietal lobe extending into the left basal ganglia. A brainstem contusion was also queried. A second CT scan, 4 days after the injury indicated diffuse axonal shearing. The duration of coma was approximately 5 days. She also sustained a depressed fracture in the left parietal area and a fracture of the zygomatic bone of the right orbit. She also incurred fractures of the left ribs and scapula. A CT scan performed approximately 6 months after injury was indicative of minimal atrophy in the frontal lobes bilaterally and showed minimal attenuation peripherally in the

right occipital lobe consistent with traumatic atrophy. At the time of admission, she presented with cognitive deficits, visual disturbances thought to be related to cranial nerve injuries, decreased balance, right foot drop, poor balance, and dysmetria on reaching tasks. She was occasionally incontinent of both bowel and bladder.

Physical Limitations

On admission to the rehabilitation program M used a manual wheelchair for mobility and walked only when supervised by staff. Her initial Berg balance score was 36/56. At discharge she was walking with a four-wheeled walker with supervision and her Berg balance score had increased to 39/56. Transfers to and from a bed, chair, and toilet had improved from minimal one-person assist to independent using grab bars and transfer poles. Tub transfers improved from needing one-person physical assistance to needing supervision and cuing only. Her Clinical Outcome Variables Scale (COVs) scores improved from 47/91 at admission to 72/91 at discharge. Her average speed measured while completing a 2-minute walk test improved from 0.3 m/sec to 0.46 m/sec.

Cognitive Limitations

Neuropsychology testing completed approximately 4.5 months after injury revealed moderate to severe impairment in all aspects of cognitive functioning.

Time Course of Rehabilitation

M was admitted into the BIRP 89 days after injury. She was enrolled in the program for a total of 410 days (13.5 months). During this period, she participated in the same circuit training program that C participated in, approximately 6 months after her accident. The overall goals for her training were similar to those of C. M completed 28 training sessions over the 14-week training period. During the aerobic training phase, the prescribed target HR was 105 bpm based on her initial incremental exercise test. However, M had considerable difficulty attaining this HR during training, which is consistent with previous research (34) that has demonstrated this in patients with acute TBI. She was unable to complete the required 20 minutes continuously and had to take several breaks. M had difficulty motivating herself to participate in the circuit training program and completed an average of only two training sessions per week.

The changes in peak aerobic fitness and body composition as a result of participating in the circuit raining program for M are presented in Tables 9.1 and 9.2, respectively. Although M did show some improvement in peak VO$_2$, the magnitude of the improvement was considerably lower that that observed in C. This is most likely because of the difficulty that M had in attaining the aerobic training prescription based on her initial fitness level. However, M demonstrated a large decrease in her peak HR after the circuit training program, despite the increase in the peak power output. It is likely that her ability to attain a higher peak power output after training was owing to increased quadriceps muscle strength and endurance rather than an increase in aerobic fitness.

Discharge from Rehabilitation Hospital

As can be seen in the chart of FAM scores in Table 9.3, M demonstrated a great improvement in her ability to ambulate. At admission, she was ambulating in a wheelchair, whereas at discharge she was able to walk a distance of 50 m independently. She also demonstrated good improvement in the ability to transfer from the bed, chair, and wheelchair and in some other areas of self-care. M demonstrated significant changes in her cognitive skills, particularly in the area of reading and writing. At discharge, her FAM scores for adjustment to limitations and safety judgment remained unchanged from admission. This represents very limited self-awareness of the significant cognitive deficits she was experiencing and their impact on her ability to live independently. At discharge, M returned to live with her family. Family members, including her mother and mother-in-law, provided assistance and supervision with household and child-rearing activities. Referrals were made to the appropriate community services to provide on-going support to M and her family.

Although these two individuals completed 33 and 28 circuit training sessions, respectively, over a period of 14 weeks, this moderately high level of participation was owing to the structure and routines established within the rehabilitation hospital. The circuit training sessions were scheduled three times per week and copies of the patient's schedules were posted on their units, made available to the patient, and were also accessible to therapists on-line. As with the regularly scheduled therapy programs, such as occupational and physical therapy, staff sought out patients who did not keep their appointments and encouraged them to participate in treatment and exercise sessions. Even when a patient initially refused, efforts were made to verbally persuade them to attend and often they would. People with TBI who live in the community would not have the same degree of external support and encouragement to attend exercise programs. Members of the rehabilitation team should include participation in regularly scheduled exercise in their discharge planning and make special efforts to facilitate access to fitness programs for individuals with TBI. Caregivers should be educated about the importance of exercise and the health implications in the TBI population.

REFERENCES

1. American College of Sports Medicine. *Guidelines for Exercise Testing and Prescription.* Philadelphia: Lippincott Williams & Wilkins; 2001.

2. Ashman TA, Gordon WA, Cantor JB, Hibbard MR. Neurobehavioral consequences of traumatic brain injury. *Mt. Sinai J Med* 2006; 73(7):999–1005.

3. Barnard P, Dill H, Eldredge P, Held JM, Judd DL, Nalette E. Reduction of hypertonicity by early casting in a comatose head-injured individual. A case report. *Phys Ther* 1984;64(10)1540–1542.

4. Bateman A, Culpan FJ, Pickering AD, Powell JH, Scott OM, Greenwood RJ. The effect of aerobic training on rehabilitation outcomes after recent severe brain injury: A randomized controlled evaluation. *Arch Phys Med Rehabil* 2001;82(2)174–182.

5. Bell SE, Hlatky R. Update in the treatment of traumatic brain injury. *Curr Treat Options Neurol* 2006;8(2)167–175.

6. Bhambhani Y, Maikala R, Farag M, Rowland G. Reliability of near-infrared spectroscopy measures of cerebral oxygenation and blood volume during handgrip exercise in nondisabled and traumatic brain-injured subjects. *J Rehabil Res Dev* 2006;43(7):845–856.

7. Bhambhani Y, Rowland G, Farag M. Effects of circuit training on body composition and peak cardiorespiratory responses in patients with moderate to severe traumatic brain injury. *Arch Phys Med Rehabil* 2005;86(2)268–276.

8. Bhambhani Y, Rowland G, Farag M. Reliability of peak cardiorespiratory responses in patients with moderate to severe traumatic brain injury. *Arch Phys Med Rehabil* 2003;84(11):1629–1636.

9. Binder S, Corrigan JD, Langlois JA. The public health approach to traumatic brain injury: An overview of CDC's research and programs. *J Head Trauma Rehabil* 2005;20(3):189–195.

10. Brain Trauma Foundation, American Association of Neurological Surgeons, Congress of Neurological Surgeons and Joint Section on Neurotrauma and Critical Care, AANS/CNS. Guidelines for the

management of severe traumatic brain injury. XIV. Hyperventilation. *J Neurotrauma* 2007;24(Suppl 1):S87–S90.

11. Brown TH, Mount J, Rouland BL, Kautz KA, Barnes RM, Kim J. Body weight-supported treadmill training versus conventional gait training for people with chronic traumatic brain injury. *J Head Trauma Rehabil* 2005;20:(5):402–415.

12. Butefisch CM. Neurobiological bases of rehabilitation. *Neurol Sci* 2006;27(Suppl 1):S18–S23.

13. Bhambhani Y, Coutts K, Gillespie M, et al. *Inclusive Fitness and Lifestyle Services of All Disabilities.* Canadian Society for Exercise Physiology; 2002.

14. Cantu RC. Posttraumatic retrograde and anterograde amnesia: Pathophysiology and implications in grading and safe return to play. *Journal of Athletic Training* 2001;36:244–248.

15. Centers for Disease Control and Prevention. *Traumatic Brain Injury in the United States: A Report to Congress.* Atlanta, Georgia: Centers for Disease Control and Prevention; 1999.

16. Coles JP. Imaging after brain injury. *Br J Anaesth* 1997;99(1):49–60.

17. Convertino VA, Bloomfield SA, Greenleaf JE. An overview of the issues: Physiological effects of bed rest and restricted physical activity. *Med Sci Sports Exerc* 1997;29(2):187–190.

18. Dault MC, Dugas C. Evaluation of a specific balance and coordination programme for individuals with a traumatic brain injury. *Brain Inj* 2002;16(3):231–244.

19. Dawes H, Bateman A, Culpan J, Scott O, Wade DT, Roach N, Greenwood R. The effect of increasing effort on movement economy during incremental cycling exercise in individuals early after acquired brain injury. *Clin Rehabil* 2003;17(5):528–534.

20. Dawes H, Scott OM, Roach NK, Wade DT. Exertional symptoms and exercise capacity in individuals with brain injury. *Disabil Rehabil* 2006;28(20):1243–1250.

21. Dawes HN, Barker KL, Cockburn J, Roach N, Scott O, Wade D. Borg's rating of perceived exertion scales: Do the verbal anchors mean the same for different clinical groups? *Arch Phys Med Rehabil* 2005;86(5):912–916.

22. Driver S, O'Connor J, Lox C, Rees K. Evaluation of an aquatics programme on fitness parameters of individuals with a brain injury. *Brain Inj* 2004;18(9):847–859.

23. Giacino JT, Kalmar K, Whyte J. The JFK Coma Recovery Scale-Revised: Measurement characteristics and diagnostic utility. *Arch Phys Med Rehabil* 2004;85(12):2020–2029.

24. Goldstein LB. Prescribing of potentially harmful drugs to patients admitted to hospital after head injury. *J Neurol Neurosurg Psychiatry* 1995;58(6):753–755.

25. Gordon WA, Zafonte R, Cicerone K, et al. Traumatic brain injury rehabilitation: State of the science. *Am J Med Rehabil* 2006;85(4):343–382.

26. Gracies JM. Physical modalities other than stretch in spastic hypertonia. *Phys Med Rehabil Clin North Am* 2001;12(4):769–792, vi.

27. Gray DS. Slow-to-recover severe traumatic brain injury: A review of outcomes and rehabilitation effectiveness. *Brain Inj* 2000;14(11):1003–1014.

28. Gray DS, Burnham RS. Preliminary outcome analysis of a long-term rehabilitation program for severe acquired brain injury. *Arch Phys Med Rehabil* 2000;81(11):1447–1456.

29. Henson MB, De Castro JM, Stringer AY, Johnson C. Food intake by brain-injured humans who are in the chronic phase of recovery. *Brain Inj* 1993;7(2):169–178.

30. Horn S, Watson M, Wilson BA, McLellan DL. The development of new techniques in the assessment and monitoring of recovery from severe head injury: A preliminary report and case history. *Brain Inj* 1992;6(4):321–325.

31. Hunter M, Tomberlin J, Kirkikis C, Kuna ST. Progressive exercise testing in closed head-injured subjects: Comparison of exercise apparatus in assessment of a physical conditioning program. *Phys Ther* 1990;70(6):363–371.

32. Irdesel J, Aydiner SB, Akgoz S. Rehabilitation outcome after traumatic brain injury. *Neurocirugia (Astur)* 2007;18(1):5–15.

33. Iverson GL, Gaetz M, Lovell MR, Collins MW. Cumulative effects of concussion in amateur athletes. *Brain Inj* 2004;18(5):433–443.

34. Jackson D, Turner-Stokes L, Culpan J, Bateman A, Scott O, Powell J, Greenwood R. Can brain-injured patients participate in an aerobic exercise programme during early inpatient rehabilitation? *Clin Rehabil* 2001;15(5):535–544.

35. Jankowski LW, Sullivan SJ. Aerobic and neuromuscular training: Effect on the capacity, efficiency, and fatigability of patients with traumatic brain injuries. *Arch Phys Med Rehabil* 1990;71(7):500–504.

36. Jankowski LW, Sullivan SJ. Aerobic and neuromuscular training: Effect on the capacity, efficiency, and fatigability of patients with traumatic brain injuries. *Arch Phys Med Rehabil* 1990;71(7):500–504.

37. Jorge RE, Robinson RG, Moser D, Tateno A, Crespo-Facorro B, Arndt S. Major depression following traumatic brain injury. *Arch Gen Psychiatry* 2004;61(1):42–50.

38. Kraus JF, McArthur DL. Epidemiologic aspects of brain injury. *Neurol Clin* 1996;14(2):435–450.

39. Laatsch L, Krisky C. Changes in fMRI activation following rehabilitation of reading and visual processing deficits in subjects with traumatic brain injury. *Brain Inj* 2006;20(13–14):1367–1375.

40. LaRoche SM, Helmers SL. The new antiepileptic drugs: Clinical applications. *JAMA* 2004;291(5):615–620.

41. Lequerica AH, Rapport LJ, Loeher K, Axelrod BN, Vangel SJ, Jr, Hanks RA. Agitation in acquired brain injury: Impact on acute rehabilitation therapies. *J Head Trauma Rehabil* 2007;22(3):177–183.

42. Lim HB, Smith M. Systemic complications after head injury: A clinical review. *Anaesthesia* 2007;62(5):474–482.

43. McKinlay WW, Watkiss AJ. Cognitive and behavioral effects of brain injury. In: Rosebthal M, Kreutzer J, Griffith E, Pentland B, eds. *Rehabilitation of the Adult and Child with Traumatic Brain Injury.* Philadelphia: FA Davis; 1999:74–86.

44. Mehrholz J, Major Y, Meissner D, Sandi-Gahun S, Koch R, Pohl M. The influence of contractures and variation in measurement stretching velocity on the reliability of the Modified Ashworth Scale in patients with severe brain injury. *Clin Rehabil* 2005;19(1):63–72.

45. Mossberg KA. Reliability of a timed walk test in persons with acquired brain injury. *Am J Med Rehabil* 2003;82(5):385–90; quiz 391–392.

46. Mossberg KA, Ayala D, Baker T, Heard J, Masel B. Aerobic capacity after traumatic brain injury: Comparison with a nondisabled cohort. *Arch Phys Med Rehabil* 2007;88(3):315–320.

47. Mossberg KA, Greene BP. Reliability of graded exercise testing after traumatic brain injury: Submaximal and peak responses. *Am J Med Rehabil* 2005;84(7):492–500.

48. Painter P, Durstine JL, Rimmer J, Morgan D, Franklin B, Pitteti K. Increasing physical activity in disabled populations. *Medicine and Science in Sports and Exercise* 1998;30(5, Suppl):S86.

49. Parnes LS, Agrawal SK, Atlas J. Diagnosis and management of benign paroxysmal positional vertigo (BPPV). *CMAJ* 2003;169(7):681–693.

50. Putnam S, Fichtenberg N. Neuropsychological examination of the patient with traumatic brain injury. In: Rosenthal M, Kreutzer J, Griffith E, Pentland B, eds. *Rehabilitation of the Adult and Child with Traumatic Brain Injury.* Philadelphia: FA Davis; 1999:147–166.

51. Raggueneau JL, Gambini D, Levante A, Riche F, de Vernejoul P, Echter E. [Monitoring of extra- and intra-cellular compartment through total body impedance (author's transl)]. *Anesth Analg (Paris)* 1979;36(9–10):439–443.

52. Ruff R. Two decades of advances in understanding of mild traumatic brain injury. *J Head Trauma Rehabil* 2005;20(1):5–18.

53. Salazar AM, Jabbari B, Vance SC, Grafman J, Amin D, Dillon JD. Epilepsy after penetrating head injury. I. Clinical correlates: A report of the Vietnam Head Injury Study. *Neurology* 1985;35(10):1406–1414.

54. Satkunam LE. Rehabilitation medicine: 3. Management of adult spasticity. *CMAJ* 2003;169(11):1173–1179.

55. Scherzer BP. Rehabilitation following severe head trauma: Results of a three-year program. *Arch Phys Med Rehabil* 1986;67(6):366–374.

56. Seel RT, Wright G, Wallace T, Newman S, Dennis L. The Utility of the FIM + FAM for Assessing Traumatic Brain Injury Day Program Outcomes. *J Head Trauma Rehabil* 2007;22(5):267–277.

57. Singer BJ, Jegasothy GM, Singer KP, Allison GT, Dunne JW. Incidence of ankle contracture after moderate to severe acquired brain injury. *Arch Phys Med Rehabil* 2004;85(9):1465–1469.

58. Taber KH, Warden DL, Hurley RA. Blast-related traumatic injury: What is known? *J Neuropsychiatry Clin Neurosci* 2006;18(2): 141–145.

59. Teasdale G, Jennett B. Assessment of coma and impaired consciousness. *Lancet* 1974;2:81–84.

60. Temkin NR, Dikmen SS, Anderson GD, et al. Valproate therapy for prevention of posttraumatic seizures: A randomized trial. *J Neurosurg* 1999;91(4):593–600.

61. Thurman DJ, Coronado V, Selassie A. The epidemiology of brain injury: Implications for public health. In: Zasler ND, Katz DI, Zafonte RD, eds. *Brain Injury Medicine, Principles and Practice.* New York: Demos Medical Publishing; 2007;13:45–55.

62. Varghese G. Heterotopic ossification. *Phys Med Rehabil Clin North Am* 1992:407–415.

63. Vaynman S, Gomez-Pinilla F. License to run: Exercise impacts functional plasticity in the intact and injured central nervous system by using neurotrophins. *Neurorehabil Neural Repair* 2005;19(4):283–295.

64. Verweij BH, Amelink GJ, Muizelaar JP. Current concepts of cerebral oxygen transport and energy metabolism after severe traumatic brain injury. *Prog Brain Res* 2007;161:111–124.

65. Vitale AE, Jankowski LW, Sullivan SJ. Reliability for a walk/run test to estimate aerobic capacity in a brain-injured population. *Brain Inj* 1997;11(1):67–76.

66. Vitale AE, Sullivan SJ, Jankowski LW. Underestimation of subjects' monitored radial pulse rates following traumatic brain injury. *Percept Mot Skills* 1995;80(1):57–58.

67. Vitale AE, Sullivan SJ, Jankowski LW, Fleury J, Lefrancois C, Lebouthillier E. Screening of health risk factors prior to exercise or a fitness evaluation of adults with traumatic brain injury: A consensus by rehabilitation professionals. *Brain Inj* 1996;10(5):367–375.

68. Wehman P, Targett P, West M, Kregel J. Productive work and employment for persons with traumatic brain injury: What have we learned after 20 years? *J Head Trauma Rehabil* 2005;20(2):115–127.

69. Wilson DJ, Powell M, Gorham JL, Childers MK. Ambulation training with and without partial weightbearing after traumatic brain injury: Results of a randomized, controlled trial. *Am J Med Rehabil* 2006;85(1):68–74.

70. Wolman RL, Cornall C. Aerobic training in brain-injured patients. *Clinical Rehabilitation* 1994;8:253–257.

71. Yamada T, Yeh M, Kimura J. Fundamental principles of somatosensory evoked potentials. *Phys Med Rehabil Clin North Am.* 2004;15:19–42.

72. Zhu XL, Poon WS, Chan CC, Chan SS. Does intensive rehabilitation improve the functional outcome of patients with traumatic brain injury (TBI)? A randomized controlled trial. *Brain Inj* 2007; 21(7):681–690.

73. Ziino C, Ponsford J. Measurement and prediction of subjective fatigue following traumatic brain injury. *J Int Neuropsychol Soc* 2005; 11(4):416–425.

Musculoskeletal Conditions

KENNETH PITETTI, *Section Editor*

More than 100 rheumatologic conditions are considered forms of arthritis. Osteoarthritis (OA), rheumatoid arthritis (RA) and fibromyalgia syndrome (FM) are three of the most common forms. Each is a very distinct condition. Although there is no cure for OA, RA, or FM, each condition can be medically and pharmacologically managed with some success. Surgical procedures have been successful, especially for patients with OA and RA. Patient education programs, including exercise, nutritional counseling, and behavior modification techniques, have also had therapeutic benefits for certain patients. These types of arthritis typically result in long-term disability to the patient. In fact, arthritis is the leading cause of disability in the United States (1). Additionally, arthritis-attributable work limitations have been reported by approximately 30% of people with arthritis (2). Therefore, many patients are interested in therapeutic treatments, especially exercise, to help them manage their disease and decrease their levels of disabilities. In general, rehabilitative exercise has been shown to have a significant impact on decreasing the impairment and disability of arthritis.

EPIDEMIOLOGY AND PATHOPHYSIOLOGY

OSTEOARTHRITIS

Osteoarthritis (OA), also known as degenerative joint disease or osteoarthrosis, is the most common type of arthritis and one of the most common chronic diseases in the United States (3), affecting approximately 27 million people (4). It is the second most common cause of long-term disability in the adult population (3,5). Contrary to popular myth, it is not a normal characteristic of aging, yet it is strongly related to age. Clinical signs and symptoms of OA are estimated to be present in 12% of people 25–75 years of age (3). OA is characterized by localized degeneration of the articular cartilage (the major pathology) and synthesis of new bone at the joint surfaces or margins. It typically affects the hips, knees, feet, spine, and hands. Risk factors for OA are age, gender, race, occupation (i.e., repetitive trauma, overuse), obesity, history of joint trauma, bone or joint disorders, genetic mutations of collagen, and a history of inflammatory arthritis (3).

The prevalence of OA differs, depending on which joints are considered and how the disease is assessed. The prevalence of OA also differs among different populations. Many individuals may show OA on x-ray, but have no symptoms. Therefore, the prevalence of OA when assessed by x-ray is much higher than when determined by the symptomatology. Of the population, 90% shows evidence of degenerative changes in weight-bearing joints (hips, knees, feet) by age 40; however, symptoms are generally not present (6). These x-ray changes and the incidence of symptomatic OA continue to progress with increasing age. OA occurs more frequently in women than men after age 50, with evidence of an increase in disease severity and the number of joints affected (7,8). This disparity becomes larger with age. Under the age of 45, however, the prevalence of OA is about the same for men and women. The incidence of OA is not well defined; however, for hip, knee, and hand OA, the incidence rises with age and is greater in women than men (9). Older women are more often diagnosed with OA of the hand and finger joints and the knees. Knee OA is more prevalent in black women than white women (10,11), as well as obese persons, nonsmokers, and those who are physically active (12). Women are more susceptible than men to the inflammatory type of OA.

Osterarthritis is classified into two major types, primary OA and secondary OA (6). Primary or idiopathic OA, the most common type, is diagnosed when no cause is known for the symptoms. Secondary OA is diagnosed when there is an identifiable cause (e.g., trauma or underlying joint disorders). Each type is further classified into subtypes. For more information on the types and subtypes of OA, see Chapter 105 by Moskowitz in *Arthritis and Allied Conditions: A Textbook of Rheumatology* (6). Specific classification criteria have also been developed by the American College of Rheumatology for OA of the hand (13), knee (14), and hip (15). The common major criterion for each is the presence of pain. Because there is no nerve supply to the articular cartilage, pain may be caused by inflammation of the synovium, medullary hypertension, microfractures in the subchondral bone, stretching of periosteal nerve endings by the osteophytes (spurs), or stretching of ligaments and spasming of muscles around the inflamed joint capsule (16).

TABLE 10.1. COMMON SIGNS AND SYMPTOMS OF OSTEOARTHRITIS (OA), RHEUMATOID ARTHRITIS (RA), AND FIBROMYALGIA (FM)

OA	RA	FM
Pain during joint use	Joint pain	Diffuse nonarticular pain
Short-term stiffness (<30 min.)	Joint swelling	Multiple tender points
Gelling in inactive joints (stiffness for several minutes)	Joint stiffness (>60 min.)	Fatigue
	Contractures	Morning stiffness
Osteophytes (bony hypertrophy)	Muscle weakness	Sleep disturbance
Cartilage destruction	Fatigue	Possibly:
Joint malalignment	Systemic inflammation:	Irritable bowel syndrome (50% of cases)
Ligament and tendon laxity	Low grade fever	Tension headaches
Movement or gait problems	Malaise	Cognitive dysfunction
Muscle weakness	Myalgias	Fine motor weakness
Activity limitation	Loss of appetite	Restless leg syndrome
Pain worse during activity; better with rest	Weight loss	Temperature and chemical sensitivities
	Other organ systems affected	Paresthesias

Two hallmark symptoms of OA are pain during joint use and short-term stiffness or gelling in inactive joints. For the common signs and symptoms of OA, see Table 10.1. Inflammation is not a typical sign of OA, but mild synovial inflammation may be present in some cases. Specific joint symptoms are instability and buckling of the knees with knee OA, groin pain and radiating leg pain with hip OA, decreased manual dexterity with hand OA, and radiating pain, weakness, and numbness (nerve root compression) in neck and low back OA (3). As pain increases on joint loading or weight bearing, physical activity and joint mobility decreases. It is not unusual for joint contractures, especially of the weight-bearing joints, to occur secondary to the decrease in joint mobility. This leads to an increase in the energy expenditure needed to participate in functional and physical activities. Inactivity because of OA may consequently lead to an increased risk of other comorbid conditions, such as heart disease, hypertension, diabetes, depression, obesity, and some cancers.

RHEUMATOID ARTHRITIS

Rheumatoid arthritis (RA) is a chronic, systemic inflammatory disease affecting the synovium of diarthrodial joints. Synovitis or inflammation of the synovial membrane is the dominant pathology. The prevalence of RA is approximately 1%–2% in the population, affecting women two to three times more often than men (3,17,18). RA affects all ethnic groups. RA is most often diagnosed between the ages of 30 and 60 years, although prevalence increases with age (3). In addition, RA tends to shorten life expectancy (19). The incidence of RA is 0.5 per 100 people per year (3). The etiology of RA is unknown; however, the progression and pattern of inflammation are both related to genetic and environmental factors (3). For example, first-degree relatives of patients with RA are at 1.5 times higher risk of developing RA than the general population. Overall heritability of RA is estimated to be 50%–60% (3).

RA can be classified in terms of the functional status of the patient. Functional status is divided into four classes (20). Please refer to Table 10.2 for a description of the RA functional status classes. When prescribing exercise for an individual with RA, functional status must be considered.

With RA, it is typical to observe symmetric and bilateral joint involvement, marked over time by structural damage and deformities (3,21). Inflammatory synovitis may result in reversible (morning stiffness, synovial inflammation) and irreversible (structural joint damage)

TABLE 10.2. RHEUMATOID ARTHRITIS (RA) FUNCTIONAL STATUS CLASSES

FUNCTIONAL CLASS	PATIENT ABILITIES CAN PERFORM INDEPENDENTLY	LIMITATIONS IN PERFORMANCE
I	Self-care activities (e.g., feeding, bathing, grooming) Recreational and leisure activities Work, school, and home activities	None
II	Self-care activities Work, school, and home activities	Recreational and leisure activities
III	Self-care activities	Work, school, and home activities Recreational and leisure activities
IV	None	Self-care activities Work, school, and home activities Recreational and leisure activities

signs and symptoms of RA. With synovial inflammation, patients commonly experience prolonged morning stiffness (>1 hour). This is unlike the morning stiffness that is experienced in OA, which typically lasts up to 30 minutes. With a remission of inflammation, the patient with RA has a decrease in morning stiffness. During active inflammatory synovitis, the affected joints are usually warm, red, and swollen. A linear relationship exists between the time of active, uncontrolled synovitis and the progression of joint structural damage (3). Joint destruction usually begins within the first 1–2 years of the disease. Prognostic variables have been identified that predict a poor outcome for patients with RA. Some of these are being female, having a strong family history of RA, a large number of swollen and tender joints, a high rheumatoid factor (RF) titer (in 75%–85% cases of RA), high anticyclic citrullinated peptide (anti-CCP) titer, persistent pain, increased erythrocyte sedimentation rate (ESR) and C-reactive protein (CRP) levels, and low socioeconomic status (3).

Common signs and symptoms of RA are joint pain, swelling, stiffness, and contractures, with concomitant muscle weakness and fatigue. The muscles and tendons that surround the inflamed joints tend to spasm and shorten, whereas the ligaments are weakened by the enzymatic breakdown of collagen. The most common joints affected are the hands, wrists, elbows, shoulders, cervical spine, hips, knees, ankles, and feet. Other nonarticular symptoms that may occur include low grade fever, malaise, myalgias, and decreased appetite and weight loss because of the systemic inflammation (3). In approximately 40%–50% of patients with RA, inflammation of other organ systems occurs. Some of these extra-articular manifestations are skin (e.g., rheumatoid nodules), ophthalmologic (e.g., keratoconjunctivitis sicca), respiratory (e.g., pleuritis), cardiac (e.g., pericarditis), gastrointestinal (e.g., gastritis, peptic ulcer), renal (e.g., interstitial renal disease), neurologic (e.g., cervical spine instability, peripheral nerve entrapment), vascular (e.g., vasculitis), and hematologic (e.g., normocytic normochromic anemia) (3). The most common extra-articular condition is Sjögren's syndrome (dry eyes and mouth), which occurs in approximately 35% of patients (3). Patients with RA have a higher incidence of myocardial infarction and stroke than the general population because of accelerated atherosclerosis as a result of chronic inflammation (3). For the common signs and symptoms of RA, see Table 10.1.

FIBROMYALGIA

Fibromyalgia (FM) is a rheumatic syndrome that presents as chronic diffuse nonarticular musculoskeletal pain, yet it does not appear to be an inflammatory process (3). It is not considered a true form of arthritis. FM is not associated with the development of joint deformities or joint disease (22–24). It is the most common rheumatic cause of chronic widespread pain (3) and affects approximately 5 million Americans (4). FM is predominantly diagnosed in women between 30 and 50 years of age (3,25). The approximate prevalence of FM in population-based studies indicates rates from 3% to 5% in women and 0.5% in men (4,26). The prevalence of FM appears to increase with age. It presents in approximately 15% of rheumatology patients and 5% of general medical patients (3). Individuals with autoimmune disease are at a higher risk of developing FM (26). The incidence of FM is unknown. FM has previously been known as fibrositis, psychogenic rheumatism, nonarticular rheumatism, primary fibromyalgia (no underlying or concomitant condition), and secondary fibromyalgia (other concomitant conditions). In 1990, however, criteria for classifying patients with FM were published by the Multicenter Committee of the American College of Rheumatology (ACR) (27) and the classifications were abandoned.

The etiology of FM is unknown. Studies have been conducted that suggest possible factors for the development of FM, however, none are conclusive. It has been suggested that the pain of FM may be caused by (a) genetic factors, including a genetic susceptibility to microtrauma of the musculature or neurohormonal dysfunction, and polymorphisms that affect the metabolism or transport of monoamines, which are important for sensory processing and responding to stress; (b) peripheral mechanisms, such as muscle tissue abnormalities and microtrauma; and (c) central mechanisms, including electroencephalographic (EEG) abnormalities during sleep, neuroendocrine abnormalities (i.e., hypothalamic-pituitary-adrenal axis, low blood serum levels of serotonin, high cerebrospinal fluid (CSF) levels of substance P and low levels of somatomedin C), immunologic factors (i.e., viral infection, Lyme disease), physical trauma, psychological distress or psychiatric disorders, regional pain conditions, and abnormalities in central nervous center (CNS) structures (i.e., thalamus and caudate nucleus) (3,25,28).

Common symptoms and features of FM are diffuse nonarticular (soft tissue) pain, multiple tender points, fatigue and morning stiffness, and sleep disturbance (3). For the common signs and symptoms of FM, see Table 10.1. Fatigue, the most limiting feature, affects 75%–80% of people with FM, and is often due to poor sleep (3). In addition, patients with FM may have concomitant osteoarthritis, RA, Lyme disease, or sleep apnea. FM symptoms may be exacerbated by inactivity, emotional stress, poor sleep, high humidity, and moderate physical activity (3). Approximately 30% of patients with FM have a diagnosis of depression as well (29).

In general, risk factors associated with all types of arthritis can be considered nonmodifiable and modifiable. The nonmodifiable risk factors are female gender (60% of all cases), genetic predisposition, and age. Although arthritis is not considered a normal part of the aging process, the risk does increase with age. Modifiable risk factors are obesity, joint injuries, infections, and certain physically demanding occupations (especially those that require repetitive knee-bending) (30).

CLINICAL EXERCISE PHYSIOLOGY

Many studies have shown that patients with OA, RA, or FM have lower neuromuscular and cardiorespiratory function, as well as physical functioning (flexibility, functional performance), than nondiseased individuals. In a very general sense, this is due to the effect that pain has on the ability of the patient to exercise and even perform activities of daily living (ADLs). These patients are less active because of the pain on movement. This leads to a neuromuscular deconditioning, followed by a generalized cardiorespiratory deconditioning, and ultimately, difficulty in performing their everyday activities. This downward spiral (loss of physiologic reserve) will continue unless appropriate treatments are given.

Many studies have shown that significant declines occur in joint range of motion (ROM) or flexibility (31–33), neuromuscular function, including EMG activity, muscle strength, muscle endurance, and muscle contraction speed (31,33–49), cardiorespiratory function, including $\dot{V}O_2$, heart rate (HR), blood pressure (BP), and exercise capacity (32,35,38,40,50–55), functional performance, including walking, climbing stairs (31,32,42, 47,49,52–55,57–64), physical fitness (65), and physical activity (47,66–69). In addition, increases in arthritis symptoms, including pain, have been documented (31,32,42,49,50,52,55–63). In general, they also show that pain and inflammation limit physical activity and performance on all physiologic and functional tests. This is most likely because of motor unit or muscle inhibition (70,71). For patients with OA, RA or FM, incorrectly prescribed or performed exercises may exacerbate arthritis symptoms, especially the pain associated with the microtrauma to the joints and/or musculature.

Many different exercise programs have been studied in the OA, RA, and FM patient groups. Most have focused on aerobic exercise, resistance exercise, or general conditioning protocols (72–84). In general, they have been successful in eliciting some level of improvement in flexibility (33,54,77,85–93), neuromuscular function (33,34,39,43–46,52,56–62,77,81,86–90,92,94–129), cardiovascular function (39,52,54,77,81,86,89,92,94,99, 100,106,107,116,129–139), functional performance (34, 43,52,56–64,88,91–93,95–97,100,104,106,108,110,114, 116,118,121,124,126,129,131–134,137,139,140–159,16 1–163), pain (44,45,52–54,56–62,64,77,87,88,90–97, 105,106,108,109,113,114,116,121,122,124,125,127–132, 134,135,138–140,142–146,149–152,154,156,158,159,161– 173), disease symptomatology (33,34,43,44,53,54,64,77, 85,88,90,92,93,99,105,106,109,110,113,114,116,118, 121,127–131,135,139,144,146,147,150–156,162,163,

165–168,171–174), exercise self-efficacy (63,114,126, 128,141,145,149,153,155,158,170,175), psychological function (i.e., depression, anxiety, quality of life) (54,63, 77,85,93,109,113,121,124,127,128,133,138,139,148– 155,162,165–167,171,174,176), and physical activity (77,115).

It is important for the exercise technician to accurately assess physiologic function and functional performance in the arthritis patient to prescribe an exercise progression that would focus on improving the patient's physiologic and functional limitations. When prescribing exercise for patients with arthritis, it is critical to carefully assess baseline exercise capacity (cardiorespiratory, neuromuscular, flexibility, and so forth) and functional performance or status to prescribe individually the most beneficial program for each patient. Individually prescribed progressive programs, based on physiologic and functional deficits, are necessary to ensure that the patients do not fail in the early stages of an exercise program. For the arthritis patient, it is useful to begin the exercise progression slowly, to allow the patient to adapt physiologically, prevent early exacerbation, and reduce the potential for noncompliance.

PHARMACOLOGY

Pain reduction or relief is the primary reason for pharmacologic treatments in OA, RA, and FM. Usually the first line of treatment for OA is simple analgesics, such as acetaminophen. At times, topical analgesics, such as capsaicin cream, may provide pain relief as well. The second line of medications for OA and the first line for RA are nonsteroidal anti-inflammatory drugs (NSAIDs). NSAIDs inhibit the synthesis of proinflammatory prostaglandins (3). Examples of these are aspirin, celecoxib, ibuprofen, naproxen, and indomethacin. Although they generally provide good pain relief, this class of drugs also is known for their increased risk of upper gastrointestinal, renal, hepatic, and central nervous system toxicity (177). Not much evidence exists that indicates that NSAIDs are effective for FM (24).

Low dose oral corticosteroids, such as prednisone, may be used. With local, severe inflammation or a joint effusion, intra-articular corticosteroid injections may be indicated for relief of the painful joint in OA and RA. Because of the high toxicity of corticosteroids, they are not used as often, and should only be used as an adjunct to other pharmacologic or nonpharmacologic therapies. Adverse reactions to corticosteroids include osteoporosis, myopathy, cataracts, hypertension, and diabetes mellitus (3,177). Intra-articular injections of hyaluronan may reduce the symptoms of early OA (3).

Another class of medications is disease modifying antirheumatic drugs (DMARDs). DMARDs are more often indicated for patients with RA and are used aggressively early in the disease process (usually within 3–6 months of disease onset) to prevent disability. Effectiveness of the DMARDs for RA is determined by their ability to change the course of RA by increasing physical function, decreasing inflammatory synovitis, and slowing structural damage. Examples of DMARDs are methotrexate, leflunomide, sulfasalazine, hydroxychloroquine, and injectable gold. Methotrexate, the most common DMARD, has been used successfully in combination with other DMARDs and biologics. As with the other arthritis medications, each DMARD has its related toxic effects. For example, long-term methotrexate use typically results in liver function complications, whereas sulfasalazine can result in gastrointestinal and CNS toxicity. Biologics, which are also considered DMARDs, specifically target the pathogenic mediators of joint inflammation and damage (e.g., tumor necrosis factor [TNF] antagonists, anti-IL-1 receptor antagonists). Common biologic agents include the TNF inhibitors (i.e., etanercept, infliximab, and adalimumab), which specifically inhibit the proinflammatory cytokine, TNF-α, and anti-IL-1 receptor antagonists (i.e., anakinra). For more severe RA, the biologics abatacept and rituximab may be needed. Side effects of the TNF inhibitors may include an increased risk of lymphoma and other malignancies, heart failure, and demyelinating disorders (3). No evidence exists that suggests that any DMARDs are effective or can modify OA.

Popular treatments for arthritis, especially OA, are glucosamine, chondroitin sulfate, or the combination of both. Their effectiveness for relieving pain is equivocal (178). It appears that they are most effective for moderate to severe knee pain (179). Currently, research is being conducted to determine the use of vitamins C and D for reducing the risk of progression of knee OA.

Specific to FM, medications are used to improve restorative sleep and mood, and decrease pain to reduce fatigue and decrease the symptomatology of FM. Some of the pharmacologic agents used for sleep include amitriptyline, cyclobenzaprine, zolpidem, and pramipexole. Medications for pain include amitriptyline, tramadol, duloxetine, and the anticonvulsants gabapentin and pregabalin. Medications prescribed to improve mood include tricyclic antidepressants (amitriptyline and cyclobenzaprine), selective serotonin reuptake inhibitors (SSRIs), such as fluoxetine and sertraline, and serotonin-norepinephrine reuptake inhibitors (SNRIs) (venlafaxine and duloxetine) (3). Recently, pregabalin was the first drug approved by the US Food and Drug Administration (FDA) for treating FM after research showed that it decreased pain and improved restorative sleep in patients with FM (180). As is typical with any medication, their effectiveness is not the same for all patients. A meta-analysis of the efficacy of treatment outcomes for FM indicates that nonpharmacologic treatments, especially exercise in combination with cognitive behavioral therapy, give the best outcomes (181). However, these can be supplemented by pharmacologic treatments to reduce pain and sleep disturbances. See Table 10.3 for the common pharmacologic treatments for OA, RA, and FM.

Each pharmacologic agent for arthritis has side effects and toxicity levels that can have an impact on different physiologic systems. In general, there does not appear to be

TABLE 10.3. SOME COMMON PHARMACOLOGIC TREATMENTS FOR OSTEOARTHRITIS (OA), RHEUMATOID ARTHRITIS (RA), AND FIBROMYALGIA (FM)

OA	RA	FM
Analgesics	**NSAIDs** (see OA list)	**Pain**
Acetaminophen (Tylenol)	**DMARDs**	Pregabalin (Lyrica)
Capsaicin (Capzasin-P)	Methotrexate (Rheumatrex)	Gabapentin (Neurontin)
NSAIDs	Leflunomide (Arava)	Duloxetine (Cymbalta)
Aspirin	Sulfasalazine (Azulfidine)	Tramadol (Ultram)
Celecoxib (Celebrex)	Hydroxychloroquine (Plaquenil)	Amitriptyline (Elavil)
Ibuprofen (Advil)	**Biologics**	**Sleep**
Naproxen (Aleve)	Etanercept (Enbrel)	Amitriptyline (Elavil)
Corticosteroids	Infliximab (Remicade)	Cyclobenzaprine (Flexeril)
Prednisone	Adalimumab (Humira)	Zolpidem (Ambien)
Viscosupplementation	Abatacept (Orencia)	Pramipexole (Mirapex)
Hyaluronan (Euflexxa)	Rituximab (Rituxan)	Pregabalin (Lyrica)
Hylan G-F 20 (Synvisc)		**Mood**
		SSRIs
		Fluoxetine (Prozac)
		Sertraline (Zoloft)
		SNRIs
		Venlafaxine (Effexor)
		Duloxetine (Cymbalta)
		Tricyclics
		Amitriptyline (Elavil)

DMARDs, disease modifying antirheumatic drugs; NSAIDs, nonsteroidal anti-inflammatory drugs; SNRIs, serotonin-norepinephrine reuptake inhibitors; SSRIs, selective serotonin reuptake inhibitors.

any more risk of these medications having an impact on exercise testing and training than any other class of medications. To find out the specific impact of each drug and its interactions, the reader is referred to the PDR (*Physicians' Desk Reference*) (182). For OA, RA, and FM, it is always recommended that the pharmacologic management be used in combination with nonpharmacologic treatments.

PHYSICAL EXAMINATION

Osteoarthritis is typically diagnosed by a history and physical examination (3). Several characteristics that may be present on physical examination (i.e., joint palpation) in a patient with OA are localized symptomatic joints, pain on motion (joint capsule irritation), tenderness at the joint margins and capsules (bony enlargements), decreased range of joint motion (osteophyte formation, contractures), joint instability, joint locking (loose bodies or cartilage fragments in joint), crepitus (irregular joint surfaces), joint malalignment (varus or valgus deformity), and local signs of inflammation (warmth, soft tissue swelling). Blood tests and synovial fluid are typically normal. A diagnosis of OA is confirmed by radiographs of the affected joints. Osteophyte formation (bony proliferation) at the joint margins is a typical finding on x-ray of a patient with OA. Other findings that indicate OA on the x-ray are asymmetric joint space narrowing, subchondral bone sclerosis, and possibly subchondral cyst formation. If bone demineralization (periarticular osteoporosis) and erosion of bone at the joint margins is visible on x-ray, the diagnosis is more likely RA than OA (3).

Rheumatoid arthritis is difficult to diagnose early on in the disease process because of the lack of definitive characteristics that are typically present. It generally takes several weeks to several months for RA to be present before it can be diagnosed. The onset is insidious. The American College of Rheumatology has described the seven criteria for classifying an individual with RA. To have a diagnosis of RA, the patient needs to have at least four of the seven criteria, and criteria one through four need to be present for a minimum of 6 weeks. See Table 10.4 for the RA classification criteria (3,183). On palpation of surface joints (fingers, elbows, knees), joint deformities may be evident. Deformities of the deeper joints (shoulders, hips) may only be evident by ROM limitations. Usually joint deformities occur in the upper extremity, especially the fingers and wrist, first, as the patient can still function adequately even with a reduced ROM and less mobility.

For a diagnosis of FM to be made, certain criteria must be met. See Table 10.5 for the FM diagnostic criteria (27).

MEDICAL AND SURGICAL TREATMENTS

Medical management of patients with OA, RA, or FM must use a multidisciplinary approach. In general, the

---

TABLE 10.4. RHEUMATOID ARTHRITIS (RA) CLASSIFICATION CRITERIA[a]

1. Morning stiffness lasting a minimum of 1 hour in and around the joints.
2. Soft tissue swelling or fluid in at least three joint areas (especially hands, wrists, elbows, knees, ankles and feet) simultaneously.
3. At least one swollen hand or wrist joint.
4. Concurrent involvement of the same joint area bilaterally.
5. Rheumatoid nodules (subcutaneous nodules that typically are located over bony prominences or extensor surfaces).
6. Abnormal amount of serum rheumatoid factor.
7. Radiographic evidence of structural changes typical of RA, such as bone erosion or decalcification in or adjacent to the involved joints (especially the hand and wrist).

[a] For a diagnosis of RA, 4 of 7 criteria must be present. Criteria 1-4 need to be present for a minimum of 6 weeks.

---

major goals for treating patients with OA, RA, and FM are fourfold. They are to relieve the arthritis symptoms (e.g., pain), maintain or increase physical functioning, limit physical disability, and avoid drug toxicity (3,184). Besides the prescription of medications, medical treatments may include referring the arthritis patient to the appropriate healthcare professionals for different nonpharmacologic treatments, such as joint protection and energy conservation techniques (including assistive devices), weight loss and maintenance, use of heat and cold modalities, patellar taping techniques (for knee OA), transcutaneous electrical nerve stimulation (TENS) for pain relief, exercise, meditation, acupuncture, biofeedback, and massage (3,16,80). In addition, for patients with RA, short-term splinting of inflamed joints (hands) may be indicated to decrease inflammation and joint trauma, as well as increase joint alignment. For those with FM, the interaction between pain, fatigue, sleep and mood disturbances, as well as general physical deconditioning, must be taken into account. In addition to exercise, electrical

---

TABLE 10.5. FIBROMYALGIA (FM) DIAGNOSTIC CRITERIA

1. Patient must have a history of widespread pain (i.e. pain on both sides of the body and above and below the waist) for at least 3 months. Patient must have pain in the axial skeletal region (i.e. cervical spine, anterior chest, thoracic spine, or low back).
2. Patient must have pain in 11 of 18 tender points (9 bilateral points) on digital palpation of approximately 4 kg or by using a calibrated dolorimeter. Tender point sites are:
   a. Occiput, at the suboccipital muscle insertions
   b. Low cervical, at the anterior aspects of the intertransverse spaces of C5-C7
   c. Trapezius, at the midpoint of the upper border
   d. Supraspinatus, above the medial border of the scapular spine
   e. Second rib, at the second costochondral junctions
   f. Lateral epicondyle, 2 cm distal to the epicondyles
   g. Gluteal, at the upper outer quadrants of the buttocks
   h. Greater trochanter, posterior to the trochanteric prominence
   i. Knee, at the medial fat pad proximal to the joint line

stimulation of the tender areas, coupled with heat (ultrasound or whirlpool), may be therapeutic for patients with FM. For patients with FM and RA, it is important to treat their underlying depression. This can typically be treated by tricyclic antidepressants, patient education, or both. It has been shown that patients who are younger and have less severe disease have better outcomes (3).

Cognitive behavioral therapies have been shown to reduce pain and disability in patients with OA, RA, and FM (24,74,167,185–189). Some of these therapies include relaxation training, activity pacing, coping skills training, reinforcement of healthy behaviors, and pain management techniques.

Surgery for OA and RA is usually not considered a treatment alternative until the patient cannot get pain relief from other methods and has significant functional impairments. Several surgical options are available for different joints. For the knee, arthroscopic debridement, lavage with meniscectomy, or both may be performed to increase joint function and decrease pain by removing loose fragments of cartilage, bone and menisci (3). Osteotomies for the knee (high tibial) and hip (femoral) may be performed to realign the joints and redistribute the loading on the joints (3). For very advanced disease, arthrodesis or joint fusion may be performed to decrease pain, and increase stability and joint alignment. This procedure is more frequently performed for the spine (cervical and lumbar), wrists, ankles, and hand and foot joints (3). Joint fusion is not typically recommended because it completely eliminates joint motion and may increase loading on the unfused joints. A surgical treatment that is successful in reducing or eliminating arthritis pain is total joint arthroplasty. This procedure is performed routinely for knees and hips. Total joint replacements, although usually successful, cannot exactly replicate natural articular cartilage and over time may need revision (3). No surgical techniques have been recommended for FM. The rate of recovery from surgery depends on the patient's condition before surgery. Therefore, it is important to try to optimize presurgical functional status (122).

DIAGNOSTIC TECHNIQUES

As mentioned in the *Physical Examination* section above, a diagnosis of OA is made by a history and physical examination and confirmed by radiographs of the affected joints. As a routine matter, standard laboratory tests are conducted; results are typically normal. In addition, tests for rheumatoid factor (RF) and erythrocyte sedimentation rate (ESR) are conducted to exclude other joint diseases (3).

No one particular test confirms RA, although inflammatory synovitis must be present. This can be determined by leukocytes in the synovial fluid or evidence of joint erosion on x-ray. As mentioned previously, the history and physical examination are important procedures to help in the diagnosis. The main factor that indicates disease activity is the number of tender and swollen joints. Other factors include degree of pain and disability, radiographic progression, and serum levels of the inflammatory biomarkers (3). Laboratory tests to determine serum RF, anti-CCP antibodies, ESR, and C-reactive protein levels are typically ordered to assist with the diagnosis of RA. ESR and C-reactive protein are good indicators of synovial inflammation. Contrary to popular myth, RF is not a diagnostic test for RA (190). Some patients with RA are not RF positive, although approximately 85% of patients with RA have RF (3). For those patients who are RF positive, their disease is usually severe and they exhibit extra-articular manifestations of RA. Imaging techniques, such as x-ray, magnetic resonance imaging (MRI), and ultrasound, are common in RA to assess the degree of joint destruction (including articular cartilage, ligaments, tendons, and bones) and inflammation (3,190). Typical changes seen with imaging are symmetrical joint space narrowing, bony erosions on the joint margins, subluxation and joint malalignment, and laxity or rupture of the ligaments or tendons. Some clinical assessments include tender and swollen joint counts, ROM measurements, walking time, duration of morning stiffness, assessment of fatigue severity, and grip strength. Other diseases or conditions that may be confused for RA are psoriatic arthritis, lupus, systemic sclerosis, Sjögren's syndrome, and hepatitis C-associated polyarthritis (3).

In general, no standard diagnostic tests are available for FM. In addition to the classification criteria for FM outlined under *Physical Examination* (above), a sleep history is typically taken from the patient. The laboratory tests that may be done include a blood chemistry panel, complete blood count, liver and kidney function tests, and tests to determine levels of inflammatory markers (CRP and ESR), thyroid-stimulating hormone, and creatine kinase (3). These tests are frequently conducted to rule out other diseases, however. Several other conditions that can mimic FM include depression, regional pain syndrome, tapering of steroids, malignancy, drug-induced myopathy (from statins), diabetes, human immunodeficiency virus (HIV), hepatitis C, metabolic myopathies, osteomalacia, lupus, RA, polymyalgia rheumatica, hyper- or hypothyroidism, sleep apnea, and chronic fatigue syndrome (3).

EXERCISE/FITNESS/ FUNCTIONAL TESTING

In general, it is important for the patient to perform the exercise or functional test protocols in the most pain-free manner possible. Therefore, the exercise technician must consider the positioning of the patient during the testing, as well as the order of the tests to ensure appropriate recovery of the different systems (e.g., cardiorespiratory, neuromuscular) and muscle groups. It is not unusual for patients with OA and RA to have joint contractures and, therefore, reduced flexibility or ROM. Care must be taken with these patients to allow for recovery from fatigue between test protocols and to adjust testing equipment and protocols in case of pain or symptom exacerbation. If it is the judgment of the exercise technician that the risks of the testing outweigh the benefits derived from the exercise program, then the patient should not be tested.

Thoughtful planning of testing procedures is important for the different types of arthritis. Usually, there is some assessment of pain, physical limitations, physical function, flexibility, muscle function, and cardiovascular function. As mentioned earlier, taking into consideration the patient's symptoms and exercise goals will allow the exercise scientist to measure the appropriate variables.

Pain and functional limitations are often measured by self-report questionnaires, such as visual analog scales for pain or marking painful areas on a diagram of the body. Several specific assessments are valid and reliable for patients with arthritis. The two major assessment tools are the Arthritis Impact Measurement Scales 2 (191) for all types of arthritis and the Western Ontario and McMaster Universities (WOMAC) Osteoarthritis Index for OA (192). The assessment tool most often used for FM is the Fibromyalgia Impact Questionnaire (FIQ) (193).

Physical function or performance can be measured in many ways, including a 6-minute walk (distance) plus pulse and rating of perceived exertion, low back flexibility (sit and reach), rising from a chair for 1 minute, climbing stairs, and a measured walk for speed. Besides the sit and reach test, flexibility can be measured with a goniometer as the subject moves the desired joints through their ranges of motion. For shoulder flexibility, a forward reach test has been shown to be valid.

Muscle function (strength, endurance, contraction speed, power) can be measured isometrically, isotonically, or isokinetically. When conducting these tests, it is important to consider the effect that a painful joint will have on the ability to produce a maximal muscle contraction. Pain will result in neural inhibition, thereby leading to a much lower measure of muscle function. In some cases, EMG activity (surface or invasive) may also be measured.

Work capacity or aerobic function is measured in multiple ways as well. In some cases, depending on the severity of the disease, it may be more practical to estimate aerobic power from a submaximal test (194). Generally, most patients with OA, RA, or FM will be able to accomplish a symptom-limited graded exercise test, where the major symptoms are pain and peripheral muscle fatigue. It is important to consider the testing equipment that will be used to conduct the test. Using a weight-bearing activity, such as walking on a treadmill, may result in an abbreviated test because of joint pain in any of the weight-bearing joints. Performing a nonweight-bearing activity, such as on a cycle ergometer, may allow a more accurate measurement of cardiovascular function if patients can perform to a higher level before they experience pain and stop the test. Because of the possibility of comorbid conditions, especially cardiovascular diseases, it is recommended that all patients be continuously monitored (ECG, heart rate, and BP) throughout the cardiovascular testing (resting, work, and recovery). For patients with FM, it is usually standard to assess their pain threshold over their tender points using a dolorimeter.

EXERCISE PRESCRIPTION AND PROGRAMMING

As has been shown throughout this chapter, OA, RA, and FM are very different forms of arthritis. Therefore, it is important to understand the type of arthritis, the characteristic symptoms and limitations, prognosis of the disease, and other comorbid conditions that the patients have when prescribing exercises. Because of the pain, inflammation, fatigue, and limitations in joint movement, these patients are usually more deconditioned peripherally than centrally. This means that the limitations to exercise are usually in the peripheral musculature. Many arthritis patients will stop an exercise test protocol because of muscle fatigue or joint pain, not usually because of dyspnea, angina, or other acute cardiorespiratory events. Therefore, the type of exercise program should focus initially on the primary limitation of each type of arthritis and then progress to more general exercises. For example, if a patient has OA of the knee joint, has pain on weight bearing, and quadriceps muscle atrophy, nonweight-bearing resistance exercises would be more appropriate than aerobic exercises initially.

In general, patients with arthritis can participate in many different types of exercises. With a properly designed program, they will reap the same benefits as anyone who exercises. When designing an exercise program for individuals with arthritis, it is important to distinguish between exercising to improve functional capabilities and exercising to achieve a level of physical fitness. It is essential for the exercise specialist to provide exercises to increase the patient's functional capabilities first and then, increase physical fitness. The goal of many patients with arthritis is to engage in their normal everyday activities without undue fatigue or pain. In many cases, they may be more focused on this outcome than achieving a level of physical fitness.

Previous research has shown that patients with OA, RA, and FM can benefit from aerobic exercises, including walking, stationary cycling, and water exercise (53, 54,64,77,78,86,92,99,100,102,107,114–117,121,122, 129,131–141,143–146,149–151,153–158,165,166,168, 172,174,176,195), but the benefits over time may be relatively short-lived (86,131,196) or sustained above baseline measures for several months (53,64,85,100,115, 116,123,125,134,139,142,151,153–155,159,171,174,175). Although there may be aerobic benefits (e.g. increase in peak oxygen consumption) and reduction in pain (53,54,64,77,92,114,116,121,129–132,139,140,144,145, 149–151,154,156,158,165,166,168,172), generally there is not as much improvement accrues in muscle strength and muscle endurance or flexibility from aerobic programs (139). Warm water exercises are recommended for patients with arthritis. Some scientific evidence has shown that they improve the patients' aerobic capacity, muscle strength or endurance (89,115,126,150), joint flexibility and overall physical function, pain, quality of life, disease symptoms, self-efficacy, and mood (63,85,91,113,124, 139,141,150–154,157,159,161,165,166,171,174).

In patients with OA, RA, and FM, research focusing on resistance exercises has shown that these patients have dramatic improvements in muscle strength, muscle endurance, and contraction speed of the muscles that support the active joints (34,39,45,52,56–58,60–62,78,86, 88,94–101,103–106,108–113,117–120,122,123,125, 127–129,133,134,143,158). This type of exercise has also been shown to provide pain relief (45,52,56–58, 60–62,88,92,93,95–97,105,106,108,109,113,122,125, 127–130,133,134,143,145,146,148,149,158,163,164,169, 174) and increases in muscular efficiency, exercise capacity, and cardiovascular performance (39,52,86,88,99, 106,110,130,133–136,143), thereby allowing patients to perform aerobic exercises at a level where they can achieve a cardiovascular and aerobic benefit. In most cases, evidence indicates that arthritis patients who participate in resistance exercises can sustain their improvements above baseline measures for several months or more after the completion of the exercise programs (34,57,100,113,120,123,125,134,149).

The best exercise prescription for individuals with arthritis appears to be a progression from flexibility exercises, especially of affected joints (to prevent contractures), to muscle function exercises (focusing on muscle strength, endurance, and contraction speed), to aerobic exercises (including nonweight-bearing and weight-bearing alternatives). Built into this prescription may be functional activities (e.g., climbing stairs, rising from a low chair, walking) and relaxation activities (e.g., Tai Chi, yoga). This same type of progression would be useful for prescribing exercise for arthritis patients to improve their everyday function, as well as for improving fitness. Using this rehabilitative strategy, the approach may be more conservative initially in order to monitor any exacerbation of symptoms, determine the rate of physiologic adaptability to the exercise, and to encourage exercise compliance and program adherence.

Table 10.6 provides a general outline of progressive exercise prescriptions for individuals with OA, RA, and FM. The prescription is basically the same for OA and RA. However, for RA, it is critical to build an appropriate rest and recovery time into the protocol so as not to cause a flare-up, exacerbation, or undo inflammation because of an intense acute bout of exercise. Appropriate rest is also critically important for FM patients.

TABLE 10.6. GENERAL AND PROGRESSIVE EXERCISE PRESCRIPTIONS FOR OSTEOARTHRITIS (OA), RHEUMATOID ARTHRITIS (RA), AND FIBROMYALGIA (FM)[a]

TYPE OF ARTHRITIS	EXERCISE	PROGRESSION	FREQUENCY	INTENSITY	DURATION
OA	Flexibility	• ROM	Daily	Active/gentle	10–15 min
	Resistance	• Strength	2–3×/wk	10%–80% max	5–10 reps
		• Endurance	2–3×/wk	10%–80% max	90–120 sec
		• Speed	2–3×/wk	10%–80% max	5–10 reps
	Aerobic	• Endurance	3–4×/wk	60%–80% peak HR	30–60 min (cumulative)
	Functional Activities		Daily	Moderate	1–5 reps
RA	Flexibility	• ROM	Daily	Active/gentle	10–15 min
	Resistance	• Strength	2–3×/wk	10%–80% max	5–10 reps
		• Endurance	2–3×/wk	10%–80% max	90–120 sec
		• Speed	2–3×/wk	10%–80% max	5–10 reps
	Aerobic	• Endurance	3–4×/wk	60%–80% peak HR	30–60 min (cumulative)
	Functional Activities		Daily	Moderate	1–5 reps
FM	Flexibility	• ROM	Daily	Active/gentle	10–15 min
	Resistance	• Isotonic/isometric	2–3×/wk	5%–80% of max	5–30 reps
		• Endurance	2–3×/wk	5%–80% of max	30–120 sec
		• Speed	2–3×/wk	5%–80% of max	5–30 reps
		• Strength	2–3×/wk	5%–80% of max	3–5 reps
	Aerobic	• Endurance	3–4×/wk	40%–80% of peak HR	10–60 min (cumulative 30 min)
	Functional Activities		Daily	Low–moderate	1–5 reps

Min, minutes; reps, repetitions; ROM, range of motion; sec, seconds.

[a]See text for explanation of progression.

FLEXIBILITY EXERCISES

A general program of flexibility and stretching exercises is important for individuals with OA, RA, and FM (33,54,92,93,118,122,149,158,172,173). It is important to gently and actively move all joints through the ROM to prevent joint contractures and to stretch the surrounding musculature. This may be performed three to five times a day. To prevent injury, the joints should never be forced through their ROM.

RESISTANCE ACTIVITIES

Resistance exercise programs have become very popular for OA (34,52,56,57,60–62,88,92,93,95–97,122,123, 125,127–129,143,145,158,163,169,173,197), RA (39,78, 79,86,98–100,103–106,108,117–120), and FM (33,43–45, 94,109,110,112,113,130,149). When prescribing resistance exercises for patients with arthritis, it is important initially to assess each patient's limitations. Whether using a strain gauge, isokinetic device, or the one repetition maximum (1-RM) technique, it is important to have a measurement of the patient's maximal capability for any given muscle or muscle group before prescribing resistance exercise. Based on the symptomatology, the progression of resistance exercises may differ for patients with FM than for patients with OA and RA. Several types of resistance exercises can be prescribed for arthritis patients (i.e. isometric, isotonic, or isokinetic), which can be used in different ways to address deficits in muscle strength, muscle endurance. or muscle contraction speed.

Strength

For OA and RA patients who have direct joint involvement, it is important to begin the resistance training with maximal voluntary isometric contractions of the muscles that support the affected joints. An isometric contraction will maximally contract the muscle without joint movement. Ideally, there is no pain. To improve strength, three to five maximal contractions of each muscle group should be performed once a day. Each contraction should be held for 5–10 seconds (progression). Patients can perform isometric exercises using a variety of methods (e.g., resistance bands, overloaded weight bench, bicycle tire or surgical tubing, another person). Strength can also be improved by progressing to higher resistance, low repetition dynamic (formally known as isotonic contractions) muscle contractions. It is recommended that the progression for resistances begins very low (approximately 10% of the patient's maximum) and progresses at a maximal rate of 10% per week. Although this may appear conservative, it allows the exercise technician to monitor the patient's progress and ability to adapt to the exercise without an exacerbation of symptoms. Patients should perform the dynamic contractions or exercises three times per week. They do not need to do more than 5–10 repetitions with any muscle group per day. For patients with FM, the initial resistances may be lower and the progression slower than for the OA and RA patients because of the potential for more widespread pain and fatigue. For these patients, performing up to 30 repetitions would be advisable before increasing the resistance. If the patients have access to a clinic with isokinetic equipment, they can perform the isometric and isokinetic exercises with supervision. In all cases, regardless of where the patients go to exercise, they need to be taught the proper mechanics of performing each exercise so as not to become injured or progress at too rapid a rate.

Endurance

Several ways exist to improve muscle endurance. Traditionally, muscle endurance has been addressed using a low resistance, high repetition model. Although this may improve the endurance of the slow twitch or type I muscle fibers, it does not train all muscle fiber types equally within the muscle. To address multiple muscle fiber types, it is important to sustain a muscle contraction over time. One way to do this is by having the patient lift the prescribed resistance (beginning at 10% of maximal and increasing by 10% each week) and holding it for a period of time. Depending on the type of arthritis, the patient may progressively increase the amount of time the resistance is held or always hold it for a predetermined amount of time. For example, patients with OA and RA can sustain the contraction for 90 seconds at each training session, whereas the FM patients may initially hold the contraction for 30 seconds and eventually work up to 90 seconds using the same resistance before increasing to a higher resistance.

Contraction Speed or Rate of Force Development

Another aspect of muscle physiology that is frequently overlooked when exercising individuals with arthritis is their ability to contract their muscles quickly. It is important to improve their muscle contraction speed or rate of force development to improve their ability to do certain functional activities (e.g., cross the street before the traffic light changes) and to help prevent falls. In many people with arthritis, their gait becomes affected over time, either because of joint deformities, pain, fatigue, and possible contralateral limb compensation strategies. Contraction speed can be improved by having the patient lift the prescribed resistances as rapidly as possible in a controlled manner through the range of joint motion. If dynamic exercises are performed without supervision, it is extremely important to teach the patient how to lift the resistances in a controlled manner to protect the arthritic joint and to prevent muscle injury and undue pain. These exercises can also be performed safely using isokinetic equipment. Patients with FM will be able to add contraction speed exercises into their exercise progression earlier in their programs than patients with OA and RA because with FM, there is not as much concern for joint effusions. It is recommended that for patients with OA and RA, contraction speed exercises should be added to the progression last, after the muscles around the affected joints have begun to adapt and help support the joint. It is recommended that this higher impact activity be performed 3 days per week and using lower resistances initially. Within 6–12 weeks, the musculature should be trained to a level where the patient starts to notice significant improvements in function and, in many cases, a reduction in pain and fatigue levels.

CARDIOVASCULAR ACTIVITIES

Once the musculature has been trained sufficiently and the muscles can be used more efficiently, it is recommended that aerobic exercises and functional activities be added to the exercise progression. Again, if the potential exists to measure the patients' maximal or peak aerobic power, this will provide the tools to prescribe the best aerobic program. An important consideration when prescribing an aerobic training program for persons with arthritis is to consider the types of aerobic activity they are comfortable doing. For instance, many individuals with OA and RA are overweight and will not do water exercises because they are uncomfortable in public wearing a bathing suit. It is also important to consider if a non-weight-bearing or weight-bearing aerobic exercise would be more appropriate. Generally, whatever exercise the patient is willing to perform regularly will suffice. It is recommended that the exercise progression begin conservatively by allowing the patient to adapt to aerobic activity by using lower target heart rate ranges and then progress up to the cardiovascular training ranges.

FUNCTIONAL ACTIVITIES

Functional activities can be defined as basic physical activities that an individual does to participate in personal daily leisure, recreational, family, and work activities. Examples of these activities are walking, climbing stairs, rising from a chair, and bending. As part of an overall exercise program, it is important to include functional activities. It has been shown that, although there is physiologic adaptation with the traditional types of exercise, it does not translate into better functioning unless individuals can use their improved physiology to increase the efficiency of their actual functional activities.

EDUCATION AND COUNSELING

Other than the medical, pharmacologic, and surgical management of the different types of arthritis, patient self-management is critical. It has been shown that arthritis patients with higher self-efficacy report less pain and

impairment during physical activities (114,126,141,145, 149,153,155,158,170,198). Group programs, combining strategies to improve fitness and flexibility with stress reduction techniques and support groups, seem to hold promise as community or outpatient programs for individuals with arthritis (114,149,150,155,167,174,199). Generally, any programs to promote physical activity and weight reduction with which the patient will comply are recommended. The Arthritis Foundation offers several community-based programs for individuals with arthritis. These include the land-based Arthritis Foundation Exercise Program (formerly known as the People with Arthritis Can Exercise [PACE] Program) (114) and the warm water-based Arthritis Foundation Aquatic program. Both programs focus on low-level flexibility, strength, and endurance activities. Other Arthritis Foundation programs include Tai Chi (Sun style) and the Walk with Ease Program, which are designed to increase quality of life and encourage regular physical activity. Another educational intervention is the Arthritis Foundation Self-Help Program. It gives the patients information on their disease, medications, and side effects, dealing with their physicians, pain management, energy conservation techniques, nutrition, and weight management, relaxation techniques, and exercise and physical activity (3,30). This program has been shown to reduce the costs associated with arthritis care as well as reduce the patients' perceptions of pain by 20% (200,201). Infrequently, patients are referred to physical or occupational therapy, unless they experience an acute disease flare.

REFERENCES

1. Centers for Disease Control and Prevention (CDC). Prevalence of disabilities and associated health conditions among adults: United States, 1999. *MMWR* 2001;50:120–5.
2. Theis KA, Murphy L, Hootman JM, Helmick CG, Yelin E. Prevalence and correlates of arthritis-attributable work limitation in the US population among persons ages 18–64:2002 National Health Interview Survey data. *Arthritis Care Res* 2007;57(3):355–63.
3. Klippel JH, Stone JH, Crofford LJ, White PH, eds. *Primer on the Rheumatic Diseases*. 13th ed. New York: Springer; 2008.
4. Lawrence RC, Felson DT, Helmick CG, et al. Estimates of the prevalence of arthritis and other rheumatic conditions in the United States. Part II. *Arthritis Rheum* 2008;58:26–35.
5. Peyron JG, Altman RD. The epidemiology of osteoarthritis. In: Moskowitz RW, Howell DS, Goldberg VM, Mankin HJ, eds. *Osteoarthritis: Diagnosis and Medical/Surgical Management*. 2nd ed. Philadelphia: WB Saunders; 1992:15–37.
6. Moskowitz RW. Clinical and laboratory findings in osteoarthritis. In: Koopman WJ, editor. *Arthritis and Allied Conditions: A Textbook of Rheumatology*. 13th ed. Baltimore: Williams & Wilkins; 1997: 1985–2011.
7. Kellgren JH, Lawrence JS, Bier F. Genetic factors in generalized osteo-arthrosis. *Ann Rheum Dis* 1963;22:237–55.
8. Felson DT, Naimark A, Anderson JJ, Kazis L, Castelli W, Meenan RF. The prevalence of knee osteoarthritis in the elderly: The Framingham Osteoarthritis Study. *Arthritis Rheum* 1987;30:914–8.
9. Felson DT. Epidemiology of the rheumatic diseases. In: Koopman WJ, editor. *Arthritis and Allied Conditions: A Textbook of Rheumatology*. 13th ed. Baltimore: Williams & Wilkins; 1997:3–34.

10. Peyron JG. Epidemiologic and etiologic approach to osteoarthritis. *Semin Arthritis Rheum* 1979;8:288–306.

11. Anderson J, Felson DT. Factors associated with knee osteoarthritis (OA) in the HANES I survey: Evidence of an association with overweight, race and physical demands of work. *Am J Epidemiol* 1988;128:179–89.

12. Felson DT, Zhang Y, Hannan MT, Naimark A, Weissman B, Aliabadi P, Levy P. Risk factors for incident radiographic knee osteoarthritis in the elderly: The Framingham study. *Arthritis Rheum* 1997;40:728–33.

13. Altman R, Alarcón G, Applerouth D, et al. The American College of Rheumatology criteria for classification and reporting of osteoarthritis of the hand. *Arthritis Rheum* 1990;33:1601–10.

14. Altman R, Asch E, Bloch D, et al. Development of criteria for classification and reporting of osteoarthritis. Classification of osteoarthritis of the knee. *Arthritis Rheum* 1986;29:1039–49.

15. Altman R, Alarcón G, Applerouth D, et al. Criteria for classification and reporting of osteoarthritis of the hip. *Arthritis Rheum* 1991;34:505–15.

16. Brandt KD. Nonsurgical management of osteoarthritis, with an emphasis on nonpharmacologic measures. *Arch Fam Med* 1995;4: 1057–64.

17. Albani S, Carson DA. Etiology and pathogenesis of rheumatoid arthritis. In: Koopman WJ, ed. *Arthritis and Allied Conditions: A Textbook of Rheumatology.* 13th ed. Baltimore: Williams & Wilkins; 1997:979–92.

18. Helmick CG, Felson DT, Lawrence RC, et al. Estimates of the prevalence of arthritis and other rheumatic conditions in the United States. Part I. *Arthritis Rheum* 2008;58:15–25.

19. Wolfe F, Mitchell DM, Sibley JT, et al. The mortality of rheumatoid arthritis. *Arthritis Rheum* 1994;37:481–94.

20. Hochberg MC, Chang RW, Dwosh I, Lindsey S, Pincus T, Wolfe F. The American College of Rheumatology 1991 revised criteria for the classification of global functional status in rheumatoid arthritis. *Arthritis Rheum* 1992;35:498–502.

21. Hale LP, Haynes BF. Pathology of rheumatoid arthritis and associated disorders. In: Koopman WJ, ed. *Arthritis and Allied Conditions: A Textbook of Rheumatology.* 13th ed. Baltimore: Williams & Wilkins; 1997:993–1016.

22. Goldenberg DL. Treatment of fibromyalgia syndrome. *Rheum Dis Clin North Am* 1989;15:61–71.

23. Buckelew SP. Fibromyalgia: A rehabilitation approach. *Am J Phys Med Rehabil* 1989;68:37–42.

24. Goldenberg DL, Burckhardt C, Crofford L. Management of fibromyalgia syndrome. *JAMA* 2004;92:2388–95.

25. Bradley LA, Alarcón GS. Fibromyalgia. In: Koopman WJ, ed. *Arthritis and Allied Conditions: A Textbook of Rheumatology.* 13th ed. Baltimore: Williams & Wilkins; 1997:1619–40.

26. Lawrence RC, Helmick CG, Arnett FC, et al. Estimates of the prevalence of arthritis and selected musculoskeletal disorders in the United States. *Arthritis Rheum* 1998;41:778–99.

27. Wolfe F, Smythe HA, Yunus MB, et al. The American College of Rheumatology 1990 Criteria for the Classification of Fibromyalgia: Report of the Multicenter Criteria Committee. *Arthritis Rheum* 1990;33:160–72.

28. Mease P. Fibromyalgia syndrome. Review of clinical presentation, pathogenesis, outcome measures and treatment. *J Rheumatol* 2005;32:6–21.

29. Burckhardt CS, O'Reilly CA, Wien AN. Assessing depression in fibromyalgia patients. *Arthritis Care Res* 1994;1:35–9.

30. Arthritis Foundation, Association of State and Territorial Health Officials, and Centers for Disease Control and Prevention. *National Arthritis Action Plan: A Public Health Strategy.* Arthritis Foundation National Office, Atlanta, GA; 1999.

31. Mannerkorpi K, Burckhardt CS, Bjelle A. Physical performance characteristics of women with fibromyalgia. *Arthritis Care Res* 1994;7:123–9.

32. Minor MA, Hewett JE, Webel RR, Dreisinger TE, Kay DR. Exercise tolerance and disease related measures in patients with rheumatoid arthritis and osteoarthritis. *J Rheumatol* 1988;15:905–11.

33. Jones KD, Burckhardt CS, Clark SR, Bennett RM, Potempa KM. A randomized controlled trial of muscle strengthening versus flexibility training in fibromyalgia. *J. Rheumatol* 2002;29(5):1041–8.

34. Hurley MV, Scott DL. Improvements in quadriceps sensorimotor function and disability of patients with knee osteoarthritis following a clinically practicable exercise regimen. *Br J Rheumatol* 1998;37:1181–7.

35. Ettinger WH Jr., Afable RF. Physical disability from knee osteoarthritis: The role of exercise as an intervention. *Med Sci Sports Exerc* 1994;26:1435–40.

36. Slemenda C, Brandt KD, Heilman DK, Mazzuca S, Braunstein EM, Katz BP, Wolinsky FD. Quadriceps weakness and osteoarthritis of the knee. *Ann Intern Med* 1997;127:97–104.

37. Tan J, Balci N, Sepici V, Gener FA. Isokinetic and isometric strength in osteoarthrosis of the knee. *Am J Phys Med Rehabil* 1995;74:364–9.

38. Beals CA, Lampman RM, Figley Banwell B, Braunstein EM, Albers JW, Castor CW. Measurement of exercise tolerance in patients with rheumatoid arthritis and osteoarthritis. *J Rheumatol* 1985;12:458–61.

39. Danneskiold-Samsøe B, Lyngberg K, Risum T, Telling M. The effect of water exercise given to patients with rheumatoid arthritis. *Scand J Rehab Med* 1987;19:31–5.

40. Ekdahl C, Broman G. Muscle strength, endurance, and aerobic capacity in rheumatoid arthritis: A comparative study with healthy subjects. *Ann. Rheum Dis* 1992;51:35–40.

41. Hsieh LF, Didenko B, Schumacher HR Jr., Torg JS. Isokinetic and isometric testing of knee musculature in patients with rheumatoid arthritis with mild knee involvement. *Arch Phys Med Rehabil* 1987;68:294–7.

42. Fisher NM, Pendergast DR. Reduced muscle function in patients with osteoarthritis. *Scand J Rehab Med* 1997;29:213–21.

43. Valkeinen H, Alen M, Hannonen P, Häkkinen A, Airaksinen O, Häkkinen K. Changes in knee extension and flexion force, EMG and functional capacity during strength training in older females with fibromyalgia and healthy controls. *Rheumatology* 2004;43: 225–8.

44. Häkkinen A, Häkkinen K, Hannonen P, Alen M. Strength training induced adaptations in neuromuscular function of premenopausal women with fibromyalgia: A comparison with healthy women. *Ann Rheum Dis* 2001;60(1):21–6.

45. Valkeinen H, Häkkinen A, Hannonen P, Häkkinen K, Alen M. Acute heavy-resistance exercise-induced pain and neuromuscular fatigue in elderly women with fibromyalgia and in healthy controls: Effects of strength training. *Arthritis Rheum* 2006;54(4): 1334–9.

46. Häkkinen K, Pakarinen A, Hannonen P, Häkkinen A, Airaksinen O, Valkeinen H, Alen M. Effects of strength training on muscle strength, cross-sectional area, maximal electromyographic activity, and serum hormones in premenopausal women with fibromyalgia. *J Rheumatol* 2002;29(6):1287–95.

47. Thyberg I, Hass UAM, Nordenskiold U, Gerdle B, Skogh T. Activity limitation in rheumatoid arthritis correlates with reduced grip force regardless of sex: The Swedish TIRA Project. *Arthritis Care Res* 2005;53(6):886–96.

48. Hakkinen A, Hannonan P, Nyman K, Hakkinen K. Aerobic and neuromuscular performance capacity of physically active females with early and long-term rheumatoid arthritis compared to matched healthy women. *Scand J Rheumatol* 2002;31:345–50.

49. Ling SM, Xue QL, Simonsick EM, Tian J, Bandeen-Roche K, Fried LP, Bathon JM. Transitions to mobility difficulty associated with lower extremity osteoarthritis in high functioning older women: Longitudinal data from the Women's Health and Aging Study II. *Arthritis Care Res* 2006; 55:256–63.

50. Mengshoel AM, Vollestad NK, Forre O. Pain and fatigue induced by exercise in fibromyalgia patients and sedentary healthy subjects. *Clin Exp Rheumatol* 1995;13:477–82.

51. Philbin EF, Groff GD, Ries MD, Miller TE. Cardiovascular fitness and health in patients with end-stage osteoarthritis. *Arthritis Rheum* 1995;38:799–805.

52. Fisher NM, Pendergast DR. Effects of a muscle exercise program on exercise capacity in subjects with osteoarthritis. *Arch Phys Med Rehabil* 1994;75:792–7.

53. Richards SCM, Scott DL. Prescribed exercise in people with fibromyalgia: Parallel group randomised controlled trial. *BMJ* 2002;325:185–9.

54. Valim V, Oliveira L, Suda A, et al. Aerobic fitness effects in fibromyalgia. *J Rheumatol* 2003;30(5):1060–9.

55. Sutbeyaz ST, Sezer N, Koseoglu BF, Ibrahimoglu F, Tekin D. Influence of knee osteoarthritis on exercise capacity and quality of life in obese adults. *Obesity* 2007;15:2071–6.

56. Fisher NM, Gresham GE, Pendergast DR. Quantitative progressive exercise rehabilitation for osteoarthritis of the knee. *Phys Med Rehabil Clin North Am* 1994;5:785–802.

57. Fisher NM, Pendergast DR, Gresham GE, Calkins E. Muscle rehabilitation: Its effects on muscular and functional performance of patients with knee osteoarthritis. *Arch Phys Med Rehabil* 1991;72: 367–74.

58. Fisher DR, Pendergast DR. Application of quantitative and progressive exercise rehabilitation to patients with osteoarthritis of the knee. *Journal of Back and Musculoskeletal Rehabilitation* 1995;5:33–53.

59. Fisher NM, Gresham GE, Abrams M, Hicks J, Horrigan D, Pendergast DR. Quantitative effects of physical therapy on muscular and functional performance in subjects with osteoarthritis of the knees. *Arch Phys Med Rehabil* 1993;74:840–7.

60. Fisher NM, Gresham G, Pendergast DR. Effects of a quantitative progressive rehabilitation program applied unilaterally to the osteoarthritic knee. *Arch Phys Med Rehabil* 1993;74:1319–26.

61. Fisher NM, Kame VD, Rouse L, Pendergast DR. Quantitative evaluation of a home exercise program on muscle and functional capacity of patients with osteoarthritis. *Am J Phys Med Rehabil* 1994;73:413–20.

62. Fisher NM, White SC, Yack HJ, Smolinski RJ, Pendergast DR. Muscle function and gait in patients with knee osteoarthritis before and after muscle rehabilitation. *Disability Rehabil* 1997;19:47–55.

63. Gowans SE, deHueck A, Voss S, Silaj A, Abbey SE, Reynolds WJ. Effect of a randomized, controlled trial of exercise on mood and physical function in individuals with fibromyalgia. *Arthritis Care Res* 2001;45:519–29.

64. DaCosta D, Abrahamowicz M, Lowensteyn I, Bernatsky S, Dritsa M, Fitzcharles MA, Dobkin PL. A randomized clinical trial of an individualized home-based exercise programme for women with fibromyalgia. *Rheumatology* 2005;44:1422–7.

65. Bennett RM, Clark SR, Goldberg L, Nelson D, Bonafede RP, Porter J, Specht D. Aerobic fitness in patients with fibrositis: A controlled study of respiratory gas exchange and [133]xenon clearance from exercising muscle. *Arthritis Rheum* 1989;32:454–60.

66. Sokka T, Hakkinen A, Kautiainen H, et al. Physical inactivity in patients with rheumatoid arthritis: Data from twenty-one countries in a cross-sectional, international study. *Arthritis Care Res* 2008;59:42–50.

67. Mancuso CA, Rincon M, Sayles W, Paget SA. Comparison of energy expenditure from lifestyle physical activities between patients with rheumatoid arthritis and healthy controls. *Arthritis Care Res* 2007;57:672–8.

68. van den Berg MH, de Boer IG, le Cessie S, Breedveld FC, Vliet Vlieland TPM. Are patients with rheumatoid arthritis less physically active than the general population? *J. Clin Rheumatol* 2007; 13:181–6.

69. Shih M, Hootman JM, Kruger J, Helmick CG. Physical activity in men and women with arthritis. National Health Interview Survey, 2002. *Am J Prev Med* 2006;30(5):385–93.

70. McNair PJ, Marshall RN, Maguire K. Swelling of the knee joint: Effects of exercise on quadriceps muscle strength. *Arch Phys Med Rehabil* 1996;77:896–9.

71. Hurley MV. The role of muscle weakness in the pathogenesis of osteoarthritis. *Rheum Dis Clinics North Am* 1999;25:283–98.

72. Jones KD, Adams D, Winters-Stone K, Burckhardt CS. A comprehensive review of 46 exercise treatment studies in fibromyalgia (1988–2005). *Health Qual Life Outcomes* 2006;4:67.

73. Gowans SE, deHueck A. Effectiveness of exercise in management of fibromyalgia. *Curr Opin Rheumatol* 2004;16:138–42.

74. Rooks DS. Fibromyalgia treatment update. *Curr Opin Rheumatol* 2007;19:111–7.

75. Busch AJ, Barber KAR, Overend TJ, Peloso PMJ, Schachter CL. Exercise for treating fibromyalgia syndrome. *Cochrane Database Syst Rev* 2008;3.

76. Mannerkorpi K. Exercise in fibromyalgia. *Curr Opin Rheumatol* 2005;17:190–4.

77. Westby MD. A health professional's guide to exercise prescription for people with arthritis: A review of aerobic fitness activities. *Arthritis Care Res* 2001;45:501–511.

78. Stenstrom CH, Minor MA. Evidence for the benefit of aerobic and strengthening exercise in rheumatoid arthritis. *Arthritis Care Res* 2003;49:428–34.

79. Mayoux Benhamou MA. Reconditioning in patients with rheumatoid arthritis. *Ann Readapt Med Phys* 2007;50(6):382–5.

80. Vliet Vlieland TPM. Non-drug care for RA—Is the era of evidence-based practice approaching? *Rheumatology* 2007;46:1397–1404.

81. van den Ende CHM, Vliet Vlieland TPM, Munneke M, Hazes JMW. Dynamic exercise therapy for treating rheumatoid arthritis. *Cochrane Database Syst Rev* 2008;3.

82. Roddy E, Zhang W, Doherty M. Aerobic walking or strengthening exercise for osteoarthritis of the knee? A systematic review. *Ann Rheum Dis* 2005;64:544–8.

83. Bartels EM, Lund H, Hagen KB, Dagfinrud H, Christensen R, Danneskiold-Samsoe B. Aquatic exercise for the treatment of knee and hip osteoarthritis. *Cochrane Database Syst Rev* 2008;3.

84. Fransen M, McConnell S, Bell M. Exercise for osteoarthritis of the hip or knee. *Cochrane Database Syst Rev* 2008;3.

85. Hall J, Skevington SM, Maddison PJ, Chapman K. A randomized and controlled trial of hydrotherapy in rheumatoid arthritis. *Arthritis Care Res* 1996;9:206–15.

86. van den Ende CH, Hazes JM, le Cessie S, Mulder WJ, Belfor DG, Breedveld FC, Dijkmans BA. Comparison of high and low intensity training in well controlled rheumatoid arthritis. Results of a randomized clinical trial. *Ann. Rheum Dis* 1996;55: 798–805.

87. Dellhag B, Wollersjo I, Bjelle A. Effect of active hand exercise and wax bath treatment in rheumatoid arthritis patients. *Arthritis Care Res* 1992;5:87–92.

88. Huang M-H, Yang R-C, Lee C-L, Chen T-W, Wang M-C. Preliminary results of integrated therapy for patients with knee osteoarthritis. *Arthritis Care Res* 2005;53:812–20.

89. Wang TJ, Belza B, Thompson FE, Whitney JD, Bennett K. Effects of aquatic exercise on flexibility, strength and aerobic fitness in adults with osteoarthritis of the hip or knee. *J Adv Nurs* 2007; 57(2):141–52.

90. Messier SP, Loeser RF, Miller GD, et al. Exercise and dietary weight loss in overweight and obese older adults with knee osteoarthritis: The Arthritis, Diet, and Activity Promotion Trial. *Arthritis Rheum* 2004;50:1501–10.

91. Wyatt FB, Milam S, Manske RC, Deere R. The effects of aquatic and traditional exercise programs on persons with knee osteoarthritis. *J Strength Cond Res* 2001;15:337–40.

92. Peloquin L, Bravo G, Gauthier P, Lacombe G, Billiard J-S. Effects of a cross-training exercise program in persons with osteoarthritis of the knee. A randomized controlled trial. *J Clin Rheumatol* 1999;5: 126–36.

93. Petrella RJ, Bartha C. Home based exercise therapy for older patients with knee osteoarthritis: A randomized clinical trial. *J Rheumatol* 2000;27:2215–21.

94. Mengshoel AM, Komnaes HB, Forre O. The effects of 20 weeks of physical fitness training in female patients with fibromyalgia. *Clin Exp Rheumatol* 1992;10:345–9.

95. O'Reilly SC, Muir KR, Doherty M. Effectiveness of home exercise on pain and disability from osteoarthritis of the knee: A randomized controlled trial. *Ann Rheum Dis* 1999;58:15–19.

96. Røgind H, Bibow-Nielsen B, Jensen B, Møller HC, Frimodt-Møller H, Bliddal H. The effects of a physical training program on patients with osteoarthritis of the knees. *Arch Phys Med Rehabil* 1998;79:1421–7.

97. Maurer BT, Stern AG, Kinossian B, Cook KD, Schumacher HR. Osteoarthritis of the knee: Isokinetic quadriceps exercise versus an educational intervention. *Arch Phys Med Rehabil* 1999;80:1293–9.

98. Machover S, Sapecky AJ. Effect of isometric exercise on the quadriceps muscle in patients with rheumatoid arthritis. *Arch Phys Med Rehabil* 1966;47:737–41.

99. Lyngberg KB, Danneskiold-Samsøe B, Halskov O. The effect of physical training on patients with rheumatoid arthritis: Changes in disease activity, muscle strength and aerobic capacity. A clinically controlled minimized cross-over study. *Clin Exp Rheumatol* 1988;6:253–60.

100. Ekdahl C, Andersson SI, Moritz U, Svensson B. Dynamic versus static training in patients with rheumatoid arthritis. *Scand J Rheumatol* 1990;19:17–26.

101. Brighton SW, Lubbe JE, van der Merwe CA. The effect of a long-term exercise programme on the rheumatoid hand. *Br J Rheumatol* 1993;32:392–5.

102. Hansen TM, Hansen G, Langgaard AM, Rasmussen JO. Long-term physical training in rheumatoid arthritis. A randomized trial with different training programs and blinded observers. *Scand J Rheumatol* 1993;22:107–12.

103. Lyngberg KB, Ramsing BU, Nawrocki A, Harreby M, Danneskiold-Samsøe B. Safe and effective isokinetic knee extension training in rheumatoid arthritis. *Arthritis Rheum* 1994;37:623–8.

104. Hakkinen A, Hakkinen K, Hannonen P. Effects of strength training on neuromuscular function and disease activity in patients with recent-onset inflammatory arthritis. *Scand J Rheumatol* 1994;23:237–42.

105. Rall LC, Meydani SN, Kehayias JJ, Dawson-Hughes B, Roubenoff R. The effect of progressive resistance training in rheumatoid arthritis. Increased strength without changes in energy balance or body composition. *Arthritis Rheum* 1996;39:415–26.

106. Komatireddy GR, Leitch RW, Cella K, Browning G, Minor M. Efficacy of low load resistive muscle training in patients with rheumatoid arthritis functional class II and III. *J Rheumatol* 1997;24:1531–9.

107. Lyngberg KK, Harreby M, Bentzen H, Frost B, Danneskiold-Samsøe B. Elderly rheumatoid arthritis patients on steroid treatment tolerate physical training without an increase in disease activity. *Arch Phys Med Rehabil* 1994;75:1189–95.

108. McMeeken J, Stillman B, Story I, Kent P, Smith J. The effects of knee extensor and flexor muscle training on the timed-up-and-go test in individuals with rheumatoid arthritis. *Physiother Res Int* 1999;4:55–67.

109. Geel SE, Robergs RA. The effect of graded resistance exercise on fibromyalgia symptoms and muscle bioenergetics: A pilot study. *Arthritis Care Res* 2002;47:82–6.

110. Rooks DS, Silverman CB, Kantrowitz FG. The effects of progressive strength training and aerobic exercise on muscle strength and cardiovascular fitness in women with fibromyalgia: A pilot study. *Arthritis Rheum* 2002;47(1):22–8.

111. Valkeinen H, Häkkinen K, Pakarinen A, et al. Muscle hypertrophy, strength development, and serum hormones during strength training in elderly women with fibromyalgia. *Scand J Rheumatol* 2005;34:309–14.

112. Kingsley JD, Panton LB, Toole T, Sirithienthad P, Mathis R, McMillan V. The effects of a 12-week strength-training program on strength and functionality in women with fibromyalgia. *Arch Phys Med Rehabil* 2005;86:1713–21.

113. Gusi N, Tomas-Carus P, Häkkinen A, Häkkinen K, Ortega-Alonso A. Exercise in waist-high warm water decreases pain and improves health-related quality of life and strength in the lower extremities in women with fibromyalgia. *Arthritis Care Res* 2006;55(1):66–73.

114. Callahan LF, Mielenz T, Freburger J, et al. A randomized controlled trial of the People with Arthritis Can Exercise Program: Symptoms, function, physical activity, and psychosocial outcomes. *Arthritis Care Res* 2008;59:92–101.

115. Stenstrom CH, Lindell B, Swanberg E, Swanberg P, Harms-Ringdahl K, Nordemar R. Intensive dynamic training in water for rheumatoid arthritis functional class II—A long-term study of effects. *Scand J Rheumatol* 1991;20:358–65.

116. Neuberger GB, Press AN, Lindsley HB, et al. Effects of exercise on fatigue, aerobic fitness, and disease activity measures in persons with rheumatoid arthritis. *Res Nurs Health* 1997;20:195–204.

117. van den Ende CHM, Breedveld FC, le Cessie S, Dijkmans BAC, de Mug AW, Hazes JMW. Effect of intensive exercise on patients with active rheumatoid arthritis: A randomised clinical trial. *Ann Rheum Dis* 2000;59:615–21.

118. Hakkinen A, Sokka T, Kotaniemi A, Hannonen P. A randomized two-year study of the effects of dynamic strength training on muscle strength, disease activity, functional capacity, and bone mineral density in early rheumatoid arthritis. *Arthritis Rheum* 2001;44(3):515–22.

119. Hakkinen A. Effectiveness and safety of strength training in rheumatoid arthritis. *Curr Opin Rheumatol* 2004;16:132–7.

120. Hakkinen A, Sokka T, Kautiainen H, Kotaniemi A, Hannonen P. Sustained maintenance of exercise induced muscle strength gains and normal bone mineral density in patients with early rheumatoid arthritis: A 5 year follow-up. *Ann Rheum Dis* 2004;63:910–6.

121. Neuberger GB, Aaronson LS, Gajewski B, Embretson SE, Cagle PE, Loudon JK, Miller PA. Predictors of exercise and effects of exercise on symptoms, function, aerobic fitness, and disease outcomes of rheumatoid arthritis. *Arthritis Care Res* 2007;57:943–52.

122. Rooks DS, Huang J, Bierbaum BE, et al. Effect of preoperative exercise on measures of functional status in men and women undergoing total hip and knee arthroplasty. *Arthritis Care Res* 2006;55:700–8.

123. Iwamoto J, Takeda T, Sato Y. Effect of muscle strengthening exercises on the muscle strength in patients with osteoarthritis of the knee. *Knee* 2007;15:224–30.

124. Hinman RS, Heywood SE, Day AR. Aquatic physical therapy for hip and knee osteoarthritis: Results of a single-blind randomized controlled trial. *Phys Ther* 2007;87:32–43.

125. Rogers MW, Wilder FV. The effects of strength training among persons with hand osteoarthritis: A two-year follow-up study. *J Hand Ther* 2007;20:244–50.

126. Foley A, Halbert J, Hewitt T, Crotty M. Does hydrotherapy improve strength and physical function in patients with osteoarthritis—A randomised controlled trial comparing a gym based and a hydrotherapy based strengthening programme. *Ann. Rheum Dis* 2003;62:1162–7.

127. Baker KR, Nelson ME, Felson DT, Layne JE, Sarno R, Roubenoff R. The efficacy of home based progressive strength training in older adults with knee osteoarthritis: A randomized controlled trial. *J Rheumatol* 2001;28:1655–65.

128. Hopman-Rock M, Westhoff M. The effects of a health educational and exercise program for older adults with osteoarthritis of the hip or knee. *J Rheumatol* 2000;27:1947–54.

129. McCain GA, Bell DA, Mai FM, Halliday PD. A controlled study of the effects of a supervised cardiovascular fitness training program

on the manifestations of primary fibromyalgia. *Arthritis Rheum* 1988;31:1135–41.

130. Martin L, Nutting A, MacIntosh BR, Edworthy SM, Butterwick D, Cook J. An exercise program in the treatment of fibromyalgia. *J Rheumatol* 1996;23:1050–3.

131. Wigers SH, Stiles TC, Vogel PA. Effects of aerobic exercise versus stress management treatment in fibromyalgia. A 4.5 year prospective study. *Scand J Rheumatol* 1996;25:77–86.

132. Mangione KK, McCully K, Gloviak A, Lefebvre I, Hofmann M, Craik R. The effects of high-intensity and low-intensity cycle ergometry in older adults with knee osteoarthritis. *J Gerontol Med Sci* 1999;54A:M184–90.

133. Minor MA, Hewett JE, Webel RR, Anderson SK, Kay DR. Efficacy of physical conditioning exercise in patients with rheumatoid arthritis and osteoarthritis. *Arthritis Rheum* 1989;32:1396–405.

134. Ekblom B, Lovgren O, Alderin M, Fridström M, Sätterström G. Effect of short-term physical training on patients with rheumatoid arthritis I. *Scand J Rheumatol* 1975;4:80–6.

135. Harkcom TM, Lampman RM, Banwell BF, Castor CW. Therapeutic value of graded aerobic exercise training in rheumatoid arthritis. *Arthritis Rheum* 1985;28:32–9.

136. Baslund BK, Lyngberg K, Andersen V, Halkjaer Kristensen J, Hansen M, Klokker M, Pedersen BK. Effect of 8 weeks of bicycle training on the immune system of patients with rheumatoid arthritis. *J Appl Physiol* 1993;75:1691–5.

137. Minor MA, Hewett JE. Physical fitness and work capacity in women with rheumatoid arthritis. *Arthritis Care Res* 1995;8:146–254.

138. Noreau L, Martineau H, Roy L, Belzile M. Effects of a modified dance-based exercise on cardiorespiratory fitness, psychological state and health status of persons with rheumatoid arthritis. *Am J Phys Med Rehabil* 1995;74:19–27.

139. Jentoft ES, Kvalvik AG, Mengshoel AM. Effects of pool-based and land-based aerobic exercise on women with fibromyalgia/chronic widespread muscle pain. *Arthritis Rheum* 2001;45:42–7.

140. Burckhardt CS, Mannerkorpi K, Hedenberg L, Bjelle A. A randomized, controlled clinical trial of education and physical training for women with fibromyalgia. *J Rheumatol* 1994;21:714–20.

141. Gowans SE, deHueck A, Voss S, Richardson M. A randomized, controlled trial of exercise and education for individuals with fibromyalgia. *Arthritis Care Res* 1999;12:120–8.

142. Deyle GD, Henderson NE, Matekel RL, Ryder MG, Garber MB, Allison SC. Effectiveness of manual physical therapy and exercise in osteoarthritis of the knee. A randomized, controlled trial. *Ann Intern Med* 2000;132:173–81.

143. Ettinger WH Jr., Burns R, Messier SP, et al. A randomized trial comparing aerobic exercise and resistance exercise with a health education program in older adults with knee osteoarthritis. The Fitness Arthritis and Seniors Trial (FAST). *JAMA* 1997;277:25–31.

144. Kovar PA, Allegrante JP, MacKenzie CR, Peterson, MG, Gutin B, Charlson ME. Supervised fitness walking in patients with osteoarthritis of the knee. A randomized, controlled trial. *Ann Intern Med* 1992;116:529–34.

145. Rejeski WJ, Ettinger WH, Martin K, Morgan T. Treating disability in knee osteoarthritis with exercise therapy: A central role for self-efficacy and pain. *Arthritis Care Res* 1998;11:94–101.

146. Perlman SG, Connell KJ, Clark A, et al. Dance-based aerobic exercise for rheumatoid arthritis. *Arthritis Care Res.* 1990;3:29–35.

147. Stenstrom CH, Arge B, Sundbom A. Dynamic training versus relaxation training as home exercise for patients with inflammatory rheumatic diseases. A randomized controlled study. *Scand J Rheumatol* 1996;25:28–33.

148. Stenstrom CH, Arge B, Sundbom A. Home exercise and compliance in inflammatory rheumatic diseases—Prospective clinical trial. *J Rheumatol* 1997;24:470–6.

149. Rooks DS, Gautam S, Romeling M, et al. Group exercise, education, and combination self-management in women with fibromyalgia: A randomized trial. *Arch Intern Med* 2007;167(20):2192–200.

150. Mannerkorpi K, Nyberg B, Ahlman M, Ekdahl C. Pool exercise combined with an education program for patients with fibromyalgia syndrome. A prospective, randomized study. *J Rheumatol* 2000; 27(10):2473–81.

151. Mannerkorpi K, Ahlmen M, Ekdahl C. Six- and 24-month follow-up of pool exercise therapy and education for patients with fibromyalgia. *Scand J Rheumatol* 2002;31(5):306–10.

152. Gowans SE, deHueck A. Pool exercise for individuals with fibromyalgia. *Curr Opin Rheumatol* 2007;19:168–73.

153. Gowans SE, deHueck A, Voss S, Silaj A, Abbey SE. Six-month and one-year follow-up of 23 weeks of aerobic exercise for individuals with fibromyalgia. *Arthritis Care Res* 2004;51(6):890–8.

154. Tomas-Carus P, Häkkinen A, Gusi N, Leal A, Häkkinen K, Ortega-Alonso A. Aquatic training and detraining on fitness and quality of life in fibromyalgia. *Med Sci Sports Exerc* 2007;39(7): 1044–50.

155. King SJ, Wessel J, Bhambhani Y, Sholter D, Maksymowych W. The effects of exercise and education, individually or combined, in women with fibromyalgia. *J Rheumatol* 2002;29(12):2620–7.

156. Schachter CL, Busch AJ, Peloso PM, Sheppard MS. Effects of short versus long bouts of aerobic exercise in sedentary women with fibromyalgia: A randomized controlled trial. *Phys Ther* 2003; 83: 340–58.

157. Eversden L, Maggs F, Nightingale P, Jobanputra P. A pragmatic randomised controlled trial of hydrotherapy and land exercises on overall well being and quality of life in rheumatoid arthritis. *BMC Musculoskelet Disord* 2007;8:23.

158. Hughes SL, Seymour RB, Campbell R, Pollak N, Huber G, Sharma L. Impact of the fit and strong intervention on older adults with osteoarthritis. *Gerontologist* 2004;44:217–28.

159. Fransen M, Nairn L, Winstanley J, Lam P, Edmonds J. Physical activity for osteoarthritis management: A randomized controlled clinical trial evaluating hydrotherapy or tai chi classes. *Arthritis Care Res* 2007;57:407–14.

160. Hurley MV, Walsh NE, Mitchell HL, et al. Clinical effectiveness of a rehabilitation program integrating exercise, self-management, and active coping strategies for chronic knee pain: A cluster randomized trial. *Arthritis Care Res* 207;57:1211–9.

161. Cochrane T, Davey RC, Matthes Edwards SM. Randomised controlled trial of the cost-effectiveness of water-based therapy for lower limb osteoarthritis. *Health Technol Assess* 2005;9(31):iii–xi,1.

162. Fransen M, Crosbie J, Edmonds J. Physical therapy is effective for patients with osteoarthritis of the knee: A randomized controlled trial. *J Rheumatol* 2001;28:156–64.

163. Topp R, Woolley S, Horuyak J, Khuder S, Kahaleh B. The effect of dynamic versus isometric resistance training on pain and functioning among adults with osteoarthritis of the knee. *Arch Phys Med Rehabil* 2002;83:1187–95.

164. van Baar ME, Dekker J, Oostendorp RA, Bijl D, Voorn TB, Lemmens JA, Bijlsma JW. The effectiveness of exercise therapy in patients with osteoarthritis of the hip or knee: A randomized clinical trial. *J Rheumatol* 1998;25:2432–9.

165. Assis MR, Silva LE, Alves AMB, et al. A randomized controlled trial of deep water running: Clinical effectiveness of aquatic exercise to treat fibromyalgia. *Arthritis Care Res* 2006;55(1): 57–65.

166. Altan L, Bingol U, Aykac M, Koc Z, Yurtkuran M. Investigation of the effects of pool-based exercise on fibromyalgia syndrome. *Rheumatol Int* 2004;24(5):272–7.

167. Lemstra M, Olszynski WP. The effectiveness of multidisciplinary rehabilitation in the treatment of fibromyalgia. A randomized controlled trial. *Clin J Pain* 2005;21:166–74.

168. Talbot LA, Gaines JM, Huynh TN, Metter EJ. A home-based pedometer-driven walking program to increase physical activity in older adults with osteoarthritis of the knee: A preliminary study. *J Am Geriatr Soc* 2003;51:387–92.

169. Quilty B, Tucker M, Campbell R, Dieppe P. Physiotherapy, including quadriceps exercises and patellar taping, for knee osteoarthritis

with predominant patello-femoral joint involvement: Randomized controlled trial. *J Rheumatol* 2003;30:1311–7.

170. Yip YB, Sit JWH, Fung KKY, Wong DYS, Chong SYC, Chung LH, Ng TP. Effects of a self-management arthritis programme with an added exercise component for osteoarthritic knee: Randomized controlled trial. *J Adv Nurs* 2007;59:20–8.

171. Stener-Victorin E, Kruse-Smidje C, Jung K. Comparison between electro-acupuncture and hydrotherapy, both in combination with patient education and patient education alone, on the symptomatic treatment of osteoarthritis of the hip. *Clin J Pain* 2004; 20(3):179–85.

172. Bautch JC, Malone DG, Vailas AC. Effects of exercise on knee joints with osteoarthritis: A pilot study of biologic markers. *Arthritis Care Res* 1997;10:48–55.

173. Thomas KS, Muir KR, Doherty M, Jones AC, O'Reilly SC, Bassey EJ. Home based exercise programme for knee pain and knee osteoarthritis: Randomised controlled trial. *BMJ* 2002;325:752–7.

174. Cedraschi C, Desmeules J, Rapiti E, et al. Fibromyalgia: A randomised, controlled trial of a treatment programme based on self management. *Ann Rheum Dis* 2004;63:290–6.

175. Buckelew SP, Conway R, Parker J, et al. Biofeedback/relaxation training and exercise interventions for fibromyalgia: A prospective trial. *Arthritis Care Res* 1998;11:196–209.

176. Thorstensson CA, Roos EM, Petersson IF, Ekdahl C. Six-week high-intensity exercise program for middle-aged patients with knee osteoarthritis: A randomized controlled trial. *BMC Musculoskel. Dis* 2005;6:27.

177. Semble EL. Rheumatoid arthritis: New approaches for its evaluation and management. *Arch Phys Med Rehabil* 1995;76: 190–201.

178. Messier SP, Mihalko S, Loeser RF, et al. Glucosamine/chondroitin combined with exercise for the treatment of knee osteoarthritis: A preliminary study. *Osteoarthritis Cartilage* 2007;15:1256–1266.

179. Clegg DO, Reda DJ, Harris CL, et al. Glucosamine, chondroitin sulfate, and the two in combination for painful knee osteoarthritis. *N Engl J Med* 2006;354(8):795–808.

180. Crofford LJ, Rowbotham MC, Mease PJ, et al.; Pregabalin 1008-105 Study Group. Pregabalin for the treatment of fibromyalgia syndrome: Results of a randomized, double-blind, placebo-controlled trial. *Arthritis Rheum* 2005;52:1264–73.

181. Rossy LA, Buckelew SP, Dorr N, et al. A meta-analysis of fibromyalgia treatment interventions. *Ann Behav Med* 1999;21: 180–91.

182. *Physicians' Desk Reference (PDR)*. 62nd ed. Montvale, NJ: Thomson Healthcare; 2007.

183. Arnett FC, Edworthy SM, Bloch DA, et al. The American Rheumatism Association 1987 revised criteria for the classification of rheumatoid arthritis. *Arthritis Rheum* 1988;31:315–24.

184. American College of Rheumatology Subcommittee on Rheumatoid Arthritis Guidelines. Guidelines for the management of rheumatoid arthritis. 2002 update. *Arthritis Rheum* 2002;46(2): 328–46.

185. Bradley LA, Young LD, Anderson KO, et al. Effects of psychological therapy on pain behavior of rheumatoid arthritis patients. Treatment outcome and six-month follow-up. *Arthritis Rheum* 1990;30:1105–14.

186. Keefe FJ, Caldwell DS, Williams DA, Gil KM, Mitchell D, Robertson C. Pain coping skills training in the management of osteoarthritis knee pain: A comparative study. *Behav Ther* 1990;21:49–62.

187. Nielson WR, Walker C, McCain GA. Cognitive behavioral treatment of fibromyalgia syndrome: Preliminary findings. *J Rheumatol* 1992;19:98–103.

188. Goldenberg DL, Kaplan KH, Nadeau MG, Brodeur C, Smith J, Schmid CH. A controlled study of a stress-reduction, cognitive-behavioral treatment program in fibromyalgia. *J Musculoskel Pain* 1994;2:53–66.

189. White KP, Nielson WR. Cognitive-behavioral treatment of fibromyalgia syndrome: A follow-up assessment. *J Rheumatol* 1995; 22:717–21.

190. Fuchs HA, Sergent JS. Rheumatoid arthritis: The clinical picture. In: Koopman WJ, editor. *Arthritis and Allied Conditions: A Textbook of Rheumatology*. 13th ed. Baltimore: Williams & Wilkins; 1997: 1041–70.

191. Meenan RF, Mason JH, Anderson JJ, Guccione AA, Kazis LE. AIMS2. The content and properties of a revised and expanded Arthritis Impact Measurement Scales health status questionnaire. *Arthritis Rheum* 1992;35:1–10.

192. Bellamy N, Campbell J, Stevens J, Pilch L, Stewart C, Mahmood Z. Validation study of a computerized version of the Western Ontario and McMaster Universities v3.0 Osteoarthritis Index. *J Rheumatol* 1997;24:2413–5.

193. Burckhardt CS, Clark CR, Bennett RM. The fibromyalgia impact questionnaire: Development and validation. *J Rheumatol* 1991;18: 728–33.

194. King S, Wessel J, Bhambhani Y, Maikala R, Sholter D, Maksymowych W. Validity and reliability of the 6 minute walk in persons with fibromyalgia. *J Rheumatol* 1999;26:2233–7.

195. Chamberlain MA, Care G, Harfield B. Physiotherapy in osteoarthritis of the knees. A controlled trial of hospital versus home exercises. *International Rehabilitation Medicine* 1982;4:101–6.

196. Sullivan T, Allegrante JP, Peterson MGE, Kovar PA, MacKenzie CR. One-year follow-up of patients with osteoarthritis of the knee who participated in a program of supervised fitness walking and supportive patient education. *Arthritis Care Res* 1998;11: 228–33.

197. Mikesky AE, Mazzuca SA, Brandt KD, Perkins SM, Damush T, Lane KA. Effects of strength training on the incidence and progression of knee osteoarthritis. *Arthritis Care Res* 2006;55:690–9.

198. Buckelew SP, Murray SE, Hewett JE, Johnson J, Huyser B. Self-efficacy, pain, and physical activity among fibromyalgia patients. *Arthritis Care Res* 1995;8:43–50.

199. Bennett RM, Burckhardt CS, Clark SR, O'Reilly CA, Wiens AN, Campbell SM. Group treatment of fibromyalgia: A 6 month outpatient program. *J Rheumatol* 1996;23:521–8.

200. Lorig K, Mazonson PD, Holman HR. Evidence suggesting that health education for self-management in patients with chronic arthritis has sustained health benefits while reducing health care costs. *Arthritis Rheum* 1993;36:439–46.

201. Kruger JMS, Helmick CG, Callahan LF, Haddix AC. Cost-effectiveness of the Arthritis Self-Help Course. *Arch Intern Med* 1998; 158:1245–9.

CHAPTER 1

Exercise and Activity for Individuals with Nonspecific Back Pain

Low back pain (LBP) is an enigma. It remains a common, complex, and controversial problem. It is one of the most widely experienced health-related problems in the world. It is incredibly costly in both human and economic terms, and its presentation and consequences are characterized by variability. LBP may be sudden or insidious in onset; result from major trauma or multiple episodes of microtrauma; have muscular, articular, nociceptive, and neuropathic components; involve single or multiple sites of pain; and persist for weeks, months, or a lifetime.

Some individuals experience an acute episode of LBP as a temporary, albeit uncomfortable, inconvenience that has little if any effect on their regular activity. Others with an apparently similar level of impairment enter a downward spiral of distress, disability, and dependence on the healthcare system (1). Most individuals with LBP adapt to, and cope with, persistent and recurrent symptoms of pain and temporary activity limitation (2). Clearly, LBP is a simple label for a complex multidimensional (biopsychosocial) problem that is managed rather than cured. Clinical guidelines now recommend that this management should be based on education, and advice to maintain or resume activity (3–8). This chapter reviews the problem of LBP and its management using an expanded conceptual framework and best available evidence.

DEFINITIONS

Impairment and disability are key terms in any discussion of LBP. In 1980, the World Health Organization (WHO) defined the terms as follows. *Impairment* is any loss or abnormality of psychological, physiological, or anatomical structure or function (e.g., decreased range of motion or strength). *Disability* is any restriction or lack (resulting from an impairment) of the ability to perform an activity in the manner or within the range considered normal (e.g., the inability to work) (9). Wang et al. (10) recognized the need for a concept that bridged impairment and disability, and proposed the term *functional limitation. Functional limitation* is defined as compromised ability to perform tasks of daily life. The authors proposed a model that illustrated the linkage from pathology,

through impairment and functional limitation to disability.

Pathology → Impairment → Functional Limitation → Disability

A shortcoming of this model is the implied unidirectional and linear progression from pathology through to disability that is not entirely accurate. Rather, each of the constructs is complex and is influenced by a myriad of factors. Depending on when and how the different constructs are measured, and on the influence of mediating factors (e.g., psychosocial factors), the relationships among the constructs (pathology, impairment, functional limitation, and disability) may be trivial. Nevertheless, the disablement model provided an expanded conceptual framework for understanding, assessing, and managing LBP. This conceptual change to an expanded model of health and disability is in line with the WHO International Classification of Functioning, Disability and Health (ICF) (11).

The ICF "mainstreams" the experience of disability and recognizes it as a universal human experience. By shifting the focus from cause to impact, the ICF takes into account the social aspects of disability and does not see disability only as "medical" or "biological" dysfunction. By including *contextual factors*, in which environmental factors are listed, ICF allows to record the impact of the environment on the person's functioning (12). Thus, the ICF is concerned with health and health-related domains in terms of body functions and structures, activities, and participation. Most evidence-based rehabilitation practices endorse the ICF and the application of the ICF framework and its principles has helped consolidate the expanded conceptual change in rehabilitation.

EPIDEMIOLOGY

The lifetime prevalence of LBP is between 58% to 70% in industrial countries (13–16) and the yearly prevalence rate is between 15% and 37% (15,17,18). Although interesting, these data do not provide much information about the nature or the effect of the problem. The data frequently do not distinguish between a single episode of mild backache that lasts less than a day and severe back pain that is permanently incapacitating. And although an episode of LBP may settle quickly, recurrence rates are about 50% in the following 12 months. Andersson (14) reported that about 2% of the population with LBP, are temporarily or chronically disabled by LBP.

Von Korff et al. (20) reported that 41% of adults aged between 26 and 44 years reported having back pain in the previous 6 months. Most had occasional episodes of pain that lasted a few days, was mild or moderate in intensity, and did not limit activities. However, 25% of individuals had back pain that limited their activity and was more often present than not. Wahlgren et al. (2) showed, in a cohort of 76 individuals with a first episode of LBP, that 78% still experienced pain at 6 months and 72% still experienced pain at 12 months. Further, 26% and 14% of individuals were disabled by LBP at 6 and 12 months, respectively, after a first episode of LBP. These results show that, although a high percentage of individuals have persistent LBP, most (75%) self-manage their problem and a few become significantly disabled by LBP. Indeed, self-management is a consistent and strong recommendation of evidence-based clinical practice guidelines.

The costs of care for the minority who enter the healthcare system are tremendous. Frymoyer and Durret (14a) estimated the costs of LBP in the United States to range between $38 and $50 billion a year. This includes the costs for approximately 50 million chiropractic visits and more than 5 million physical therapist visits each year (14). There are also about 300,000 operations annually (21), back and neck operations being the third most common form of surgery in the United States (22).

Despite the cost and extent of healthcare for those with LBP who seek professional care, little consensus and less evidence support the many specific treatment techniques and regimens for most cases of LBP. Indeed, treatment regimens have been based on historical tradition, practitioners' knowledge, skills, and biases; available resources; and payers' regulations, rather than the needs of the individual (21–26).

In recent years, clinical guidelines (see recommended readings) have been published in the United States, the United Kingdom, New Zealand, and the Netherlands (3–5,7,8,27–29). The guidelines are based on systematic reviews and consensus statements and focus on the assessment and management of back pain in primary care. Most guidelines promote the use of a screening assessment "red flags" to identify serious physical pathology (Table 11.1), promote the use of a psychosocial screening assessment "yellow flags" to identify those at risk of chronic disability (Figure 11.1 and Table 11.2). All guidelines promote the use of patient education and exercise in the management of LBP. The newer guidelines (5,7,30) also emphasize and promote self-management, whereas older guidelines reflect a balance between traditional healthcare and self-management. This difference may reflect cultural differences, but essentially reflect the evidence available when the guidelines were produced

TABLE 11.1. RED FLAGS FOR POTENTIALLY SERIOUS CONDITIONS

- Features of cauda equine syndrome (especially urinary retention, bilateral neurologic symptoms and signs, saddle anesthesia)—this requires very urgent referral
- Significant trauma
- Weight loss
- History of cancer
- Fever
- Intravenous drug use
- Steroid use
- Patient over 50 years of age
- Sever, unremitting nighttime pain
- Pain that gets worse when patient is lying down

and the contemporary conceptual maturity of the problem (i.e., a recognition of the problem of low back pain as a biopsychosocial problem not just a biomedical or impairment problem of the spine). Although, a gap remains between this knowledge, clinical guidelines based on this knowledge, and clinical practice (31–40). Outcomes are better when activity-based guidelines are followed (41).

RISK FACTORS

A myriad of personal, physical, and psychosocial factors are associated with the presence, the report, and the impact of LBP. This is evidence of the multidimensional nature of the problem. Personal factors associated with LBP include age and gender, some anthropometric characteristics (e.g., height and body build), spinal abnormalities, and previous history of low back problems. The latter remains one of the most reliable predictors of subsequent back problems. None of the foregoing factors are modifiable, whereas other personal risk factors (e.g., weight, physical fitness, and smoking) are. In a 1-year longitudinal survey of 2,715 adults, Croft et al. (42) reported that poor general health was the strongest predictor of a new episode of LBP. They also noted, however, that self-reported low level of physical activity was not consistently linked with subsequent LBP.

A number of social or work-related factors are also associated with LBP. These include physical factors such as heavy physical work, lifting and forceful movements, awkward postures, and whole body vibration. Work-related risk factors account for 28%–50% of the low back problem in an adult population.

Although no evidence suggests that psychological factors predict the initial occurrence of LBP, these factors do predict the impact of LBP and the response to treatment. Therefore, practitioners need to understand and address such treatment confounders. Overattention to the biological domain at the expense of psychological and sociological domains is destined to lead to treatment failure and frustration for patient and practitioner. Factors predictive

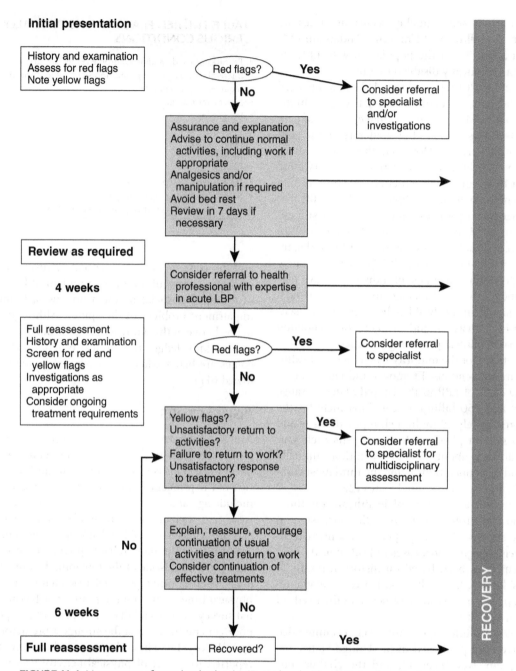

FIGURE 11-1. Management of acute low back pain. (Reproduced with permission from the Accident Rehabilitation and Compensation Insurance Corporation of New Zealand and the National Health Committee, Wellington, New Zealand, 1997.)

of disability or poor outcome include depressed mood, negative or passive coping strategies, catastrophic thinking (43), and fear of pain and reinjury (44). Social factors predictive of negative outcome include dissatisfaction with current work, low educational level, and solicitous behavior of significant others (44).

TYPES

Diagnostic terms used in LBP are usually descriptive, anatopathologic or physiologic, whereas classification of LBP is usually based on duration of trouble, signs and

symptoms, treatment or consequences (45). A variety of diagnostic labels are applied to LBP (e.g., facetogenic, myofascial, discogenic, muscle strain, and sprain). The labels are based on hypothesized injuries or pathologies of specific structures. Most, however, are not verifiable owing to problems with the sensitivity and specificity of clinical assessment and imaging measures. Grazier et al. (45) estimated that of the 11 million outpatient visits made to physicians for LBP each year, 9 million were soft tissue problems, "diagnosed" as strains and sprains. However, Nachemson et al. (46) estimated that a specific *verifiable* diagnosis is possible in less than 5% of

TABLE 11.2. YELLOW FLAGS FOR POTENTIAL RISK OF CHRONIC INCAPACITY, DISTRESS, AND WORK LOSS

Attitudes and Beliefs About Back Pain
- Belief that pain is harmful or disabling, resulting in fear and avoidance of movement
- Belief that all pain must be abolished before return to normal activity or work
- Expectation of increased pain with activity or work, lack of ability to predict capability
- Catastrophising, thinking the work, misinterpreting bodily symptoms
- Belief that pain is uncontrollable
- Passive attitude toward rehabilitation

Behaviors
- Use of extended rest
- Reduced activity level with significant withdrawal from activities of daily living
- Irregular participation with physical exercise, poor pacing
- Avoidance of normal activity and progressive substitution of lifestyle away from productive activity
- Report of extremely high intensity of pain
- Excessive use on the use of aids or appliances
- Sleep quality reduced since onset of back pain
- Smoking

Compensation/Litigation Issues
- Lack of financial incentive to return to work
- Delay in accessing income support and treatment costs, disputes over eligibility
- History of claims for other claims management
- Previous experience of ineffective claims management

Diagnostic and Treatment
- Health professional sanctioning disability, not providing interventions that will improve function
- Experience of conflicting diagnoses or explanations for back pain, leading to confusion
- Diagnostic language leading to catastrophising and fear
- Dramatization of back pain by health professional producing dependency on treatments, and continuation of passive treatment
- Number of visits to health professionals in the previous year
- Expectation of a quick fix
- Lack of satisfaction with previous treatment for back pain
- Advice to withdraw from job

Emotions
- Fear of increased pain with activity or work
- Depression, loss of sense of enjoyment
- More irritable than usual
- Anxiety about and heightened awareness of body sensations
- Feeling under stress and unable to maintain a sense of control
- Presence of social anxiety or disinterested in social activity
- Feeling useless and not needed

Family
- Overprotective partner or spouse, emphasizing fear of harm (usually well-intentioned)
- Solicitous behavior from spouse
- Socially punitive behavior from spouse
- Extent to which family members support return to work
- Lack of support person to talk about problems

Work
- History of manual work
- Work history, frequent job changes, dissatisfaction, poor relationships with peers, lack of vocational direction
- Belief that work is harmful
- Unsupported or unhappy work environment
- Low educational background, low socioeconomic status
- Job involves significant biomechanical demands, such as lifting and handling heavy items, extended sitting, extended standing, driving, vibration, inflexible work schedule
- Shift work or unsociable hours
- Minimal availability or unsatisfactory implementation of selected duties and graduated return to work pathways
- Negative experience of workplace management of back pain
- Absence of interest from employer

acute cases. A newer approach to "diagnosis and management" or at least subgrouping of patients with LBP has focused on pain experienced during specific movements (47–49).

Regardless of such diagnostic or subgrouping issues, it is unlikely that injuries are as tissue specific as many diagnostic labels imply. Tissue injury leads to an increased sensitivity of both the injured and adjacent tissues, thereby confounding a tissue specific "diagnosis." If significant or definitive spinal (e.g., fracture, spinal stenosis, nerve root compression) or visceral pathologies (i.e., "red flags") have been ruled out, a generic term such as "nonspecific" LBP is probably the most useful and accurate diagnostic term. The term does not conjure worrisome images of spinal disintegration for patients, and does not provide a false sense of diagnostic knowledge to practitioners.

The U.S. clinical practice guidelines recommended the use of three categorizations based on medical history and clinical findings (3). These are (a) potentially serious spinal condition (e.g., spinal tumor, infection, fracture, or cauda equina syndrome); (b) sciatica: back-related lower limb symptoms suggesting nerve root compromise; and (c) nonspecific back symptoms, symptoms occurring primarily in the back that suggests neither nerve root compromise, nor a serious underlying condition. Nonspecific back pain includes, but is not limited to, pain of muscular origin.

Grouping individuals with LBP based on pain distribution and duration is the simplest and the most reliable classification method. Individuals are grouped according to whether they have (a) back pain alone, (b) back pain with radiating pain into the thigh, and (c) back pain with pain radiating into the leg below the knee (50). Pain distribution has been shown to influence levels of pain, disability, and physical performance (51, 52). In regard to duration of the problem, individuals are usually grouped as follows: (a) acute, <6 weeks; (b) subacute, 6–12 weeks; and (c) chronic, >12 weeks of continuous symptoms (50). Duration of symptoms can be a problematic basis for classification because of the recurrent, episodic nature of LBP. However, the problem can be ameliorated by the inclusion of a "recurrent" category. Thus the New Zealand LBP guidelines classify LBP as acute, chronic or recurrent. Recurrent LBP is defined as episodes of acute low back problems lasting less than 3 months but recurring after a period of time without low back symptoms sufficient to restrict activity or function (27). Bekkering et al. (53) examined many different prognostic factors for outcomes and used a variety of statistical modeling techniques. The most stable predictor of prognosis in LBP was the duration of the current episode (53).

PROBLEMS

The primary problems of individuals with LBP are pain, physical dysfunction, and concerns about pain and physical dysfunction. Treatment interventions usually include strategies to reduce pain, improve physical function, and correct any catastrophic misconceptions about LBP. It is axiomatic that optimal management is predicated on an adequate understanding of the fundamental problems.

PAIN

Pain is a multidimensional (biopsychosocial) experience that is one of the most misunderstood and mismanaged problems (1,21,25,44). A comprehensive review of the complex physiologic mechanisms (e.g., transduction, central processing, modulation, and neural plasticity), psychological factors (e.g., personality characteristics, emotional states, and cognitive processes), and social circumstances (e.g., family and work interactions) involved in the pain experience is beyond the scope of this chapter. This chapter focuses simply on some of the key elements and common misconceptions about the pain of LBP, especially as this relates to the relationship—or lack thereof—between tissue injury, pain and physical dysfunction, and the ameliorating role of activity and exercise.

NEUROBIOLOGICAL FACTORS AND PAIN

An extensive plexus of nerve fibers supplies the spine (osseous and nonosseous tissues), the surrounding facet joints, soft tissues (muscle and ligaments), and the neurovascular tissues. The extensive plexus is one reason why the source of pain is frequently enigmatic. Any innervated structure can trigger a nociceptive signal, and most structures in the back are well innervated, relatively small, and in close proximity to each other. The sensory system that transmits nociceptive signals includes sensory receptors in the periphery, processing circuits in the dorsal horn and ascending pathways in the spine to the brain where the signal is interpreted.

Imaging studies implicate many brain regions involved in nociception (54). However, a nociceptive signal may or may not be interpreted as painful because a myriad of factors, such as past experience, current mood, expectancy, and social context all influence interpretation. Thus an important distinction exists between nociception and pain.

Nociception refers to neural events and reflex responses evoked by noxious stimuli that are potentially sufficient to cause tissue injury. Pain is more complex, it is an unpleasant sensory and emotional experience, usually (but not always) associated with actual or potential tissue injury (55). Tissue injury, nociception, and pain are not synonymous. Indeed, the relationship among them may be trivial, especially in chronic pain, because nociceptive signals persist even after tissue has healed. Moreover, the nociceptive signal is modified during transmission and the interpretation of the signal is influenced by a myriad of psychological and social factors, further weakening the relationship.

Nociception is usually initially triggered by actual or impending tissue injury. The noxious stimulus may be mechanical, electrical, or chemical. Regardless of stimulus type, acute tissue injury is followed by inflammation, which essentially involves an endogenous biochemical cascade. A variety of substances are released from the injured tissue, from blood vessels, and from primary afferent nerve fibers in the injured area (54). Many of these substances (e.g., prostaglandins, leukotrienes, bradykinin, histamine, sustance P calcitonin gene-related peptide) either sensitize or directly stimulate receptors involved in nociception, including "silent nociceptors." Silent nociceptors are normally unresponsive to mechanical stimuli, but following tissue injury, they respond to mechanical stimuli (even very weak mechanical stimuli). Silent nociceptor sensitization accounts for the increased sensitivity (hyperalgesia) to noxious and non-noxious stimuli in the directly injured tissues and in adjacent tissues. Hence accurate location of specifically injured tissue is difficult and error prone. Although the *area* of injury can be identified with confidence, this confidence is misplaced in regard to the accurate location of a specifically injured tissue.

Persistent or intense noxious input also leads to sensitization of cells in the central nervous system. Nociceptive neurons in the dorsal horn are classified as nociceptive specific (NS) and wide dynamic range (WDR) neurons, based on their response characteristics. As their name suggests, nociceptive neurones respond to noxious input, whereas WDR neurons respond to both noxious and non-noxious input. Persistent noxious input to WDR neurons leads to a progressive increase in their response, processes known as "wind-up" and central sensitization. Wind-up is largely mediated through N-methyl-D-aspartate (NMDA) glutamate receptors, whereas central sensitization is largely mediated through excitatory amino acids, and substance P and can last for hours (54).

Central sensitization also leads to enhanced responses of spinothalmamic tract neurons. In essence, peripheral nociceptive input results in a cascade of activity throughout the neural system. The threshold for nociceptive signals is decreased and, once generated, nociceptive signals can persist even after the initiating noxious stimulus is removed (56). This aberrant nociceptive sensitivity and enhanced nociceptive signaling make it difficult to ifentify accurately the injured tissue based on location of pain or on specific provocative movements that may be used as part of a clinical assessment.

Finally, the neural system is plastic. Persistent nociceptive input leads to neuroplastic changes throughout the neural system and these changes help account for persistent or chronic pain that is no longer associated with ongoing tissue injury. *Thus, chronic pain is not simply acute pain that lasts a long time. Indeed, chronic pain is a pathologic condition in and of itself (similar to epilepsy).* Acute pain should be managed appropriately in an effort to inhibit neuroplastic changes that contribute to persistent and disabling chronic pain.

Psychological Factors and Pain

Clearly, the nociceptive signal that arrives at the cortex is distinctly different from that generated in the periphery. Whether the signal is enhanced or inhibited depends on the relative strength of the opposing neuromodulatory processes. Whether the signal is interpreted as painful or not, however, it is influenced by a myriad of psychological and social factors. The individual's expectancy, mood, attention, sense of control, current activity, past experience, and the social and environmental context in which the signal is received influence the interpretation of that signal. Indeed, the meaning that the individual attaches to the pain will influence his or her emotional response and subsequent behavior and that behavior outlasts the sensory signal and contributes to disability. (See the excellent review by Vlaeyen and Linton, on this topic [57]).

The beliefs that individuals has about their pain will influence what they do about it. Some individuals will consider the pain a minor inconvenience and attempt to ignore it, whereas others will worry about its meaning and even think the pain is catastrophic and immediately seek professional help. If pain is aggravated by activity, they may avoid activities that are painful and even those that they anticipate will be painful. Although this action may be appropriate in the short term for acute pain it is not appropriate for the long term and indeed will aggravate the problem.

An important point to consider in this context is that pain, mood, stress, and exercise or activity all have neurobiochemical bases. The interactions among these constructs are complex and not well understood, either at the molecular or the person level. It is intriguing to consider whether such central mechanisms account for the reported nonspecific effects of specific exercise regimens (58,59).

In summary, LBP is a multidimensional experience. It has sensory, emotional, cognitive, and behavioral components. The relative magnitude of each component helps determine how an individual's problem should be managed (i.e., modify sensory input, address misunderstandings about the meaning of the pain and the relationship to injury, and address anxieties about pain and activity). The simple adage "let pain be the guide" belies the complexity of the construct.

For a significant acute back injury (where pain and injury are related) it is reasonable to reduce activity for a day or two, treat the pain (e.g., with analgesic medication a physical modality, such as ice, or both) and be guided by pain intensity and duration as normal activity is resumed (1–2 days). The period of inactivity should be limited by time not pain, however. An early return to normal activities should be encouraged and expected. *Any advice to rest must be accompanied by advice on activity resumption.*

For chronic or recurrent LBP, this approach is inappropriate and even harmful. Pain is not indicative of ongoing tissue injury and it is likely to persist, therefore it cannot be used to guide the amount of activity. Practitioners must be sensitive to the degree of pain and to its effect on an individual's psychological and physical state.

Measurement of pain and disability caused by LBP using reliable and valid assessment tools is an essential component of LBP management. *You cannot manage what you do not measure.* This does not imply that practitioners should focus on pain and pain behavior. It does mean that practitioners should acknowledge the presence of pain, and address misconceptions or fears about pain, tissue injury, and activity. Most importantly, practitioners should provide appropriate reassurance (19) and advise patients on resumption of activity. The reassurance must include recognition and acknowledgement of the patient's problems. Patronizing reassurance without perceived understanding or acknowledgement of the individual's problems is likely to aggravate rather than alleviate the problem.

Pain Assessment

Pain is a subjective phenomenon, therefore self-report should be the primary form of assessment. Pain assessment should focus not only on pain intensity, but also on pain affect and pain distribution.

Pain intensity and pain affect can easily be measured using numeric rating scales (NRS) or visual analogue scales (VAS). Numerous studies provide support for the reliability, validity, and responsiveness of these measures (60). For a measure of pain intensity using an NRS, the individual is asked to select a number between 0 and 10 that best describes the intensity of the pain, 0 = no pain and 10 = most severe pain imaginable. A VAS consists of a 10-cm line with descriptors at the endpoints (e.g., 0 = no pain and 10 = most severe pain imaginable). The individual places a mark on the line to indicate the intensity of the pain. A pain intensity score is computed by measuring the distance from the 0 point to the mark made by the individual.

A second important dimension of the pain experience is pain affect. Pain affect refers to the unpleasantness of pain. It can be measured at the same time as pain intensity using 0–10 NRS or 10-cm. VAS, with different endpoint words. Endpoints for pain affect are, 0 = not at all unpleasant and 10 = most unpleasant pain imaginable. Pain intensity and affect are related but certain treatments, including some medications and physical therapies, can have their effect through a reduction in pain affect rather than pain intensity (61).

Pain location is most easily assessed using a body map, which is an outline of a human figure, on which the individual is asked to shade the painful area.

FUNCTIONAL ASSESSMENT

Low back pain can have a major impact on a person's functional ability. Standard clinical assessments of LBP are traditionally limited to measures of impairment. Although restoration of function is one of the most common aims of treatment (62), function is not always directly assessed but is inferred from the level of impairment. In the last two decades it has become increasingly obvious that impairment does not have a strong or stable relationship with functional limitation or disability. This is partly because of the complexity of the constructs and partly because of the difficulties in measuring them. Functional measures assess at the level of the person, whereas impairment measures (e.g. range of motion, muscle strength) assess at the level of the "part."

Traditional assessments based on impairment measures are now often complemented with functionally based measures. They assess the impact of any impairment and, in that respect, they are more meaningful to the patient. The assessment methods include patient self-report questionnaires and clinician measured tasks (63).

An advantage of questionnaires is that they sample a range of different activities, including mobility and the performance of household chores and other work-related activity. They can be relatively quick, simple, and practical to administer and score. They are widely used, norms are available, and clearly they have superior face validity when compared with health professionals' estimates of function. The most commonly used self-report questionnaires for LBP are the Oswestry Disability Questionnaire (64), Roland and Morris Questionnaire (65), and the SF-36 (66). The SF-36 is a multidimensional measure of general health status, whereas the Oswestry and Roland and Morris Questionnaires are both LBP specific.

Simmonds et al. (67) developed, tested, and refined a comprehensive, but simple battery of performance tests to complement the functional assessment of individuals with LBP. Performance on the task battery is generally measured on the basis of how quickly a task can be performed, or how far a subject can reach forward (an indirect measure of spinal load) because individuals with LBP have difficulty withstanding spinal loads (compressive and shear), and velocity and acceleration of motion is generally slower compared with pain-free individuals (61,67,68). The timed tasks include repeated trunk bending, sit to stand, 50-foot speed walk; the distance tasks include a 5-minute walk and the distance reached forward while holding a 4.6-kg weight.

All measures have excellent inter-rater reliability. Intraclass correlation coefficients (ICC1,1) were all equal or greater than 0.95. Face validity, convergent, discriminant, and predictive validity have also been established (67). Noteworthy is that in 66 patients with LBP, physical performance measures outperformed impairment factors as predictors of disability ($R2 = 0.61$) compared with ($R2 = 0.47$) (69).

EXERCISE AND ACTIVITY

A consequence of LBP, regardless of its genesis, is a temporary or permanent reduction in activity. Physical inactivity can have a detrimental effect on the cardiovascular and musculoskeletal systems. It can also have a detrimental effect on psychosocial well-being (70). It has now been well established that deconditioning neither contributes to back pain nor indeed is it a consequence of it (71–74). It is also well established that physical activity is beneficial for those with or without back pain. Therefore, maintenance of, or early return to, normal activity is a fundamental aim of management. What is less clear is whether any particular exercise or activity regimen will facilitate resumption of normal activity and, if so, whether the specific mechanisms of effects are biological, psychological, sociological, or all of those.

Physical activity is an umbrella term that includes concepts such as fitness, exercise, training, and conditioning (75). Essentially any bodily movement that increases energy expenditure above the resting level is physical activity (76). Exercise is frequently used interchangeably with physical activity. However, exercise and exercise training is purposeful activity specifically designed to improve or maintain a particular component of physical fitness (e.g. flexibility, strength, or endurance—cardiovascular or musculoskeletal).

In the case of LBP, a variety of different treatment regimens and specific types and intensity of exercise have been used in clinical practice to prevent or treating LBP and its consequences. Most regimens have been based on a biomedical impairment model and have thus focused on improving specific trunk strength, endurance, flexibility, and aerobic fitness (59,62,77). The implied rationale of this assessment and management approach is that trunk muscles are weak and the spine is stiff. Trunk strength and mobility, however, neither predict LBP (77–80) nor disability (69,80). Moreover, these measures frequently do not discriminate between individuals with and without LBP because of the large range of interindividual variability (81).

Other treatment regimens focus on general exercises and aerobic conditioning. Jette et al. (62) reported that endurance exercises were included in 52% of treatment plans of 739 individuals with LBP. Again, the implied and the stated rationale (82) is that individuals with LBP are deconditioned or become deconditioned because of LBP. The evidence supporting that notion is weak and contradictory (76,83), however. In 1994, the Agency for Health Care Policy and Research (AHCPR) recommended the use of low-stress aerobic, endurance, and conditioning exercises (3). The report acknowledged, however, that the evidence supporting that recommendation was moderate to weak.

Although the AHCPR guidelines were associated with political and scientific controversy following their release, the guidelines served to shake clinical complacency regarding the evidence, or lack thereof, supporting common clinical practice for LBP. One result has been systematic investigations into the *mechanisms* of action, the *efficacy*, and the *effectiveness* of specific exercise regimens in acute, subacute, and chronic nonspecific LBP.

A serious review and critique of the literature on LBP is a daunting task, but a number of scientific groups have conducted systematically reviews of the literature (5,28,84–98). The literature is voluminous and highly variable in terms of scientific quality. Moreover, the natural history of the condition and the many methodologic differences among studies make it difficult to compare study outcomes.

For example, subjects are heterogeneous or are not well described; exercise interventions are often inadequately described in terms of type, intensity, or duration; and outcome measures vary from specific impairment measures (e.g., pain reduction) to social measures, such as return to work. Although the latter is a very important outcome, it is influenced more strongly by the individuals' beliefs about their back problem, their education, and job skills, and by the unemployment rate than by the severity of their LBP. Finally, studies differ in their length of follow-up that may vary between immediate postintervention or up to 2 years postintervention. The length of follow-up is an important consideration in LBP because of its recurrent nature. Also, individuals seek healthcare when symptoms are at their worst, therefore natural history and regression to the mean favor early resolution, or at least reduction in symptoms, despite any treatment intervention. Long-term follow-up is difficult, but essential to establish the effectiveness of an exercise intervention.

Given the voluminous and variable nature of the literature, the lag between research and the clinical application of research findings is understandable. This is why government agencies, scientific societies, and research groups have formed task forces (clinicians and researchers) to appraise the evidence and publish treatment guidelines (7). Dissemination of findings to key decision makers, and consumers of healthcare services is expected to assist healthcare professionals and managers to ensure that their practice reflects best available evidence. Research, however, has shown problems with the implementation of guidelines in clinical practice. For clinical guidelines to be useful, they must be known by the target group and used. Many guidelines are not used after development and dissemination (32,40,98,99). Moreover, standard implementation activities frequently produce only moderate improvement (40) despite that adherent care is related to better clinical outcomes and lower costs (41, 101). Research on guideline adherence has shown that for guidelines to be used, they must be meaningful to clinicians and they must be simple and easy to use. Ironically, it is also necessary that guidelines do not deviate too much from current clinical practice.

The final section of this chapter reviews the evidence and discusses the guidelines regarding exercise for nonspecific LBP. Acute and chronic LBP will be discussed because chronic LBP cannot be optimally managed without a good understanding of (*a*) how the condition became chronic and (*b*) whether the acute phase was managed appropriately. Moreover, all patients with chronic LBP will have recurrent episodes of acute LBP. Indeed, that may be the time at which they seek professional care. Therefore, practitioners must understand the role of exercise in all phases of nonspecific LBP.

EXERCISE FOR ACUTE LOW BACK PAIN

Acute nonspecific LBP is defined as symptoms <6 weeks in duration, with no evidence of serious pathology or nerve root irritation. The history rather than the physical examination provides the most useful categorization information to the clinician (3,101). Several investigative teams have examined the effects of rest, exercise, education, and other interventions in individuals with acute LBP (102–104). Others have conducted systematic or critical reviews of the evidence (29,105,106).

The AHCPR guidelines were published in 1994. They contained three recommendations against the use of bedrest for acute LBP (two of which were supported by moderate evidence), and six recommendations regarding exercise for acute LBP (all of which were supported by limited or no research evidence). The recommendations and the evidence that supported them are as follows.

1. Low stress aerobic exercise can prevent debilitation caused by inactivity and may help return patients to the highest level of function appropriate to their circumstances. *Strength of evidence: Limited (at least one adequate scientific study).*
2. Aerobic (endurance) exercise programs, which minimally stress the back (walking, biking, or swimming) can be started during the first 2 weeks for most patients with acute low back problems. *Strength of evidence: No research basis.*
3. Conditioning exercises for trunk muscles (especially back extensors), gradually increased, are helpful for patients with acute back pain. *Strength of evidence: Limited (at least one adequate scientific study).*
4. Back-specific exercises on machines provide no benefit over traditional exercise. *Strength of evidence: No research basis.*
5. Stretching exercises (of back muscles) are not recommended. *Strength of evidence: No research basis.*
6. Exercises using quotas yield better outcomes than exercises using pain as a guide to progression. *Strength of evidence: Limited (at least one adequate scientific study).*

Thus, consensus and evidence indicate that rest is detrimental for LBP. Based on that evidence, it seems reasonable to believe that exercise is beneficial for LBP. The guideline recommendations regarding exercise are primarily based on consensus rather than evidence. Subsequent systematic reviews (29,105,106), a report from the International Paris Task Force (107), and the European

Guidelines (8) do not support the use of specific exercise regimens in acute LBP. They promote reassurance and advice to remain active but no specific exercise regimens. Faas et al. (106) identified four randomized, controlled trials on acute LBP that met the criteria for inclusion in their systematic review. They reported that the trials with the highest method score reported no efficacy of flexion or extension exercises. For example, Detorri et al. (59) compared outcomes in 149 individuals with LBP assigned to a trunk flexion exercise group, a trunk extension exercise group, or a no exercise group. They reported no differences in outcomes (impairment, pain and disability) at 8 weeks between the exercise groups. Moreover, no differences were seen in recurrence rates between any of the groups at 6 and 12 months. A finding that questions the value of exercise in preventing LBP, albeit evidence suggests that physical activity mediates disability caused by LBP (108).

In contrast, Faas et al. (106) reported that the trials with the lowest method score reported positive results from McKenzie type exercise. In a later (2000) Cochrane review, Van Tulder et al. (109) reported that for acute LBP, strong evidence indicates that exercise therapy was not more effective than any inactive or other active treatments it had been compared with. Effectiveness was judged on the basis of reduction in pain intensity, increase in self-report of functional status, overall improvement, and return to work.

Although specific exercises are not useful, advice to continue ordinary activity is (102). The United Kingdom guidelines assert that there are "generally consistent findings in the majority of acceptable studies. . . ." that ". . . .advice to continue ordinary activity can provide for a *faster* symptomatic recovery from an acute episode. . . ."

Most people with nonspecific LBP are expected to recover within days or weeks, regardless of management strategy. Analgesics and anti-inflammatory medication are appropriate to control symptoms and allow people to remain reasonably active. An important component of acute care is to provide reassurance, promote self-care, and identify individuals at risk of disability (110). The New Zealand guidelines suggest that a preliminary screen for psychosocial yellow flags is appropriate at the time of initial presentation. Others suggest the screen be used for those individuals with LBP who still have significant pain and disability after about 4 weeks. Finally, excess disability can result from the attitude and beliefs of the treatment provider as well as those of the patient. "Reliance on a narrow medical model of pain; passive treatments, discouragement of self care strategies and failure to instruct the patient in self management; sanctioning of disability and not providing interventions that will improve function; and over-investigation and perpetuation of belief in the 'broken part hypothesis'" will contribute to chronic disabling LBP (27).

EXERCISE FOR CHRONIC LOW BACK PAIN

Chronic nonspecific LBP is characterized by the persistence of symptoms beyond 12 weeks. However, with the exception of sharing a minimal time of symptom duration, individuals with chronic LBP are characterized by heterogeneity. Most individuals with chronic and persistent symptoms of LBP do not seek healthcare, they have little disability, continue to work, and are generally not distressed about their back pain. Those who do seek professional care vary widely in terms of the total duration of symptoms, symptom severity, disability level, distress, and overall physical condition resulting from those symptoms. Clearly, the approach to management has to be individualized, holistic, and rational, with consideration given to biological, psychological, and sociological factors.

Clinical guidelines now address the assessment and management of chronic LBP (7). Also, in the United Kingdom, the Clinical Standards Advisory Group (4) has suggested that as LBP becomes chronic, psychological factors become more important and purely physical management should be avoided in favor of active exercise and multidisciplinary rehabilitation based on a biopsychosocial model. These recommendations are essentially concordant with the European Guidelines for the Management of Chronic Nonspecific Low Back Pain (7): education, cognitive behavioral therapy, supervised activity, and active multidisciplinary biopsychosocial treatment. Although the Guidelines suggest that a short course of mobilization can be considered, physical modalities (i.e., heat, cold, laser, transcutaneous electrical nerve stimulation [TENS], massage, corsets) are not recommended. The 2000 report from the International Paris Task Force on Back Pain (107) recommends the prescription of physical, therapeutic, or recreational exercise in cases of chronic nonspecific back pain.

A number of randomized, controlled trials and systematic reviews have addressed exercise and activity in individuals with chronic nonspecific LBP. It seems clear that exercise and activity are beneficial for individuals with LBP because they can reduce the perception of pain and enhance the sense of well-being. It is less clear whether the type, intensity, frequency, or duration of exercise or activity is important. The Paris Task Force recommends that exercise programs should combine strength training, stretching and fitness, whereas other guidelines are less prescriptive. But perhaps the most effective exercise or activity regimen is that which is done.

In individuals with LBP, barriers to, and motivators of, physical activity are similar to those in the general population (e.g., lack of time, inclement weather, and family commitments) (111). However, it is interesting that back problems are identified as both barriers to, and motivators of, activity. In a qualitative study Keen et al. (111) interviewed 27 individuals who were participants in a randomized, controlled trial of a progressive exercise program. They reported that some individuals believed that being more physically active helped ease their back pain and made them feel better. They were worried about stopping exercise for fear that their back pain would return. Others did not exercise on a regular basis but resumed exercise when reminded to by their backache. Still others avoided physical activity for fear of an aggravation of their LBP. Although all subjects identified the avoidance of some physical activity (e.g., lifting and gardening), not all were fearful or anxious about such activity. It appears that those individuals in the latter category, reported that their confidence was restored over time through (a) reassurance and advice from health professionals, (b) modifying the way an activity was done (e.g., less vigorous), and (c) a progressive exercise program (111). It appears that a change in behavior led to a change in belief about the ability to be active.

Participation in exercise or activity is essential if benefits are to accrue, whether those benefits are physical or attitudinal. Friedrich et al. (112) conducted a double-blind, randomized study and evaluated the effect of a motivation program on exercise compliance (adherence) and disability. A total of 93 patients with LBP were randomly assigned to either a standard exercise program (n = 49) group or a combined exercise and motivation group (n = 44). The exercise program consisted of an individual submaximal gradually increased training session. Each patient was prescribed 10 sessions that each lasted about 25 minutes. The specific exercises were aimed at "improving spinal mobility, as well as trunk and lower limb muscle length, force, endurance, and coordination, thereby restoring normal function." Flexibility exercises for the trunk and lower limbs preceded strengthening exercises for the trunk. The motivation program consisted of five sessions that included counseling, information about LBP and exercise, reinforcement, forming a treatment contract between patient and therapist, and keeping an exercise diary.

The combined exercise and motivation group increased the rate of attendance and reduced disability and pain in the short term (4 and 12 months). However, there was no difference in exercise adherence in the long term. Long-term adherence to exercise is an acknowledged problem in the general population and is no different in those with LBP. In the case of LBP, when exercise benefits may not be immediate or even apparent, and when recurrence of LBP is inevitable anyway, it is hardly surprising that adherence to exercise is problematic. For some individuals, encouraging and facilitating them to have a more active lifestyle may be more beneficial for them than prescribing a specific exercise regimen that they do not do. That no evidence supports the notion that specific regimens are differentially more effective for nonspecific back pain supports this position. Some evidence, however, indicates that supervised activity is more effective than nonsupervised activity (103,104). The mechanisms through which supervision is effective are not established and may not be as obvious as they seem. Supervision, however, ensures that the prescribed exercises and activities are carried out. The nonspecific effects (e.g., reduction of anxiety) have not been ruled out.

A number of studies have shown that individuals in exercise programs do better than control subjects. No clear indication exists of any superiority of any specific exercise regimen. The Paris Task force reviewed 10 scientifically rigorous randomized, controlled trials of exercise for chronic LBP. Patients did better than control subjects in 7 of the 10 trials. However, the regimens were characterized by variability of type, intensity and duration. Moreover, some treatment programs included additional components, such as education or behavior modification.

For example, Frost et al. (103) tested a supervised general fitness program composed of 81 individuals with chronic LBP, who were randomized to a fitness program or a control group. Both groups were taught exercises and attended an educational program on LBP. The exercise group also attended eight sessions of a supervised fitness program that extended over 4 weeks. Cognitive behavioral principles and a normal model of human behavior rather than a disease model was followed. Participants were encouraged to compare themselves with sports participant who had been laid off from training and who needed to get back to previous activity level. They were also reminded that unaccustomed exercise might lead to muscle aches, and that pain and injury (hurt and harm) was not synonymous. Finally, participants were encouraged to improve their own performance record (not compete with others) and to complete an activity diary. The fitness program is included in Table 11.3. A mean reduction

of 7.7% (pain and disability) was obtained in the exercise group compared with a 2.4% reduction in the control group. This difference was statistically significant and was maintained at the 2-year follow up. However, the authors note that the confidence interval of the differences between groups was large, indicating a wide variation in treatment effect. Moreover and mathematically, the use of percentage change always biases results in favor of individuals with an initial low level of pain and disability. It is not possible to determine from the article whether those who responded optimally were, in fact, those with a relatively low level of pain and disability at baseline.

It is not surprising that in studies comparing relatively active and relatively passive intervention, the active intervention appears more effective. However, in a recent Volvo Award Winning study, Mannion et al. (58) compared three active therapies for chronic LBP. In this study, 148 subjects were randomly assigned to (*a*) an active physiotherapy program, (*b*) a muscle reconditioning program using training devices, or (*c*) a low-impact aerobics program. Subjects attended their program twice a week for 3 months. All programs led to a reduction in pain and disability that were maintained at 6 months. That no differences were seen between groups suggested a lack of treatment specificity.

In summary, it appears that the specific type of exercise or exercise regimen is much less important than once thought. Although the notion may be an anathema to traditional thinking clinicians with a more narrow structurally focused biomedical (impairment) model, it is less surprising to those who recognize the biopsychosocial nature of chronic LBP. Exercises targeted at a specific biological or structural impairment may effect changes in impairment, but the actual impairment may contribute relatively little to the individual's LBP problem. Although speculative at present, it is plausible to suggest that exercise is beneficial for those with chronic LBP because it reduces psychosocial distress (70), leads to improvement in mood, reduces anxieties about the LBP, and changes the perception of self as disabled. Thus, the primary benefits of exercise or activity for individuals with chronic LBP are central rather than peripheral or structural.

SUMMARY

The title of Waddell's book, "The Back Pain Revolution," captured the profound change in the conceptualization and, thus, assessment and management of LBP that began in the last decade (25). Recognition of a broad psychosocial model of health, the positive role of activity, the reliance on clinical evidence, and the application of clinical guidelines has the potential to transform the assessment and management of LBP into one that has a more rational basis (113). Primary management of LBP must include education and advice on staying active. The approach should be individualized, holistic, and rational, with

TABLE 11.3. FITNESS PROGRAM CIRCUIT OF EXERCISE

1. Static cycling; gradually increase resistance, not speed
2. Free arm weights while in lying down; increase and record weight
3. Alternate knee raise while in standing (right knee toward left hand and vice versa. Progress by lifting legs higher toward the opposite elbow).
4. Repeated sit-to-stand
5. Press-ups against wall, progressing through half press-ups to full press-ups on a mat
6. Bridging
7. Setp-ups
8. Medicine ball lifts while in lying down
9. Jogging on a bouncer
10. Rounding and hollowing back in four-point kneeling
11. Walking—back and forth between two markers on the floor; gradually increase speed
12. Arm raising while in standing; gradually increase speed
13. Straight leg lifting while in lying down
14. Abdominal crunch while in lying down
15. Skipping with a rope

consideration given to biological, psychological, and sociological factors.

Clearly it is not possible to recommend evidence-based specific exercise or activity regimens for individuals with nonspecific LBP. The exercise and activity principles are essentially no different from those applied to individuals without LBP. Perhaps the enigma of LBP is the no enigma exists after all.

REFERENCES

1. Pither C, Nicholas M, eds. *The Identification of Iatrogenic Factors in the Development of Chronic Pain Syndromes: Abnormal Treatment Behaviour?* Proceedings of the Vith World Congress on Pain. Bond M, Charlton J, Woolf C, eds. Netherlands: Elsevier Science: 1991: 429–434.

2. Wahlgren D, Atkinson JH, Epping-Jordan JE, et al. One-year follow-up of first onset low back pain. *Pain* 1997;73:213–221.

3. Bigos S, et al. Acute low back problems in adults. *Clinical Practice Guideline No. 14.* Rockville, MD: 1994 Agency for Health Care Policy and Research, Public Health Service, U.S. Department of Health and Human Services.

4. Clinical Standards Advisory Group C. *Back Pain: Report of a CSAG Committee on Back Pain.* London: His Majesty's Stationary Office; 1994.

5. Chou R, Huffman LH Nonpharmacologic therapies for acute and chronic low back pain: A review of the evidence for an American Pain Society/American College of Physicians clinical practice guideline. *Ann Intern Med* 2007;147(7):492–504.

6. Philadelphia Panel evidence-based clinical practice guidelines on selected rehabilitation interventions for low back pain. *Phys Ther* 2001;81(10):1641–1674.

7. Airaksinen O, et al. European guidelines for the management of chronic nonspecific low back pain. *Eur Spine J* 2006;15(Suppl 2):S192–S300.

8. van Tulder M, et al. European guidelines for the management of acute nonspecific low back pain in primary care. *Eur Spine J* 2006;15(Suppl 2):S169–S191.

9. O'Brien K, et al. Progressive resistive exercise interventions for adults living with HIV/AIDS. *Cochrane Database Syst Rev* 2004(4): CD004248.

10. Nagi SZ. Disability concepts revisited: implications for prevention. In: AM Pope, AR Tarlov, eds. *Disability in America: Towards a National Agenda for Prevention.* Washington, DC: Division of Health Promotion and Disease Prevention. Institute of Medicine, National Academy Press; 1991:309–327.

11. WHO. International Classification of Functioning, Disability and Health (ICF) Online. 2006 (cited September 1, 2006); Available from: www.who.int/classifications/icf/en. Accessed 10/27/2008.

12. WHO. International Classification of Functioning, Disability and Health (ICF). 2006 (cited 2006; Available from: http://www3.who.int/icf/onlinebrowser/icf.cfm. Accessed 10/27/2008.

13. Papergeorgiou A, et al. Estimating the prevalence of low back pain in the general population. Evidence from the South Manchester back pain Survey. *Spine* 1995;20:1889–1894.

14. Andersson G. The epidemiology of spinal disorders. In: Frymoyer J, ed. *The Adult Spine: Principles and Practice,* 2nd ed. Philadelphia: Lippincott-Raven: Philadelphia; 1997:93–142.

14a. Frymoyer JW, Durret CL. The economics of spinal disorders. In: JW Frymoyer, ed. The *Adult Spine: Principles and Practice,* 2nd ed. Philadelphia: Lippincott-Raven; 1997:143–150.

15. Walsh K, Cruddas M, Coggon D. Low back pain in eight areas of Britain. *J Epidemiol Community Health.* 1992;46:227–230.

16. Skovron M, et al. Sociocultural factors in and back pain. A population based study in Belgian adults. *Spine* 1994;19:129–137.

17. Mason V. The prevalence of back pain in Great Britain. In: Office of Population Censuses and Surveys, 1994, Social Survey Division. London: HMSO; 1994:1–24.

18. Anderson J, Felson D. Factors associated with osteoarthritis of the knee in the first national Health and Nutrition Examination Survey (HANES I). Evidence for an association with overweight, race, and physical demands of work. *Am J Epidemiol* 1988;128: 179–189.

19. Croft P, ed. *Low Back Pain.* Oxford: Radcliffe Medical Press, 1997.

20. Von Korff M, et al. An epidemiologic comparison of pain complaints. *Pain* 1988;32:173–183.

21. Waddell G. Low back pain: A twentieth century health care enigma. *Spine* 1996;21(24):2820–2825.

22. Cherkin D, et al. An international comparison of back surgery rates. *Spine* 1994;19:1201–1206.

23. Jette AM, et al. Physical therapy episodes of care for patients with low back pain. *Phys Ther* 1994;74(2):101–10; discussion 110–115.

24. Wennburg J. Practice variations and the challenge to leadership. *Spine* 1996;21:910–916.

25. Waddell G. *The Back Pain Revolution.* Edinburgh: Churchill Livingstone; 1998.

26. Battie M. et al. Managing low back pain: Attitudes and treatment preferences of physical therapists. *Phys Ther* 1994;74:219–226.

27. New Zealand acute low back pain guide, and Guide in assessing psychosocial yellow flags in acute low back pain. Wellington, NZ: Accident Rehabilitation and Compensation Insurance Corporation of New Zealand and the National Health Committee; 1997.

28. Chou R. Evidence-based medicine and the challenge of low back pain: Where are we now? *Pain Pract* 2005;5(3):153–178.

29. Van Tulder M. Evidence-based physical therapy for low back pain: A promising future. *Dutch Journal of Physical Therapy* 1999;109: 29–32.

30. van Eijk FA, Chavannes AW, Gubbels JW. A randomized trial of exercise therapy in patients with acute low back pain. Efficacy on sickness absence. *Spine* 1995;15:941–947.

31. Dahan R, et al. The challenge of using the low back pain guidelines: A qualitative research. *J Eval Clin Pract* 2007;13(4): 616–620.

32. Fullen BM, et al. Adherence of Irish general practitioners to European guidelines for acute low back pain: A prospective pilot study. *Eur J Pain* 2007;11(6):614–623.

33. Bekkering, G.E., et al. Implementation of clinical guidelines on physical therapy for patients with low back pain: Randomized trial comparing patient outcomes after a standard and active implementation strategy. *Phys Ther* 2005;85(6):544–555.

34. Espeland A, Baerheim A. Factors affecting general practitioners' decisions about plain radiography for back pain: Implications for classification of guideline barriers—A qualitative study. *BMC Health Serv Res* 2003;3(1):8.

35. Armstrong MP, McDonough S, Baxter GD. Clinical guidelines versus clinical practice in the management of low back pain. *Int J Clin Pract* 2003;57(1):9–13.

36. Koes BW, et al. Clinical guidelines for the management of low back pain in primary care: An international comparison. *Spine* 2001;26(22):2504–2513; discussion 2513–2514.

37. Foster NE, et al. Management of nonspecific low back pain by physiotherapists in Britain and Ireland. A descriptive questionnaire of current clinical practice. *Spine* 1999;24(13):1332–1342.

38. Bekkering GE, et al. Effect on the process of care of an active strategy to implement clinical guidelines on physiotherapy for low back pain: A cluster randomised controlled trial. *Qual Saf Health Care* 2005;14(2):107–112.

39. Burgers JS, et al. Characteristics of effective clinical guidelines for general practice. *Br J Gen Pract* 2003;53:15–19.

40. Grol R. Successes and failures in the implementation of evidence-based guidelines for clinical practice. *Med Care* 2001;39(8 Suppl 2):II-46–II-54.

41. Fritz JM, Cleland JA, Brennan GP. Does adherence to the guideline recommendation for active tTreatments improve the quality of care for patients with acute low back pain delivered by physical therapists? Med Care 2007;45(10):973–980.

42. Croft P et al. Short-term physical risk indicators for new episodes of low back pain. *Spine* 1999;24:1556–1561.

43. Sullivan MJ, Rodgers WM, Kirsch I. Catastrophizing, depression and expectancies for pain and emotional distress. *Pain* 2001; 91(1–2):147–154.

44. Turk D. The role of demographic and psychosocial factors in transition from acute to chronic pain. In: Jensen T, Turner J, Wiesenfeld-Hallin Z, eds. *Proceedings of the 8th World Congress on Pain, Progress in Pain Research and Management*. Seattle: IASP Press; 1997:185–213.

45. Grazier KL, et al. The frequency of occurrence, impact, and cost of musculoskeletal conditions in the United States. Chicago: American Academy of Orthopedic Surgeons; 1984.

46. Nachemson A, ed. Exercise, fitness and back pain. *Scientific Proceedings of the International Conference on Exercise, Fitness and Health*. Champaign, IL: Human Kinetics; 1998.

47. Fritz JM, Cleland JA, Childs JD. Subgrouping patients with low back pain: Evolution of a classification approach to physical therapy. *J Orthop Sports Phys Ther* 2007;37(6):290–302.

48. Cleland JA, et al. Development of a clinical prediction rule for guiding treatment of a subgroup of patients with neck pain: Use of thoracic spine manipulation, exercise, and patient education. *Phys Ther* 2007;87(1):9–23.

49. Fritz JM, et al. An examination of the reliability of a classification algorithm for subgrouping patients with low back pain. *Spine* 2006;31(1):77–82.

50. Spitzer W, et al. Scientific approach to the assessment and management of activity-related spinal disorders. *Spine* 1987;7S:S1–S55.

51. Selim A, et al. The importance of radiating leg painin assessing health outcomes among patients with low back pain: Results from the Veterans Health Study. *Spine* 1998;23:470–474.

52. Simmonds M, Lee C, Jones S. Pain distribution and physical function in patients with low back pain. In: *13th International Congress of World Confederation for Physical Therapy*. Yokohama, Japan; 1999.

53. Bekkering GE, et al. Prognostic factors for low back pain in patients referred for physiotherapy: Comparing outcomes and varying modeling techniques. *Spine* 2005;30(16):1881–1886.

54. Willis W, ed. Introduction to the basic science of pain and headache for the clinician: physiological concepts. In: Max M, ed. Pain 1999—An Updated Review. Seattle; IASP Press; 1999: 561–572.

55. International Association for the Study of Pain: Subcommittee on Taxonomy. Pain Terms: A list with definitions and notes on usage. *Pain* 1980;8:249–252

56. Tillman D. Heat response properties of unmyelinated nociceptors. Baltimore, MD: Johns Hopkins University; 1992.

57. Vlayen J,Linton S. Fear-avoidance and its consequences in chronic musculoskeletal pain: A state of the art. *Pain* 2000;85:317–332.

58. Mannion AF, et al. A randomized clinical trial of three active therapies for chronic low back pain. *Spine* 1999;24(23):2435–2448.

59. Dettori J, et al. The effects of spinal flexion and extension exercises and their associated postures in patients with acute low back pain. *Spine* 1995;20:2303–2312.

60. Jensen M, Karoly P. Self-report scales and procedures for assessing pain in adults. In: Turk D, Mlezack R, eds. Handbook of Pain Assessment. D. Turk and R. Melzack. New York: Guilford Press; 1992:135–151.

61. Simmonds MJ, Claveau Y. Measures of pain and physical function in patients with low back pain. *Physiother Theory Pract* 1997;13: 53–65.

62. Jette A, et al. Physical therapy episodes of care for patients with low back pain. *Phys Ther* 1994;74:101–115.

63. Lee CE, et al. Self-reports and clinician-measured physical function among patients with low back pain: A comparison. *Arch Phys Med Rehabil* 2001;82(2):227–231.

64. Fairbank J, et al. The Oswestry low back pain disability questionnaire. *Physiotherapy* 1980;66:271–273.

65. Roland M, Morris R. A study of the natural history of back pain. Part I: Development of a reliable and sensitive measure of disability in low-back pain. *Spine* 1983;8(2):141–144.

66. Ware J, Sherbourne C. The MOS 36-item short-form health survey (SF-36). I. Conceptual framework and item selection. *Med Care* 1992;30:473–483.

67. Simmonds MJ, et al. Physical performance tests: are they psychometrically sound and clinically useful for patients with low back pain? *Spine* 1998;23(22):2412–2421.

68. Marras W, Wongsamm P. Flexibility and velocity of normal and impaired lumbar spine. *Arch Phys Med Rehabil* 1986;67:213–217.

69. Simmonds M, et al. Disability prediction in patients with back pain using performance based models. In: Joint Meeting North American Spine Society and American Pain Society, 1998; Charleston, South Carolina.

70. Simmonds MJ, Kumar S, Lechelt E. Psychological factors in disabling low back pain: causes or consequences? *Disabil Rehabil* 1996;18(4):161–168.

71. Smeets RJ, et al. The association of physical deconditioning and chronic low back pain: A hypothesis-oriented systematic review. *Disabil Rehabil* 2006;28(11):673–693.

72. Smeets RJ, et al. Do patients with chronic low back pain have a lower level of aerobic fitness than healthy controls? Are pain, disability, fear of injury, working status, or level of leisure time activity associated with the difference in aerobic fitness level? *Spine* 2006;31(1):90–97; discussion 98.

73. Wittink H, et al. The association of pain with aerobic fitness in patients with chronic low back pain. *Arch Phys Med Rehabil* 2002;83: 1467–1471.

74. Wittink H, et al. Aerobic fitness testing in patients with chronic low back pain: Which test is best? *Spine* 2000;25(13):1704–1710.

75. Protas E. Physical activity and low back pain. In: Max M, ed. Pain 1999—An updated review. Seattle: IASP Press 1999:145–152.

76. U.S. Department of Health and Human Services. *Physical Activity and Health: A report of the Surgeon General*. Atlanta: U.S. Department of Health and Human Services, Centers for Disease Control and Prevention, National Center for Chronic Disease Prevention and Health Promotion; 1996.

77. Helewa A, et al. Does strengthening the abdominal muscles prevent low back pain—A randomized controlled trial. *J Rheumatol* 1999;26:1808–1815.

78. Battie M, et al. The role of spinal flexibility in back pain complaints within industry. *Spine* 1990;15:768–773.

79. Nelson R. NIOSH Low back atlas of standardized tests and measures. Springfield, VA: National Technical Information Service; 1988.

80. Waddell G. A new clinical model for the treatment of low back pain. *Spine* 1987;12:632–644.

81. Newton M, et al. Trunk strength testing with Iso-machines. Part 2: Experimental evaluation of the Cybex II Back testing system in normal subjects and patients with chronic low back pain. *Spine* 1993;18(7):812–824.

82. Mayer T, Gatchel R. *Functional Restoration for Spinal Disorders: The Sports Medicine Approach*. Philadelphia: Lea and Febiger; 1988.

83. Protas E. Aerobic exercise in the rehabilitation of individuals with chronic low back pain: a review. *Critical Reviews in Physical and Rehabilitation Medicine* 1996;8:283–295.

84. Bronfort G, et al. Efficacy of spinal manipulation and mobilization for low back pain and neck pain: A systematic review and best evidence synthesis. *The Spine Journal* 2004;4:335–356.

85. Clare HA, Adams R Maher CG. A systematic review of efficacy of McKenzie therapy for spinal pain. *Aust J Physiother* 2004;50:209–216.

86. van der Roer N, et al. What is the most cost-effective treatment for patients with low back pain? A systematic review. *Best Pract Res Clin Rheumatol* 2005;19(4):671–684.

87. Ostelo RW, et al. Behavioural treatment for chronic low-back pain. *Cochrane Database Syst Rev* 2005(1):CD002014.

88. Staal JB, et al. Return-to-work interventions for low back pain: A descriptive review of contents and concepts of working mechanisms. *Sports Med* 2002;32(4):251–267.

89. van Tulder MW, et al. Behavioral treatment for chronic low back pain: A systematic review within the framework of the Cochrane Back Review Group. *Spine* 2001;26(3):270–281.

90. van Tulder M, et al. Exercise therapy for low back pain: A systematic review within the framework of the cochrane collaboration back review group. *Spine* 2000;25(21):2784–2796.

91. van Tulder MW, et al. (Chronic low back pain: Exercise therapy, multidisciplinary programs, NSAID's, back schools and behavioral therapy effective; traction not effective; results of systematic reviews). *Ned Tijdschr Geneeskd* 2000;144(31):1489–1494.

92. Hancock MJ, et al. Systematic review of tests to identify the disc, SIJ or facet joint as the source of low back pain. *Eur Spine J* 2007.

93. Liddle SD, Gracey JH, Baxter GD. Advice for the management of low back pain: A systematic review of randomised controlled trials. *Man Ther* 2007;12(4):310–327.

94. Gulich M, et al. (Development of a guideline for rehabilitation of patients with low back pain. Phase 2: Analysis of data of the classification of therapeutic procedures). *Rehabilitation (Stuttg)* 2003;42(2):109–117.

95. Pengel HM, Maher CG, Refshauge KM. Systematic review of conservative interventions for subacute low back pain. *Clin Rehabil* 2002;16(8):811–820.

96. Koes BW, et al. Spinal manipulation for low back pain. An updated systematic review of randomized clinical trials. *Spine* 1996;21(24):2860–2871; discussion 2872–2873.

97. Engers A, et al. Patient education for low-back pain. *Cochrane Database Syst Rev* 2003(1).

98. Baker R, Lecouturier J, Bond S. Explaining variation in GP referral rates for x-rays for back pain. *Implementation Science* 2006;1:15.

99. Negrini S, et al. General practitioners' management of low back pain: impact of clinical guidelines in a non-English-speaking country. *Spine* 2001;26(24):2727–2733; discussion 2734.

100. Feuerstein M, et al. Evidence-based practice for acute low back pain in primary care: Patient outcomes and cost of care. *Pain* 2006;124(1–2):140–149.

101. Jackson D, Llewelyn-Philips H, Klaber-Moffett J. Categorization of back pain patients using an evidence based approach. *Musculoskeletal Management* 1996;2:39–46.

102. Malmivaara A, et al. The treatment of acute low back pain—Bed rest, exercises, or ordinary activity? *N Engl J Med* 1995;332: 351–355.

103. Frost H, et al. A fitness programme for patients with chronic low back pain: 2-year follow-up of a randomized controlled trial. *Pain* 1998;75:273–279.

104. Tortensen T, et al. Efficiency and costs of medical exercise therapy, conventional physiotherapy, and self-exercise in patients with chronic low back pain. *Spine* 1998;23:2616–2624.

105. Maher C, Latimer, J. Refshauge K. Prescription of activity for low back pain: What works? *Aust J Physiother* 1999;45:121–132.

106. Faas A, Battie M, Malmivaara A. Exercises: Which ones are worth trying for which patients and when? *Spine* 1996;21:2874–2879.

107. Abenhaim L, et al. The role of activity in the therapeutic management of back pain. Report of the International Paris Task Force on Back Pain. *Spine,* 2000;25(4 Suppl):1S–33S.

108. Videman T, et al. The long-term effects of physical loading and exercise lifestyles on back-related symptoms, disability, and spinal pathology among men. *Spine* 1995;20:699–709.

109. van Tulder M, et al. Exercise therapy for low back pain (Cochrane Review). The Cochrane Library. Oxford: Update Software, 2000(2).

110. van Tulder M, et al. European Guidelines for the management of acute nonspecific low back pain in primary care. In COST B13 Working Group on Guidelines for the Management of Acute Low Back Pain in Primary Care. European Commission, Research Directorate-General, Department of Policy, Co-ordination and Strategy;2004. Available at www.backpaineurope.org.

111. Keen S, et al. Individuals with low back pain: How do they view physical activity? *Fam Pract* 1999;16:39–45.

112. Friedrich M, et al. Combined exercise and motivation program: Effect on the compliance and level of disability of patients with chronic low back pain: A randomized controlled trial. *Arch Phys Med Rehabil* 1998;79(5):475–487.

113. Simmonds MJ, et al. Physical therapy assessment: Expanding the model. In: *Proceedings of the 9th World Congress on Pain. Progress on Pain.* Progress in Pain Research and Management, vol 16. Dever M, Rowbotham MC, Wiesenfield-Hallin. IASP Press, Seattle: 2000; 1013–1030.

Osteoporosis

EPIDEMIOLOGY AND PATHOPHYSIOLOGY

Osteoporosis is the most common disease that affects the skeleton. It is estimated that 10 million women in the United States today have osteoporosis and approximately 34 million have low bone mass, placing them at increased risk for osteoporosis (77). It is estimated that >2 million osteoporotic fractures occurred in the United States in 2005. The distribution of fractures included 27% vertebral fractures, 19% wrist fractures, 14% hip fractures, 7% pelvic fractures, and 33% "other" fractures (14). Fractures of the hip and spine result in disability, decreased independence and quality of life, and increased risk of death (19). The incidence of osteoporotic fractures rises sharply in the fourth decade of life. A 50-year-old woman has a lifetime fracture risk of 54%. Her risk of sustaining a spinal fracture is 32%–35%, 16%–18% for a hip fracture, and 15%–17% for a wrist fracture. Most hip fractures are a consequence of traumatic falls, making falls the number 1 cause of accidental death in people over the age of 75. Approximately 50,000 deaths result from complications from hip fractures each year. Currently, osteoporosis-related fractures occurring in the United States cause a direct medical cost of $17 billion per year (14,20). Nonvertebral fractures account for 73% of the fractures and 94% of the cost. Men comprise 30% of osteoporosis-related fractures and 25% of the cost. By the year 2025, it is projected that the annual number of fractures will surpass 3 million and the direct cost will increase to approximately $25 million (14). In addition, it is predicted that the nonwhite (mainly Hispanic) population will have a rapidly increasing share of the disease burden over time.

DEFINITION, CLASSIFICATION

Osteoporosis is defined as a disease characterized by low bone mineral density (BMD, also referred to as bone mass), microarchitectural deterioration of bone tissue with a consequent increase in bone fragility and susceptibility to fracture (83). The two categories of osteoporosis are primary osteoporosis and secondary osteoporosis. Primary osteoporosis is caused by a disruption in the normal cycle of bone turnover. Postmenopausal osteoporosis

(type I) is categorized as primary osteoporosis. Other types of primary osteoporosis are senile osteoporosis (type II) and idiopathic osteoporosis. Secondary osteoporosis occurs when bone loss is a consequence of diseases such as Cushing's disease, hyperthyroidism, and prolonged treatment with corticosteroids.

BONE PHYSIOLOGY

Bone tissue has three main functions. First, bones provide structural and mechanical support for soft tissues, serving as attachment points for skeletal muscle and acting as levers for locomotion. Second, the skeleton is responsible for maintaining calcium homeostasis, as well as serving as a storage site for phosphate, magnesium, potassium, and bicarbonate. Finally, the skeleton is the primary site of blood cell formation (97).

The two types of bone tissue are cortical bone and trabecular bone. Cortical bone, also known as compact bone, is found in the shafts of the long bones and it comprises approximately 80% of the skeleton. Trabecular, or cancellous bone, constitutes the remaining 20% of the skeleton. Trabecular bone, which is arranged in a honeycomb pattern of trabeculae, is found in the flat bones, such as the pelvis and vertebral bodies, and in the ends of the long bones, such as the head and neck of the femur. Trabecular bone is more metabolically active with an annual bone turnover rate of 25% compared with cortical bone with an annual bone turnover rate of 2%–3% (16). Therefore, trabecular bone is more sensitive to changes in biochemical, hormonal, and nutritional status and thus more susceptible to being lost. For this reason, most osteoporotic fractures occur in areas with a large proportion of trabecular bone: the spine, proximal hip (femoral neck and greater trochanter), and distal radius and ulna.

The adult skeleton is a dynamic organ that undergoes a constant process of resorption and deposition, referred to as *bone remodeling*. Bone remodeling serves to maintain the architecture and strength of the bone, maintain mineral homeostasis, and prevent fatigue damage. Remodeling is also important during periods of growth when most of adult bone mass is laid down.

Bone resorption is carried out by osteoclasts, large multinucleated cells originating from stem cells in the bone marrow. Resorption involves the dissolving of a predetermined volume of bone mineral over 1–2 weeks by proteolytic enzymes and organic acids released from the osteoclasts (16,45). The result is a cavity of approximately 60 μm within the surface of the bone. Deposition of new bone matrix in the cavity created by the osteoclasts is carried out by osteoblasts. Bone matrix is composed of collagen fibers and calcium salts known as hydroxyapatite. The complete remodeling cycle takes several months and leaves a new Haversian system in cortical bone and a new "packet" of bone in cancellous bone (16).

Osteoporosis results a disruption occurs at any point during the remodeling cycle of resorption and deposition. During young adulthood, these two processes are balanced and bone loss is minimal with peak bone mass being attained by the end of the second decade (16). During perimenopause, women lose bone mass at a rate of approximately 1% per year. At menopause, when ovarian function ceases, estrogen deficiency ensues and results in rapid bone loss for up to 5 years after menopause (29,52,52). Some age-related bone loss (approximately 0.5%–1.0% per year) is experienced by both men and women (36,37,37,52), although the exact age of onset of this loss is not really known.

RISK FACTORS AND PATHOPHYSIOLOGY

Several risk factors are associated with osteoporosis, some of which are immutable and others over which we have some control. Immutable risk factors include family history of osteoporosis, female sex, advanced age, race, menstrual history, hysterectomy, and nulliparity (never given birth). Risk factors that can be controlled to some extent include dietary factors, inadequate physical activity, smoking, gonadal hormone insufficiency, and use of certain medications.

As with many other diseases, including cancer and cardiovascular disease, osteoporosis tends to run in families. Peak bone density and rate of bone loss are dependent on genetic components as well as shared environmental factors. Women are at greater risk than men for developing osteoporosis. This is mostly because of the postmenopausal loss of estrogen, but also partly because women tend to be less physically active than men and most women also have inadequate calcium intakes. Women can lose up to 15% of bone mass within 5–10 years of menopause (40). Men do not experience the same rapid drop in testosterone, which is responsible for bone mass in males. In addition, it has also been shown that bone density in the femur declines 0.95% per year in women compared with only 0.5% per year in men (81). The continual expected loss of bone further increases the risk of osteoporosis as people age.

Currently, white, Asian, Native American, and Hispanic women are at risk for osteoporosis. The National Health and Nutrition Examination Survey (NHANES) III data indicate that the highest prevalence of osteoporosis is in older white women, followed by Hispanic women, then black women (70). However, the National Osteoporosis Risk Assessment (NORA) study found that Native Americans were similar to white women in terms of osteoporosis risk. It was also demonstrated that Asian and Hispanic women had increased risk of osteoporosis and black women had a decreased risk for osteoporosis compared with white women (109). Although the risk for osteoporosis is much higher in women than in men, the mortality rate after a fracture is higher in men, most likely because osteoporosis develops later in life in men (9).

A woman's menstrual history can affect her risk of osteoporosis. A late onset of the menstrual cycle (119) or an early onset of menopause can negatively affect the BMD related to the decreased amount of time estrogen circulates in the body. A woman who has a hysterectomy is also at an increased risk for the same reasons. It has also been found that women who are nulliparous have decreased BMD (111).

Dietary factors that can influence the risk of osteoporosis for an individual include inadequate calcium and vitamin D intake, excessive consumption of alcohol and caffeine, and consumption of colas. Adequate calcium intake is necessary for the attainment of peak bone mass as well as being effective in reducing postmenopausal bone loss. Vitamin D is required for calcium absorption from the gut and for the maintenance of bone calcium. A recent meta-analysis recommended minimum doses of 1,200 mg of calcium and 800 IU of vitamin D to aid in the prevention of osteoporosis in people 50 years of age or older (113). An early study determined that caffeine causes a short-term increase in urinary calcium loss and is associated with an increased risk of hip fracture in elderly women (57). Further investigation revealed that caffeine had no harmful effect on bone provided that individuals took the recommended daily allowances of calcium (46). A recent study concluded, however, that a daily intake of 330 mg of caffeine (4 cups of coffee) or more may be associated with a modest increase in risk of fractures (41). In addition, the increased risk of fractures was greater in women with lower intakes of calcium.

Similar to caffeine, alcohol is associated with increased urinary loss of calcium and excessive alcohol intake may reduce absorption of calcium from the intestine. Alcohol is also known to be toxic to osteoblasts (45). Recent studies have found that a moderate intake of alcohol has a positive effect on BMD in men and women (75,129). Excessive alcohol intake, however, continues to increase the risk of fractures, especially in men (75), and is still considered to be a risk factor for osteoporosis and fractures (53,75).

Intake of colas is also considered a risk factor for osteoporosis. A recent study determined that intake of cola by women, but not other types of carbonated beverages, is associated with low BMD in the hip but not the spine (118). The findings were similar for diet colas but were weaker when the colas were decaffeinated.

Lower body weight is directly correlated to lower bone density (3,98) and is a determinant of bone density in adults (34). Smoking is associated with low BMD (91), an increased risk of fracture (54), decreased levels of vitamin D (121), and decreased calcium absorption (91). It is thought that smoking also interferes with estrogen metabolism (114). The gonadal hormones, particularly estrogen, are essential for maintaining bone mass. Estrogen directly affects bone turnover by binding to estrogen receptors on the osteoblasts. Estrogen also enhances calcium absorption from the intestines (16). Several medications, in particular the glucocorticoids, have adverse effects on the skeleton. These include increased urinary excretion and decreased intestinal absorption of calcium, reduced levels of gonadal hormones, inhibition of osteoblast function, and increased bone resorption (16).

Another risk factor for osteoporosis is decreased activity level. It is well known that increased activity level and exercise will aid in maintaining or improving BMD. In a recent study it was determined that among many lifestyle risk factors, high school sports participation appeared to have the greatest influence on BMD levels in the femoral neck (3). This supports the need for physical activity, especially during adolescence, for accruing and improving bone mass.

Several of these risk factors are interrelated. For example, peak bone mass is largely determined by genetic factors; however, failure to reach one's genetic potential is often the result of inadequate calcium intake and exercise (45). Also, risk of osteoporosis increases with advancing age, particularly after menopause in women, with early menopause, either natural or surgical, causing an even greater risk. Postmenopausal bone loss is largely the result of estrogen deficiency, but pharmacologic therapy can dramatically attenuate postmenopausal bone loss.

CLINICAL EXERCISE PHYSIOLOGY

Bone density does not respond to acute exercise bouts and cardiovascular responses to acute exercise have not been well studied in osteoporotic populations. Lombardi et al. (69) examined physical capacity during exercise in women with osteoporosis, with and without vertebral fracture, and compared their responses with those of women without osteoporosis. Very few differences were found in measures of physical capacity during walking exercise at 3 or 4 mph ($\dot{V}O_2$, metabolic equivalents [METs], heart rate) although energy expenditure was positively associated with the degree of kyphosis (69). The primary purposes of acute exercise testing are typically to aid in the diagnoses of coronary artery disease (CAD) and to determine appropriate levels of exercise training. Osteoporosis can sometimes mask the presence

of CAD if it prevents an individual from achieving the adequate heart rate and blood pressure necessary for accurate diagnoses. In addition, severe thoracic kyphosis can impair respiration and limit the test (24). Nonetheless, no specific recommendations from the American College of Sports Medicine (ACSM) would suggest that osteoporosis is an absolute contraindication to exercise testing (1). If an exercise stress test is to be used in patients with osteoporosis, one utilizing a bicycle protocol would probably be the best choice, because that would involve the least trauma and impact on the bones. Caution, however, must still be taken when utilizing a bike protocol. An upright posture should be maintained by the patient at all times because spinal flexion is contraindicated in people with osteoporosis. Treadmill protocols can be utilized if need be, but a walking protocol should be used and care should be taken to ensure the patient does not trip or fall.

Bone mass responses to chronic exercise in the osteoporotic population and in postmenopausal women have been well studied (11,26,43,64,78,89,120). The primary purpose of prescribing exercise in these populations would be to increase both BMD and overall fitness and balance to aid in fall prevention (62). In this regard, most studies have shown positive results. A number of studies in postmenopausal women have shown that exercise can increase BMD or prevent further bone loss when compared with nonexercising controls (11,26,64,78).

Although bone mass responds positively to chronic exercise in adults, the use of exercise as a treatment for older adults with low bone mass is limited (61) because increases in BMD with exercise are generally small (2% or less). A better utilization of exercise may lie in prevention of osteoporosis by improving peak bone mass. Recent reviews of the literature highlight the importance of exercise in establishing optimal levels of bone mineral during the growing years when bone may respond better to chronic exercise (4,6). Further, the timing of exercise intervention in childhood has been demonstrated to affect bone mineral status in adulthood. Female tennis and squash players who started their playing careers before or at menarche were found to have a two- to threefold greater dominant arm bone mineral content than those who had started playing more than 15 years after menarche (55). So, the chronic responses of bone to exercise would appear to differ, depending at what point in life the exercise is initiated.

PHARMACOLOGY

Most women diagnosed with osteoporosis, and postmenopausal women in general, likely will be taking some form of calcium and vitamin D supplements. Other common drugs available that may be used for treatment of osteoporosis include estrogen alone or in combination with progesterone, bisphosphonates, calcitonin, and selective estrogen receptor modulators (SERM). Other less common agents include isoflavones (natural and synthetic), sodium fluoride, and parathyroid hormone. The effects of any of these drugs or nutrients on exercise performance or cardiovascular responses to acute or chronic exercise have not been well studied, but any effect is likely minimal. In one long-term study looking at the interaction of alendronate and exercise on BMD, $\dot{V}O_2$ and leg strength were not affected by alendronate (120). Calcitonin has been shown to increase β-endorphin levels, but any effect of that on exercise performance has not been evaluated. Estrogen has acute vasodilator action and has been shown to increase blood flow during exercise (59). Despite the increased blood flow, peak exercise responses ($\dot{V}O_2$, total exercise time, heart rate) were not altered (59).

PHYSICAL EXAMINATION

The physical assessment of the patient with osteoporosis should include a detailed medical history with an inquiry about all medications, vitamins, and minerals taken. A pain history also provides useful information along with careful assessment of height and observation of posture.

PAIN ASSESSMENT

Although osteoporosis frequently presents with no pain until a fracture has occurred, pain history is an important part of the physical examination of the patient with osteoporosis. The most common fractures that occur in individuals with osteoporosis are hip, wrist, and vertebral fractures. Fractures of the hip and wrist are easily identified on x-ray film and usually occur as a result of a fall. Vertebral fractures, however, often cannot be visualized on x-ray film, and frequently occur during routine daily activity, such as lifting a grocery bag or sneezing. Sharp and persistent back pain may be the only physical finding to suggest vertebral fracture. Although a bone scan can be performed to confirm the fracture, the nature of the pain experienced and circumstances leading up to the pain are often considered sufficient to make the diagnosis of vertebral fracture. History of any previous fractures should also be noted, along with the mechanics and circumstances leading up to these fractures.

ASSESSMENT OF STATURE

Loss of height that may range from 1 inch to as much as 4 or 5 inches is an important physical finding because a loss of height occurs with each spinal compression fracture sustained by the patient with osteoporosis. In a compression fracture of the vertebra, the bone within the vertebral body collapses resulting in a loss of height of the vertebra. An individual can sustain multiple fractures to the same vertebra or fractures to multiple vertebrae that can result in several inches of lost height. These compression fractures may be accompanied by severe pain or little pain that may be ignored by the individual. In any case, loss of height is always a significant finding and should be monitored closely. The use of a stature board allows precise measurement of height and is useful in monitoring changes.

POSTURAL ASSESSMENT

Often, spinal compression fractures occur specifically in the anterior portion of the vertebral body. When the anterior portion of the vertebral body collapses, the loss in vertebral height anteriorly results in a wedge-shaped vertebra (hence the name, wedge fracture). Wedge fractures cause a change in the overall curvature of the spine that is seen as an increased thoracic kyphosis, sometimes referred to as "dowager's hump." As the thoracic kyphosis progresses, the head is thrust forward and the ribs approach the pelvic bones, resulting in further loss of height. Additionally, as the kyphosis progresses, there is less room for lung expansion. If the kyphosis is sufficiently severe, respiration will be affected. In this case, pulmonary function tests may be indicated; if these are unavailable, a simple tape measure assessment of chest wall expansion with full inspiration (taken at the 4th intercostal space) is useful for assessing baseline status and progression or reduction of the impairment (21,24,103). Standardized procedures for taking this measurement, as well as normative values for different age groups, are presented elsewhere (66). Degree of forward head, thoracic kyphosis, and lumbar lordosis should be noted in the postural assessment. Additionally, simple tools exist that can be used to obtain objective measurements of thoracic kyphosis and lumbar lordosis. A surveyor's flexicurve provides a simple, inexpensive method of assessing thoracic kyphosis and lumbar lordosis (25). The flexicurve is a plastic "ruler" that bends in one plane and holds its shape. It can be molded to a subject's spine, then lifted and laid on a ruled sheet to be traced. Objective measurements can then be obtained from the tracing.

MEDICAL TREATMENTS

Several nonpharmacologic and pharmacologic agents are available to increase, or slow the loss of bone mass. These include calcium and vitamin D supplementation, estrogen (or hormone) replacement therapy, SERMs, bisphosphonates, parathyroid hormone (PTH), and calcitonin. Pharmacologic therapies are shown in Table 12-1. A brief review of the approved therapies are presented here; more extensive reviews can be found elsewhere (38,68).

Both calcium and vitamin D alone and in combination have been used in patients with osteoporosis, although their effectiveness for increasing BMD is equivocal. The evidence suggests that calcium is necessary for bone structure, but its role is more passive depending on

TABLE 12.1. PHARMACOLOGIC THERAPIES AVAILABLE IN THE TREATMENT OR PREVENTION OF OSTEOPOROSIS

DRUG CLASS	NAME OF DRUG	BRAND NAME
Antiresorptive Medications		
Estrogens (ERT)	Several available	Several
Estrogen + Progestin (HRT)[1]		
Calcitonin[2]	Synthetic Salmon	Miacalcin
	Calcitonin	Calcimar
		Fortical
Bisphosphonates[3]	Alendronate	Fosamax
	Risedronate	Actonel
	Ibandronate	Boniva
SERM[4]	Raloxifene	Evista
Bone Formation Medications		
Parathyroid Hormone[5]	Teriparatide	Forteo

ERT, estrogen replacement therapy; HRT, hormone replacement therapy; SERM, selective estrogen receptor modulator. [1]Both ERT and HRT have US Food and Drug Administration (FDA) approval for prevention of postmenopausal osteoporosis. [2]All calcitonins have FDA approval for treatment of postmenopausal osteoporosis. [3]All bisphosphonates have FDA approval for both prevention and treatment of osteoporosis. Alendronate and risedronate are approved for treatment of osteoporosis in men. [4]Raloxifen is FDA approved for prevention and treatment of osteoporosis. [5]Teriparatide is FDA approved for treatment of osteoporosis in postmenopausal women and to increase bone mass in men with primary osteoporosis.

adequate hormonal regulation. The effect of calcium intake in postmenopausal women may depend on their stage in menopause. Despite the unclear role of calcium and vitamin D in osteoporosis prevention, recent meta-analyses indicate calcium and vitamin D supplementation have small positive effects on bone density and also result in significant reductions in fracture risk (105,113). Recent prospective studies using vitamin D have also found reductions in fracture or fracture risk (31,116). Another important finding regarding vitamin D is that it has been shown to reduce the number of falls a person has, presumably by increasing musculoskeletal function (7). In addition, the effectiveness of other therapies (bisphosphonates, calcitonin) may be reduced without the use of calcium or vitamin D supplementation (96).

Most of the current drugs with US Food and Drug Administration (FDA) approval for osteoporosis are considered antiresorptive therapy. They halt the loss of bone or even increase bone mass by inhibiting bone resorption, while having no effect on bone formation. Estrogen replacement therapy (ERT, estrogen alone) and hormone replacement therapy (HRT, estrogen in combination with progestin) have been used for several years in the treatment and prevention of osteoporosis in postmenopausal women. Studies have shown that ERT or HRT can halt the loss of and often increase bone mass (49,63,124). Studies have also demonstrated reductions in fracture risk with HRT, but most were observational or retrospective studies (51,122). The Women's Health Initiative (WHI) is one of the few large-scale, randomized clinical trials done with ERT and HRT. Results from the WHI indicated a significant reduction in both vertebral and hip

fracture risk with the use of both HRT and ERT (2,99). The major finding of the WHI was, however, that both HRT and ERT resulted in an increased risk of cardiovascular disease and HRT also increased the risk for certain cancers (2,99). As a result, the recommendation of HRT in the treatment of osteoporosis must be reconsidered.

Bisphosphonates are probably the most powerful of the antiresorptive drugs available and are now the preferred drug therapy for osteoporosis (68). Currently, three different bisphosphonates have FDA approval for prevention and treatment of osteoporosis (Table 12-1). Both randomized clinical trials and several meta-analyses have indicated the effectiveness of each of the bisphosphonates in reducing bone loss and decreasing fracture risk in postmenopausal women (10,28,73,80) and in men (72,74,92,94,95,102,115,127).

Calcitonin and SERM are the other antiresorptive agents approved for treatment or prevention of osteoporosis. Randomized controlled trials and meta-analyses have shown antifracture efficacy for both calcitonin (18,23) and the SERM raloxifene (27,104) and each can increase bone mass, although typically not to the same extent as bisphosphonates. The advantages of SERMs are that they have favorable effects on lipids, but they do not have the stimulatory effect on breast or endometrial tissue as seen with estrogen (56). Calcitonin has been shown to reduce the back pain often associated with vertebral compression fractures (60).

Teriparatide, a derivative of parathyroid hormone, is currently the only FDA approved treatment that has an anabolic action on bone. Increases in BMD seen with the use of teriparatide are a result of increased bone formation (15). Both increased BMD and reductions in fracture risk have been demonstrated in studies with teriparatide (17,65). The increases in BMD are generally larger than seen with antiresorptive medications (5%–6% vs. 2%–4%, respectively). The major drawback to teriparatide is that treatment requires daily subcutaneous administration and the cost is up to 10 times higher than bisphosphonates (68).

DIAGNOSTIC TECHNIQUES

Diagnosis of osteoporosis involves the measurement of bone mineral density. Several methods for measuring BMD have been used in the past, including radiogrammetry, single-photon absorptiometry, and dual-photon absorptiometry. These techniques, however, lacked the precision and accuracy necessary for broad clinical use. Dual-energy x-ray absorptiometry (DXA), quantitative computer tomography (QCT), and ultrasound are now used for the measurement of BMD.

Dual-energy x-ray absorptiometry is the most commonly used technology for measuring BMD. DXA uses low dose x-ray to emit photons at two different energy levels. BMD is calculated based on the amount of energy attenuated by the body. DXA measurements are reported in grams per square centimeter (g/cm^2), so they are not a true density, but rather area density measurements. DXA is capable of differentiating between bone and soft tissue and so can also be used to measure regional and total body composition. The advantages of DXA are that it is capable of measuring small changes in BMD over time, has a precision of 0.5%–2.0%, requires short examination times (5–10 minutes), and provides low radiation exposure.

Quantitative computer tomography has two distinct advantages over DXA. First, QCT provides a precise three-dimensional anatomic localization for direct measurement of true bone density. Second, QCT is capable of differentiating between trabecular and cortical bone and is used to examine the anatomy of trabecular regions within the spine. QCT, however, is less practical than DXA for routine screening owing to expense and higher radiation exposure.

Quantitative ultrasound measures the velocity and attenuation of sound waves as they pass through bone and soft tissue. In addition to providing a measure of bone mass, ultrasound assesses qualitative factors such as bone elasticity. The advantages of ultrasound are that it does not use radiation and ultrasound units are compact, making them ideal for use in field settings.

Bone mineral density is reported not only in grams per square centimeter (DXA) or grams per cubic centimeter (g/cm^3; QCT), but also in terms of standard deviations, or T-scores. The likelihood of sustaining a fracture increases 1.5 to 3-fold for each standard deviation decrease in BMD. The World Health Organization Consensus Development Conference has developed diagnostic criteria for osteoporosis based on this relationship (128). Normal BMD is that which is less than 1.0 standard deviation below the mean for young adults. A BMD that is between 1.0 and 2.5 standard deviations below the young adult mean is considered low bone mass or osteopenia. Osteoporosis is defined as BMD more than 2.5 standard deviations below the young adult mean, and is considered "severe" if accompanied by one or more fragility fractures. These criteria were originally developed for diagnosis of osteoporosis at the proximal femur in postmenopausal women, and recent recommendations from the International Society for Clinical Densitometry (ISCD) suggest that T-scores not be used with all populations (67). Instead z-scores and other criteria should be used; z-scores indicate the number of standard deviations below the age-matched mean.

EXERCISE, FITNESS, AND FUNCTIONAL TESTING

Exercise recommendations for patients with osteoporosis or those who are at risk for developing osteoporosis generally include an aerobic weight-bearing program and a resistive exercise program to promote bone health (8,62,87). Additionally, if an individual has been diagnosed with osteoporosis, that individual is at increased risk for fracturing a bone. Because falls are associated with most hip and wrist fractures, and are a leading cause of injury in older adults, a balance training program (62,87) and a falls intervention program should be instituted in all older adults who are diagnosed with osteoporosis. The following exercise testing should be conducted to provide an individual with a safe, effective training program.

AEROBIC FITNESS TESTING

Although osteoporosis occurs in young amenorrheic women, it is still a disease that primarily occurs in older women and men. Currently, the American College of Sports Medicine recommends that anyone at high risk for cardiac disease who wants to begin a moderate or vigorous exercise program should have a medically supervised stress test (1). For osteoporotic adults not at high risk who simply want to begin a moderate intensity walking or resistance training program, this recommendation may be both impractical and unnecessary. Careful screening should be undertaken to identify which individuals might need further evaluation by a physician (79).

MUSCLE STRENGTH TESTING

Muscle strength testing is used to determine training intensity for the resistance exercise program. The one-repetition maximum (RM) is frequently used for strength assessment in the apparently healthy individual and has been used safely to assess and progress very elderly women on resistance training programs (32,78,93). No studies have yet investigated the use of 1-RM to determine training intensity in women who are known to have osteoporosis. Therefore, use of the 1-RM assessment is generally discouraged in the patient with osteoporosis because of safety concerns. Assessment of the 6, 8, or 10-RM is recommended for the osteoporotic patient, although no consensus exists on which is most desirable. A dose-response relationship between resistance exercise and bone health has not yet been determined (112).

Because deficits in lower extremity muscle strength are associated with an increased incidence of falls (39,125,126), maximal isometric muscle strength assessment is used to identify muscle strength deficits as part of the overall evaluation of fall risk. Handheld dynamometry provides an objective measurement of isometric strength and is useful for identifying muscle strength impairments as well as for monitoring change in muscle strength in response to an exercise program. Strength assessment of the hip flexors, extensors, and abductors as well as knee extensors and plantarflexors should be conducted (117).

BALANCE TESTING

A deficit in balance has also been shown to be a predictor of falls (39), and is therefore a critical component in the evaluation of fall risk. A simple test of static balance, such as timed ability to stand on one leg (single stance time), when compared with established performance norms can be used (13). Although force platform systems can provide more information about the nature of the balance impairment, single stance time has been shown to distinguish fallers from nonfallers among the elderly (22,35,44,47) and is a useful measure (47).

FALL RISK ASSESSMENT

Considerable evidence indicates that the most effective way to reduce falls is the use of systematic fall risk assessments with targeted interventions (33,100,101). No consensus, however, exists on a specific method for assessing fall risk and a discussion of the various tools designed to determine fall risk is outside of the scope of this textbook.

FLEXIBILITY TESTING

General flexibility tests, such as the sit-and-reach and shoulder elevation tests, are not performed in patients with osteoporosis. Primarily, flexibility of muscles that have the potential to adversely affect posture should be assessed. Decreases in length of muscles that cross more than one joint have the greatest potential to cause problems in posture (e.g., hamstrings and hip flexors). Insufficient length in the hamstrings or hip flexors will produce a posterior pelvic tilt or anterior pelvic tilt, respectively. Such postural alterations affect how weight is borne through the bones in the spine and lower extremities. Other muscles that frequently lose flexibility and can lead to postural problems include the pectoral muscles and the gastrocnemius muscles. Flexibility is assessed by measuring joint range of motion (ROM) when the muscle is fully elongated over each joint crossed by that muscle simultaneously. For example, flexibility of the gastrocnemius muscle is assessed by measuring dorsiflexion of the ankle when the knee is kept fully extended and hamstrings can be assessed by measuring hip flexion ROM when the knee is kept fully extended.

EXERCISE PRESCRIPTION AND PROGRAMMING

Although studies have shown that several forms of exercise training have the potential to increase BMD, the optimal training program for skeletal integrity has yet to be defined. Based on current experimental knowledge and recommendations from ACSM, it has been proposed that an osteogenic exercise regimen should have load-bearing activities at high magnitude (force) with a small number of repetitions, create versatile strain distributions throughout

the bone structure (load the bone in directions to which it is unaccustomed), and be long term and progressive in nature (8,62,110,112). Resistance training (weightlifting) probably offers the best opportunity to meet these criteria on an individual basis; it requires little skill and has the added advantage of being highly adaptable to changes in both magnitude and strain distribution. In addition, strength and muscle size increases have been demonstrated following resistance training, even in the elderly (42).

No known studies have specifically examined cardiovascular adaptations in osteoporotic patients, but older adults can increase their cardiovascular fitness levels 10%–30% with prolonged endurance training (79). Many older women and men with osteoporosis will have some form of cardiovascular disease. Because exercise endurance training can decrease cardiovascular disease risk factors (e.g., high blood pressure and cholesterol), it should probably be recommended for the osteoporotic patient (79).

Thus, resistance training combined with some sort of cardiovascular training, stationary cycling or walking, is the best recommendation for an exercise program for a patient with osteoporosis. Walking is probably the preferred mode of aerobic exercise because it offers a greater weight-bearing component than does bicycling. Not only will such a program increase overall fitness and help maintain bone mass, it will aid greatly in reducing the risk of falling (79), which is one of the primary causes of fracture in osteoporosis.

Certain exercises are quite beneficial for the patient with osteoporosis. These would include exercises designed to help with balance and agility to reduce falls. Clear guidelines for the type of exercise and the frequency and duration of balance training are not available (79). Exercises that strengthen the quadriceps, hamstrings, and gluteal muscles should be helpful in that regard. Although squats with free weights should be avoided in some patients with osteoporosis, the squat is a functionally important exercise for older adults. A modification that is safe and effective for most individuals is to rise out of a chair without pushing with the hands. Another specific activity that is helpful is standing on one foot for 5 to 15 seconds while touching the hands to a counter for balance. This will help build hip and low back strength as well as improve balance. The osteoporotic patient should also be encouraged to do spine extension (but NOT spinal flexion) exercises (107). Spine extension exercises can be performed in a chair and can help strengthen the back muscles, which should help reduce the development of a dowager's hump and possibly reduce the risk of vertebral fracture (108). These and all exercises done by patients with osteoporosis should be performed with slow and controlled movements and jerky, rapid movement should be avoided. More complete information on these and other exercises for the osteoporotic patient can be found elsewhere (106,107).

For patients with osteoporosis just beginning an exercise program, goals should include an increase in cardiovascular fitness, increased muscular strength and balance, and an increase (or at least no decrease) in BMD. Heart disease remains the number one killer of adults by a wide margin. So, the goal of all adults should be to increase their physical activity to reduce the risk of heart disease. The recent position stand by ACSM and the American Heart Association recommends at least 30 minutes of moderate intensity activity for a minimum of 5 days/week or 3 days/week if the activity is vigorous (79). This would be a worthwhile goal for all adults, including those with osteoporosis. If the patient with osteoporosis is just beginning an exercise program, however, multiple bouts of physical activity ($\geq$10 min) as opposed to a continuous bout might be needed initially to allow time for adjustment to the exercise (79). As the person's fitness level increases, the amount of time exercising can be increased. For the patient with osteoporosis, a walking program should provide the needed benefits along with being a safe mode of exercise.

For increases in muscular strength and bone density, weight training offers the most benefits in that regard. Current recommendations for older adults suggest a single set of 15 repetitions of 8–10 exercises performed at least 2 days/week (62,79) depending on the health of the individual. Again, this is a worthwhile goal for the person with osteoporosis, but a less strenuous program may be needed initially. Care should be taken to avoid exercises that are dangerous for individuals with osteoporosis. In addition, some resistance training exercises have a tendency to cause spinal flexion, especially those for the upper and lower extremities, so it is important that during resistance training all exercise be done in an upright posture.

A program to increase flexibility can also be useful to the osteoporotic patient because decreased flexibility can cause problems with posture. Muscles, such as the hamstring, that cross more than one joint are particularly important, although spinal flexion must be avoided when doing hamstring exercises. Little consensus exists on the optimal training program for increasing flexibility but good suggestions are available from many sources (123). Flexibility training has been shown to be beneficial (58) and ACSM recommends at least 10 minutes of flexibility training on most days of the week (79).

Participation in athletics also has the potential for increasing BMD in both young and older populations. Indeed, a number of studies, both cross-sectional and longitudinal, have found positive effects on bone health in all age groups from the training associated with sports participation (30,71,79,82,85,86). Sufficient evidence does not yet exist that suggests one type of athletic activity is better than another in regard to their osteogenic effect. It does appear that those sports which involve a high degree of impact (gymnastics or volleyball) are more beneficial to bone than those sports without impact loading (swimming or cycling) (30,84,110).

Thus, exercise may be useful both for increasing bone density to help prevent osteoporosis and using as a therapeutic modality for those patients in whom osteoporosis is already present. The major benefit of exercise for those with osteoporosis is probably more related to fall prevention than any major effect on bone density. Caution must be observed in the type of exercise program to be used and the specific exercises done. Persons with severe osteoporosis who are just beginning an exercise program should be supervised until it is determined that they can properly perform the exercises without danger to themselves. A suggested exercise program is summarized in Table 12.2, but keep in mind that no optimal training program for the skeleton has been identified.

TABLE 12.2. SUGGESTED EXERCISE PROGRAM FOR CLIENTS WITH OSTEOPOROSIS

TRAINING METHOD	MODE	FREQUENCY, INTENSITY, AND TIME	PROGRESSION	GOALS	SPECIAL CONSIDERATIONS/ COMMENTS
Aerobic	Walking or stationary cycling	4–5 times per week at a moderate intensity; start at 20 min/session if the patient has a minimal history of exercise	Increase speed and distance gradually after initial 2 weeks	30–45 min at $\geq$3.0 mph for walking; $\geq$70 rpm for cycling	No jogging, avoid activities that increase risk of falling (e.g., step aerobics)
Strength	Resistance training	Start at 1–2 days/week depending on the client; 15 repetitions of 8–10 exercise (may require less strenuous program initially)	Add a set after initial 2 weeks	3–4 days/week at 10–12 repetitions/set	Avoid spinal flexion during all exercises; use slow and controlled movements; target legs and back
Range of Motion	Stretching	5–7 days/week for 10–12 minutes; hold each stretch for approximately 15–20 seconds		Increase or maintain range of motion	Stretching exercises involving spinal flexion should be avoided

CONTRAINDICATIONS FOR EXERCISE

High-impact exercises, such as jumping, running, or jogging, are contraindicated in people who have osteoporosis (76). These exercises cause high compressive forces in the spine and lower extremities, and can cause fractures in weakened bones. High-impact exercises, such as two-footed jumping, however, have been shown to be effective for maintaining BMD in nonosteoporotic women and can be used to help prevent osteoporosis (5).

Another activity that absolutely should not be done by persons with osteoporosis is spinal flexion, especially when combined with a resistive or twisting movement (107). Spinal flexion and twisting motions at the waist drastically increase the forces on the spine, increasing the likelihood of a fracture (12). For this reason, exercises such as toe touches, sit-ups, or rowing machines, should be avoided in people with osteoporosis (76). Other activities that should be avoided are those that may increase the chance of falling, such as trampolines, step aerobics, skating (ice or in-line), or exercising on slippery floors (76). Resistive exercises are not contraindicated in people with osteoporosis, but resistance should be used cautiously when the osteoporosis is severe (79).

EDUCATION AND COUNSELING

ACTIVITY/EXERCISE

It is important to follow instructions in an appropriate exercise program, emphasizing the following points to encourage patient compliance with the recommended exercise program.

- Gains made in bone density will only be maintained as long as the exercise is continued (62).
- Approximately 9 months to 1 year are required to detect a significant change in bone mass (16,62).
- Whether or not significant gains in bone density are achieved, participating in a regular exercise program is still beneficial for reducing cardiovascular risk factors, improving muscle strength and balance, reducing the risk for falling, and improving posture.

SAFETY HAZARDS IN THE HOME

As mentioned, falls are a frequent cause of fracture and thus it is important to prevent them in the person with osteoporosis. The reasons falls occur are varied, but identified risk factors include environmental hazards, muscle weakness, poor balance, and medication-related side effects (126). By eliminating as many of these risk factors as possible, the danger of falling can be reduced. A discussion of safety hazards in the home and suggestions for removal of these hazards is an integral part of any falls prevention program. Filling out a fall risk assessment can help identify hazards in the home. The examiner may

then make suggestions on how to remove the hazards or how to modify the home to make it safer. These suggestions may be as simple as moving a telephone to within reach of the bed to avoid falls when getting up in the dark to answer it. Other possible hazards, such as slippery floors or bathtubs, can also be eliminated (50,90). Although these efforts seem like common sense, many people may not recognize a telephone out of reach as a hazard until after an accident happens. Muscle weakness and balance can be improved at any age with the use of a properly structured exercise program. Educating persons on the side effects of medications, such as those that cause dizziness, is also an important step in fall prevention. Although many fall risk assessment tools are available and have been shown to be useful for identifying fall hazards (88), no consensus exists on which is most useful. Selection of a fall risk assessment tool should be based largely on the patient's characteristics (e.g., whether the individual is an active older adult residing in the community versus a frail adult residing in an institution) as well as prior determination that the assessment tool possesses diagnostic accuracy and reliability.

ACTIVITY MODIFICATION

Although proper body mechanics during lifting should be encouraged in all individuals, it is absolutely critical for those who have osteoporosis. Attempting to lift an object with the back flexed is a common mechanism of vertebral fracture in people with osteoporosis. Instructions must be provided on how to bend the knees and keep the back straight while reaching an object to be picked up from the floor.

Daily activities, such as sweeping, vacuuming, or mopping, can also present problems for people with osteoporosis because these activities are typically performed by using a lot of bending and twisting of the spine. These activities, however, can be modified to avoid spinal twisting and bending, and instead provide beneficial loading to the spine and hips. People with osteoporosis should be encouraged to mop, sweep, or vacuum by placing one foot in front of the other, and shifting weight from one foot to the other in a rocking motion (76). The knees are bent and the back is kept straight during this rocking motion. The rocking motion from one foot to the other takes the place of bending and twisting of the spine to reach forward when mopping, sweeping, or vacuuming.

DIETARY MODIFICATIONS AND CALCIUM SUPPLEMENTS

Individuals diagnosed with osteoporosis or osteopenia should be educated regarding dietary modifications and calcium supplementation. Education should begin with a review of foods that are a good source of calcium along with instructions on how to read food labels. Food labels do not tell how much calcium is in a given food. Instead, labels tell you what percentage of the recommended daily requirement is provided by the food item. These percentages, however, are based on the inaccurate assumption that the recommended daily requirement is 1,000 mg for everybody, regardless of age or gender. Patients can be easily educated on how to convert the percentages to actual quantity of calcium in milligram by adding a zero to the end of the percentage number. For example, if a container of yogurt has 30% of the recommended calcium per serving, then there are 300 mg of calcium per serving.

Patients should also be instructed about which types of food provide the best source of calcium. Dairy products are the best source of calcium; however, some individuals cannot eat dairy products. Other types of food that are rich in calcium are dark green leafy vegetables, such as collard greens; almonds, and canned salmon with bones. In addition, many foods (e.g., orange juice and cereal) are now fortified with calcium. It has been shown that individuals can only absorb 500–600 mg of calcium at one time. Therefore, it is beneficial to instruct patients to eat calcium throughout the day rather than at just one meal.

Finally, a discussion of the different types of calcium supplements is valuable because people often take their supplements incorrectly and therefore reduce their effectiveness. Calcium comes in many different forms, but the two most common forms are calcium citrate (e.g., Citracal), and calcium carbonate (e.g., Os-Cal, Caltrate, Viactiv). Studies show that calcium citrate is more readily absorbed (48), but has less calcium per tablet than calcium carbonate. That means more tablets of calcium citrate must be taken per day to attain the recommended requirement of 1,200 or 1,500 mg. In any case, individuals who choose calcium carbonate because of being able to take fewer tablets per day, they should take part of their requirement after each meal. Taking calcium carbonate after a meal improves the absorption, but it still will not be absorbed as well as calcium citrate. Finally, it is important that calcium supplementation is taken in smaller doses (500–600 mg) throughout the day and not just once daily to aid in the ability of the body to absorb more calcium.

CASE STUDY

Jane is a 53-year-old white woman diagnosed with osteoporosis at the femoral neck (t = −2.53) and osteopenia at the lumbar spine (L2-4) (t = −1.48) in April, 1998. Jane has no family history of osteoporosis or history of amenorrhea; she has been physically active throughout childhood and adulthood and never abused alcohol or consumed excessive caffeine. She has never smoked, but as a flight attendant for 32 years she was exposed to secondhand smoke from 1967 to 1997. She has supplemented her diet with 1,000 mg of calcium for 20 years. At age 43, Jane initiated HRT after having a hysterectomy. Immediately following diagnosis, Jane increased her calcium supplementation to 1,500 mg daily. She also increased her walking program from 30 minutes, 3–4 days/week to 50 minutes, 7 days/week and began performing isometric exercises for the abdominals and upper back twice daily. Jane also began a resistance training program consisting of 10 free weight and machine exercises performed in two sets of 8–15 repetitions, 2–3 days/week. Six months after diagnosis, Jane began treatment with 10 mg alendronate daily. In 18 months of resistance training, Jane has experienced an average increase in strength of 250%. Follow-up bone density scans in October 1999, revealed an increase in BMD of 9.28% at the femoral neck (t = −1.99) and 10.49% at the lumbar spine (t = −0.88). Based on Jane's outcome, it appears that the inclusion of an aggressive resistive and weight-bearing exercise regimen in the treatment of osteoporosis may be effective for increasing BMD above that expected from calcium supplementation and antiresorptive therapy.

REFERENCES

1. American College of Sports Medicine. *American College of Sports Medicine's Guidelines for Exercise Testing and Prescription.* 7th ed. Baltimore (MD): Lippincott Williams & Wilkins; 2006. 366 p.
2. Anderson GL, Limacher M, Assaf AR, et al. Effects of conjugated equine estrogen in postmenopausal women with hysterectomy: the Women's Health Initiative randomized controlled trial. *JAMA.* 2004;291:1701–12.
3. Bainbridge KE, Sowers M, Lin X, et al. Risk factors for low bone mineral density and the 6-year rate of bone loss among premenopausal and perimenopausal women. *Osteoporos Int.* 2004;15:439–46.
4. Bass SL. The prepubertal years: a uniquely opportune stage of growth when the skeleton is most responsive to exercise? *Sports Med.* 2000;30:73–8.
5. Bassey EJ, Ramsdale SJ. Weight-bearing exercise and ground reaction forces: a 12-month randomized controlled trial of effects on bone mineral density in healthy postmenopausal women. *Bone.* 1995;16:469–76.
6. Beck BR, Snow CM. Bone health across the lifespan—exercising our options. *Exerc Sport Sci Rev.* 2003;31:117–22.
7. Bischoff-Ferrari HA, Dawson-Hughes B, Willett WC, et al. Effect of vitamin D on falls: a meta-analysis. *JAMA.* 2004;291:1999–2006.

8. Bonaiuti D, Shea B, Lovine R, et al. Exercise for preventing and treating osteoporosis in postmenopausal women. *Cochrane Database Syst Rev.* 2002(2), CD000333.

9. Bonnick SL. Osteoporosis in men and women. *Clin Cornerstone.* 2006;8:28–39.

10. Bonnick SL, Saag KG, Kiel DP, et al. Comparison of weekly treatment of postmenopausal osteoporosis with alendronate versus risedronate over two years. *J Clin Endocrinol Metab.* 2006;91: 2631–7.

11. Borer KT, Fogleman K, Gross M, et al. Walking intensity for postmenopausal bone mineral preservation and accrual. *Bone.* 2007;41:713–21.

12. Bouxsein ML, Myers ER, Hayes WC. Biomechanics of age-related fractures. In: Marcus R, Feldman D, Kelsey JL, editors. *Osteoporosis.* San Diego (CA): Academic Press, Inc; 1996. p. 373–93.

13. Briggs RC, Gossman MR, Birch R, et al. Balance performance among noninstitutionalized elderly women. *Phys Ther.* 1989;69: 748–56.

14. Burge R, Dawson-Hughes B, Solomon DH, et al. Incidence and economic burden of osteoporosis-related fractures in the United States, 2005–2025. *J Bone Miner Res.* 2007;22:465–75.

15. Canalis E, Giustina A, Bilezikian JP. Mechanisms of anabolic therapies for osteoporosis. *N Engl J Med.* 2007;357:905–16.

16. Chavassieux P, Seeman E, Delmas PD. Insights into material and structural basis of bone fragility from diseases associated with fractures: how determinants of the biomechanical properties of bone are compromised by disease. *Endocr Rev.* 2007;28: 151–64.

17. Chen P, Miller PD, Delmas PD, et al. Change in lumbar spine BMD and vertebral fracture risk reduction in teriparatide-treated postmenopausal women with osteoporosis. *J Bone Miner Res.* 2006;21: 1785–90.

18. Chesnut CH, Silverman S, Andriano K, et al. A randomized trial of nasal spray salmon calcitonin in postmenopausal women with established osteoporosis: the prevent recurrence of osteoporotic fractures study. *Am J Med.* 2000;109:267–76.

19. Chrischilles EA, Butler CD, Davis CS, et al. A model of lifetime osteoporosis impact. *Arch Intern Med.* 1991;151:2026–32.

20. Chrischilles EA, Shireman T, Wallace R. Costs and health effects of osteoporotic fractures. *Bone.* 1994;15:377–85.

21. Cimen OB, Ulubas B, Sahin G, et al. Pulmonary function tests, respiratory muscle strength, and endurance of patients with osteoporosis. *South Med J.* 2003;96:423–6.

22. Cowley A, Kerr K. A review of clinical balance tools for use with elderly populations. *Crit Rev Phys Rehabil Med.* 2003;15: 167–206.

23. Cranney A, Tugwell P, Zytaruk N, et al. Meta-analyses of therapies for postmenopausal osteoporosis. VI. Meta-analysis of calcitonin for the treatment of postmenopausal osteoporosis. *Endocr Rev.* 2002;23:540–51.

24. Culham EG, Jimenez HA, King CE. Thoracic kyphosis, rib mobility, and lung volumes in normal women and women with osteoporosis. *Spine.* 1994;19:1250–5.

25. Cutler WB, Friedmann E, Genovese-Stone E. Prevalence of kyphosis in a healthy sample of pre- and postmenopausal women. *Am J Phys Med Rehabil.* 1993;72:219–25.

26. Dalsky GP, Stocke KS, Ehsani AA, et al. Weight-bearing exercise training and lumbar bone mineral content in postmenopausal women. *Ann Intern Med.* 1988;108:824–8.

27. Delmas PD, Ensrud KE, Adachi JD, et al. Efficacy of raloxifene on vertebral fracture risk reduction in postmenopausal women with osteoporosis: four-year results from a randomized clinical trial. *J Clin Endocrinol Metab.* 2002;87:3609–17.

28. Ensrud KE, Black DM, Palermo L, et al. Treatment with alendronate prevents fractures in women at highest risk: results from the Fracture Intervention Trial. *Arch Intern Med.* 1997;157: 2617–24.

29. Ensrud KE, Palermo L, Black DM, et al. Hip and calcaneal bone loss increase with advancing age: longitudinal results from the study of osteoporotic fractures. *J Bone Miner Res.* 1995;10:1778–87.

30. Fehling PC, Alekel L, Clasey J, et al. A comparison of bone mineral densities among female athletes in impact loading and active loading sports. *Bone.* 1995;17:205–10.

31. Feskanich D, Willett WC, Colditz GA. Calcium, vitamin D, milk consumption, and hip fractures: a prospective study among postmenopausal women. *Am J Clin Nutr.* 2003;77:504–11.

32. Fiatarone MA, Marks EC, Ryan ND, et al. High-intensity strength training in nonagenarians: effects on skeletal muscle. *JAMA.* 1990;263:3029–34.

33. Flemming PJ. Utilization of a screening tool to identify homebound older adults at risk for falls: validity and reliability. *Home Health Care Serv Q.* 2006;25:1–26.

34. Forsmo S, Hvam HM, Rea ML, et al. Height loss, forearm bone density and bone loss in menopausal women: a 15-year prospective study. The Nord-Trondelag Health Study, Norway. *Osteoporos Int.* 2007;18:1261–9.

35. Gehlsen GM, Whaley MH. Falls in the elderly. Part II: Balance, strength, and flexibility. *Arch Phys Med Rehabil.* 1990;71: 739–41.

36. Gennari L, Bilezikian JP. Osteoporosis in men: pathophysiology and treatment. *Curr Rheumatol Rep.* 2007;9:71–7.

37. Glynn NW, Meilahn EN, Charron M, et al. Determinants of bone mineral density in older men. *J Bone Miner Res.* 1995;10: 1769–77.

38. Grey A. Emerging pharmacologic therapies for osteoporosis. *Expert Opin Emerg Drugs.* 2007;12:493–508.

39. Guralnik JM, Ferrucci L, Simonsick EM, et al. Lower-extremity function in persons over the age of 70 years as a predictor of subsequent disability. *N Engl J Med.* 1995;332:556–61.

40. Guthrie JR, Lehert P, Dennerstein L, et al. The relative effect of endogenous estradiol and androgens on menopausal bone loss: a longitudinal study. *Osteoporos Int.* 2004;15:881–6.

41. Hallstrom H, Wolk A, Glynn A, et al. Coffee, tea and caffeine consumption in relation to osteoporotic fracture risk in a cohort of Swedish women. *Osteoporos Int.* 2006;17:1055–64.

42. Harridge SD, Kryger A, Stensgaard A. Knee extensor strength, activation, and size in very elderly people following strength training. *Muscle Nerve.* 1999;22:831–9.

43. Hatori M, Hasegawa A, Adachi H, et al. The effects of walking at the anaerobic threshold on vertebral bone loss in postmenopausal women. *Calcif Tissue Int.* 1993;52:411–4.

44. Hawk C, Hyland J, Rupert R, et al. Assessment of balance and risk for falls in a sample of community-dwelling adults aged 65 and older. *Chiropractic & Osteopathy.* 2006;14:3.

45. Heaney RP. Pathophysiology of osteoporosis. *Am J Med Sci.* 1996; 312:251–6.

46. Heaney RP. Effects of caffeine on bone and the calcium economy. *Food Chem Toxicol.* 2002;40:1263–70.

47. Heitmann DK, Gossman MR, Shaddeau SA, et al. Balance performance and step width in noninstitutionalized, elderly, female fallers and nonfallers. *Phys Ther.* 1989;69:923–31.

48. Heller HJ, Stewart A, Haynes S, et al. Pharmacokinetics of calcium absorption from two commercial calcium supplements. *J Clin Pharmacol.* 1999;39:1151–4.

49. Hillard TC, Whitcroft SJ, Marsh MS, et al. Long-term effects of transdermal and oral hormone replacement therapy on postmenopausal bone loss. *Osteoporos Int.* 1994;4:341–8.

50. Hornbrook MC, Stevens VJ, Wingfield DJ. Seniors' program for injury control and education. *J Am Geriatr Soc.* 1993;41: 309–14.

51. Hundrup YA, Ekholm O, Hoidrup S, et al. Risk factors for hip fracture and a possible effect modification by hormone replacement therapy. The Danish nurse cohort study. *Eur J Epidemiol.* 2005;20:871–7.

52. Jones G, Nguyen T, Sambrook P, et al. Progressive loss of bone in the femoral neck in elderly people: longitudinal findings from the Dubbo osteoporosis epidemiology study. *BMJ*. 1994;309:691–5.

53. Kanis JA, Johansson H, Johnell O, et al. Alcohol intake as a risk factor for fracture. *Osteoporos Int*. 2005;16:737–42.

54. Kanis JA, Johnell O, Oden A, et al. Smoking and fracture risk: a meta-analysis. *Osteoporos Int*. 2005;16:155–62.

55. Kannus P, Haapasalo H, Sankelo M, et al. Effect of starting age of physical activity on bone mass in the dominant arm of tennis and squash players. *Ann Intern Med*. 1995;123:27–31.

56. Khovidhunkit W, Shoback DM. Clinical effects of raloxifene hydrochloride in women. *Ann Intern Med*. 1999;130:431–9.

57. Kiel DP, Felson DT, Hannan MT, et al. Caffeine and the risk of hip fracture: the Framingham Study. *Am J Epidemiol*. 1990;132:675–84.

58. King AC, Pruitt LA, Phillips W, et al. Comparative effects of two physical activity programs on measured and perceived physical functioning and other health-related quality of life outcomes in older adults. *J Gerontol A Biol Sci Med Sci*. 2000;55:M74–M83.

59. Kirwan LD, MacLusky NJ, Shapiro HM, et al. Acute and chronic effects of hormone replacement therapy on the cardiovascular system in healthy postmenopausal women. *J Clin Endocrinol Metab*. 2004;89:1618–29.

60. Knopp JA, Diner BM, Blitz M, et al. Calcitonin for treating acute pain of osteoporotic vertebral compression fractures: a systematic review of randomized, controlled trials. *Osteoporos Int*. 2005;16:1281–90.

61. Kohrt WM. Aging and the osteogenic response to mechanical loading. *Int J Sport Nutr Exerc Metab*. 2001;11(Suppl):S137–S142.

62. Kohrt WM, Bloomfield SA, Little KD, et al. American College of Sports Medicine Position Stand: physical activity and bone health. *Med Sci Sports Exerc*. 2004;36:1985–96.

63. Kohrt WM, Snead DB, Slatopolsky E, et al. Additive effects of weight-bearing exercise and estrogen on bone mineral density in older women. *J Bone Miner Res*. 1995;10:1303–11.

64. Korpelainen R, Keinanen-Kiukaanniemi S, Heikkinen J, et al. Effect of impact exercise on bone mineral density in elderly women with low BMD: a population-based randomized controlled 30-month intervention. *Osteoporos Int*. 2006;17: 109–18.

65. Kung AW, Pasion EG, Sofiyan M, et al. A comparison of teriparatide and calcitonin therapy in postmenopausal Asian women with osteoporosis: a 6-month study. *Curr Med Res Opin*. 2006;22:929–37.

66. LaPier TK. Chest wall expansion values in supine and standing across the adult lifespan. *Physical and Occupational Therapy in Geriatrics*. 2002;21:65–81.

67. Leslie WD, Adler RA, El Hajj FG, et al. Application of the 1994 WHO classification to populations other than postmenopausal Caucasian women: the 2005 ISCD Official Positions. *J Clin Densitom*. 2006;9:22–30.

68. Levine JP. Pharmacologic and nonpharmacologic management of osteoporosis. *Clin Cornerstone*. 2006;8:40–53.

69. Lombardi I, Oliveira LM, Monteiro CR, et al. Evaluation of physical capacity and quality of life in osteoporotic women. *Osteoporos Int*. 2004;15:80–5.

70. Looker AC, Orwoll ES, Johnston CC, Jr., et al. Prevalence of low femoral bone density in older U.S. adults from NHANES III. *J Bone Miner Res*. 1997;12:1761–8.

71. Lynch NA, Ryan AS, Evans J, et al. Older elite football players have reduced cardiac and osteoporosis risk factors. *Med Sci Sports Exerc*. 2007;39:1124–30.

72. McClung M, Clemmesen B, Daifotis A, et al. Alendronate prevents postmenopausal bone loss in women without osteoporosis. A double-blind, randomized, controlled trial. *Ann Intern Med*. 1998;128:253–61.

73. McClung MR, Geusens P, Miller PD, et al. Effect of risedronate on the risk of hip fracture in elderly women. Hip Intervention Program Study Group. *N Engl J Med*. 2001;344:333–40.

74. Mortensen L, Charles P, Bekker PJ, et al. Risedronate increases bone mass in an early postmenopausal population: two years of treatment plus one year of follow-up. *J Clin Endocrinol Metab*. 1998;83:396–402.

75. Mukamal KJ, Robbins JA, Cauley JA, et al. Alcohol consumption, bone density, and hip fracture among older adults: the cardiovascular health study. *Osteoporos Int*. 2007;18:593–602.

76. National Osteoporosis Foundation. Boning up on osteoporosis: A guide to prevention and treatment. 2000. Washington, DC: National Osteoporosis Foundation.

77. National Osteoporosis Foundation. America's bone health: The state of osteoporosis and low bone mass. 2002. Washington, DC: National Osteoporosis Foundation.

78. Nelson ME, Fiatarone MA, Morganti CM, et al. Effects of high-intensity strength training on multiple risk factors for osteoporotic fractures. A randomized controlled trial. *JAMA*. 1994;272:1909–14.

79. Nelson ME, Rejeski WJ, Blair SN, et al. Physical activity and public health in older adults: recommendation from the American College of Sports Medicine and the American Heart Association. *Med Sci Sports Exerc*. 2007;39:1435–45.

80. Nguyen ND, Eisman JA, Nguyen TV. Anti-hip fracture efficacy of biophosphonates: a Bayesian analysis of clinical trials. *J Bone Miner Res*. 2006;21:340–9.

81. Nguyen TV, Kelly PJ, Sambrook PN, et al. Lifestyle factors and bone density in the elderly: implications for osteoporosis prevention. *J Bone Miner Res*. 1994;9:1339–46.

82. Nichols DL, Sanborn CF, Bonnick SL, et al. The effects of gymnastics training on bone mineral density. *Med Sci Sports Exerc*. 1994;26:1220–5.

83. NIH Consensus Development Panel on Osteoporosis Prevention DaT. Osteoporosis Prevention, Diagnosis, and Therapy. *JAMA*. 2001;285:785–95.

84. Nikander R, Sievanen H, Heinonen A, et al. Femoral neck structure in adult female athletes subjected to different loading modalities. *J Bone Miner Res*. 2005;20:520–8.

85. Nordstrom A, Karlsson C, Nyquist F, et al. Bone loss and fracture risk after reduced physical activity. *J Bone Miner Res*. 2005;20:202–7.

86. Nordstrom A, Olsson T, Nordstrom P. Sustained benefits from previous physical activity on bone mineral density in males. *J Clin Endocrinol Metab*. 2006;91:2600–4.

87. Pedersen BK, Saltin B. Evidence for prescribing exercise as therapy in chronic disease. *Scand J Med Sci Sports*. 2006;16(Suppl 1):3–63.

88. Perell KL, Nelson A, Goldman RL, et al. Fall risk assessment measures: an analytic review. *J Gerontol A Biol Sci Med Sci*. 2001;56:M761–M766.

89. Prince RL, Smith M, Dick IM, et al. Prevention of postmenopausal osteoporosis: a comparative study of exercise, calcium supplementation, and hormone-replacement therapy. *N Engl J Med*. 1991;325:1189–95.

90. Province MA, Hadley EC, Hornbrook MC, et al. The effects of exercise on falls in elderly patients. A preplanned meta-analysis of the FICSIT Trials. Frailty and Injuries: Cooperative Studies of Intervention Techniques. *JAMA*. 1995;273:1341–7.

91. Rapuri PB, Gallagher JC, Balhorn KE, et al. Smoking and bone metabolism in elderly women. *Bone*. 2000;27:429–36.

92. Reid IR, Wattie DJ, Evans MC, et al. Continuous therapy with pamidronate, a potent bisphosphonate, in postmenopausal osteoporosis. *J Clin Endocrinol Metab*. 1994;79:1595–9.

93. Rhodes EC, Martin AD, Taunton JE, et al. Effects of one year of resistance training on the relation between muscular strength and bone density in elderly women. *Br J Sports Med*. 2000;34:18–22.

94. Ringe JD, Dorst A, Faber H, Ibach K. Alendronate treatment of established primary osteoporosis in men: 3-year results of a prospective, comparative, two-arm study. *Rheumatol Int*. 2004;24:110–3.

95. Ringe JD, Faber H, Farahmand P, et al. Efficacy of risedronate in men with primary and secondary osteoporosis: results of a 1-year study. *Rheumatol Int.* 2006;26:427–31.

96. Ringe JD, van der Geest SA, Moller G. Importance of calcium co-medication in bisphosphonate therapy of osteoporosis: an approach to improving correct intake and drug adherence. *Drugs Aging.* 2006;23:569–78.

97. Rodan GA. Introduction to bone biology. *Bone.* 1992;13:S3–S6.

98. Rollins D, Imrhan V, Czajka-Narins DM, et al. Lower bone mass detected at femoral neck and lumbar spine in lower-weight vs normal-weight small-boned women. *J Am Diet Assoc.* 2003;103:742–4.

99. Rossouw JE, Anderson GL, Prentice RL, et al. Risks and benefits of estrogen plus progestin in healthy postmenopausal women: principal results From the Women's Health Initiative randomized controlled trial. *JAMA.* 2002;288:321–33.

100. Rubenstein LZ. Falls in older people: epidemiology, risk factors and strategies for prevention. *Age Ageing.* 2006;35(Suppl 2):ii37–ii41.

101. Rubenstein LZ, Josephson KR. Falls and their prevention in elderly people: what does the evidence show? *Med Clin North Am.* 2006;90:807–24.

102. Sawka AM, Papaioannou A, Adachi JD, et al. Does alendronate reduce the risk of fracture in men? A meta-analysis incorporating prior knowledge of anti-fracture efficacy in women. *BMC Musculoskelet Disord.* 2005;6:39.

103. Schlaich C, Minne HW, Bruckner T, et al. Reduced pulmonary function in patients with spinal osteoporotic fractures. *Osteoporos Int.* 1998;8:261–7.

104. Seeman E, Crans GG, Diez-Perez A, et al. Anti-vertebral fracture efficacy of raloxifene: a meta-analysis. *Osteoporos Int.* 2006;17:313–6.

105. Shea B, Wells G, Cranney A, et al. Calcium supplementation on bone loss in postmenopausal women. *Cochrane Database Syst Rev.* 2004CD004526.

106. Sinaki M. Postmenopausal spinal osteoporosis: physical therapy and rehabilitation principles. *Mayo Clin Proc.* 1982;57:699–703.

107. Sinaki M, Mikkelsen BA. Postmenopausal spinal osteoporosis: flexion versus extension exercises. *Arch Phys Med Rehab.* 1984;65:593–6.

108. Sinaki M, Wollan PC, Scott RW, et al. Can strong back extensors prevent vertebral fractures in women with osteoporosis? *Mayo Clin Proc.* 1996;71:951–6.

109. Siris ES, Miller PD, Barrett-Connor E, et al. Identification and fracture outcomes of undiagnosed low bone mineral density in postmenopausal women: results from the National Osteoporosis Risk Assessment. *JAMA.* 2001;286:2815–22.

110. Snow CM. Exercise and bone mass in young premenopausal women. *Bone.* 1996;18:51S–5S.

111. Sowers M. Pregnancy and lactation as risk factors for subsequent bone loss and osteoporosis. *J Bone Miner Res.* 1996;11: 1052–60.

112. Suominen H. Muscle training for bone strength. *Aging Clin Exp Res.* 2006;18:85–93.

113. Tang BM, Eslick GD, Nowson C, et al. Use of calcium or calcium in combination with vitamin D supplementation to prevent fractures and bone loss in people aged 50 years and older: a meta-analysis. *Lancet.* 2007;370:657–66.

114. Tansavatdi K, McClain B, Herrington DM. The effects of smoking on estradiol metabolism. *Minerva Ginecol.* 2004;56: 105–14.

115. Thiebaud D, Burckhardt P, Kriegbaum H, et al. Three monthly intravenous injections of ibandronate in the treatment of postmenopausal osteoporosis. *Am J Med.* 1997;103:298–307.

116. Trivedi DP, Doll R, Khaw KT. Effect of four monthly oral vitamin D3 (cholecalciferol) supplementation on fractures and mortality in men and women living in the community: randomised double-blind controlled trial. *BMJ.* 2003;326:469.

117. Trudelle-Jackson EJ, Jackson AW, Morrow J. Muscle strength and postural stability in healthy, older women: implications for fall prevention. *J Phys Act Health.* 2006;3:

118. Tucker KL, Morita K, Qiao N, et al. Colas, but not other carbonated beverages, are associated with low bone mineral density in older women: The Framingham Osteoporosis Study. *Am J Clin Nutr.* 2006;84:936–42.

119. Tudor-Locke C, McColl RS. Factors related to variation in premenopausal bone mineral status: a health promotion approach. *Osteoporos Int.* 2000;11:1–24.

120. Uusi-Rasi K, Kannus P, Cheng S, et al. Effect of alendronate and exercise on bone and physical performance of postmenopausal women: a randomized controlled trial. *Bone.* 2003;33:132–43.

121. Valimaki MJ, Laitinen KA, Tahtela RK, et al. The effects of transdermal estrogen therapy on bone mass and turnover in early postmenopausal smokers: a prospective, controlled study. *Am J Obstet Gynecol.* 2003;189:1213–20.

122. Vestergaard P, Rejnmark L, Mosekilde L. Fracture reducing potential of hormone replacement therapy on a population level. *Maturitas.* 2006;54:285–93.

123. Weir JP, Cramer JT. Principles of musculoskeletal exercise programming. In: American College of Sports Medicine, editors. *ACSM's Resource Manual for Guidelines for Exercise Testing and Prescription*, Baltimore (MD): Lippincott Williams & Wilkins; 2006. p. 350–365.

124. Wells G, Tugwell P, Shea B, et al. Meta-analyses of therapies for postmenopausal osteoporosis. V. Meta-analysis of the efficacy of hormone replacement therapy in treating and preventing osteoporosis in postmenopausal women. *Endocr Rev.* 2002;23:529–39.

125. Whipple RH, Wolfson LI, Amerman PM. The relationship of knee and ankle weakness to falls in nursing home residents: an isokinetic study. *J Am Geriatr Soc.* 1987;35:13–20.

126. Wickham C, Cooper C, Margetts BM, et al. Muscle strength, activity, housing and the risk of falls in elderly people. *Age Ageing.* 1989;18:47–51.

127. Wimalawansa SJ. A four-year randomized controlled trial of hormone replacement and bisphosphonate, alone or in combination, in women with postmenopausal osteoporosis. *Am J Med.* 1998; 104:219–26.

128. World Health Organization. *Assessment of Fracture Risk and Its Application to Screening for Postmenopausal Osteoporosis.* Geneva: World Health Organization; 1994.

129. Wosje KS, Kalkwarf HJ. Bone density in relation to alcohol intake among men and women in the United States. *Osteoporos Int.* 2007;18:391–400.

Vertebral Disorders

Clinical exercise practitioners may work with individuals who experience acute, subacute, or chronic spinal pain. Because the spine is critical in posture, movement, and protection, pain and loss of function hinders an individual's ability to perform routine activities. As with any complex structure, the potential for problems is great. Although "vertebral disorders" can occur in any part of the spine (cervical, thoracic, lumbar, sacral, and coccygeal), most vertebral disorders are lumbar. Lumbar disorders result in the highest medical, financial, legal, and psychosocial costs to society. Consequently, lumbar disorders have attracted international medical, scientific, economic, and popular attention. This chapter is not necessarily intended to help readers diagnose or treat back pain. Individuals experiencing new or worsening low back pain should be referred back to the appropriate clinician for diagnosis and treatment. This chapter, therefore, focuses on lumbar disorders, and specifically, on what is termed *nonspecific, mechanical* low back pain.

EPIDEMIOLOGY AND IMPACT

Low back pain is defined as "pain, muscle tension, or stiffness localized below the costal margin and above the inferior gluteal folds, with or without leg pain (sciatica)" (1, p. 134). Low back pain afflicts nearly everyone at some stage in life. Reported prevalence rates vary according to study methodology used, but a 60%–80% individual lifetime prevalence of low back pain is often reported (2–4). The prevailing notion is that episodes of low back pain are short-lived (<1 month). Evidence suggests, however, that 42%–75% of people still have symptoms after 1 year (5), although, these individuals are not necessarily seeking or receiving treatment. A disturbing statistic is that the recurrence rate after an episode of low back pain is estimated at 60% within the first year (6) and the lifetime recurrence rate may be as high as 85% (7). Consequently, low back pain is one of the most prevalent and costly health problems in industrialized countries. In 1990, direct medical costs for low back pain exceeded $24 billion. When disability costs are included, the total annual cost for low back disorders is estimated at $50 billion (8,9). Low back pain is among the leading reasons people seek healthcare and, coupled with neck problems, is the second leading cause of disability in the United States (10).

Despite that, by definition, nonspecific low back pain does not involve perceptible structural changes, it can cause limitations in function, activities, and participation as defined within the "biopsychosocial" framework of the World Health Organization's (WHO) International Classification of Functioning, Disability and Health (ICF) (11). The ICF model can be used to visualize the impact of low back pain on both populations and individuals (12). An example of the potential impact of nonspecific low back pain on an individual using the integrated ICF model is shown in Figure 13.1.

PATHOPHYSIOLOGY

Pain is considered "an unpleasant sensory and emotional experience associated with actual or potential tissue damage or described in terms of such damage" (13). Nociceptive nerve endings (pain fibers) are activated with mechanical, thermal, or chemical stimuli. *Mechanical pain* is caused by deformation of tissues and varies with physical activity. That is, certain movements or positions make mechanical pain worse and other movements or positions relieve mechanical pain. *Specific low back pain* has an identifiable cause, such as fractures, cancer, or infection. Approximately 90% of back pain has no identifiable cause and is termed *nonspecific* (1).

In general, pain can be *somatic* (arising from stimulation of nerve endings in a musculoskeletal site [joint, muscle, ligament, bone]), *visceral* (arising from a body organ), *neurogenic* (arising from irritation of the axons or cell bodies of peripheral nerves, spinal nerves, or nerve roots), or *psychogenic*. Pain resulting from irritation of spinal nerves or roots is more specifically called *radicular pain*. Furthermore, pain can be referred to, and perceived in, an area remote from the source of the pain. Pain referred elsewhere from the viscera is called *visceral referred pain*, and pain from somatic sources is described as *somatic referred pain* (14). An example of a visceral referred pain is the arm pain sometimes associated with a myocardial infarction. An example of somatic referred pain is diffuse pain in the buttock or leg associated with low back pain.

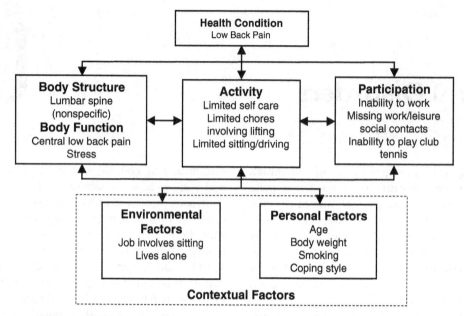

FIGURE 13-1. Example of impact of low back pain on the individual illustrated within the biopsychosocial model for health and disability of the World Health Organization (WHO) International Classification of Functioning, Disability and Health (ICF).

The etiology of spinal pain is frequently elusive. As Bogduk (14) points out, any structure with nociceptors is capable of producing irritation that manifests as the perception of pain. These structures in the spine include, but are not limited to, the intervertebral discs, zygapophysial joints, bone, muscles, ligaments, dura mater, dorsal and ventral ramus, and mixed spinal nerves. Of these anatomic sources of pain, the most common are likely the intervertebral discs and the zygapophysial joints (15,16).

Given the various anatomic sites that can be associated with spinal pain, a number of labels, or diagnoses, for vertebral disorders have evolved. Some frequently used diagnoses for specific and nonspecific vertebral disorders are as follows: low back pain, fractures, ligamentous sprains, spondylolysis, spinal stenosis, strain, zygapophysial joint locking, sacroiliac dysfunction, trigger points, zygapophysial osteoarthritis, disc degeneration, spondylolisthesis, scoliosis, instability, and herniated discs, or herniated nucleus pulposus. The latter, intervertebral disc lesions, have been further subclassified based on the extent that the nuclear material has herniated, or externalized. In one classification system, these disc pathologies have been called disc *protrusions* (bulges with no migration of nuclear material and no neural compromise), *prolapses* (migration of the nucleus, with no externalization, that can manifest with neural and dural signs), *extrusions* (externalized nuclear material with neurologic deficit), and *sequestrations* (extruded nuclear material fragmented into the spinal canal; the size and location of the fragment determines the clinical findings). Another classification system merely divides disc lesions

into those contained within the outer layer of the disc (the annulus) and those not contained within the annulus. Contained lesions usually cause minimal neurologic deficits and uncontained disc lesions tend to demonstrate greater neurologic deficits (17).

Spinal pain is rarely the result of a single event or emanates from a single tissue-type. As Sahrmann (18) points out, the question is not the source of the pain, but what caused the tissues to become painful. Frequently, the precipitating event was preceded by accumulated incidents of microtrauma from sustained or repetitive loading. As noted, lumbar disorders are typically nonspecific and theoretically result from a combination of events leading to dysfunction.

Degenerative changes have been associated with vertebral disorders. Biomechanical and biochemical changes and genetics have been implicated in the degenerative process, but the mechanisms are unclear. Kirkaldy-Willis (19) proposed a three-stage degenerative cascading process that begins with injury and cumulative trauma and leads to changes in the intervertebral disc, zygapophysial joints, supporting ligaments, joint capsules, and vertebral end plates that ultimately results in the pain and dysfunction. Stage 1 of this process (the stage of dysfunction) is characterized by joint synovitis, subluxation, early cartilage degeneration, radial and linear annular tears within the disc, local ischemia, sustained local muscle hypertonicity, and ligamentous strain. Stage 2 (the stage of instability) manifests in further cartilage degeneration and capsular laxity that permits increased rotational movement and further annular disruption and joint stress. Typical osteoarthritic changes, including joint space narrowing, fibrosis, osteophyte (bone spur) formation, and loss of joint cartilage, characterize stage 3 (the stage of stabilization). These changes can contribute to central and spinal stenosis. This degenerative cascade model helps explain the age-related incidences of spinal disorders. Discogenic sources of pain are more common in the fourth and fifth decades (stages of dysfunction and instability), and stenosis is more common in the sixth and seventh decades (stage of stabilization).

Thus, a pathoanatomic diagnosis is often not possible. Indeed, the symptoms are frequently caused by movement disorders rather than structural, morphologic disorders. Because back pain is difficult to diagnose, various classification systems have evolved. Waddell (20) suggested a three-category triage system consisting of "simple backache," "nerve root pain," and "serious spinal pathology." Simple (i.e., nonspecific, low back pain) includes a variety of disorders and is the most common type of back pain. Nerve root pain could be attributable to disorders such as disc prolapse or spinal stenosis and is present less than 5% of the time. Serious spinal pathology (and red flags) includes diseases such as tumors, infections, and inflammatory disorders, such as ankylosing spondylitis, and represents less than 1% of the persons presenting with low back pain. The value of further subclassifying low back pain will be discussed later in this chapter.

RISK FACTORS

Because low back pain is a multifactorial disorder with a number of potential causes, determining risk factors is difficult. Hence, a multitude of risk factors linked to nonspecific low back pain has been identified. None of these factors is considered causal and the strength of the evidence supporting each factor is variable, depending on the sources of the data. Overall risk factors can be divided into risk factors for primary occurrences and risk factors associated with chronicity. Risk factors can be further subcategorized generally into individual, psychosocial, health behavior, and occupational risk factors. Table 13.1 lists commonly identified risk factors associated with low back pain (1,5,21–23).

CLINICAL PICTURE

Typically, individuals with vertebral disorders present with one or more of the following physical complaints: back pain, leg pain, stiffness, muscle tension, neurologic symptoms, and spinal deformity. Pain is usually the primary complaint.

According to Waddell (20) persons with "simple backache" are usually healthy individuals, between 20 and 55 years of age, who present with pain in the lumbosacral region, buttocks, or thighs. Pain varies in intensity and may be produced, aggravated, or relieved with general or specific spinal movements, activities, positions, and time.

TABLE 13.1. POTENTIAL RISK FACTORS *ASSOCIATED* WITH THE OCCURRENCE OF NONSPECIFIC LOW BACK PAIN AND WITH CHRONICITY (1,12,23,74)

FACTORS	OCCURRENCE	CHRONICITY
Individual	Heredity/genetic[a] Age[a] Prior back pain history[a] Sex Anatomic/biomechanical variations General health status High birth weight (males)	Educational level Unemployment High levels of pain/disability Socioeconomic status
Psychosocial	Stress Depression[a] Pain behavior Anxiety	Distress Depression Fear-avoidance behavior Somatization
Health Behaviors	Smoking Obesity/Body Mass Index[a] Strength of trunk musculature Physical fitness level	Obesity/Body Mass Index[a]
Occupational	Heavy physical work Lifting, bending and twisting Monotonous tasks Whole-body vibration Static work postures Job dissatisfaction Night shifts Control at work	Unavailability of light duty Daily repetitive lifting Job dissatisfaction
Other		Healthcare provider attitudes

[a]Predictors with stronger evidence.

Morning stiffness or pain is common, and pain may worsen over the course of the day. A lateral spinal shift can be present, where the spine is pulled to one side, and the lordotic lumbar curve can be lost. Persons presenting with specific spinal conditions, such as "nerve root pain," complain of unilateral leg pain that is worse than their back pain, pain that radiates below the knee, numbness or altered sensation in the same distribution, nerve root signs (e.g., a positive straight leg raise [SLR] test), and motor, sensory, or reflex changes in one nerve root. Frank nerve root compression signs are reflex changes, muscle weakness, muscle atrophy, and sensory loss over a defined area. Spinal stenosis is a condition where the spinal canal or nerve root formina becomes narrowed (usually because of degenerative changes) and compresses the spinal cord or nerve roots. This compression, depending on location, can cause low back pain, leg pain in one or both legs, and weakness and numbness of the legs. These symptoms are characteristically aggravated by walking and relieved by sitting, lying and bending forward. *Red*

TABLE 13.2. RED FLAGS POTENTIALLY SUGGESTIVE OF MORE SERIOUS PATHOLOGY AND NEED FOR MEDICAL CONSULTATION OR REFERRAL

Saddle (anal, genital or perineum) anesthesia[a]
Unsteadiness, gait disturbances, fainting spells, or falling[a]
Urinary retention, bladder dysfunction, or fecal incontinence[a]
Progressive weakness or incoordination in arms or legs[b]
Poor general health[c]
- Unexplained weight loss
- Loss of appetite
- Unusual fatigue or general malaise
- Chest pain or heaviness
- Frequent or severe abdominal pain
- Nausea and vomiting
- Fever
- Severe headaches or dizziness
- Shortness of breath
- Unusual lumps, growths, or unexplained swelling
- Changes in vision, hearing, swallowing, or speech

Onset before 20 or after 55 years of age
Severe trauma (e.g., falls, motor vehicle accidents)
Constant, progressive nonmechanical pain
Unrelenting night pain
Thoracic pain
History of cancer, systemic steroids, osteoporosis, recent infections, rheumatologic disorders, human immunodeficiency virus (HIV), intravenous drug use
Major persisting spinal deformity
Severe spasm
Severe lumbar flexion limitation
Psychologic overlay (yellow flags: prognostic of chronic disability)
Inflammatory disorders[d]
- Gradual onset before age 40
- Marked, prolonged morning stiffness
- Persisting limitations in spinal movement in all directions
- Peripheral joint involvement
- Iritis, skin rashes, colitis, urethral discharge
- Family history

[a]Urgent referral: combination of signs suggests cauda equina lesion.
[b]Urgent referral: suggests serious spinal pathology.
[c]May require urgent referral depending on findings (e.g., cardiac).
[d]Early diagnosis of some inflammatory disorders (e.g., rheumatoid arthritis) is essential for effective treatment.

flags for "potential serious pathology" are presented in Table 13.2.

Pain involves more than the transmission of sensory input. In addition to one or more of the physical complaints, people with low back pain can also present with varying degrees of anxiety, fear, anger, frustration, preoccupation with bodily sensations, irritability, decreased concentration, fatigue, and depression *secondary to the physical disorder and pain*. These emotions are common and *normal responses* to pain. However, these same emotions can become harmful and perpetuate symptoms if they become prolonged or excessive. Pain, fear, anxiety, and depression seem particularly interrelated. Response to the stress of back pain often influences the response to intervention. Therefore, these emotions need to be considered and dealt with appropriately in any care plan. The Fear-Avoidance Beliefs Questionnaire (24) and the Beck Depression Inventory (25) may help identify the severity of the emotional response. Pain reinforced by secondary gain, inappropriate treatment, job dissatisfaction, pending litigation, and workers' compensation can manifest in symptom-magnification behaviors and total disability.

Another important consideration is the *stage of the disorder*. Symptoms vary within the same low back pain episode over the course of time. "Acute" to the patient frequently means "intense." To the healthcare provider, *acute* is usually defined in terms of the duration of symptoms in months, weeks, days, and even hours. Most commonly, *acute* typically describes pain lasting less than 6 weeks. Presumably, the acute stage reflects the characteristics of the inflammatory process accompanying the disorder. Acute pain may be present at rest, aggravated by most activities, and felt over a diffuse area.

The *subacute* stage is considered as the period of time between 6 and 12 weeks after the event. Pain in the subacute stage is more localized, associated with specific movements, and not present at rest. Notably, some clinicians do not distinguish between acute and subacute stages and consider the acute stage as lasting less than 3 months.

Chronic pain is defined as continuous pain lasting longer than 3 months, or beyond the expected recovery time. Some people have frequent recurrences, such that the condition appears chronic, but might be better classified as *recurrent* (26) versus chronic. "True" chronic pain is modulated differently within the nervous system and becomes dissociated from the original physical disorder. Chronic pain can be intractable and self-perpetuating. Chronic pain is usually not amenable to the same kinds of treatment interventions used in the acute, subacute, or recurrent stages. Patients with chronic pain can become depressed and manifest with symptom-magnification and chronic pain-related disability.

Considering the stage of the disorder is important when developing a treatment regimen. However, as noted, intermittent exacerbations of symptoms and recurrent episodes cloud the distinction among stages. An alternative approach may be to consider the irritability (ease or difficulty of provoking symptoms) of the condition rather than the length of time that the condition has persisted.

A distinction should also be made between pain with temporary dysfunction and pain with permanent, total disability. Disability is the inability or restricted capacity to perform activities and participate in life situations (11). Disability refers to patterns of behavior that have emerged over time during which functional limitations could not be overcome to maintain usual role performance (27). Persons seeking medical attention often present with at least temporary limitations in activities (including postures) or participation. Patients and some healthcare providers assume that functional limitations will be eliminated when the pain impairment is relieved. Notably, pain does not always lead to disability, nor does the reported intensity of pain reflect the amount of perceived disability (28). Pain intensity does not necessarily signal that tissue damage is occurring (i.e., pain can occur in structurally normal tissues). Simply put, *hurt* does not always mean *harm*. Stretching one's hamstrings can be uncomfortable, but is not typically harmful. Patients and clinicians need to make this distinction to help prevent chronic pain behavior and permanent disability by keeping patients generally active and functioning during their recovery or rehabilitation.

DIAGNOSTIC TECHNIQUES

Accurate diagnosis is, of course, the cornerstone of effective intervention. But, as previously pointed out, in the case of low back pain, diagnosis rarely identifies the pathologic source of the pain (29,30). In addition, evidence suggests that using specific anatomic diagnoses does not improve outcomes for most patients (31). Waddell's (20) triage system gives a broad clinical picture of low back pain and offers a screening system that can be used to guide in further diagnostic testing. A similar three-category initial triage was also recommended in a recent clinical guideline jointly developed by the American College of Physicians/American Pain Society Low Back Pain Guidelines Panel (31). In general the categories are "nonspecific low back pain," "back pain potentially associated with radiculopathy or spinal stenosis," or "back pain potentially associated with another specific spinal cause." The key points in diagnosing low back pain are determining whether the pain is indeed coming from the spine, ruling out specific disorders and potentially serious disorders, and acquiring information necessary to develop a care plan. Diagnostic procedures always include a *clinical examination and evaluation* (31) and may include *movement system, diagnostic imaging, electrodiagnostic,* and *laboratory testing* when further information is needed. Each of these diagnostic techniques is discussed briefly in the following paragraphs.

CLINICAL EXAMINATION AND EVALUATION

The primary diagnostic procedure in the case of low back pain is the clinical examination and evaluation. The clinical examination consists of two parts, the subjective examination, or history, and the objective examination, or physical. Based on the results of the examination, the clinician evaluates (or assesses) the findings of the examination and either makes a diagnosis or determines the need for further testing. Typical components of a clinical examination are outlined in Table 13.3.

HISTORY

The history, or subjective examination, consists of gathering information from patient reports in five major

TABLE 13.3. OUTLINE OF TYPICAL COMPONENTS OF A CLINICAL EXAMINATION OF A PATIENT WITH LOW BACK PAIN[a]

CLINICAL EXAMINATION
History
(Subjective Examination)

Present Condition
Mechanism and date of onset or duration
Location of symptoms
Nature, quality and intensity of pain (assessed using a pain scale)
Behavior of symptoms (better and worse)
Types of limitations/disabilities (including use of a standardized, condition-specific outcome measure [e.g., Oswestry])

Previous Incidents
Including prior treatment and outcomes

Medical and Surgical History
Including medications

Personal Information
Demographic
Occupational
Social
Living environment

Patient Goals
Using the Patient Specific Functional Scale

Physical Examination[a] (Part 1 & Part 2)
(Objective Examination)

PART 1: SYSTEMS REVIEW/MEDICAL SCREENING

Systems Review and Observations
General appearance
Communication ability, affect and behavior
Gross symmetry, structure, and skin integrity
Locomotion, balance, and transitional movements
Heart and respiratory rate and blood pressure
Height, weight, body mass index (BMI)
Other

PART 2: REGIONAL TESTS AND MEASURES TO VERIFY LUMBAR SPINE INVOLVEMENT AND GENERAL NATURE OF INVOLVEMENT

Posture/Alignment
Movement Examination: Active, Passive, and Resistive Lumbar Movements
Quantity (range) of movement
Quality and pattern of movement
Effect of movement on symptoms
Neurologic Screening Lower Quarter
Cutaneous sensation in dermatomes
Myotome (groups of muscles supplied by a single nerve root) testing
Deep tendon reflexes
Upper motor neuron screen (e.g., pathologica reflexes)
Neurodynamic tests (e.g., straight leg raising, dural mobility tests)
Vascular Screening of Lower Quadrant
Pulses, for example
Peripheral and Sacroiliac Joint Screening
Special Tests
As indicated, based on symptoms (e.g., prone instability test, active straight raise leg test)
Palpation
Temperature
Tenderness
Tissue condition: tension, texture, thickness, and so forth
Intervertebral Joint Movement Testing
Movement and end feel
Functional Assessment Screening
Task performance ability

[a]Content and extent of the physical examination varies with the practitioner's discipline, background, and experience, the results of the subjective examination, and the purpose of the examination.

areas: the present condition, previous incidents, medical and surgical history, personal information, and patient goals.

Information about the present condition can be further subdivided into information about the mechanism and date (or time period) of onset, location of symptoms, nature and intensity of pain, behavior of the symptoms, and types of functional limitations. Each of these sources of information is discussed in the following paragraphs.

The *onset* of pain could be an injury or a gradual onset with no discernable precipitating event. A gradual onset might be triggered by predisposing activities, such as a change in habits, work duties, work environment, new chair, and so forth. The *date or time frame* suggests the stage of the disorder. The *location* (or anatomic distribution) of symptoms directs the extent and type of examination. Particularly important is whether the pain is centrally located (i.e., in the back), peripherally located (in the extremities, especially if below the knee), or both.

The *nature, or quality*, of the symptoms is helpful in determining the general source of the problem. Different sources of pain give rise to different types of sensation. For example, as noted previously, somatic referred pain is typically deep, diffuse, achy, hard to localize, and varying in intensity. *Pain intensity, or severity*, is typically assessed either verbally or diagrammatically using a pain scale. When using a numeric pain scale, the patient is asked to express the intensity of the usual pain from 0 to 10 with 0 being no pain and a 10 suggesting that the pain is as bad as it could possible be, or a need to go to an emergency room. A visual analog scale (VAS) of pain intensity can also be used. A VAS typically consists of a 100-mm line with the extremes of pain denoted at each end of the line (i.e., no pain to the worst possible pain). The patient is then asked to mark the pain intensity on the line, which can then be measured and "quantified" using a ruler. Alternatively, the patient may be asked to circle adjectives describing the nature of the pain.

The *behavior of the symptoms* is especially important in helping to rule out more serious pathology, in gauging the intensity of the physical examination, and in ultimately developing an intervention strategy. Specifically, the patient is asked to describe what eases the pain and what worsens it. When evaluating mechanical pain, the clinician is particularly interested in the postures, movements, and activities that affect the nature, location, and intensity of the pain.

Other information needed about the present condition is knowledge of any functional limitation or disability the patient is encountering because of the low back pain. The patient can simply be asked about his or her activity restrictions or a functional status questionnaire can be used. Typical assessment includes inquiry about bending, lifting, standing, walking, sitting, sleeping, dressing, sexual activity, traveling, and performing household chores, childcare, work, leisure, and social activities. Urinary incontinence

has also been reported in women with low back pain (32). Two of the more widely used standardized, region-, or condition-specific measures of low back disability are the Oswestry (33) and the Roland-Morris (34) questionnaires.

The patient is also asked about the nature, duration, and frequency of any previous episodes of low back pain. Medical history questions are generally designed to identify red flags suggestive of more serious pathology and to alert the clinician to factors that may confound the problem or that need to be considered in treatment (e.g., diabetes). Personal questions include questions about age, occupation, leisure activities, and social history. Lastly, the patient is asked about his or her goals and expected outcome of care. The Patient Specific Functional Scale (PSFS) (35) is designed to complement condition-specific outcome measures. The scale is a useful and validated instrument to gather a patient's current ability level and goals in a structured way and then to monitor the results of treatment. The patient is asked to identify three activities that he or she is having difficulty performing because of pain and to rate the ability to perform these tasks on a 0 to 10 scale (0 indicates an inability to perform the task and 10 indicates ability to perform the activity as before the vertebral disorder). The minimal detectable change (MDC) of the scale for use with a single activity score is "3." That is, a positive change of greater than 3 units on the scale suggests improvement.

The examiner usually makes a *preliminary* diagnosis based on the history. In addition, the examiner judges the *irritability* of the disorder, that is, how easy or how difficult it is to provoke the symptoms (high, moderate, or low). A highly irritable condition will be easy to reproduce and may require a gentle physical examination. A less irritable condition can be difficult to evoke and may require a more extensive, vigorous physical examination.

Physical Examination

The second part of the clinical examination is the physical, or objective examination. The physical examination is used to confirm or refute the *preliminary* diagnosis by reproducing the "comparable, or asterisk, sign." The comparable or asterisk sign is the collection of signs and symptoms that reproduce *the* pain or dysfunction that caused the patient to seek the services of a healthcare provider. The content and extent of the physical examination varies with the practitioner's discipline, background and experience, the results of the subjective examination, and the purpose of the examination. A physician may need only to decide whether the patient has nonspecific low back pain, a specific spinal disorder, pain from a source other than the spine, or red flags signaling potential serious pathology. This may be sufficient information to decide on a course of action. However, a diagnosis of nonspecific low back pain (or one of the many diagnostic labels suggesting essentially the same thing (e.g., sprain or strain, degenerative disc or joint disease) is insufficient for a physical therapist, for example, to initiate intervention. A physical therapist needs detailed information about the quality and quantity of active and passive movements and the effect of movements and positions on pain and function as well as the results of several selected special tests. Assessment of the movements and postures affecting the problem is used in conjunction with other information to direct treatment.

Potential components of a physical examination are outlined in Table 13.3. The examination consists of two parts. The first part is the *systems review* (also called, medical screening or scan examination), which is used primarily to confirm or refute any red flags suggested by the history. The second part of the examination is to determine the presence of signs of nerve irritation, decide whether the pain actually involves the lumbar spine, and obtain further clarifying information to make a differential diagnosis and develop a care plan. The general intent of the physical examination is to reproduce the comparable (or asterisk) sign through selected tests, measures, and patient responses, and to determine the nature and extent of impairments, function, and disability (activity limitations and participation restrictions).

Evaluation

Based on evaluation (interpretation) of the results of the history and physical examinations, the clinician can usually decide on one of two courses of action:

- Diagnose the disorder (see section entitled, *The Medical & Clinical Diagnosis*), make a prognosis, design and implement the care plan, or
- Tentatively diagnose the disorder and determine the need for further testing to confirm or refute this working diagnosis. Trial treatment, based on the tentative diagnosis, may or may not be initiated at this time.

If further diagnostic procedures are indicated, this testing might consist of more in-depth movement system testing, diagnostic imaging, electrodiagnostic testing, or laboratory testing to clarify the diagnosis. The tests depend on the discipline and background of the practitioner and on the needs of the patient.

MOVEMENT SYSTEM TESTING

Movement is a physiologic system with several contributing components. Movement system impairments are theorized to lead to pain, functional limitations, disability, and to pathology (36). Thorough movement system testing is performed when the systems review scan examination does not yield an adequate specific medical diagnosis or additional information on movement system impairments is needed to make a clinical diagnosis and develop a care plan. *Impairments* are defined as alter-

ations in anatomic, physiologic, or psychologic structures or functions (27). For the purposes of this discussion, movement dysfunctions are as follows: reduced motion, excessive motion, aberrant motion, uncoordinated movement, or atypical recruitment patterns or timing. Movement dysfunctions can occur because of impairments in elements of the movement system at the base (musculoskeletal) level (e.g., extensibility, mobility, strength, endurance), modulator (nervous system) level (e.g., muscle recruitment, feedback, feed forward), biomechanical level (e.g., statics, dynamics), support level (e.g., cardiac, pulmonary, metabolic), or a combination (36). The movement system evaluation is used to determine which elements or which combination of these elements is causing or perpetuating the pain and dysfunction. Examples follow.

The routine clinical examination may have included screening of passive physiologic intervertebral mobility as listed in Table 13.3. If indicated by the screen, more in-depth and specialized testing of articular (joint) mobility (termed a *biomechanical examination* by Meadows [37]) may be needed. When restricted physiologic intervertebral movements are found, specific passive arthrokinematic (movement at the level of the joint surface) intervertebral movement tests are used to detect articular dysfunctions potentially amenable to manipulation or mobilization. When excessive or aberrant movement is detected with physiologic intervertebral movement testing, segmental stability is examined to test for articular integrity using one or more specific stability tests, such as a torsion test or the prone instability test. Clinical instability (38) is potentially amenable to stabilization exercises, which are discussed later in this chapter. Clinical instability can involve uncoordinated movement, aberrant movement, or movement with atypical recruitment patterns or timing (dynamic instability).

Movement system impairments occurring primarily at the musculoskeletal and neuromuscular levels (e.g., problems with muscle strength, muscle extensibility, muscle length-tension properties, endurance, mobility, alignment, stability, coordination, or muscle recruitment patterns) can also cause movement-related disorders. More in-depth movement system testing is likely to include examination and evaluation of the impairments hypothesized to relate to the patient's functional limitations and disability. This testing might consist of traditional testing of muscle force or torque capacity, such as with a dynamometer, and mobility testing using goniometry, and so on (see section on *Exercise, Fitness, and Functional Testing*). Or, regional, integrated, standardized movement impairment assessment protocols, such as that developed by Sahrmann (39), can be used to identify interrelationships among systems that affect movement quality and to detect the offending "directional susceptibility to movement (DSM)". Specific movement system disorders are corrected with individualized exercise and retraining programs.

DIAGNOSTIC IMAGING

Diagnostic imaging may be indicated in certain circumstances (e.g., in the presence of progressive neurologic deficit) and in recommended time frames. Imaging studies are not routinely, initially recommended in patients with nonspecific low back pain (31). Because anatomic anomalies and changes associated with aging will be present on diagnostic images, the patient's clinical findings must be correlated with radiologic findings. Typical imaging used to assist in diagnosis and treatment planning might include one or more of the following: plain film radiography, myelography, computerized tomography, bone scans, discography, fluoroscopy, magnetic resonance imaging, and rehabilitation ultrasound imaging. Each of these procedures is briefly discussed.

Plain film radiography (x-ray) is a primary means of diagnostic imaging for musculoskeletal disorders. The main purpose of plain film radiography is to rule out fractures, infection, serious disease, and structural abnormalities. Disc space narrowing of the lumbar vertebra appears more strongly associated with back pain than other radiographic findings, such as degenerative disc disease and facet joint arthritis (40). Radiographs poorly differentiate most soft-tissue structures.

Computed tomography (CT) scans produce cross-sectional images taken at specific levels and axial projections. Based on the amount of radiation absorbed by different structures from multiple angles, 2- or 3-dimensional images are reconstructed. CT is particularly useful for visualizing bone and has good resolution of soft tissue structures, such as the paravertebral muscles. CT scans can detect disc protrusions, spinal stenosis, joint disease, tumors, epidural scarring after surgery, and fractures.

Bone scans (radionuclide imaging) consist of intravenous injections of radioactive tracers (isotopes) to localize specific areas of high level turnover of bone. These areas of high turnover are then detected, usually with radiographs, as "hot spots." Bone scans are used to detect bone loss, active bone disease, fracture, infection, arthritis, and tumors. Bone scans are sensitive to bone abnormalities, but do not identify the specific abnormality.

Discography is an invasive and less common technique that involves injecting radiopaque dye into the nucleus pulposus of an intervertebral disc under radiographic guidance. Discography is used to determine internal disc derangement, especially when magnetic resonance imaging and myelography findings are normal. Discography is also used to determine whether the injection reproduces the patient's symptoms.

Myelography is an invasive imaging procedure used to visualize soft tissues within the spine. A radiopaque dye is injected into the epidural space and allowed to flow to different levels of the spinal cord. A plain film or CT scan is then taken. The procedure is used to detect such disorders as disc herniation, spinal stenosis, osteophytes, tumor, and nerve root entrapment. Magnetic resonance imaging (MRI) has largely replaced myelography, which can have a number of side effects. Myelography, however, is used as a surgical screen when the MRI or CT is equivocal.

Fluoroscopy is an infrequently performed technique used to show motion in joints using x-ray imaging. Fluoroscopy is frequently used, however, to direct the needle in injection therapy.

Magnetic resonance imaging (MRI) is a noninvasive, multiplanar imaging technique that uses exposure to magnetic fields to image bone and soft tissue. MRI has the advantage of no exposure to x-ray. Delineation of soft tissues is greater with MRI than with CT. MRI is the preferred technique for imaging disc disease. MRI can be used to detect tumors, disc pathology, infection, and soft tissue lesions. MRI can also be used with contrasts, for example, to enhance imaging of intrathecal nerve roots. Emerging developments in MRI, including imaging in weight-bearing positions, such as standing, and use of cinematographic MRI, may yield even more sophisticated diagnostic capabilities for low back disorders, especially for identifying movement disorders.

Rehabilitation ultrasound imaging (RUSI), or real-time or musculoskeletal, ultrasound imaging, is a radiation-free imaging modality that uses sound-wave technology to reflect off soft tissues. RUSI can be used to examine and measure selected structure and form properties of muscles. In patients with low back pain, RUSI has emerged as a tool useful for determining altered muscular control and function, particularly of the deep stabilizing musculature. RUSI can also be used as biofeedback in helping patients activate the stabilizing muscles.

ELECTRODIAGNOSTIC TESTING

Electrodiagnostic testing (e.g., electromyography [EMG] and nerve conduction velocity [NCV] studies) is sometimes indicated to localize dysfunction along lower motor neurons. Specifically, disease processes can be localized to the level of the anterior horn cell, nerve root, plexus, or peripheral nerve, neuromuscular junction, or muscle. Kinesiologic EMG can be used to determine the function and coordination of muscles during activities.

LABORATORY TESTING

Sometimes laboratory-screening tests, such as erythrocyte sedimentation rate (ESR), blood count, or urinalysis, are requested when there are clinical red flags suggesting disease or infection. Otherwise, use of laboratory tests in the case of low back pain is not common.

THE MEDICAL AND CLINICAL DIAGNOSIS

A diagnosis, even one made on interpretation of the most reliable and valid tests and measures, is largely provisional and subject to change. A diagnosis is both a process and a product. A *medical diagnosis* is the identification of a patient's pathology or disease from the symptoms, signs, and test results. Physicians diagnose and treat diseases and pathologies. Frequently, however, no significant underlying disease or pathology can be identified, or the identified disease or pathology may be insufficient on which to develop an intervention strategy. As noted, sometimes a diagnosis is simply "low back pain." In these cases, a *clinical diagnosis* is made. A clinical diagnosis is a classification, or a label, encompassing a cluster of signs and symptoms commonly associated with a disorder, syndrome, or category of impairment, functional limitation, or disability (27). Subclassifying patients with nonspecific low back pain based on diagnostic classification paradigms is essential in determining appropriate interventions and outcomes.

CLINICAL DIAGNOSIS OR CLASSIFICATION OF LOW BACK DISORDERS

Because of the recognized need to develop classifications to characterize low back pain, a number of these systems have evolved. The Quebec classification system is one such diagnostic classification system (41). Sahrmann (39) proposed a movement impairment-based classification system for clinically diagnosing clusters of impairments in movement quality. Other efforts have been aimed at developing treatment-based, clinical diagnoses that direct interventions, such as specific exercises, stabilization exercises, and manipulation (42). Delitto et al. (43) published a treatment-based classification system specifically for conservative management of persons with low back syndrome that has been substantively revised and is being substantiated with a series of clinical prediction rule (CPR) studies (44–46). Results of these studies have produced preliminary evidence for clinicians to use in matching patient's signs and symptoms to interventions that optimize chances for successful outcomes. Further information about the results of these clinical prediction rule studies is provided later in this chapter. Such classification systems are based on the concept that, although most patients with low back pain are without a specific diagnosis, they are not a homogeneous population. Clinically differentiating patients generally categorized with nonspecific low back pain is prerequisite to determining effective intervention and successful, cost-controlled outcomes. Otherwise, decisions about conservative intervention for low back pain are largely "hit or miss." Despite the recent progress, much work remains in refining and validating treatment-based classification systems for low back and other vertebral disorders.

PROGNOSIS AND PLAN OF CARE

Once a diagnosis is determined, the expected optimal level of improvement in the desired outcomes is predicted, and the amount of time required to reach these outcomes is estimated. Based on the diagnosis, stage and severity of the disorder, prognosis, and patient goals, an individualized care plan is developed specifying the goals, outcomes, specific interventions, and the proposed timing for managing the disorder. The *general* anticipated goals and expected outcomes may be one or more of the following: affect pathology or pathophysiology, reduce function-related impairments (including pain), restore function, prevent disability, reduce risk, prevent recurrences, promote health, activity and participation, and satisfy patients, all accomplished in a measurable, timely, and cost-effective manner. Interventions can be generally classified as medical, pharmacologic, physical, educational and counseling, complementary and alternative, and surgical. Of course, several intervention strategies can be used concurrently, or specific interventions may follow the successful or unsuccessful outcome of previous interventions.

MEDICAL, PHARMACOLOGIC, PHYSICAL, EDUCATIONAL AND COUNSELING, COMPLEMENTARY AND ALTERNATIVE, AND SURGICAL INTERVENTIONS

Management of spinal pain depends on the presumed cause or clinical classification, severity, stage of the disorder, the presence of comorbid conditions, practitioner experience and judgment, and individual patient factors (e.g., age, values, motivation, activity level, goals). A discussion of the management of nerve root disorders and serious spinal pathology (e.g., inflammatory diseases, cauda equina syndrome, spinal tumors) is beyond the scope of this chapter. *The focus in this section is on intervention strategies for nonspecific, activity-related, or mechanical, back pain.*

The strength of evidence for different intervention strategies varies; however, none of the evidence is overwhelmingly strong. Therefore, it should be noted that no intervention has been shown unequivocally effective in the treatment of nonspecific acute and chronic low back pain. Some of the people are helped, some of the time. As noted, part of the problem in determining effectiveness is lack of adequate methodology for subclassifying this large heterogeneous population of persons with nonspecific low back pain. To research the effectiveness of various interventions, more homogeneous groupings are needed. To expand on Kane (47), the ultimate key to successful intervention and patient outcome at all levels is to do the right things, for the right people, at the right time, and to do them well. We just do not yet know with certainty the right things, the right people, the right time, or perhaps, even the right way.

MEDICAL INTERVENTION

Medical intervention typically consists of dispensing information, advice, reassurance and psychological support, making referrals, and managing pharmacologic intervention. Dispensing information, advice, reassurance, and psychological support are discussed in the subsection on educational and counseling interventions. Recognizing the need for appropriate referrals is essential for each practitioner dealing with persons with low back pain. Pharmacologic intervention is discussed in the next subsection.

PHARMACOLOGIC INTERVENTION

Pharmacologic intervention is common for reducing the symptoms of low back pain and for maintaining function. Drugs may be nonprescription or prescription, oral, topical, or injected. Medication types used in the treatment of low back pain are anti-inflammatories (nonsteroidal anti-inflammatory drugs [NSAIDS], and steroids), muscle relaxants, analgesics (opioid and nonopioid), antidepressants, anticonvulsants, and anesthetics. Patients need to understand, however, that medications do not cure low back pain, but medications may be useful in assisting them in tolerating activity.

Commonly used nonprescription medications are acetaminophen (Tylenol), aspirin, Aleve, and ibuprofen (Motrin and Advil). Acetaminophen is a simple analgesic with strong evidence for effectiveness in relieving the symptoms of low back pain and promoting activity and participation (12). The other medications mentioned are anti-inflammatory analgesics (NSAIDS).

Widely prescribed for acute and chronic low back pain (48), NSAIDs purportedly reduce swelling and inflammation and promote healing. Examples of prescription NSAIDs are Dolobid, Naprosyn, Relafen, Ansaid, Voltaren, and Celebrex (Cox-2 inhibitor). NSAIDs have a number of potentially serious adverse drug reactions (ADRs), especially gastrointestinal tract irritation and renal effects. Cox-2 inhibitors have been associated with risk of stroke and myocardial infarction. Both prescription and nonprescription NSAIDs must be used with discretion. Even use of over-the-counter NSAIDs is not recommended for more than 10 days. NSAIDs are sometimes augmented with acetaminophen and a muscle relaxant (49) (e.g., Flexeril, Soma, Valium) to relieve muscle spasms in acute low back pain. Drowsiness is a common side effect of muscle relaxants. Oral steroids (e.g., Prednisone, Medrol) are strong anti-inflammatory medications and are occasionally used short term (1–2 weeks) for more severe inflammation. Ultram (tramadol) is a narcotic-like analgesic used to treat moderate to severe pain. A short course of narcotic analgesics (e.g., Darvocet, Tylenol with Codeine, Vicodin, OxyContin) is occasionally prescribed for more severe pain, but less likely with nonspecific low back pain. Narcotic analgesics are addictive and usually avoided. Antiseizure medications, such as Neurontin, and antidepressants are sometimes used to help control symptoms of chronic low back pain.

In addition, injection therapy is sometimes used for symptom control. Typical injections consist of myofascial trigger point, intra-articular (facet), or epidural injections and nerve blocks. Myofascial trigger points can be injected with an anesthetic to relieve pain and spasm. Intra-articular injections, epidural injections, and nerve blocks consist of local injections of a mixture that typically includes steroids and anesthetics into a specific area under x-ray (fluoroscopy) guidance. These injections are used both diagnostically and as therapy. That is, if the symptoms are relieved, the injection was treatment. If the symptoms were not affected, then presumably the injection sites were not the sources of pain. Intra-articular injections are made directly into the offending lumbar joints relieve pain and inflammation. Epidural injections consist of injecting into the epidural space close to the affected area. Epidural injections are used for patients with nerve root irritation, or compromise, and presumably decrease inflammation of nerve roots and relieve pain. A lumbar sympathetic nerve block involves injecting around the sympathetic nerves to "block" neuropathic pain. Blocks can also be selective nerve root blocks for specific spinal roots. In severe cases, injections are used to permanently destroy nerves to relieve pain. The efficacy of injection therapy is inconclusive (13).

PHYSICAL INTERVENTION

Physical intervention consists of a broad range of treatments that might be categorized as thermal modalities, electrotherapeutic modalities, mechanical modalities, orthotics, protective and supportive devices, manual therapy, and exercise. In general, the evidence supporting use of various physical interventions is inconclusive or found to be useful only during specific stages (i.e., acute or chronic) and for patients who fit well into current treatment-based classifications. The Philadelphia Panel Evidence-Based Clinical Guideline on Selected Rehabilitation Interventions for Low Back Pain (50) provided the status of the information on the effectiveness of various management strategies for use with adults with low back pain, but did not include evidence for the effectiveness of manipulation in their review.

Thermal modalities are physical agents that use heat, cold, sound or light energy to decrease pain, increase tissue extensibility, reduce soft inflammation, decrease swelling, remodel scar tissue, and so forth. Ultrasound (which has both thermal and mechanical effects), hydrotherapy, hot packs, and cold packs are examples of thermal modalities used in treatment of low back pain. Typically, thermal agents, if used, are used in the acute stages of low back pain or as adjunctive interventions to other physical interventions, such as using heat combined with stretching. Generally, the effectiveness of thermal therapy has not been substantiated.

Electrotherapeutic modalities consist of physical agents that use electricity to decrease pain, reduce soft tissue inflammation, decrease muscle spasm and guarding, and assist in muscle re-education. Examples of electrotherapeutic modalities include alternating direct and pulsed current, transcutaneous electrical nerve stimulation (TENS), low level laser, neuromuscular electrical stimulation (NMES), and surface electromyography (SEMG). Again, electrotherapeutic modalities, if used, are typically used in conjunction with other physical interventions. However, evidence is insufficient to make recommendations for usage.

Mechanical modalities include traction, compression, taping, and continuous passive motion. Mechanical modalities are typically intended to decrease pain, stabilize or mobilize an area, apply distraction or compression, or increase range of motion. The effectiveness of mechanical modalities has not been adequately studied.

Orthotics, protective and supportive devices, used in treating low back pain consist primarily of shoe inserts or lifts and various back supports, corsets, and braces. Corrective foot orthotics are sometimes prescribed for patients who have back pain in standing or walking and who do so for long periods. Shoe lifts might be used to correct a fairly large leg length discrepancy. Back supports, corsets, and braces can be used as adjunctive treatment to restrict movement and provide support. The selection of the type of brace depends on the degree of immobilization required and the region of the spine requiring stabilization. Evidence for use functional immobilization has not been demonstrated (12).

Manual therapy consists of several techniques including, but not limited to, spinal manipulation or mobilization, muscle energy technique, myofascial release, exercise, and soft tissue mobilization or massage. Manual therapy is used by a number of different practitioners, primarily osteopathic physicians, physical therapists, and chiropractors. Massage therapists also may perform some deep-tissue techniques. **Manipulation, or mobilization,** is defined as a continuum of skilled passive movements to joints and related soft tissues that are applied at varying speeds and amplitudes. *Manipulation* is typically thought of as a localized thrust of high velocity, small amplitude therapeutic movement (27); whereas, *mobilization* is usually considered a nonthrust technique. The general objectives of manipulation and mobilization are to regain pain-free movement and restore function. Evidence suggests that manipulation is effective treatment for selected patients with a recent onset (<16 days) of low back pain, especially patients who have no symptoms distal to the knee, demonstrate hypomobilitiy with intervertebral (spring) testing, and have low Fear Avoidance Behavior Questionnaire scores (42,44,45). Use of manipulation with patients with radiculopathy is controversial. **Muscle energy technique** is an active procedure in which the patient helps correct a movement by contracting

muscle in a controlled direction against a counterforce supplied by a clinician. Muscle energy technique can be used to mobilize joints, and relax, lengthen, or strengthen muscle (51). **Myofascial release and soft tissue mobilization** may serve as a prelude to other procedures. These techniques are intended to mechanically stretch skin, fascia, and muscle to improve extensibility, increase circulation, and decrease muscle guarding and spasm.

Exercise includes physical activities to increase mobility, stability, muscle performance, balance, coordination, posture, neuromuscular control, cardiovascular and muscular endurance, and movement patterns. Exercises are used to relieve pain; to improve physical function, health status, activity and participation; and to prevent complications and future impairments or functional loss. Exercise is also believed to reduce fear-avoidance behavior and facilitate function despite continued pain (1,52). Exercises will be considered in more detail in the section about exercise prescription and programming, below.

In summary, in general, well-designed randomized, controlled trials for whether to use, or not use, many physical interventions are lacking. Clinically important benefits have been demonstrated for continuing normal activity and for therapeutic exercise for subacute, chronic and postsurgical patients (50). In addition, evidence supports the use of manipulation for selected patients in the acute stage of the disorder (45), and for stabilization exercises with selected findings (46).

EDUCATIONAL AND COUNSELING INTERVENTION

Educational and counseling interventions can take many forms: informal or formal, group or individual, verbal or written, solicited or unsolicited, individualized or generic, to name a few. Nonspecific low back pain may seem common and routine for the clinician, but the patient can fear pain, damage, harm, and permanent functional limitations and disability. Information is critical in allaying these fears that naturally accompany low back pain. Another key aspect of relieving fear is providing reassurance, comfort, and caring. Pain, after all, is a sensory and emotional experience for people, not their spines.

The Joint Clinical Practice Guideline from the American College of Physicians and the American Pain Society (31) recommended that patient education include evidence-based explanations about the diagnosis, expected course of the disorder, prognosis, safe and effective methods of symptom control, use of diagnostic procedures, general course of care, and recommendations to stay active (53). Advice can also consist of the use, discontinued use, or presumed effectiveness of various treatments or products (e.g., supports, mattresses, herbals), and the *Dos and Don'ts* of general, occupational, social, and leisure activity modifications. Bedrest is not recommended for most cases of simple, nonspecific backache (54). If used, rest should not exceed 2 days for persons without neuromotor deficits (55).

To paraphrase a saying attributed to Hippocrates, "healing is often a matter of time and opportunity." Modifying various positions and activities is frequently recommended as a means of providing the opportunity for healing. It is difficult to heal that which is constantly being irritated. Patients may need *individualized* guidance on the position and activity modifications appropriate to their disorder, behavior and severity of symptoms, age, general health, and typical physical demands. For example, merely teaching a patient who experiences pain with spinal extension when returning to upright from spinal flexion to initiate movement from the hips versus the spine, may relieve all symptoms associated with that activity. Some positions and activities may be deemed irritating and, therefore, temporary or permanent lifestyle changes may be recommended.

Specific position and activity modifications are based primarily on the patient's report of the behavior of the symptoms and on known mechanical spine stressors, such as lifting. For example, if patients complain of pain *during* sitting, they may be advised to temporarily limit or interrupt periods of sitting. Likewise, if patients complain of pain *during* running, they may be advised to limit running. However, patients complaining of symptoms *after* running, may be able to continue running, but may need to modify the activity they do after running, that is, when they feel the pain (frequently sitting). Patients are generally encouraged to continue routine activities and working and to gradually increase their physical activities over a period of a few days or weeks (54).

Although evidence supporting effectiveness is limited, another area of patient education focuses on ergonomic and work and home site recommendations. Patients may need information on types of chairs and adjustments, sitting supports (e.g., lumbar rolls), pillows, shoes, standing surfaces, seating positions, desk arrangements, computer heights, lifting, and so on. Providing patient-specific information based on his or her report of "what aggravates" and "what eases," is presumably more effective than providing generic information.

Structured patient education through back schools has been somewhat effective in the workplace (53) and may include work site-specific education. Behavioral interventions, cognitive therapies, and pain management clinics are more often recommended for patients dealing with chronic pain syndrome.

In addition to individualized and group education, various pamphlets, books, magazines, and information from relatives, friends, strangers, and websites are readily available. Frequently, patients need help in interpreting this information relative to their situation and in judging the quality of the information.

COMPLEMENTARY AND ALTERNATIVE INTERVENTION

An ever-increasing number of complementary and alternative medical (CAM) interventions for treating low back pain have evolved, largely based on anecdotal and extrapolated evidence, and on real or perceived failures of conventional medical care. Some of the more common complementary interventions (i.e., used with conventional medical care) and alternative interventions (i.e., used instead of conventional medical care) for low back pain at this time are acupuncture, acupressure, biomagnets, selected mind–body techniques, herbs (e.g., devil's claw, white willow bark), and supplements (e.g., glucosamine-chrondroitin sulfates, omega-3 fatty acids). Increased popular use of these complementary and alternative interventions has sparked interest in scientific circles. At this time, most of these interventions have inadequate high-quality evidence to warrant recommendation.

SURGICAL INTERVENTION

Surgical intervention is not typically indicated for nonspecific low back pain, but is indicated with progressive neurologic deficit and with some serious disorders. Surgery is also used in some cases of severe pain and in cases with significant neurologic deficit. A number of different surgical approaches and techniques are available and constantly evolving. Common types of surgeries are fusions, artificial disc replacements, and decompressions. A trend now exists to perform more minimally invasive spine surgeries, which consist of performing selected surgeries through small incisions usually with endoscopic visualization. The advantages are less muscle-related damage and speedier recoveries.

Spinal fusion is performed to eliminate motion at one or more vertebral segments. Spinal fusion involves adding bone graft to an area of the spine that then grows between the segments to eliminate motion. Fusions may also be instrumented, that is augmented by implanting fixation implements, such as screws and rods, to further stabilize the area. Interbody fusions are common and consist of a fusion through the disc spaces. This can be accomplished by an anterior lumbar interbody fusion (ALIF), laterally using an extreme lateral interbody fusion, or posteriorly with a transforaminal interbody fusion (TLIF) or posterior lumbar interbody fusion (PLIF). Other techniques are posterior or posterolateral, anterior-posterior, and lumbar cage fusions. Fusions can be performed for conditions such as degenerative disc disease, iatrogenic segmental instability, and spondylolisthesis.

Artificial disc replacement surgery (ADR) can be used to replace degenerated discs while preserving spinal motion. Currently, ADR surgery is used mostly for patients with one symptomatic disc without bone disease (e.g., osteoporosis) or other selected disorders. An additional type of experimental spine surgery is the *prosthetic* *disc nucleus* (PDN) that also restores disc height and permits movement, but replaces only the nuclear material and not the entire disc.

The general purpose of **decompressive spinal surgery** is to relieve neural impingement by creating more space. Foraminotomy is used to increase the size of the neural foramen to relieve nerve compression. Decompressive laminectomy is a common procedure to treat lumbar spinal stenosis. Two examples of decompressive surgeries for neural impingement caused by disc herniation are microdiscectomies and discectomy (removal of the herniated disc material) via laminectomy. Percutaneous and endoscopic disectomies and intradiscal electrothermal therapy (IDET) are other less invasive surgical techniques for lumbar disc herniation.

OUTCOMES OF INTERVENTION

Successful outcomes from management of an episode of low back pain are typically measured using minimally clinically important differences (MCID) on standardized pain and disability scales, with patient-specific functional scales and with patient satisfaction questionnaires. Scales should be validated for individuals as well as groups. Given the high rate of recurrence, patients should be provided with knowledge of warning signs and self-management strategies, or first aid (e.g., ice, specific movements), for future episodes. In addition, patients should be taught individualized risk reduction (Table 13.1) and preventive strategies (see section on *Preventing Low Back Pain*). Exercise and cognitive interventions that boost confidence and reduce fear avoidance behaviors may provide improved outcomes for patients on the path toward chronic pain syndrome. Ideal success would be happy, fully functioning and actively participating individuals without recurrence or future reliance on the healthcare system.

EXERCISE, FITNESS, AND FUNCTIONAL TESTING

A variety of testing exists for measuring exercise, fitness, and function for patients with low back pain. The reliability, validity, specificity, sensitivity, likelihood ratios, and responsiveness of these tests and measures vary and, in all cases, are population-specific. As indicated, some tests are valid for individuals and others are only valid for groups. Therefore, the selection of tests should be based on the purpose of the test and applicability to the patient. Selected tests and measures associated with low back disorders are presented in Table 13.4.

CLINICAL EXERCISE PHYSIOLOGY

To understand the exercise prescription and programming, a brief description of trunk muscle function is included, followed by a brief description of acute and chronic responses to exercise.

Functionally, the lumbopelvic muscles can be divided into local stabilizing (or deep) muscles and global stabilizing muscles. Two of the primary, so-called, local stabilizing muscles are the transversus abdominis and the multifidis. These muscles have been hypothesized to contribute to lumbar spine stiffness and to control intersegmental motion. A contraction of the transversus abdominis reportedly precedes movement of an extremity (56,57). Onset of premovement activity in the transversus abdominis has been shown to be delayed in patients with low back pain. Evidence suggests that poor endurance of the multifidus and segmental fibers of the erector spinae may be a predictor for recurrent low back pain (58). Further, and importantly, the multifidi apparently do not automatically recover full strength after the first episode of low back pain without directed exercise (59).

In addition to the suspected key roles of the transversus abdominis and the multifidis in trunk stability, the pelvic floor muscles (PFM) may also be a critical component. Neumann and Gill (60) confirmed a synergistic relationship between the PFM and the deep abdominal muscles. The PFM may be necessary for developing intra-abdominal pressure (IAP). Further work on the role of the PFM is ongoing. Likewise, the diaphragm, as the upper muscular component in the torso, may also be important in spinal stability.

Muscles of the global stabilizing system consist of the erector spinae, quadratus lumborum, rectus abdominis, and internal and external obliques. These muscles not only move the spine, but also function to transfer external loads applied to the trunk to minimize load on the lumbar spine and its segments. The global stabilizing system needs strength and endurance; however, the global muscles presumably cannot control shear forces at the segmental level. Overemphasis on exercising the global system in the presence of an inadequate local stabilizing system may create a potentially harmful imbalance (61). Evidence suggests that stabilization exercise programs should be based on assessment of need and should target the appropriate stabilizing system or systems (62). Furthermore, the rectus abdominis is primarily a trunk flexor and of less importance in rehabilitating patients with low back pain.

Acute and chronic responses to exercise are usually not altered by nonspecific low back pain without concomitant diseases. However, the stage of the disorder, severity of symptoms, goals, and positions for exercising are important considerations. Certain exercises may aggravate the symptoms, especially in the first 2–3 weeks after onset of low back pain. Nonetheless, patients should be kept as active as possible to prevent debilitation secondary to inactivity. Notably, "exercise therapy" does not equal "staying active." Exercise guidelines are discussed in the next section.

TABLE 13.4. POTENTIAL TESTS AND MEASURES FOR DETERMINING EXERCISE, FITNESS, FUNCTION, ACTIVITY, AND PARTICIPATION OF PATIENTS WITH NONSPECIFIC, MECHANICAL LOW BACK PAIN

TESTS	MEASURES	COMMENTS
Aerobic Capacity and Endurance • Treadmill • Cycle (bike or recumbent) • Arm ergometer • 6- or 12-minute walk test • 10-m walk test	• 12-lead ECG, heart rate, RPE, blood pressure • Distance walked • Time	• Testing may be warranted if risk of, or symptoms of, CAD • Usually select low- impact test methods. • Choice of test method may be dictated by patient's symptoms. • Testing is usually not applicable within the first 2–6 weeks of onset when activity may be curtailed. • Fitness indicators
Posture and Anthropometry • Alignment and position (dynamic and static) • Body composition • Height and weight	• Symmetry, curvature, flexicurve measures • Body mass index or calipers • Stadiometer and scale	
Extremes/Range of Motion *Spinal* • Dual goniometry • BROM (In FN) • Tape measure *Extremities* • Goniometry	• Lumbar extremes of motion (deg) • Schober's Lumbar Flexion Method; Attraction Extension Method (cm) • Joint angle	
Flexibility/Extensibility • Goniometry	• Joint angle	• Especially two-joint muscles in lower extremities
Strength (Trunk & Extremities) • Isometric, isotonic or isokinetic dynamometry • Weight lifted	• Peak torque/force • One RM	
Muscular Endurance • Isometric, isotonic or isokinetic dynamometry • Weight lifted • Trunk extensor endurance	• Maximum repetitions at 60% peak torque/force or 10 RM • Specific timed trunk extensor endurance tests (e.g., Sorenson's, Ito's)	• Isometric tests need a minimum 5-sec holding contraction.
Articular Stability/Mobility • Spring testing • Prone instability test • Torsion testing	• Segmental mobility/stability	
Neuromuscular • Gait analysis • Locomotion • Stability (balance) • Transitional movements (e.g., sit-and-stand) • Motor control	• Observational analysis • Observations, ADL scales • Balance scales, force platforms, timed tests • Observations, ADL scales and indexes • Observations of recruitment patterns, substitutions, movement quality, compensations • Kinesiologic EMG • Real-time ultrasound	

(continued)

TABLE 13.4. POTENTIAL TESTS AND MEASURES FOR DETERMINING EXERCISE, FITNESS, FUNCTION, ACTIVITY, AND PARTICIPATION OF PATIENTS WITH NONSPECIFIC, MECHANICAL LOW BACK PAIN (*Continued*)

TESTS	MEASURES	COMMENTS
Functional Performance • Ergonomics • Body mechanics • Functional capacity • ADL • Lifting • Sports performance • Functional status	• Work simulations, impairment ratings, task analysis • ADL scales, observations • FCEs • ADL scales and indexes • Lift capacity (with different types of lifts) and projections • Screening, simulations, observations, task analysis • Roland-Morris Questionnaire, Oswestry Low Back Pain Disability Questionnaire, Patient-Specific Functional Scale	• Useful for determining work capacity, estimating job or sport restrictions
Psychosocial	• Beck Depression Index • Fear Avoidance Behavior	

Special Considerations
- Testing may not be reliable in the presence of pain owing to submaximal patient effort.
- Testing may need to be modified owing to age, stage of the disorder, comorbid conditions, pain severity, and patient needs.
- Testing may need to be terminated or deferred in the presence of increasing pain.
- Testing should be terminated with progressive sensory or motor deterioration.
- Timing of testing postoperatively is at the surgeon's discretion based on patient status and type of surgery.

ADL, activities of daily living; BROM, back range of motion; ECG, electrocardiogram; EMG, electromyelogram; FCE, functional capacity evaluation; RM, repetition maximum; RPE, rating of perceived exertion.

EXERCISE PRESCRIPTION AND PROGRAMMING

A consumer publication survey (63) of 46,000 readers reported that 66% of the respondents with back pain had tried exercise and ranked exercise "among the treatments receiving the highest marks for back pain." Interestingly, a systematic review of the use of exercise in acute, nonspecific low back pain (64), did not find that exercise was successful in relieving low back pain. Certainly, this is not the first time that popular opinion differed from research-based evidence. However, exercise is apparently helping some people. The lack of evidence of the effectiveness of exercise because of methodologic flaws in studies is not equivalent to proof of the lack of effectiveness of exercise. In addition to inappropriate design and limited, or diverse outcome measures, the problem is also one of differing definitions and lack of clarity and specificity (i.e., "back pain" is generic, "exercise" is generic, and "relieving" is generic).

What exactly is *back pain*? As discussed in the section on pathophysiology, spinal pain has numerous causes and may even arise from different areas: lumbar, thoracic, or sacral. The diagnosis of low back pain includes a heterogeneous group of disorders, and we know that not all causes of spinal pain can be helped by exercises. To further complicate the problem, the effectiveness of exercise interacts with the stage of the disorder. Abdominal strengthening may not help relieve acute low back pain,

but a chronic problem might be helped. And what is *exercise*? Exercise could be walking, weight training, stretching, self-manipulation, a standardized routine (e.g., William's flexion exercises), stabilization exercises, a self-directed program, or a specifically prescribed regimen. And, as noted, exercises appropriate for one type of disorder may not be appropriate for another. Further, exercises appropriate for the disorder, but applied at the inappropriate time in the stage of the disorder may not be effective. Compliance also affects the reported success of exercise. And finally, what is *relief*? Is relief the absence of pain, occasional pain not interfering with activities, or even continued pain but the ability to return to work and leisure activities? Is the goal of exercise only to relieve pain, or is it also to restore function, prevent disability, and promote health? We have a lot to learn. The question, then, is not only does exercise work or not, but also on whom, to what extent, and under what conditions?

Treatment of persons with certain red flags (e.g., inflammatory conditions) and some nerve root involvement may at times include exercise. However, the exercise intervention for people with these conditions should be relegated to practitioners with specific knowledge and expertise. Exercise for patients with nonspecific, mechanical low back pain is based on patient needs, severity of symptoms, and functional limitations (Table 13.5).

Patients with nonspecific low back pain need subclassifying, staging, and individualizing to design an appropriate

TABLE 13.5. GENERAL GUIDELINES FOR EXERCISE PRESCRIPTION FOR LOW BACK PAIN

GENERAL CATEGORIZATION	GENERAL RECOMMENDATION
Red flagged serious conditions	Follow exercise recommendations by qualified practitioners
Specific spinal conditions (nerve root pain/stenosis)	Follow exercise recommendations by qualified practitioners
Nonspecific, mechanical low back pain	Consider stage, irritability, acuteness, degree of severity, functional limitations, functional capacity, and individual patient needs, but, in general, continue and gradually increase activity[a]

[a] See Table 13.6

intervention; therefore, general exercise intervention strategies are difficult to describe. Further, in the absence of better guidelines, the clinician is required to "integrate" information from a number of sources, each diverse, yet similar, and each with varying scientific and empiric support. Figure 13.2 presents this author's composite algorithm for exercise intervention for patients with nonspecific low back pain. The algorithm was compiled and integrated from several sources (20,26,39,42,43,65) in an attempt to reconcile and consider seemingly different approaches, all of which appear to offer credible (all-be-it still somewhat limited) evidence for clinical effectiveness. Not all patients need to proceed through each stage of rehabilitation. Patients should "enter" the model at their appropriate stage. Therefore, guidelines to staging, based loosely on Fritz and George (66) will be discussed first.

STAGING NONSPECIFIC LOW BACK PAIN

With the current absence of evidence-based criteria for accurate staging, appropriate staging is mostly a matter of patient self-assessment and clinician-judgment. Although insurance company representatives and others prefer to consider stages as merely the passage of time, passage of time is not the sole consideration. This is analogous to advancing students in school based on passage of time (i.e., grade levels) without meeting the criteria for passing the grade level. Patients may need to learn to control somatic symptoms (stage I) regardless of the duration of their symptoms. Perhaps "graduating" from each stage (*if needed*) is necessary to decrease the recurrence rate of low back pain. The length of time a patient spends in each stage varies according to severity and the speed with which the patient accomplishes the goals of each stage. Some people need only spend a few days in each stage. Three stages of rehabilitation have been identified: Stage I: Symptom-Control; Stage II: Reactivation; and Stage III: Restoration (Figure 13.2) (43). Persons with chronic pain syndrome with dissociated symptoms and symptom-magnifying behaviors need a different type of intervention program from that presented in this chapter.

Stage I (Symptom-Control) **can** correspond to the "acute" stage in the sense of passage of time and with persons presenting with higher symptom severity, greater symptom irritability, and more major functional limitations. Persons in Stage I **might** have problems performing basic activities of daily living (ADLs), such as sitting, standing, bending, and walking. They may demonstrate consistent direction-specific symptoms with active or passive movements or with prolonged positions of the spine or extremities. *Stage II* (Reactivation) **might** include persons with medium symptom severity and more moderate functional limitations. With regard to duration, this stage **might** represent the early part of the "subacute" or "recurrent stage." However, again, passage of time may not be an important consideration. Persons in stage II **might** have difficulty performing more demanding home, occupational, and recreational activities (e.g., vacuuming, lifting, gardening). Stage II may include persons with difficulty with local static trunk ("core") stabilization and control. *Stage III* (Restoration) **can** be chronologically in the latter part of the "subacute" or "recurrent" stage. Persons in Stage III **can** have low symptom severity (and typically more intermittent symptoms), less symptom irritability, and more minor functional limitations. Exercises in stage III are started as the goals of stage II are accomplished to help patients return to full activity and participation.

GOALS AND EXERCISES FOR EACH STAGE

Providers or clinicians, for the most part, are ethically responsible for judging their own qualifications for subclassifying and staging cases of low back pain and for determining their ability to prescribe, assess, and progress exercise. Persons presenting with high symptom severity and major functional limitations (stage I) may need referral to clinicians with specific training. Stage, classification of low back pain, the general goals for each stage, and examples of exercises for selected stages are provided in Table 13.6

Stage I: Symptom-Control Exercises

The goals of exericises for persons in stage I are to relieve symptoms, increase function, prevent disability, and progress to stage II exercises. Stage I interventions include self-performed movements and specific exercises to centralize peripheral symptoms if the centralization phenomenon is present, manipulation for selected movement restrictions, if present, or stabilization via supports and specific exercises for clinical instability, if present. A common thread among interventions in stage I is that they are direction-specific, that is, specific movements and positions tend to aggravate symptoms and others ease symptoms. As the goal at this stage is more symptom relief, repetitions and prolonged holding of stabilizing muscle contractions are typically emphasized versus loading or resistance training for persons with clinical instability.

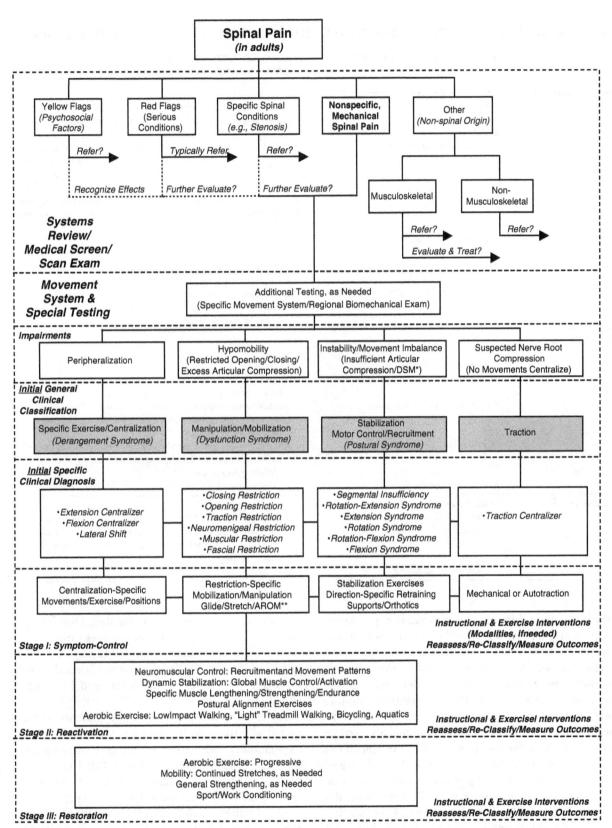

FIGURE 13-2. A composite algorithm for clinical diagnosis and intervention for persons with nonspecific, mechanical low back pain.
*DSM = Directional Susceptibility to Movement; ** AROM = Active Range of Motion
Adapted primarily from Delitto (43), DeRosa (26), Flynn (45), Fritz (42), Hicks (46), McKenzie (65), Sahrmann (39), Waddell (20) and their colleagues.

TABLE 13.6. EXAMPLES OF VARIOUS EXERCISES BY REHABILITATION STAGES AND GENERAL GOALS

STAGE	SUBCLASSIFICATION, GENERAL GOALS AND EXAMPLES	EXAMPLES OF POTENTIAL EXERCISES AND PROGRESSIONS
I. Symptom Control	**Specific Exercise Centralization**	
	• Extension	Prone lying, prone-on-elbows, press-ups, and standing backbends
	• Flexion	Supine single and double knees-to-chest, sitting flexion
	Stabilization	
	• Extension-Rotation (39)	Must be individualized to impairments, but might include an abdominal progression starting supine with leg sliding with abdominal stabilization, supine bent knee fall-outs with abdominal stabilization, side-lying hip lateral rotation with stationary pelvis, prone knee flexion with abdominal stabilization, quadruped backward rocking with movement correction, wall slides with abdominal stabilization (39)
	Segmental stabilization (local muscles) (61)	
	• Recruit transversus abdominis	Abdominal drawing in or hollowing, hollowing with arm and leg movements, hollowing with bridging
	• Recruit lumbar multifidi	Quadruped co-contraction with transversus abdominis, quadruped with single arm/leg lifts, quadruped with opposite arm/leg lifts
II. Reactivation	**Stabilization**	
	Incorporation of motor skill into light functional tasks (62)	
	• Recruit quadratus lumborum	Horizontal side support lifts with abdominal hollowing knees flexed, progress to knees extended
	• Recruit oblique abdominals	Horizontal side support lifts with abdominal hollowing, bent knee fall-outs, curl-ups with trunk rotation, leg lowering, hanging leg lifts
	Hip flexibility	Static stretching with neutral spine (co-contraction) as needed for hamstrings, hip flexors, and so on. Standing flexion from hip with neutral spine
	Aerobic conditioning	Low impact: walking or cycling
III. Restoration	**Stabilization**	
	Dynamic stabilization: Incorporation of motor skill into heavier functional tasks (62)	Neutral spine (co-contraction) with progressive gymnastic ball exercises, e.g., arm and/or leg lifts, bridging on ball, upper back lifts over ball, etc. Can be combined with weights, pulleys.
	Work/sport conditioning	Simulations

With patients exhibiting the centralization phenomenon, pain or paresthesia is abolished or moves from the periphery toward the spine with specific movement and exercises, usually spinal flexion or extension. The test movements are part of the musculoskeletal scan examination and consist of the effect of standing, supine, prone, and perhaps quadruped movements on symptoms. Movements that centralize symptoms are used as the patient's initial exercise program. For example, if extension movements centralize symptoms from the leg to the lumbar spine, prone-lying, or prone press-ups may be prescribed. The patient's response to the movements determines the exercises and the progression. Exercises that centralize the symptoms are continued and those that cause peripheralization to the leg, in this example flexion, are initially avoided. In other cases, flexion movements may centralize the symptoms and extension is initially avoided. Flexion movements might consist of double knees to the chest, progressing to flexion in sitting and finally to flexion in standing. Once symptoms are centralized, the patient can progress through the initially offending movements and on to stage II. For more information on centralization and mechanical treatment, the reader is referred to McKenzie and May (65) and Donelson et al. (67).

As mentioned previously, some patients in stage I, specifically those with symptoms for less than 16 days, hypomobility with spring testing, no symptoms distal to the knee, and low Fear Avoidance Belief Questionnaire scores will benefit from manipulation (42). Manipulative techniques are beyond the scope of this chapter.

Other patients will benefit from stabilization exercises and movement system rebalancing exercises to restore alignment and precise movement of specific segments to relieve musculoskeletal pain (39). Test movements of the spine and extremities during the movement system examination will identify the primary movement impairment. These movement impairment syndromes are subclassified in the overall category of stabilization by this author (Figure 13.2), because, although the identified movement impairments can be caused by stiff, short, weak, or imbalanced muscles or by poor patterns of muscle recruitment and motor control, the pain is presumably caused by the clinical instability or the area of compensatory movement (i.e., the directional-susceptible movement [DSM]) (68). Further information on the diagnosis and treatment of movement impairment syndromes can be found in Sahrmann's text (39).

Hicks et al. (46) performed a clinical prediction rule study to determine those persons with low back pain who may best respond to stabilization exercises using the deep stabilizing muscles (transversus abdominis and the lumbar multifidi). Based on current evidence, factors favoring success with these segmental stabilization exercises appear to all or some of the following: younger age (<40 years), greater general flexibility (average SLR >91 degrees), a positive prone instability test, aberrant motions during lumbar flexion and extension range of motion, hypermobility with spring testing, three or more episodes of low back pain, and increasing frequency of episodes (42).

Static stabilization is retraining the local stabilizing muscles, primarily the transversus abdominis, the multifidi, and maybe the PFM. According to Richardson and Jull (69), functional demands suggest that isometric exercise (a prolonged tonic holding at a low maxima voluntary contraction [MVC]) is most beneficial for re-educating these local stabilizing muscles. Initial positions used to recruit these muscles are quadruped and prone.

Asking the patient to "draw in," or hollow, the lower abdomen activates the transversus abdominis. No movement of the spine, ribs, or pelvis should occur, and the patient should be able to breathe normally. The multifidus is thought to co-contract when the patient is able to maintain the normal lumbosacral curve during the exercise. Asking the patient to "swell out," or contract, the muscles in the lumbar spine while the practitioner palpates the multifidi can encourage further, isolated contraction of the multifidi. Substitution of global muscles, such as breath-holding and spinal movement, should be corrected. Exercise for the local stabilizing muscles is to be repeated several times a day. The progression is to first increase the holding time of the co-contraction (arbitrarily to 10 seconds) and to increase the number of repetitions to at least 10.

Stage II: Reactivation Exercises

The goals for cases of stage II are to further develop trunk stabilization and endurance of the local stabilizing muscles, learn the neutral spine position, control the stabilizing muscles during progressive hip mobility and limb movements, return to low-impact aerobic conditioning activities, increase function, prevent disability, and

progress to stage III activities. The progression of stabilization exercises is to perform them with gradually increasing external loads, and then to co-contract the deep muscles during dynamic functional movements of the trunk.

When the patient can perform these contractions in quadruped and prone, this retraining is practiced in other positions (e.g., standing, during low levels of leg loading) and in light functional tasks. Examples of exercises might be supine bent-knee fall-outs, supine single or double leg sliding in supine, bridging, and opposite arm and leg lifts from a quadruped position while maintaining the neutral spine position. Patients also learn to contract these deep stabilizing muscles while performing trunk movements that usually aggravate their pain.

Again, the noteworthy implication, reported previously, is that activating the global muscles with poor local muscle control actually inhibits the deep stabilizing muscles and is potentially harmful. This finding suggests that performing exercises using the global muscles without proper local stabilization is actually contraindicated (61).

After patients have developed adequate lumbar stabilization, hip stretching (e.g., of the hip flexors, hamstrings.) may be added while the patient activates the deep stabilizing muscles. In other words, traditional stretching techniques can be used, but the patient is taught to perform the stretches with the spine maintained in the neutral posture.

Additional stage II exercises may include continuation, progression, or initiation of the movement rebalancing exercises from stage I, postural alignment, and additional stabilizing exercises emphasizing the static stabilizing elements. For example, exercises to recruit the quadratus lumborum and the oblique abdominals (also stabilizing muscles), such as the horizontal side support lifts, can be initiated. In this exercise, the patient lies on the side with knees bent and the upper body supported on the elbow and forearm. The patient incorporates the "drawing in" contraction of the transversus abdominis and then lifts the body upward from the surface. Extending the knees increases the difficulty of the exercise. Oblique abdominal exercises can gradually be incorporated and might consist of curl-ups with trunk rotation and unilateral or bilateral leg lowering.

Low-impact aerobic activities, such as walking, "light," or de-weighted, treadmill walking (i.e., using a harness system to reduce the amount of compressive forces during walking), bicycling, and aquatic exercises are encouraged. Even at this stage, the choice of activities may have some directionality. For example, if symptoms occurred with sitting, bicycling may not be the best choice for an aerobic activity. Likewise, not all patients can tolerate walking because of the more extended lumbar spine. The guidelines for aerobic exercises in this stage are similar to those of a healthy individual resuming an activity or for individuals new to aerobic exercise.

Stage III: Restoration Exercises

Persons with low back pain have been shown to have deficits in dynamic control of the trunk, such as decreased spinal proprioception, increased reaction time, and increased postural sway (70). The goals of stage III are to develop dynamic trunk stabilization and trunk strength using the local and global stabilizing muscles, use the neutral spine position in dynamic activities, progress aerobic conditioning activities, prevent disability, and return to full function, if possible. In stage III, isometric exercises for the deep stabilizing lumbar muscles are combined with dynamic exercise for other parts of the body, that is, local muscle retraining is incorporated into more dynamic activities that require both local and global trunk muscles. Dynamic stabilization programs often use unstable surfaces, such as large gymnastic balls. Here again the patient should maintain the neutral spine by contraction ("drawing in") of the transversus abdominis during all exercises. The patient can sit on the ball and perform arm and leg movements maintaining the neutral spine. Additionally, the patient can lie supine on a surface and put his or her legs on the ball and bridge, or the patient can maintain a bridging position lying with his or her back on the ball and feet on the floor. Catching and throwing activities, wobble boards, and trampolines can be used. Activities should also incorporate patient-specific sport, leisure, or work activities, such as lifting and weight training.

Evidence suggests that it may take several months to accomplish the goals of an exercise program and, further, that low back exercises may be more effective when performed daily (71).

PREVENTING LOW BACK PAIN

Interestingly, just as much of the evidence for clinical care of persons with low back pain is of unsubstantiated effectiveness, interventions to prevent primary (first episode) or recurrent low back pain are also of unsubstantiated effectiveness. We know a little about what has not been found helpful. In a review article, Krismer and van Tulder (12) reported that pharmacologic treatment has no demonstrated effect in preventing nonspecific low back pain or preventing it from becoming chronic. Likewise, the use of lumbar supports in preventing low back pain has not been effective.

Investigators have associated higher levels of cardiovascular fitness with a decreased incidence of low back pain (72) and with effective interventions for both acute and chronic low back pain (53,73). Therefore, patients are typically encouraged to continue with an aerobic exercise program. This may or may not reduce the likelihood of recurrence, but does provide general health benefits. In addition, some individuals should be encouraged to continue other specifically selected exercises based on

their individual movement impairments, and encouraged to use the protective neutral spine position, especially in activities that stress the lumbar spine, such as lifting.

Other recommendations (based on associated versus causal data) that may be helpful in preventing low back pain are to quit smoking, change positions frequently, lose weight, and to comply with safe lifting standards and general ergonomic guidelines.

SUMMARY

General recommendations for treatment of *adults with acute or recurrent low back* currently consist of individualized patient education, acetaminophen, NSAIDs, spinal manipulation for patients without radiculopathy, activity modifications, rest for up to 2 days for patients without leg pain, gradual resumption of activity, trunk exercises, and aerobic activities. General nonpharmacologic recommendations for *adults with chronic low back* pain currently consist of supervised, individualized general exercise programs that incorporate stretching and strengthening. Intensive interdisciplinary rehabilitation may be justified. Although evidence from large randomized. controlled trials indicating the role of particular exercises in the treatment and *prevention of low back pain* is increasing, it is still limited and fairly general. Research in this area is a high priority because of the exorbitant cost of low back pain and findings that suggest that surgery may not be the better option in a large number of cases.

Thus far, the key points with respect to exercise programs seem to be to (*a*) relieve symptoms with individualized direction-specific exercises, manipulation, or stabilization exercises; (*b*) retrain and increase the endurance of the core stabilizing muscles, as needed; (*c*) introduce more dynamic stabilization activities only after successfully training and recruitment the deep stabilizing muscles; (*d*) maintain a neutral spine position with co-contraction of the rectus abdominis, pelvic floor, and lumbar multifidi during activities that stress the spine; (*e*) develop extremity mobility and flexibility and strength; and (*f*) condition aerobically.

Meanwhile, we continue our quest for the right thing, for the right person, at the right time, done the right way.

REFERENCES

1. Manek NJ, MacGregor AJ. Epidemiology of back disorders: prevalence, risk factors, and prognosis. *Curr Opin Rheumatol* 2005;17: 134–40.
2. Andersson GB. Epidemiology of low back pain. *Acta Orthop Scand Suppl* 1998;281:28–31.
3. Frymoyer JW, Cats-Buril WL. An overview of the incidences and cost of low back pain. *Orthop Clin North Am* 1991;22:263–71.
4. Walker BF. The prevalence of low back pain: A systematic review of the literature 1966 to1998. *J Spinal Disor* 2000;13:205–17.
5. Hestbaek L, Leboef-Yde C, Manniche C. Low back pain: what is the long term cause? A review of studies of general patient populations. *Eur Spine.* 2003;12:149–65.

6. Troup JD, Martin JW, Lloyd DC. Back pain in industry: A prospective survey. *Spine* 1981;6:61–9.

7. Anderson RA. A case study in integrating medicine: alternate theories and the language of biomedicine. *J Altern Complement Med* 1999;5:165–73.

8. Frymoyer JW. Can low back pain disability be prevented? *Baillieres Clin Rheumo* 1992;6:595–606.

9. National Institute of Neurological Disorders and Stroke. Web site [Internet]. NIH, Bethesda, MD: National Institute of Neurological Disorders and Stroke. Low back pain fact sheet; [cited 2007 Aug 12]. Available from: http://www.ninds.nih.gov/disorders/backpain/detail_backpain.htm

10. Center for Disease Control and Prevention. Prevalence of disabilities and associated health conditions among adults: United States, 1999. *MMWR* 2001;50:120–5.

11. World Health Organization Web site [Internet]. Geneva: Towards a Common language for Functioning, Disability and Health ICF; 2002. Available from: http://www.who.int/classifications/icf/site/beginners/bg.pdf.

12. Krismer M, van Tulder M, The Low Back Pain Group of the Bone and Joint Health Strategies for Europe Project. Low back pain (nonspecific). *Best Pract Res Clin Rheumatol* 2007;21:77–91.

13. Nelemans PJ, deBie RA, deVet HCW, Sturmans F. Injection therapy for subacute and chronic benign low back pain. *Cochrane Database Syst Rev* 2000(2):CD001824.

14. Bogduk N. *Clinical Anatomy of the Lumbar Spine and Sacrum,* 3rd ed. New York: Churchill Livingstone; 1997:187–213.

15. Kuslich SD, Ulstrom CL, Michael CJ. The tissue origin of low back pain and sciatica: a report of pain response to tissue stimulation during operations on the lumbar spine using local anesthesia. *Orthop Clin North Am* 1991;22:181–7.

16. Schwarzer, AC, Aprill CN, Derby R, et al. The relative contributions of the disc and zygapophyseal joint in chronic low back pain. *Spine* 1994;19:801–6.

17. Jönsson B, Strömqvist B. Clinical appearance of contained and non-contained lumbar disc herniation. *J Spinal Disord* 1996;9:32–8.

18. Sahrmann SA. *Diagnosis and Treatment of Movement Impairment Syndromes.* St. Louis: Mosby; 2001:6.

19. Kirkaldy-Willis WH. Three phases of the spectrum of degenerative disease. In: Kirkaldy-Willis WH, Burton CV, eds. *Managing Low Back Pain,* 3rd ed. New York: Churchill-Livingstone; 1992: 105–19.

20. Waddell G. *The Back Pain Revolution.* Edinburgh: Churchill Livingstone; 1998:9–25.

21. Hurwitz EL, Morgenstern H. Correlates of back problems and back related disability in the United States. *J Clin Epidemiol* 1997;50: 669–81.

22. Kopec JH, Sayre EC, Esclaile JM. Predictors of back pain in a general population cohort. *Spine* 2004;79:70–7.

23. Manchikanti L. Epidemiology of low back pain. *Pain Physician* 2000;3:167–92.

24. Waddell G, Newton M, Henderson I, et al. A Fear-Avoidance Beliefs Questionnaire (FABQ) and the role of fear-avoidance beliefs in chronic low back pain and disability. *Pain* 1993;52:157–68.

25. Beck AT, Ward CH, Mendelson M, et al. An inventory for measuring depression. *Arch Gen Psychiatry* 1961;4:53–63.

26. DeRosa CP, Porterfield JA. A physical therapy model for the treatment of low back pain. *Phys Ther* 1992;72:261–9.

27. American Physical Therapy Association. Guide to physical therapist practice, 2nd ed. *Phys Ther* 2001;81:9–744.

28. Cassidy JD, Carroll LJ, Cote P. The Saskatchewan health and back pain survey. The prevalence of low back pain and related disability in Saskatchewan adults. *Spine* 1998;23:1860–6.

29. Abenhaim L, Rossignol M, Gobeille D, et al. The prognostic consequences of making the initial medical diagnosis of work-related back injuries. *Spine* 1995;20:791–5.

30. Lawrence RC, Helmick CG, Arnett FC, et al. Estimates of the prevalence of arthritis and selected musculoskeletal disorders in the United States. *Arthritis Rheum* 1998;41:778–99.

31. Chou R, Qaseem A, Snow V, et al. Diagnosis and treatment of low back pain: A joint clinical practice guideline from the American College of Physicians and the American Pain Society. *Ann Intern Med* 2007;147:478–91.

32. Eliasson K, Elfving B, Nordgren B, et al. Urinary incontinence in women with low back pain. *Man Ther* 2008;13:206–12.

33. Fairbank JC, Couper J, Davies JB, et al. The Oswestry low back pain disability questionnaire. *Physiotherapy* 1980;66:271–3.

34. Roland M, Morris R. A study of the natural history of back pain. Part I: development of a reliable and sensitive measure of disability in low back pain. *Spine* 1983;8:141–4.

35. Stratford P, Gill C, Westaway M, et al. Assessing disability and change on individual patients: A report of a patient specific measure. *Physiother Can* 1995;47:258–63.

36. Sahrmann SA. *Diagnosis and Treatment of Movement Impairment Syndromes.* St. Louis: Mosby; 2001:9–50.

37. Meadows JTS. *Orthopedic Differential Diagnosis in Physical Therapy: A Case Study Approach.* New York: McGraw-Hill; 1999:4.

38. Panjabi MM. The stabilizing system of the Spine. Part II: Neutral zone and instability hypothesis. *J Spinal Dis* 1992;5:390–7.

39. Sahrmann SA. *Diagnosis and Treatment of Movement Impairment Syndromes.* St. Louis: Mosby; 2001:51–119.

40. Pye SR, Reid DM, Smith R, et al. Radiographic features of lumbar disc degeneration and self-reported back pain. *J Rheumatol* 2004; 31:753–8.

41. Scientific approach to the assessment and management of activity-related spinal disorders. A monograph for clinicians. Report of the Quebec Task Force on Spinal Disorders. *Spine* 1987;12:S1–59.

42. Fritz JM, Cleland JA, Childs JD. Subgrouping patients with low back pain: Evolution of a classification approach to physical therapy. *J Orthop Sports Phys Ther* 2007;37:290–302.

43. Delitto A, Erhard RE, Bowling RW. A treatment-based classification approach to low back syndrome: Identifying and staging patients for conservative treatment. *Phys Ther* 1995;75:470–85.

44. Childs JD, Fritz JM, Flynn TW, et al. A clinical prediction rule to identify patients with low back pain most likely to benefit from spinal manipulation: A validation study. *Ann Intern Med* 2004;141: 920–8.

45. Flynn T, Fritz J, Whitman J, et al. A clinical prediction rule for classifying patients with low back pain who demonstrate short-term improvement with spinal manipulation. *Spine* 2002;27:2835–43.

46. Hicks GE, Fritz JM, Delitto A, et al. Preliminary development of a clinical prediction rule for determining which patients with low back pain will respond to a stabilization exercise program. *Arch Phys Med Rehabil* 2005;86:1753–62.

47. Kane RL. Looking for physical therapy outcomes. *Phys Ther* 1994;74: 425–9.

48. van Tulder MV, Scholten RJ, Koes BW, et al. Nonsteroidal anti-inflammatory drugs for low back pain: A systematic review within the Cochrane Collaboration Back Review Group. *Spine* 2000;25:2501–13.

49. Cherkin DC, Wheeler KJ, Barlow W, et al. Medication use for low back pain in primary care. *Spine* 1998;23:607–14.

50. Philadelphia Panel evidenced-based clinical practice guidelines on selected rehabilitation interventions for low back pain. *Phys Ther* 2001;81:1641–74.

51. Greenman PE. *Principles of Manual Medicine.* Baltimore: Williams & Wilkins; 1989:88–93.

52. Klaber Moffett JA, Carr J, Howarth E. High fear-avoiders of physical activity benefit from an exercise program for patients with back pain. *Spine* 2004;29:1167–72.

53. Bigos S, Bower O, Braen G, et al. *Acute Low Back Pain in Adults.* US Department of Health and Human Services. Public Health Service. Agency for Health Care Policy and Research Guideline No. 14. AHCPR Publication No. 97-N012. Rockville, MD, February 1997.

54. Waddell G, Feder G, Lewis M. Systematic reviews of bed rest and advice to stay active for acute low back pain. *Br J Gen Pract* 1997; 47:647–52.

55. Deyo RA, Diehl AK, Rosenthal M. How many days of bed rest for acute low back pain? A randomized clinical trial. *N Engl J Med* 1986;23:1064–70.

56. Hodges PW, Richardson CA. Contraction of the abdominal muscles associated with movement of the lower limb. *Phys Ther* 1997;77: 132–42.

57. Hodges PW, Richardson CA. Feedforward contraction of the transversus abdominis is not influenced by the direction of arm movement. *Exp Brain Res* 1997;114:362–70.

58. Sihvonen T, Lindgren KA, Airaksinen O, et al. Movement disturbances of the lumbar spine and abnormal back muscle electromyographic findings in recurrent low back pain. *Spine* 1997;22:289–95.

59. Hides JA, Richardson CA, Jull GA. Multifidus muscle recovery is not automatic after resolution of acute, first-episode low back pain. *Spine* 1996;21:2763–9.

60. Neumann P, Gill V. Pelvic floor and abdominal muscle interaction: EMG activity and intra-abdominal pressure. *Int Urogynecol J* 2002; 13:125–32.

61. Richardson C, Jull G, Hodges P, et al. *Therapeutic Exercise for Spinal Segmental Stabilization in Low Back Pain: Scientific Basis and Clinical Approach.* Edinburgh: Churchill Livingstone; 1999:17.

62. Richardson C, Jull G, Hodges P, et al. *Therapeutic Exercise for Spinal Segmental Stabilization in Low Back Pain: Scientific Basis and Clinical Approach.* Edinburgh: Churchill Livingstone; 1999:105–23.

63. The mainstreaming of alternative medicine. *Consumer Reports.* May 2000:17–25.

64. van Tulder MV, Malmivarra A, Esmail R, et al. Exercise therapy for low back pain (Cochrane Review). In: *The Cochrane Library*, Issue 2, 2001. Oxford: Update Software.

65. McKenzie RA, May S. *The Lumbar Spine: Mechanical Diagnosis and Therapy.* Vol. 1. Waikanae, New Zealand: Spinal Publications New Zealand Ltd; 2003:139–80.

66. Fritz JM, George S. The use of a classification approach to identify subgroups of patients with acute low back pain. Interrater reliability and short-term treatment outcomes. *Spine* 2000;25:106–14.

67. Donelson R, Silva G, Murphy K. Centralization phenomenon. Its usefulness in evaluating and treating referred pain. *Spine* 1990;15:211–3.

68. Sahrmann SA. *Diagnosis and Treatment of Movement Impairment Syndromes.* St. Louis: Mosby; 2001:4.

69. Richardson CA, Jull GA. Muscle control–pain control. What exercises would you prescribe? *Man Ther* 1995;1:2–10.

70. Gill KP, Callaghan MJ. The measurement of lumbar proprioception in individuals with and without low back pain. *Spine* 1998;23: 371–7.

71. McGill SM. Low back exercises: Evidence for improving exercise regimens. *Spine* 1998;78:754–65.

72. Cady LD, Bischoff DP, O'Connell ER, et al. Strength and fitness and subsequent back injuries in firefighters. *J Occup Med* 1979;21: 269–72.

73. van Tulder MV, Koes BW, Bouter LM. Conservative treatment of acute and chronic nonspecific low back pain. A systematic review of randomized controlled trials of the most common interventions. *Spine* 1997;22:2128–56.

74. Rubin DI. Epidemiology and risk factors for spine pain. *Neurol Clin* 2007;25:353–71.

SUGGESTED READING

Liemohn W. *Exercise Prescription and the Back.* New York: McGraw-Hill; 2001.

Low Back Pain Exercise Guide. American Academy of Orthopedic Surgeons. http://orthoinfo.aaos.org/topic.cfm?topic=A003302. Accessed 05/29/2008.

NIAMS National Institute of Arthritis and Musculoskeletal and Skin Diseases, National Institutes of Health, Departement of Health and Human Services. http://www.niams.nih.gov/Health_Info/Back_Pain/default.asp. Accessed 05/29/2008.

SUGGESTED RESOURCES

Agency for Healthcare Research and Quality
540 Gaither Road
Rockville, MD 20850
Phone: 301-427-1364
Website: http://www.ahrq.gov

American Academy of Orthopedic Surgeons (AAOS)
P.O. Box 2058
Des Plains, IL 60017
Toll Free: 1-800-824-BONE (2663)
E-mail: pemr@aaos.org
Website: http://www.aaos.org

American College of Rheumatology (ACR)
1800 Century Place, Suite 250
Atlanta, GA 30347-4300
Phone: 404-633-3777
Website: http://www.rheumatology.org

American Physical Therapy Association
1111 North Fairfax Street
Alexandria, VA 22314-1488
Toll Free: 1-800-999-2782
Website: www.apta.org

Arthritis Foundation
P.O. Box 7669
Atlanta, GA 30357-0669
Toll Free: 1-800-283-7800
Website: http://www.arthritis.org

National Institute of Arthritis and Musculoskeletal and Skin Diseases (NIAMS)
Information Clearing House
National Institutes of Health
1 AMS Circle
Bethesda, MD 20892-3675
Toll Free: 1-877-22NIAMS (226-4267)
Phone: 1-301-495-4484
TTY: 301-565-2966
Fax: 301-718-6366
E-mail: NIAMSinfo@mail.nih.gov
Website: http://www.niams.nih.gov

National Institute of Neurological Disorders and Stroke (NINDS)
NIH Neurological Institute
P.O. Box 3801
Bethesda, MD 20824
Toll Free: 1-800-352-9424
Phone: 1-301-496-5751
TTY: 1-301-468-5981
Website: http://www.ninds.nih.gov

North American Spine Society (part of AAOS)
22 Calendar Court 2nd Floor
Le Grange, IL 60525
Toll Free: 1-877-SPINEDR (774-6337)
Website: http://www.spine.org

Amputation

EPIDEMIOLOGY AND PATHOPHYSIOLOGY

Amputations have historically been described in two major categories: upper extremity and lower extremity. Most (80%) of lower-extremity (LE) amputations are the direct result of peripheral vascular disease and diabetes (1), with trauma (e.g., vehicular accidents or job-related accidents) being the second most prevalent cause. Major causes of upper-extremity (UE) amputations are vehicular accidents, severe lacerations from tools or machinery, and frostbite. Curative treatment of tumors, such as a malignant osteogenic sarcoma that has not yet metastasized, and congenital limb anomalies are additional causes for both upper- and lower-extremity amputations. Amputations caused by infection have been significantly reduced since the advent of antibiotics, improved aseptic surgical techniques, and sepsis control.

LOWER-EXTREMITY AMPUTATIONS

Major lower extremity amputations are classified into the following categories:

- Syme's (transsection of distal tibia and fibula through cancellous bone with preservation of the calcaneal fat pad)
- Transtibial, previously known as below-knee (amputation through the tibia and fibula)
- Transfemoral, previously known as above-knee (amputation through the femur)
- Hip disarticulation (separation of femur from the acetabulum)
- Transpelvic amputation, previously known as hemipelvectomy (removal of any portion of the pelvis and all distal parts)
- Translumbar amputation, previously known as hemicorporectomy (removal of the entire pelvis and all distal tissue)

Lower extremity amputations, as well as upper eextremity amputations, can be further classified as involving one limb (unilateral) or both limbs (bilateral). For instance, a person could have a unilateral transtibial amputation (one leg, below-knee) or bilateral transtibial-transfemoral amputations (one leg below-knee, one leg above knee).

It is important to note that the energy expenditure when walking with a prosthesis is greater and walking speed slower for LE amputees when compared with persons with intact extremities, and the increased energy cost is directly related to the level and cause of amputation (2–6). That is, the more LE involved (transtibial versus transfemoral, unilateral versus bilateral) and if the cause of amputation was vascular (i.e., not traumatic), the greater the energy expended at a given walking speed and the slower the walking speed. It has been demonstrated, however, that energy expenditure of ambulation can be lowered when LE amputees are involved in an exercise program that improves cardiovascular fitness (7).

UPPER-EXTREMITY AMPUTATIONS

Amputations of the upper extremity are commonly categorized as either below-elbow or above-elbow amputation. Within these two major categories are several subcategories that are listed in Table 14.1. Upper-extremity amputations have little effect on the individual's ambulatory capacity and, therefore, have much less effect on activity level. Upper-extremity amputees have no greater risk of cardiovascular disease, hypertension, obesity, or adult-onset diabetes than able-bodied individuals (8,9).

CLINICAL EXERCISE PHYSIOLOGY

Risks and complications from amputations are divided into **preprosthetic** (or postoperative) and **postprosthetic** types. Preprosthetic complications include delayed healing, which can be caused by inappropriate amputation-level selection, suboptimal operative technique, inadequate postoperative management, and infection. The closure site of the amputation must have an adequate amount of soft-tissue envelope to decrease the risk of the underlying bone adhering to the skin on the residual limb (i.e., stump). The risk of flexion contractions increases when the patient maintains a flexed limb posture for long periods, which is generally the position of comfort. Flexure contracture of the knee and hip is common for both below-knee amputations and above-knee amputations, respectively. Contracture of the shoulder to a position of glenohumeral adduction and forward flexion is common in UE amputees. Flexion contracture of the

TABLE 14.1. SUBCATEGORIES OF BELOW-ELBOW AND ABOVE-ELBOW AMPUTATIONS

CATEGORY AND SUBCATEGORY	DESCRIPTION
Below Elbow	
Partial hand	One or more digits, could include the radial or ulnar borders of the hand
Wrist disarticulation	Removal of all portions of the hand distal to the radioulnar joint
Long below-elbow	Residual limb approximately 8–10 inches from center of the lateral epicondyle
Medium below-elbow	Residual limb approximately 6–8 inches in length
Short below-elbow	Residual limb approximately 2–4 inches from the center of the lateral epicondyle
Above Elbow	
Elbow disarticulation	Spares the entire length of the humerus
Long above-elbow	Residual limb 50%–90% original length of humerus
Short above-elbow	Residual limb 30%–50% original length of humerus
Shoulder disarticulation	Amputation of the arm from 30% of length of original humerus through the shoulder

elbow is common in a below-elbow amputation. Early, aggressive range-of-motion (ROM) exercises must be instituted, as soon as the postoperative pain has decreased to a tolerable level, to prevent these contractures. If postoperative pain is not controlled early, pain medications may be warranted to allow the patient to gain valuable ROM in this critical time period.

It is important to improve muscular strength of the residual limb to prepare for the prosthesis. This can be done by manual resistive isometric and isotonic training. In most cases, it is best to begin treatment with a static isometric hold techniques, alternating isometrics, progressing to submaximal isotonic exercise. Isotonic exercise training allows the patient to move the residual limb through the full ROM as the assistant provides manual hand resistance to the movement. This improves muscular strength at the knee and hip or at the elbow and shoulder for all movements required of the below-knee and above-elbow amputations, respectively.

Postprosthetic complications can be the result of residual limb pain, adherence of skin to bone, insensitive skin leading to overuse and tissue breakdown, poor prosthetic fit, and body or bone overgrowth in children. These complications for LE amputations present a major obstacle for weight-bearing movements and, therefore, limit activities of daily living (ADL). Although these complications may only be temporary (i.e., days to weeks), the patient's overall physical capacities (aerobic power, muscle flexibility, muscle strength, and endurance of uninvolved limbs) could significantly deteriorate. It is recommended that, in addition to ROM exercises, limited or partial weight-bearing exercises (e.g., upper or lower-

body ergometers, such as the Schwinn Air-Dyne, arm crank ergometers, swimming) be performed to prevent overall physical deconditioning during recovery times.

Prosthetic use for UE amputation is encouraged as soon as pain is tolerable to enable the individual to have prehension (grabbing or seizing of an object) from the involved extremity and ultimately to restore body image. Functional use of the upper extremity is paramount to most UE amputees. Normal functioning of the involved upper extremity, including dexterity and coordination of the prosthetic arm and hand, involves daily training and practice. In addition to dexterity and coordination, the ability to learn tactile sensation, proprioception, pressure, and position sense of the involved limb is equally important. As with LE amputations, the greater the length of the UE residual limb, the better the prosthetic fit and, therefore, more functional ability is maintained. Therefore, a patient with a below-elbow amputation will fare better than a patient with an above-elbow amputation.

One biomechanical problem of concern for the amputee is the change in his or her center of gravity. The center of gravity is the one single point in the body where every portion of body mass is equally distributed. This point for an able-bodied adult is positioned slightly anterior to the second sacral vertebra (10). The loss of a limb will shift this position to the contralateral side of the body (i.e., the side opposite the amputated limb). This shift in the center of gravity will require greater muscular strength and endurance as well as better balance on the opposite side of the body to compensate for this shift. Balance and proprioception exercises will assist with center of gravity changes and help with gait. Weight shifting (side-to-side, forward-backward, and diagonal) will allow patients to better assess their balance limits as well as gain independence for activities, such as walking independently. Advanced activities, such as timed single-leg stance, side-stepping, braiding (carioca), and forward and backward walking all enhance ambulation abilities.

Regardless of the level of amputation, therapeutic exercise is needed to help decrease pain and swelling; increase residual limb muscular strength, endurance, and ROM; and maintain neuromuscular patterns, kinesthesis, proprioception, and balance.

Therapeutic exercise for LE amputations that incorporates the involved extremity should be performed for cardiovascular endurance, muscular strength, and endurance and for ROM, proprioception, and balance. An LE amputation will hinder, to varying extents, the amputee's ability to run or jog, and, in some cases, walk. Therefore, cardiovascular fitness is generally more affected by an LE amputation than by a UE amputation because the UE amputee still has full function of his or her lower extremities. LE amputees who find it difficult to perform LE cardiovascular exercise with a prosthesis can perform such modes of exercise as swimming, combined upper- and lower-body cycle ergometers, or arm ergometry.

One of the most important, yet most overlooked, regions of the body, which also needs strength and ROM exercises for LE amputees, includes the lower back, abdomen, hip–pelvic girdle, and upper thigh musculature. A recent study found that chronic low back pain was found amoung 89.6% of 37 patients following lower limb amputation (11). The strength of this body region is crucial for LE amputations because it provides a base that maintains both static and dynamic stability. Without proximal stability of the abdomen, hips, and upper thighs, coordinated or noncompensated movements of the distal extremities will be limited. Therefore, during both pre- and postprosthetic phases, stretching and strengthening exercises for these areas of the body are essential. Stretching of the lower back and hip muscles can be performed using the single and double knee-to-chest stretches, lower trunk rotation stretch, and hip flexor, quadriceps, and hamstring stretches. Trunk and hip stability and strength can be gained by performing partial abdominal curl-ups, pelvic tilt, straight-leg raise, and any other core stability training exercise. Proprioception and balance training can be performed initially on a stable base, then progress to a moveable surface, such as a dynadisk (i.e., wobble board) or theraball (i.e., big bouncy Swiss-ball). Exercises can also incorporate devices, such as elastic tubing, medicine balls, or manual resistance movements, with the therapist. Excellent resources that describe balance, agility, coordination, endurance, stretching, and strengthening exercises for LE amputees are found in the following three texts: *Stretching and Strengthening for Lower Extremity Amputees* (12); *Balance, Agility, Coordination and Endurance for Lower Extremity Amputees* (13); and *Home Exercise Guide for Lower Extremity Amputees* (14). Therapeutic exercises of this type may appear easy, but to the LE amputee recovering from trauma or surgery, they can be very fatiguing. Therefore, sufficient recovery time should be included between daily exercise sessions.

Coordinated movement of the arms for the UE amputee depends on the shoulder girdle. These joints include the sternoclavicular joint, acromioclavicular joint, scapulothoracic joint, and the glenohumeral joint. With the exception of a shoulder disarticulation amputation, all four of these joints remain intact with most UE amputations. Initially, full active ROM must be provided through stretching exercises for all the joints listed to ensure adequate excursion of the prosthetic equipment. Exercises to increase muscular strength surrounding these joints include rows, shrugs, overhead press, bench press, and dips. Rotator cuff exercises with elastic tubing can include shoulder abduction, flexion, extension, and internal and external rotation. These exercises can be performed in straight-plane patterns or diagonal patterns. The diagonal pattern will help increase neuromuscular

timing and coordination. Common exercises for muscles of the elbow for below-elbow UE amputees include elbow curls and elbow extensions. As with all of the above exercises, they can initially begin as isometrics, progressing to isotonic strengthening.

PHARMACOLOGY

Most LE amputations are a direct result of peripheral vascular disease and diabetes, and many amputees take drugs specific to these diseases. The kinds of medication usually taken and the effect these medications have on exercise capacity (15) will not be addressed in this chapter.

Most amputees experience the phenomenona called "phantom pain" (i.e., pain emitting from their amputated limb) and "phantom limb" (i.e., the feeling that the amputated limb is still present). Phantom pain is covered in the *Education and Counseling* section of this chapter. Phantom pain from phantom limbs can range from an inconvenience to excruciating in nature. Amputees often obtain relief from this pain by using drugs that are also given to counteract epilepsy or depression, but will have little or no effect on their response to exercise. Some amputees find that their phantom pain is eased by a combination of antidepressants and narcotics (e.g., methadone). An amputee who is taking a narcotic for this phenomenon should consult with his or her physician before beginning an exercise program.

PHYSICAL EXAMINATIONS

The physical examination should start by observing the stump. Skin of the stump is susceptible to problems owing to conditions caused by shear and stress forces or damp or wet stump socks (i.e., caused by perspiration) while wearing the prosthesis (16). Soap, lotion, or topical preparations, as well as the sock or liner used with the prosthesis itself, can cause skin irritation (17). Observation of the skin can reveal numerous problems, such as acroangiodematitis (caused by chronic venous insufficiency), contact dermatitis, bullous deseases (caused by subepidermal bullous autoimmune disease against autoantigens in epidermal basement membrane zone), eczema, epidermal cysts, epidermal hyperplasia, bacterial and fungal infections, discoloration, scarring, or drainage.

Second, different sensations should be tested over dermatone regions. This evaluation should be performed with the patient's eyes closed. A light sweep of the examiner's hands across the skin of the involved limb will determine if the individual can feel light sensation. Vials of warm and cold water should be used to determine temperature sensation, and tactile sensation to a sharp object can be assessed with a paper clip or pinwheel.

Third, the active and passive ROM of the residual limb should be assessed, with special consideration of the proximal joints (which are critical to optimal function of the limb) using a goniometer. Active ROM gives the examiner an indication of the muscles' ability to move the joint, the ROM of that joint, and the patient's willingness to move the extremity. During passive ROM, the examiner moves the extremity through the available ROM while the patient is relaxed. Passive ROM assesses inert structures, such as ligaments, bursa capsules, and cartilage.

Flexibility of the muscles should also be examined because flexibility measurements do differ from ROM measurements. Flexibility measurements place the extremity in specific patterns of movement in an attempt to stretch a specific muscle. These measurements are important, for instance, for an LE amputee who is at risk of developing contracture of the anterior hip musculature, which results in the hip remaining in a slightly flexed position at all times.

And last, manual muscle testing should be assessed to determine the relative strength of the residual limb and the proximal joint. Generally, the manual muscle testing is performed in a static position so that inert tissues will not be involved. Manual muscle testing is usually graded with a 5/5 indicating full strength to 0/5 indicating no strength at all (18).

MEDICAL AND SURGICAL TREATMENTS

The recommended resource for this section is *Atlas of Limb Prosthetics: Surgical, Prosthetic and Rehabilitation Principles* (19).

DIAGNOSTIC TECHNIQUES

Diagnostic techniques pertain to amputees with vascular, hematologic, or metabolic (i.e., diabetes) conditions, and not necessarily to the amputation. Therefore, this is not within the scope of this chapter.

EXERCISE/FITNESS/ FUNCTIONAL TESTING

The basic principles for exercise testing stated in *ACSM's Guidelines for Exercise Testing and Prescription* (20) provide the foundation for this section and the section on, *Exercise Prescription and Programming*. When not otherwise stated, these principles will apply. Special situations created by amputation will be covered in this section.

LOWER-EXTREMITY AMPUTATION

Cardiovascular

For those with unilateral transtibial and transfemoral amputations, bilateral amputations involving both legs below-

knee, and bilateral amputations involving one leg above-knee and one leg below-knee the recommendation for all is to use an ergometer that involves both upper- and lower-body musculature as a mode of testing to determine aerobic fitness. The Schwinn Air-Dyne ergometer would be an example of such a mode. Depending on comfort, above-knee amputees can perform the test with their prosthesis on or off.

The amputee should first practice at work levels of 25 W (150 kpm) and 50 W (300 kpm) for 2 minutes at each level, or until the amputee feels comfortable with the movement. Amputees with peripheral vascular disease, diabetes, deconditioning, or other secondary conditions should start their initial workload at 25 W for 2 minutes, then increase incrementally 12.5 W every minute until volitional exhaustion. Younger or older physically fit amputees can begin at 50 W for 2 minutes and increase incrementally 25 W every minute until volitional exhaustion.

The recommended mode of testing for bilateral, above-knee amputees is the arm crank ergometer (ACE). The ACE should be positioned so that the pedal shaft is level with the amputee's acromioclavicular joint and the ergometer is placed sufficiently far from the patient to allow slight flexion of the elbow at the furthest point of the pedal stroke. If the amputee is deconditioned, owing to a sedentary lifestyle, initial workload should start at 0 W at a constant cadence of 50 rpm for 2 minutes (warm-up) with increases of 5 W every 2 minutes until volitional exhaustion. Younger or more active bilateral above-knee amputees should begin at 5 W for 2 minutes with increases of 5 W every 2 minutes until volitional exhaustion.

Unilateral amputees with peripheral vascular disease (PVD), especially those whose amputation was the results of PVD, may have difficulty with any mode of exercise that involves their lower extremities. ACE has been shown to be a safe and effective alternative for these individuals in detection of coronary artery disease and prescribing safe levels of exercise (21). The same method of testing should be followed as outlined above for bilateral above knee amputees.

Strength, Range-of-Motion, and Endurance Testing

Most upper-body measurement techniques, used (*a*) to assess range-of-motion, and upper-body strength and endurance test protocols and (*b*) to evaluate able-bodied individuals, can be performed by LE amputees. It is suggested that the LE amputee be seated or lie on a bench to allow the amputee to concentrate on his or her performance without concern of maintaining balance while standing. Variations for LE testing protocols depend on the level of amputation and leg involvement. For instance, a unilateral amputee could perform most test protocols used to evaluate able-bodied individuals. Knee flexion and extension tests can be measured for most below-knee amputations, depending on the length of stump, but not above-knee. Except for complete hip disarticulation, hemipelvectomy, or shortness of stump, most hip measurements (e.g., flexion, extension, adduction, abduction) used to evaluate able-bodied individuals can also be used for LE amputees. For upper-body measurements, the amputee should be sitting (as in knee or hip flexion and extension measurements) or prone (as in leg press) to maintain balance. Standing test measurements, such as a squat, should be performed with caution for unilateral amputees and are contraindicated for bilateral amputees.

UPPER-EXTREMITY AMPUTATION

Cardiovascular

As with able-bodied individuals, the treadmill and bicycle protocols outlined in ACSM's Guidelines (20) are applicable to UE amputees.

Strength, Range-of-Motion, and Endurance Testing

A UE amputation presents the opposite situation as with an LE amputation. Most ROM measurements and strength and endurance tests that are used to evaluate able-bodied individuals can be used for UE amputees. The same considerations and limitations are applied to UE amputees for upper extremities as are applied to LE amputees with one exception: The feet and legs for the UE amputee are paramount for balance and stability when performing upper-extremity measurements. Therefore, UE amputees should perform upper-extremity measurements while standing and, if sitting, allow their feet to be in contact with the floor.

EXERCISE PRESCRIPTION AND PROGRAMMING

LOWER-EXTREMITY AMPUTATIONS

Few studies have been published concerning the effects of exercise for LE amputees, but those few do report positive results. James (22) reported that, for healthy male unilateral above-knee amputees, one-legged (noninvolved leg) bicycle ergometry training improved cardiovascular fitness of the participants. Improvement in cardiovascular fitness was also seen for healthy unilateral below- and above-knee amputees, and bilateral below- and above-knee amputees using a Schwinn Air-Dyne ergometer (7). Additionally, following a treadmill training program, a 63-year-old bilateral below-knee amputee with class IV cardiac and restrictive-obstructive pulmonary disease improved cardiovascular fitness, improved cardiac class IV to class II, and therapeutically improved from class E (bedrest) to class C (moderate exercise restriction). An exercise protocol using ACE for LE amputees with PVD was shown to be a safe and effective method in improving upper body work capacity (23). This suggests that amputees, healthy or with secondary disabilities, can improve their fitness levels with exercise using different modes of exercise.

An essential resource for any professional involved in training LE amputees for sport or health is the publication by the Department of Veterans Affairs, *Physical Fitness: A Guide for Individuals with Lower Limb Loss* (24). The publication represents a guide for prescribing exercises that will improve all aspects of physical fitness, including cardiovascular, flexibility, muscular strength and endurance, and motor skills. The publication includes illustrations for calisthenics, stretching exercises, as well as specific muscle strength and endurance exercises for arms, shoulders, legs, abdominals, chest, and back. It also includes training programs for walking, running, aerobic dance, swimming, cycling, rowing, crosscountry skiing, and a variety of sports (e.g., basketball, hockey, soccer, squash). Another good resource for sports and recreation for those with LE amputation is the publication by Kegel (25).

The prescribed number of sets and repetitions for muscle strengthening should be adjusted to the needs of the amputee. The proper frequency, duration, and intensity of cardiovascular exercises should follow those prescribed by ACSM Guidelines (20).

It is important that an amputee have a comfortable prosthetic limb that is suited for the activity or exercise. Activities or exercises such as walking, bicycling, rowing, StairMaster, Body Trec, and other aerobic machines do not require special adaptations to standard artificial limbs. Such activities and exercises, such as running, sprinting, and swimming, do require special adaptations, and these special adaptations are addressed in the text by Burgess and Rappoport (24). It is recommended that amputees work with their prosthetist to obtain any adaptation needed for their prosthetic device.

UPPER-EXTREMITY AMPUTATION

Upper-extremity amputees, because of their intact lower extremities, are not as limited to modes of exercise as LE amputees. All activities and exercises involving the lower extremities that can be performed by able-bodied individuals are applicable to UE amputees.

EDUCATION AND COUNSELING

Phantom limb pain is pain (burning, electric shocks, stabbing sensations) coming from the lost limb; *residual limb pain* is ongoing discomfort at the amputation site; and *phantom limb sensation* is the feeling that the missing limb is still there. Phantom limb sensation is not painful, but sometimes uncomfortable, such as tingling and itching.

Study designs using retrospect surveys have reported that most amputees suffer from this phenomenon, whether the amputation was owing to trauma, surgery, or congenital limb deficiency (26–28). Phantom pain is a part of "the luggage" that comes with amputation for most amputees. Amputees know the difference between pain emitting from the stump (i.e., residual pain) and phantom pain. Pain from the stump usually occurs owing to hair follicle infections, skin or scar tissue breakdown, or from excessive pressure from the prosthetic device. Pain from the stump is recognized by the sensory cerebral hemisphere as pain *from the stump*, not from that portion of the anatomy that has been amputated. Indeed, the sensory cerebral hemisphere recognizes phantom pain as actually originating from the amputated areas of the limb (29).

Although the cause of phantom pain remains an enigma for the amputee, the phenomenon is very real, and it is more common in LE amputations than in UE amputations and more common in proximal than in distal amputations. Amputees have identified exercise, objects approaching the stump, and cold weather as the primary triggers of phantom sensation (27). For instance, LE amputees are more likely to have phantom pain on days when the amputee has used his or her prothesis (e.g., standing, walking, mowing the lawn) for long periods of time. These activities might also intensify phantom pain. However, aerobic exercises using such non–weight-bearing exercise modes as swimming, stationary bicycle ergometry, and rowing ergometry should not cause or intensify phantom pain (author's [KHP] personal experience). If weight-bearing modes of exercise (e.g., jogging, fast walking, StairStepper) are increasing the incidence of phantom pain, it is suggested to substitute non–weight-bearing modes of exercise in their place. Of importance is the need for the LE amputee not to use phantom pain as a reason for eliminating exercise from his or her lifestyle.

Depression has been related to a higher incidence of phantom pain and, therefore, can be a potential barrier to exercise. In a study by Lindesay (30), it was found that many of the amputees with long-standing phantom pain were more depressed when compared with a group of amputees that did not report problems with phantom pain.

Skin breakdowns (blisters) or **hair follicle infections** can significantly affect the activity level of any amputee. Practicing good hygiene for both the residual limb (stump) and the inside lining of the prosthetic limb will help prevent skin problems. Stump socks should be changed daily, and determining the right size and number of stump socks for proper fit is essential to prevent skin irritations and blisters. Amputees have found that the use of nylon sheaths can significantly reduce friction between the skin and the wool or cotton stump sock. Socks should always be changed when damp or wet. Managing body weight is also important to minimize stress on stump and weight-bearing surfaces.

CASE STUDY   Jessica C. Roberts

The following patient was referred for exercise testing for functional assessment and evaluation for a prosthesis. She is a 15-year-old girl who was diagnosed with osteogenic sarcoma. She had a left-arm, above-the-elbow amputation 6 months before the assessment and is currently receiving chemotherapy and radiation treatments. Her stump is still healing, and she has had continuous phantom pains since the operation. She frequently complains of fatigue, has a poor appetite, and spends most of her time in her room watching TV or sleeping.

Throughout her childhood and adolescent years, she participated in organized softball and basketball and, before her diagnosis and operation, had been looking forward to playing for her high school softball and basketball teams.

RESTING DATA

An ECG showed normal sinus rhythm, with a heart rate of 72 bpm and a blood pressure of 118/76 mm Hg.

EXERCISE RESPONSE

The patient performed a modified Bruce Protocol (2-min stages), and the test was terminated after 9 minutes, 13 seconds when the patient reported fatigue and wanted to stop.

The maximal heart rate was 160 bpm and maximal blood pressure was 150/82 mm Hg with normal sinus rhythm.

INTERPRETATION

Although the treadmill test did not identify any cardiac anomalies, the patient is experiencing significant adjustment issues following her diagnosis, amputation, and cancer treatment. The patient has lost 10 pounds, her hair has fallen out, and she has become increasingly withdrawn from her family and friends. It has been determined by her medical staff that the patient has several psychosocial issues to resolve secondary to her amputation. The patient expresses little interest in being fitted for a prosthetic arm because of her concern how friends would respond to the prosthetic device (i.e., altered body image). The patient continues to keep her stump covered in public and in the presence of her family, even though it has healed. She has expressed concerns that people look at her as a "freak" when she is in public because she feels that everyone stares at her amputated arm.

Clinical Implications

The patient's clinical presentation suggests several areas that should be addressed. The patient is experiencing significant grief and loss issues secondary to her amputation and may be clinically depressed. Referral to a pediatric psychologist to work on these adjustment issues is indicated. The patient's difficulties with changed body image place her at risk of rejecting the use of an artificial limb. It is recommended that her physical therapist help her accept the changed body image by allowing the patient to unwrap and manipulate her stump during physical therapy sessions. This will increase her exposure to,

and acceptance of, her changed physical appearance. The physical therapist will also play a crucial role in educating her concerning the importance of maintaining upper-body strength and ROM by prescribing a "training schedule" that will maintain the muscle tone, muscle strength, and flexibility of (a) the shoulder and upper arm to prevent flexion contracture of the shoulder; and (b) the hip on her involved side to maintain posture and upper-body control. Also, the "training schedule" should incorporate balance exercises designed to help her reestablish her center of gravity.

The patient's adjustment to her amputation can be facilitated by introducing her to other adolescents and young adult amputees. Support groups, sports specific for amputees (e.g., paralympics), and written or visual materials about the many options that amputees have in life could help lay the groundwork for a positive transition to prosthetic use. All of these will help the patient come to a realistic evaluation of her situation and will provide her with role models in coping with the challenges in the areas of sports and vocation.

REFERENCES

1. Dillingham TR, Pezzin LE, Mackenzie EJ. Limb amputations and limb deficiency: Epidemiology and recent trends in the United States. *South Med J* 2002;95:875–883,

2. Gonzalez EG, Edelstein JE. Energy expenditure during ambulation. In: Gonzalez EG, Myers SJ, Edelstein JE, et al., eds. *Downey & Darling's Physiological Basis of Rehabilitation Medicine.* Boston: Butterworth Heinemann; 2001:413–446

3. Gailey RS, Wenger MA, Raya M et al. Energy expenditure of transtibial amputees during ambulation at self-selected pace. *Prosthet Orthot Int* 1994;18:84–91.

4. Jaegers SMHJ, Vos LD, Rispens P, et al. The relationship between comfortable and most metabolically efficient walking speed in person with unilateral above-knee amputation. *Arch Phys Med Rehabil* 1993;74:521–525.

5. Nowroozi F, Satonelli MI, Gerber LH. Energy expenditure in hip disarticulation and hemipelvectomy. *Arch Phys Med Rehabil* 1983; 64:300–303.

6. Waters RL, Mulroy SJ. Energy expenditure of walking in individuals with lower limb amputation. In: Smith DG, Michael JW, Bowker JH, eds. *Atlas of Amputations and Limb Deficiencies.* Rosemont, IL: American Academy of Orthopedic Surgeons; 2004:400–403.

7. Pitetti KH, Snell PG, Stray-Gunderson J. Aerobic training exercise for individuals who had amputation of the lower limb. *J Bone Joint Surg* 1987;69:914–921.

8. Hrubec Z, Ryder RA. Traumatic limb amputation and subsequent mortality from cardiovascular disease and other causes. *J Chronic Dis* 1978;33:239–250.

9. Rose HC, Schweitzer P, Charoenkul V, et al. Cardiovascular disease risk factors in combat veterans after traumatic leg amputation. *Arch Phys Med Rehabil* 1987;68:20–23.

10. Braune W, Fischer O. *On the Center of Gravity of the Human Body.* Berlin, Germany: Springer-Verlag; 1984.

11. Kusljugic A, Kapidzic-Durakovic S, Kudumovic Z, et al. Chronic low back pain in individuals with lower-limb amputation. *Bosn J Basic Med Sci* 2006;6(2):67–70.

12. Gailey RS, Gailey AM. *Stretching and Strengthening for Lower Extremity Amputees.* Miami, FL: Advanced Rehabilitation Therapy; 1994. (Correspondence: Advanced Rehabilitation Therapy, Inc., 7641 SW 126th Street, Miami, FL 33156.)

13. Gailey RS, Gailey AM. *Balance, Agility, Coordination and Endurance for Lower Extremity Amputees.* Miami, FL: Advanced Rehabilitation Therapy; 1994.

14. Gailey RS, Gailey AM, Sendelbach SJ. *Home Exercise Guide for Lower Extremity Amputees.* Miami, FL: Advanced Rehabilitation Therapy; 1995.

15. American College of Sports Medicine. *ACSM's Exercise Management for Persons with Chronic Diseases and Disabilities.* Champaign, IL: Human Kinetics; 2003:374.

16. Meulenbelt HEJ, Geertzen JHB, Kijkstra PU, et al. Skin problems in lower limb amputees: An overview by case reports. *J Eur Acad Derm Venereol* 2007;21:147–155.

17. Edelstein JE. Amputations and prostheses. In: Cameron MH, Monroe LG, eds. *Physical Rehabilitation. Evidence-Based Examination, Evaluation, and Intervention.* Philadelphia: Saunders-Elsevier; 2007:267–299.

18. Kendall FP, McCreary EK, Provance PG, et al. *Muscles: Testing and Function.* 5th ed. Baltimore, MD: Lippincott Williams & Wilkins; 2005:4–47.

19. Bowler JH, Michael JW. *Atlas of Limb Prosthetics: Surgical, Prosthetic and Rehabilitation Principles.* American Academy of Orthopaedic Surgeons. St. Louis, MO: Mosby-Year Book; 1992:930.

20. American College of Sports Medicine. *ACSM's Guidelines for Exercise Testing and Prescription.* 6th ed. Philadelphia: Lippincott Williams & Wilkins; 2000.

21. Priebe M, Davidoff G, Lampman RM. Exercise testing and training in patients with peripheral vascular disease and lower extremity amputation. *West J Med* 1991;154:598–601.

22. James U. Effect of physical training in healthy male unilateral above-knee amputees. *Scand J Rehabil Med* 1973;5:88–101.

23. Davidoff G, Lampman R, Westbury L, et al. Exercise testing and training of dysvascular amputees: Safety and efficacy of arm ergometry. *Arch Phys Med Rehabil* 1992; 73:334–338.

24. Burgess EM, Rappoport A. *Physical Fitness: A Guide for Individuals with Lower Limb Loss*. Washington, DC: Department of Veterans Affairs; 1991:245.

25. Kegel B. Physical fitness: Sports and recreation for those with lower limb amputation or impairment. *J Rehabil Res Dev Clin Suppl* 1985; 1:1–125.

26. Machin P, de C Williams AC. Stiff upper lip: Coping strategies of World War II veterans with phantom limb pain. *Clin J Pain* 1998; 14(4):290–294.

27. Wilkins KL, McGrath PJ, Finley GA, et al. Phantom limb sensations and phantom limb pain in child and adolescent amputees. *Pain* 1998;78(1):7–12.

28. Wartan SW, Hamann W, Wedley JR, et al. Phantom pain and sensation among British veterans amputees. *Br J Anaesth* 1997;78(6):652–659.

29. Schmid HJ. Phantom limb after amputation—Overview and new knowledge. *Schweiz Rundsch Med Prax* 2000;89(3):87–94.

30. Lindesay JE. Multiple pain complaints in amputees. *J R Soc Med* 1985;78(6):452–455.

SECTION

III

Neoplastic, Immunologic, and Hematologic Conditions

DAVID NIEMAN, *Section Editor*

PATHOPHYSIOLOGY

Cells that grow out of control and form a mass are called a tumor or neoplasm (i.e., "new growth"). Some tumors, referred to as *benign*, grow and enlarge only at the site where they began. Other tumors, called *malignant* or *cancerous*, have the potential to invade and destroy the normal tissue around them and to spread throughout the body. Cancer is not a single disease, but rather a collection of many different diseases. What cancer cells typically share, however, is changes in the genes that regulate cell division, programmed cell death, and cell mobility. These genetic changes lead to the characteristic features of cancer, namely (*a*) accumulation of abnormal cells, (*b*) invasion of nearby tissues, and (*c*) spread to distant sites. Cancers are classified into several groups, depending on the kind of normal cell from which they arise. The most common cancers develop from epithelial cells that line the body's surfaces. These cancers are called *carcinomas* and they include prostate, breast, colon, lung, and cervical cancers. Cancers can also arise from the cells of the blood (i.e., leukemias), the immune system (i.e., lymphomas), and bone and connective tissues (i.e., sarcomas).

EPIDEMIOLOGY

More than 1.4 million Americans will be diagnosed with cancer in 2007 (Table 15.1) (1). The lifetime probability of being diagnosed with cancer in the United States is about 42% (Table 15.2) (1). Moreover, cancer is the second leading cause of death in the United States after heart disease, with about 560,000 deaths from cancer expected in 2007. The four most common cancers—prostate, lung, breast, and colorectal—account for more than 50% of all new cancer cases and deaths (Table 15.1) (1). In terms of disease burden, men are slightly more likely to develop and die from cancer than women, and older adults are significantly more likely to develop and die from cancer than children or younger adults (Table 15.2) (1). More specifically, about 80% of all cancers are diagnosed in persons aged 60 and older.

Early detection and improved treatments for some cancers have resulted in increased survival rates over the last few decades (1). The current 5-year relative survival rate (adjusted for normal life expectancy) is estimated to be about 66%, although this figure varies considerably, depending on the type of cancer and stage of the disease at diagnosis (Table 15.3) (1). For example, if detected early, the 5-year relative survival rate is more than 90% for common cancers, such as prostate, breast, and colorectal. The high incidence and good survival rates have resulted in more than 10 million cancer survivors in the United States. As defined by the National Coalition for Cancer Survivorship, a cancer survivor is any person diagnosed with cancer, from the time of diagnosis and for the balance of life.

ETIOLOGY AND RISK FACTORS

Although the causes and risk factors for human cancer are diverse—ranging from genetics, to behavior, to the environment—lifestyle factors appear to be paramount. The Harvard Report on Cancer Prevention (2) concluded that nearly two-thirds of cancer mortality in the United States can be linked to tobacco use, poor diet, and lack of exercise (2). Moreover, only 5%–10% of most types of cancer are caused by defects in single genes that run in families, and only a similar small percentage are because of occupational and environmental exposures.

Physical inactivity as a risk factor for cancer has received increased research attention based on a number of plausible biological mechanisms. Over the past decade, mounting evidence has indicated that physical activity may significantly reduce the risk of some cancers (3). The general consensus is that physical activity is (*a*) convincingly associated with the reduced risks of developing colon (4) and breast (5) cancers, (*b*) probably associated with the reduced risk of endometrial cancer (6), and (*c*) possibly associated with the reduced risks of prostate (7) and lung (8) cancers. Moreover, evidence is also available to suggest that physical activity may have a protective effect against ovarian (9), kidney (10), and pancreatic (11) cancers, although definitive conclusions cannot be made at this time. Evidence for other cancers (e.g., lymphomas, testicular, stomach) is currently too sparse to make even tentative conclusions.

TABLE 15.1. ESTIMATED NEW CANCER CASES AND DEATHS FOR THE MOST COMMON CANCERS IN THE UNITED STATES BY SEX

SITE	ESTIMATED NEW CASES			ESTIMATED NEW DEATHS		
	TOTAL	MALE	FEMALE	TOTAL	MALE	FEMALE
All Sites	1,444,920	766,860	678,060	559,650	289,550	270,100
Prostate	218,800	218,890	–	27,050	27,050	–
Lung and Bronchus	213,380	114,760	98,620	160,390	89,510	70,880
Breast	180,510	2,030	178,480	40,910	450	40,460
Colon	112,340	55,290	57,050	52,180	26,000	26,180
Rectum	41,420	23,840	17,580			
Urinary Bladder	67,160	50,040	17,120	13,750	9,630	4,120
Melanoma	59,940	33,910	26,030	8,110	5,220	2,890
Non-Hodgkin lymphoma	63,190	34,200	28,990	18,660	9,600	9,060
Uterine Corpus	39,080	–	39,080	7,400	–	7,400
Ovarian	22,430	–	22,430	15,280	–	15,280

Note: Excludes basal and squamous cell skin cancers and in situ carcinomas except urinary bladder. (Adapted from the American Cancer Society. *Cancer Facts & Figures 2007*. Atlanta, GA: American Cancer Society; 2007.)

COMMON SIGNS AND SYMPTOMS

Because cancer is not one disease, the common signs and symptoms of cancer are not generic but rather are cancer-specific. Most of the signs and symptoms of cancer, however, are similar to those of other medical conditions, and so their presence is not necessarily indicative of cancer. Nevertheless, when these symptoms do occur, it is important to have them checked by a physician. Table 15.4 (12) summarizes the major signs and symptoms for the most common cancer sites.

SCREENING AND DIAGNOSIS

A key to improving survival rates from cancer is early detection of the disease. Screening is the process of identi-

fying disease in people who are asymptomatic. The major advantage of screening is that it can identify abnormalities that may be cancer at an early stage before physical signs and symptoms develop. Screening tests are available for many of the most common types of cancer, including breast, colorectal, prostate, and uterine. No effective screening tests currently exist for lung cancer. The recommended screening procedures for cancer in general and for the most common cancers in particular are provided in Table 15.5(12).

Screening tests for breast cancer include mammography, clinical breast examination (CBE), and breast self-examination (BSE). The most definitive test, called mammography, is a special type of x-ray procedure. Screening tests for colorectal cancer include digital rectal examination (DRE), fecal occult blood (stool blood) test, flexible

TABLE 15.2. PERCENTAGE OF THE UNITED STATES POPULATION DEVELOPING THE MOST COMMON INVASIVE CANCERS OVER SELECTED AGE INTERVALS BY SEX

SITE		BIRTH TO 39	40–59	60–69	70+	BIRTH TO DEATH
All Sites	Male	1.42	8.69	16.58	39.44	45.31
	Female	2.03	9.09	10.57	26.60	37.86
Prostate	Male	0.01	2.59	7.08	13.38	17.12
Lung	Male	0.03	1.09	2.61	6.76	8.02
	Female	0.04	0.85	1.84	4.25	6.15
Breast	Female	0.48	3.98	3.65	6.84	12.67
Colorectal	Male	0.07	0.93	1.67	4.92	5.79
	Female	0.07	0.73	1.16	4.45	5.37
Urinary	Male	0.02	0.41	0.96	3.41	3.61
Bladder	Female	0.01	0.13	0.26	0.96	1.14
Melanoma	Male	0.13	0.53	0.56	1.32	2.04
	Female	0.21	0.42	0.29	0.63	1.38
Non-Hodgkin lymphoma	Male	0.14	0.45	0.57	1.56	2.14
	Female	0.08	0.32	0.44	1.30	1.83
Uterine corpus	Female	0.06	0.70	0.81	1.28	2.49

Note: Excludes basal and squamous cell skin cancers and in situ carcinomas except urinary bladder. (Adapted from the American Cancer Society. *Cancer Facts & Figures 2007*. Atlanta, GA: American Cancer Society; 2007.)

TABLE 15.3. FIVE-YEAR RELATIVE SURVIVAL RATES FOR THE MOST COMMON CANCERS IN THE UNITED STATES BY STAGE AT DIAGNOSIS

SITE	ALL STAGES (%)	LOCAL (%)	REGIONAL (%)	DISTANT (%)
Prostate	99.9	100	—	33.3
Lung	15.0	49.3	15.5	2.1
Breast	88.5	98.1	83.1	26.0
Colorectal	64.1	90.4	68.1	9.8
Urinary bladder	80.8	93.7	46.0	6.2
Melanoma	91.5	99.0	64.9	15.3
Uterine corpus	83.2	95.7	66.9	23.1
Ovarian	44.7	93.1	69.0	29.6

Note: Rates are adjusted for normal life expectancy and are based on cases diagnosed from 1996 to 2002 followed through 2003. (Adapted from the American Cancer Society. *Cancer Facts & Figures 2007*. Atlanta, GA: American Cancer Society; 2007.)

sigmoidoscopy, double contrast barium enema, and colonoscopy. The most definitive test for colorectal cancer is a colonoscopy, which involves visualizing the internal surface of the rectum and large bowel using a flexible fiberoptic tube. Screening tests for prostate cancer include DRE and prostate-specific antigen (PSA) testing. PSA, a substance produced only by the prostate, is measured by a blood test.

Screening tests are only suggestive of cancer; they do not diagnose it. An actual diagnosis of cancer requires analysis of a tissue sample. By examining cells under the microscope, a trained pathologist can almost always distinguish malignant cells from their benign (i.e., nonmalignant) counterparts. The pathologist looks for cells that are frequently dividing, are invading normal surrounding tissue, or have unusual cellular features, such as large and disorganized nuclei. Increasingly, it is possible to prove

TABLE 15.4. SIGNS AND SYMPTOMS FOR THE MOST COMMON CANCERS

CANCER SITE	SIGNS AND SYMPTOMS
Breast	Breast lump, thickening, swelling, distortion, or tenderness; skin irritation or dimpling; and nipple pain, scaliness, or retraction.
Colorectal	Rectal bleeding, blood in the stool, or a change in bowel habits.
Lung	Persistent cough, sputum (spit or phlegm) streaked with blood, chest pain, and recurring pneumonia or bronchitis.
Prostate	Weak or interrupted urine flow; inability to urinate, or difficulty starting or stopping the urine flow; the need to urinate frequently, especially at night; blood in the urine; pain or burning on urination; continuing pain in lower back, pelvis, or upper thighs.

(Adapted from the American Cancer Society. *Cancer Prevention and Early Detection Facts & Figures 2007*. Atlanta, GA: American Cancer Society; 2007.)

that suspicious cells are truly malignant by identifying cancer-related genetic mutations using the techniques of molecular biology.

STAGING

After the initial diagnosis, it is important to learn the extent to which the disease has spread or progressed. Cancer staging is essential in determining the choice of therapy and assessing prognosis. Cancer stage is determined by patient history, physical examination, laboratory testing, and diagnostic imaging (e.g., chest radiography, computed tomography [CT], magnetic resonance imaging [MRI]). A number of different staging systems are currently used to classify tumors, but the most common is the Tumor (T), Node (N), Metastasis (M) system (13). The TNM system stages cancer based on the size of the primary tumor (T), the involvement of regional lymph nodes (N), and the presence or absence of distant metastases (M). Once the T, N, and M are determined, a "stage" can be assigned, generally ranging from I (least advanced) through IV (most advanced) and often including many substages (e.g., Ic, IIa, IIb, IIIa, etc.). In general, regionally confined cancers are stage I and II, locally advanced cancers are stage III, and cancers with overt distant metastases are stage IV.

MEDICAL AND SURGICAL TREATMENTS

Cancer treatments may be used to cure cancer, to prolong life when a cure is not possible, or to improve symptom management and quality of life. The three primary cancer treatment modalities are surgery, radiation therapy, and systemic therapy (i.e., drugs). Surgery is the oldest and most frequently used modality in cancer therapy and is the treatment of choice for most localized carcinomas and sarcomas. Cancer operations can be classified as either radical or conservative. Radical resections, which attempt to encompass all gross and microscopic tumor in a single operation, are performed with curative intent. These operations commonly involve excision of tumor and draining regional lymph nodes as a single specimen. Conservative surgeries are usually performed to minimize the volume of tissue removed and preserve organ function. In general, conservative surgeries require additional nonsurgical treatment with radiotherapy, systemic therapy, or both to eradicate residual cancer cells. Some common cancer operations and their sequelae are described in Table 15.6.

Radiation therapy is the treatment of cancer using ionizing radiation. It is considered a local-regional treatment, with the goal to irradiate the known tumor volume while sparing adjacent radiation-sensitive tissues. Several types of radiation are used in the clinic, but most radiotherapy treatments are external beams of high-energy photons produced by linear accelerators or from the decay of

TABLE 15.5. SUMMARY OF THE AMERICAN CANCER SOCIETY'S RECOMMENDATIONS FOR THE EARLY DETECTION OF CANCER IN ASYMPTOMATIC PEOPLE

SITE	RECOMMENDATION
General	During regular health examinations, a cancer-related portion should include health counseling and, depending on a person's age, might include examinations for cancers of the thyroid, oral cavity, skin, lymph nodes, testes, and ovaries, as well as for some nonmalignant diseases.
Breast	Women 40 and older should have an annual mammogram, an annual clinical breast examination (CBE) by a healthcare professional. The CBE should conducted close to the scheduled mammogram. Women ages 20–39 years should have a CBE by a healthcare professional every 3 years and should know self-breast examinations are an option. Woman with increased risk should have additional tests, more frequent tests, or tests done at a younger age.
Colorectal	Men and women aged 50 or older should follow one of three examination schedules: (1) an annual fecal occult blood test and a flexible sigmoidoscopy every 5 years, (12) a colonoscopy every 10 years, or (49) a double-contrast barium enema every 5–10 years. A digital rectal examination (DRE) should be done at the same time as sigmoidoscopy, colonoscopy, or double-contrast barium enema. People who are at moderate or high risk for colorectal cancer should talk with a doctor about a different testing schedule.
Prostate	A prostate-specific antigen (PSA) blood test and a DRE should be offered annually to men 50 and older who have a life expectancy of at least 10 years and to younger men (i.e., 45 years) who are at high risk.
Uterus	*Cervix:* All women who are or have been sexually active or who are 21 and older should have an annual Pap test and pelvic examination. After three or more consecutive satisfactory examinations with normal findings, the Pap test may be performed less frequently; however, given certain risk factors, a Pap test may need to be performed more frequently. *Endometrium:* At the time of menopause woman should be informed of the risk of endometrial cancer. Annual screening using an endometrial biopsy beginning at age 35 for woman at risk for hereditary nonpolyposis colon cancer.

(Adapted from the American Cancer Society. Cancer Prevention and Early Detection *Cancer Facts & Figures 2007.* Atlanta, GA: American Cancer Society; 2007.)

cobalt. These photons penetrate into tissue and produce ionized (electrically charged) particles that damage DNA. This DNA damage usually inhibits cell replication and often leads to cell death. Radiation therapy is delivered in repeated small doses over an extended period of time to kill cancer cells without undue damage to normal cells. A total dose of 60 grays (Gy), for example, may be "fractionated" into 2 Gy every weekday for 6 weeks in the treatment of breast cancer. A full course of external beam radiotherapy can range from 8 weeks of low-fraction therapy administered each weekday (given with curative intent) to a single high-dose treatment (given to palliate a

TABLE 15.6. COMMON CANCER OPERATIONS AND THEIR SEQUELAE

OPERATION	DESCRIPTION TYPE	SEQUELAE
Pulmonary lobectomy	Removal of one lobe of one lung Conservative	Reduced lung capacity and function, dyspnea, deconditioning
Pneumonectomy	Removal of one entire lung Radical	Reduced lung capacity and function dyspnea, deconditioning
Radical neck dissection	Removal of cervical lymphatics Radical	Reduced neck ROM and muscle strength; occasional CN XI palsy
Mastectomy and axillary node dissection	Removal of entire breast and Radical	Chest wall pain, reduced arm ROM, draining lymphatics; occasionally arm lymphedema
Lumpectomy and axillary node dissection	Removal of breast tumor and Conservative	Reduced arm ROM, occasional arm sparing remaining breast, arm lymphedema
Radical prostatectomy	Removal of prostate, seminal Radical	Urinary incontinence, erectile dysfunction vesicles, and ampullae of vesa are common, deconditioning deferentia
Abdominoperineal resection	Removal of rectum and draining Radical	Patient may require ostomy, deconditioning lymphatics
Hemicolectomy	Removal of involved colon and Radical	Patient occasionally requires ostomy, draining lymphatics; deconditioning, diarrhea
Limb amputation	Removal of tumor with margin of normal tissue Radical	Occasional chronic pain syndromes, deconditioning
Limb-sparing surgery	Removal of tumor and some tissue Conservative	Post operative casing leads to decreased joint ROM and muscle atrophy, occasional chronic pain syndromes, deconditioning

CN, cranial nerve; ROM, range of motion.

TABLE 15.7. COMMON ADVERSE EFFECTS OF RADIATION THERAPY

RADIATION SITE	COMMON CANCERS	COMMON SIDE EFFECTS
Skin	All cancers	Redness, pain, blistering, and reduced elasticity
Brain	Brain cancers and metastases	Nausea and vomiting, fatigue, loss/thinning of hair
Pharynx	Upper respiratory cancers	Mouth ulceration
Salivary gland	Upper respiratory cancers	Xerostomia (dry mouth)
Thorax	Breast, lung, lymphoma	Some degree of irreversible lung fibrosis, heart *may* receive radiation causing pericardial inflammation or fibrosis; premature atherosclerosis; cardiomyopathy
Abdomen	Pancreas, stomach, lymphoma	Vomiting and/or diarrhea
Pelvis	Prostate, uterine cervix	Diarrhea, pelvic pain, bladder scarring, and occasionally incontinence and sexual dysfunction
Joints	Sarcomas, bone metastases	Connective tissue and joint capsule fibrosis; may decrease range of motion

patient with a painful bone metastasis). Although malignant cells are typically more radiosensitive than normal cells, normal tissue toxicity does occur and is entirely dependent on what part of the body is irradiated (Table 15.7).

Because cancer cells frequently metastasize beyond the primary site and regional lymph nodes, systemic therapy (i.e., drugs) is prescribed for many advanced solid tumors. Moreover, systemic therapy is the mainstay of curative treatment for leukemia and lymphoma, where cancer cells are only rarely regionally confined. Cancer chemotherapy exploits biological differences between normal and malignant cells to preferentially kill malignant cells. Most of the currently used chemotherapy drugs have been selected to be toxic to proliferating cells (Table 15.8). However, newer anticancer drugs are being developed for their abilities to kill more slowly growing tumors. Increasingly, it is being realized that anticancer drugs trigger apoptosis—programmed cell death—and that cancer cells may be more susceptible to these triggers than normal tissues.

In general, curative chemotherapy requires combinations of several chemotherapy drugs, given in repeated courses or cycles 2–4 weeks apart, for 3–6 months. Adult cancers often cured by chemotherapy include acute leukemias, Hodgkin lymphoma, some non-Hodgkin lymphomas, and testicular cancers. Because the goal of treatment is cure, most patients are willing to accept the mul-

TABLE 15.8. CLASSES OF SYSTEMIC THERAPY FOR CANCER AND THEIR COMMON ADVERSE EFFECTS

CLASS	EXAMPLES	COMMON ADVERSE EFFECTS
Antimetabolite chemotherapy (intravenous)	Methotrexate, fluorouracil, gemcitabine	Fatigue, anorexia, nausea, anemia, neutropenia, thrombocytopenia
Antitubulin chemotherapy (intravenous)	Taxol, taxotere, vinorelbine, vincristine	Fatigue, muscle pain, sensory and motor peripheral neuropathy, ataxia, amenia, neutropenia, thrombocytopenia
Alkylator chemotherapy	Cyclophosphamide, chlorambucil	Fatigue, anorexia, nausea, anemia, neutropenia, thrombocytopenia
Anthracycline chemotherapy (intravenous)	Doxorubicin (Adriamycin), Mitoxantrone	Fatigue, cardiotoxicity (cardiac failure in < 5% of patients), nausea, vomiting, amenia, neutropenia, thrombocytopenia
Platinum salt chemotherapy (intravenous)	Cisplatin, carboplatin	Fatigue, nausea, sensory and motor peripheral neuropathy, anemia neutropenia, thrombocytopenia
High-dose chemotherapy with bone marrow/stem	Combinations of 2–4 chemotherapy drugs in cell transplantation	Loss of muscle mass, deconditioning, maximally tolerated doses nausea, vomiting, neuropathy, anemia, neutropenia, thrombocytopenia, infection
Glucocorticoid hormonal therapy (oral)	Dexamethasone (Decadron), prednisone	Fat redistribution (truncal and facial obesity); proximal muscle weakness, osteoporosis, edema, infection
Antiestrogen hormonal therapy (oral)	Tamoxifen	Weight gain, fatigue, hot flashes
Antiandrogen hormonal therapy (oral)	Flutamide	Weight gain, fatigue, loss of muscle mass, hot flashes, osteoporosis
Leutenizing hormone-releasing hormone agonists (subcutaneous injection)	Goseralin, buserelin	Weight gain, fatigue, hot flashes, osteoporosis

tiple side effects of systemic treatment. If these particular cancers recur after standard chemotherapy, treatment with high-dose chemotherapy (requiring bone marrow or stem cell transplantation to restore the blood-forming system) can provide long-term survival.

About 20% of cancers in males and about 40% in females arise in hormone-sensitive organs—prostate, breast, and uterus. The hormonal environment of the body can directly stimulate the growth of established cancers. Depriving an established prostate, breast, or uterine cancer of its sustaining hormones cannot only halt growth but may also actually induce regression of the tumor. For example, a patient with metastatic breast cancer treated with an antiestrogen may have partial or complete disappearance of the metastatic lesions. Similarly, patients with advanced prostate cancer derive substantial benefit from depletion of testosterone. Although surgical removal of the ovaries or testes will, respectively, deplete estrogen or testosterone, drug treatment with luteinizing hormone-releasing hormone (LHRH) agonists also stops sex hormone production without the need for surgery.

Glucocorticoid agents are cytotoxic to some leukemic and lymphoma cells and are used at high doses for these cancers. Additionally, glucocorticoids are commonly given to prevent and treat chemotherapy-induced nausea, reduce cancer-related pain and anorexia, and to treat and prevent allergic reactions from chemotherapy drugs. Use of these agents, however, causes muscle loss, proximal muscle weakness, fat accumulation in the trunk and face, osteoporosis, and an increased susceptibility to infection.

Increasingly, combinations of the main cancer treatment modalities (surgery, radiotherapy, and systemic therapy) are being used to treat cancer. The major advantages of combined modality treatment include (a) disease missed by locoregional therapy may be treated by systemic therapy, (b) tumor shrinkage by radiotherapy or systemic therapy can allow conservative surgery and thereby preserve organ function, and (c) tumors may respond more dramatically to combined therapy. Combined modality therapy is now the standard of care for high-risk or locally advanced solid tumors, including breast, lung, colon, rectal, cervical, ovarian, prostate, and esophageal carcinomas, as well as many sarcomas. Hodgkin lymphoma and aggressive non-Hodgkin lymphomas are commonly treated with combination chemotherapy and radiotherapy.

EFFECTS OF CANCER/TREATMENTS ON PHYSICAL FUNCTIONING AND HEATH

Cancer and its treatments can damage healthy tissue in addition to destroying cancer cells, which can disrupt the body systems over the course of treatment. This can result in a wide array of side effects that can have a negative impact on the physiologic and psychological well-being of cancer survivors resulting in significant reductions in quality of life. Some of the common psychological sequelae that may result from cancer treatments include depression, anxiety, and stress (14). The physical and functional effects of cancer treatments may include reduced cardiovascular, immune, and pulmonary function; muscle weakness, wasting, and atrophy, and weight change; difficulty sleeping; and fatigue, nausea, vomiting, and pain (15,16). Although these side effects tend to peak during treatment, therapy-related symptoms can persist months or even years following treatment (17). More recently, it has been recognized that cancer treatments can also result in long-term chronic effects (i.e., effects that remain even after cancer treatments are stopped) and late effects (i.e., effects that only emerge many months or years after the treatments are stopped) (18). Table 15.9 (18) summarizes some of the most common late effects of cancer treatments that will be important to exercise professionals working with cancer survivors who have completed treatments. The above evidence suggests that it is possible that all of the health-related fitness components of the cancer survivors may be negatively impacted at some point after diagnosis.

Cardiorespiratory fitness may be reduced by the effects of cancer treatments on the cardiovascular, respiratory, and musculoskeletal systems of the body in combination with deconditioning owing to periods of reduced physical activity (15,16,18) (Table 15.9) (18). Cancer treatments can have a negative impact on body composition in a number of ways, including an increased fat mass, decreased lean (i.e., muscle) mass known as cachexia, and decreased bone density. Approximately 50%–96% of female breast cancer patients experience weight gain following diagnosis, consisting of an increase in fat mass and a decrease in lean mass (19). Men diagnosed with prostate cancer and receiving androgen deprivation therapy have also been shown to gain fat mass and lose lean mass (20). To contrast, cachexia affects approximately 50% of all cancer survivors and can result in the loss of both fat and lean mass (21). Cancer survivors may be at risk for bone mineral density loss caused by the cancer itself and its treatments (18,22). Cancers involving the bone and some hematologic malignancies can affect the quality of the bone (15). Androgen deprivation therapy, some chemotherapies, selective estrogen-receptor modulators, aromatase inhibitors, glucocorticoids, stem cell transplantation, and radiation have all been associated with bone loss (22). This loss of bone mineral can lead to functional limitations, osteopenia or osteoporosis, and a greater risk of fracture and poorer recovery in cases of fracture (15).

Muscle wasting and weakness can occur during cancer treatments, which can reduce both muscular strength and endurance. The causes of this loss in lean mass can include cachexia, neuropathy, steroid treatments, and de-

TABLE 15.9. POSSIBLE LATE EFFECTS OF RADIOTHERAPY AND CHEMOTHERAPY

ORGAN SYSTEM	LATE EFFECTS/SEQUELAE OF RADIOTHERAPY	LATE EFFECT/SEQUELAE OF CHEMOTHERAPY	CHEMOTHERAPEUTIC DRUGS RESPONSIBLE
Bone and Soft Tissue	Short stature; atrophy, fibrosis, osteonecrosis,	Avascular necrosis	Steroids
Cardiovascular	Pericardial effusion; pericarditis, CAD	Cardiomyopathy, CHF	Anthracylines, Cyclophosphamide
Pulmonary	Pulmonary fibrosis; decreased lung volumes	Pulmonary fibrosis, Interstitial pneumonitis	Bleomycin, BCNU, Methotrexate, Anthracylines
Central Nervous System	Neuropsychological Deficits, structural changes, hemorrhage	Neuropsychological deficits, structural changes, hemiplegia; seizure	Methotrexate
Peripheral Nervous System	—	Peripheral neuropathy, hearing loss	Platinum analogues, Vinca alkaloids
Hematological Renal	Cytopenia, myelodysplasia, decreased creatinine clearance; hypertension	Myelodyplastic syndromes, decreasedcreatinine clearance, Inc. creatinine; renal failure, delayed renal failure	Platininum analogues, Methotrexate, Nitrosoureas
Genitourinary	Bladder fibrosis, contractures	Bladder fibrosis; Hemorrhagic cystitis	Cyclophosphamide
Gastrointestinal	Malabsorption; stricture, Abnormal LFT	Abnormal LFT; hepatic fibrosis, cirrhosis	Mathotrexate
Pituitary	Growth hormone deficiency; pituitary deficiency	—	—
Thyroid Gonadal	Hypothyroidism; nodules. Men: risk of sterility, Leydig cell dysfunction. Women: ovarian failure, early menopause	Men: sterility Woman: sterility, premature menopause	Alkylating agents Procarbazine
Dental and Oral Health	Poor enamel and root formation; dry mouth	Tooth decay	multiple
Opthalmological	Cataracts; retinopathy	Cataracts	Steroids

CAD, coronary artery disease; CHF, congestive heart failure; LFT, liver function tests.
(Reprinted with permission from Aziz, N; 2007.

conditioning owing to physical inactivity (15,16,21). Surgery and radiation can affect flexibility through soft tissue damage, temporary or permanent nerve damage, fibrosis, or pain, which can result in impaired mobility and function of the specific joint or area of the body that was treated (23). Impaired shoulder function is often seen following mastectomy and axillary dissection and radiation for breast cancer (23) and is also a well-recognized surgical complication of neck dissection procedures (24).

It is probable that a combination of the above decrements in all of the fitness components over the course of cancer treatments contributes to a reduced level of physical functioning often described in cancer survivors (25). More recently, Bennett at al. (25) have suggested the importance of a multidimensional representation to conceptualize and measure physical functioning in cancer survivors. Their model attempts to encompass the interactions between cancer itself and its treatments, the effect of these treatments on subjective and objective physical function and the health-related fitness components, and the relationship between physical function and fitness components. This stresses the importance of considering the cancer survivor's en-tire experience in examining the health-related fitness components.

THE CANCER CONTROL CONTINUUM

Exercise interventions can take place at various time points across the cancer control continuum (26). We will discuss the potential role of exercise during four distinct postdiagnosis time points: pretreatment, treatment, survivorship, and end of life. Pretreatment includes the period after a definitive cancer diagnosis until first treatment is initiated, which can range from weeks to several years for some cancers (e.g., watchful waiting in non-Hodgkin lymphoma or prostate cancer). The treatment period usually includes the primary cancer treatments, such as surgery, radiation therapy, chemotherapy, and biologic therapies. The time spent in the treatment phase can last months or years. Survivorship is the period following first diagnosis and primary treatments and before the development of a recurrence or death. The end of life time period focuses on those survivors with a limited life expectancy receiving palliative care. The goals, motives, barriers, benefits, risks, types, volumes, progression, periodization, and context of exercise are all likely to vary across the cancer control continuum.

CLINICAL EXERCISE PHYSIOLOGY

Recent research is beginning to dispel many of the early fears over the safety, efficacy, and feasibility of exercise during and following cancer treatment. Mounting evidence now indicates that exercise can have a positive impact on body composition, cardiorespiratory fitness, muscular fitness, flexibility, and quality of life (QOL) for cancer survivors, both during and following treatment. Schmitz et al. (16) completed a systematic review and meta-analysis addressing exercise as an intervention for cancer survivors during and following treatment (16). In total, 32 controlled trials were included, 27 of which were randomized. A variety of physiologic and psychosocial outcomes were analyzed in 12 studies during cancer treatment and 20 studies following cancer treatment. During treatment, physical activity interventions demonstrated small to moderate positive improvements on physical activity behavior, cardiorespiratory fitness, physiologic outcomes, symptoms or side effects, and immune variables (16).

A recent large scale, multicenter randomized controlled trial investigated the effects of different types of exercise training in 242 patients with breast cancer initiating adjuvant chemotherapy (27). Usual care was compared with supervised resistance training or supervised aerobic training. Results showed that aerobic training was superior to usual care for improving self-esteem, aerobic fitness, and percent body fat. Resistance training was superior to usual care for improving self-esteem, muscular strength, lean body mass, and chemotherapy completion rate. Although no significant improvements were noted in the patient-rated outcomes of QOL, fatigue, depression, or anxiety, the changes favored the exercise groups. Further, no lymphedema or adverse events were caused by exercise training and aderence to the intervention was around 70%.

Segal et al. (20) studied the effect of resistance training in 155 men with prostate cancer receiving androgen deprivation therapy. In this randomized, controlled trial, fatigue, QOL, and muscular fitness were evaluated. Following the 12 weeks of supervised resistance training three times a week, men in the exercise group experienced significantly improved health-related QOL as well as fatigue compared with the usual care group. Further, the exercise group had significantly higher upper and lower body muscular fitness than the control group. These differences remained regardless of whether men were treated with curative or palliative intent, or whether androgen deprivation therapy had been received for less than or greater than 1 year.

Following treatment, physical activity has been found to have a positive impact on cardiorespiratory fitness, vigor and vitality, body image, confusion, body size (avoiding arm volume gain), and multiple constructs of mental health (16). Among these, strong consistent evidence is found of the positive effect of physical activity on cardiorespiratory fitness and QOL.

A recent randomized, controlled trial examined the effect of an 8-week aerobic exercise intervention when compared with exercise-placebo or usual care in 108 breast cancer survivors 1–3 years after treatment (28). Following 8 weeks of training, the exercise group had significantly, and clinically meaningful, higher QOL than the usual care group. The exercise-placebo group did not report meaningful improvement in QOL compared with the usual care group. Significant improvements in several psychological health outcomes, such as depression, were also evident with both exercise training and exercise-placebo. These improvements in psychological health remained at the 24-week follow-up.

The issue of whether postdiagnosis exercise may influence tumor growth, disease progression, recurrence, or survival remains an open question. Preliminary evidence indicates, however, that exercise following cancer treatment is associated with better clinical outcomes for certain cancers, such as breast (29,30) and colorectal (31,32). In a prospective cohort study, colorectal cancer survivors with higher levels of postdiagnosis exercise were shown to have a significant reduction in cancer recurrence and overall mortality (31). Research in breast cancer has shown that women who are physically active following breast cancer diagnosis, walking 3–5 hours/week at an average pace, had a reduced risk of death from breast cancer (29).

Although current research in exercise and cancer is promising, a paucity of research has been done in some areas of the cancer continuum, such as pretreatment, long-term survivorship, and end of life. High-quality research trials are required before clear conclusions about the effects and efficacy of exercise can be made in these groups.

EXERCISE AND FUNCTIONAL TESTING

Before the completion of any exercise testing, it is prudent that each cancer survivor undergo a comprehensive medical evaluation. This should include a complete medical history to determine any preexisting health issues (i.e., comorbid conditions) and a thorough cancer history (time since diagnosis, type and stage of disease, type of surgery and adjuvant therapy, and known or suspected side effects of treatment), a physical examination to determine current health status, and physician clearance to undergo the fitness assessment (15). This medical evaluation will ensure the safety of the cancer survivor, identify those who require further diagnostic testing before completing fitness assessments, and assist in choosing the appropriate type and mode of testing for each individual. We recommend that, at a minimum, the initial exercise testing of a cancer survivor be medically supervised. This is in line with recommendations for fitness assessments in individuals with other chronic illnesses for which extensive guidelines have been laid out (33–35). These guidelines provide an outline that may be helpful when completing exercise testing in cancer survivors. Furthermore, exercise testing in cancer patients and survivors requires special precautions and considerations (15). These special precautions arise from the significant morbidity experienced by cancer patients during and following individual or combined modality therapies.

Exercise testing to assess the health-related fitness components at specific times across the cancer control continuum can serve a number of purposes (15). At the time of diagnosis and before any cancer treatment, exercise testing may provide insight to the impact (if any) of the development of cancer on any of the components by comparing values with age and gender specific norms. Testing at the completion of treatment would allow for quantification of the impact of cancer treatments on the fitness components. Further assessment(s) following the completion of cancer treatments would allow for the determination of recovery (or lack) of the fitness components, and also the impact of any long-term or late treatments effects. In more general terms, exercise testing of cancer survivors at any stage of the continuum can provide their current physical and functional status, aid in prescribing an exercise program to maintain or improve fitness, possibly elicit any underlying comorbid conditions (either preexisting or treatment related) that may preclude further exercise testing or training (15), and determine the fitness benefits of a prescribed exercise program. To obtain a comprehensive physical and functional assessment of the cancer survivor, it is ideal to assess each of the health-related fitness components, especially because they may all have been impacted by cancer treatments (16). As an exercise professional, this will also allow prescribing an exercise program aimed at maintaining or improving each of the components and will result in the greatest overall benefit for the cancer survivor (15). However, if assessment of all of the components is not possible, particular attention should be paid to those that are known or likely to be directly affected by the particular cancer treatment.

The gold standard test to determine cardiorespiratory fitness is the assessment of maximal oxygen consumption ($\dot{V}O_2max$) (33). If direct measurement of ($\dot{V}O_2max$) is not possible, however, a number of indirect methods are available. These include a number of submaximal and field testing protocols designed to indirectly estimate $\dot{V}O_2max$ by the use of varying testing modes and protocols (33,36). It is important to note that many submaximal tests are limited because they rely on the assumption of "normal" exercise responses for an accurate maximal estimation, which may not be accurate for cancer survivors who currently are, or have already have, completed chemotherapy (15,33). Whichever test is chosen to assess cardiorespiratory fitness, it is desirable that it stresses the cancer survivor to the intensity that will be experienced in any subsequent exercise training to ensure that any symptoms that arise do so in a medically supervised situation (15).

When assessing muscular strength, the one repetition maximum testing (1-RM), which is the heaviest weight that can be lifted one time for a particular exercise with proper technique is often used (33,34). If safety of the 1-RM is a concern, submaximal testing such as 6- or 10-RM tests can be performed to estimate an individual's 1-RM. A number of options to assess muscular endurance exist, including maximal repeated contraction, standard load, and static contraction tests (33,34). Classic maximal repeated contraction tests are the sit-up and push-up tests. The standard load test determines the number of repetitions completed at a fixed submaximal load for a given exercise, and sometimes matched to a specific cadence (33,34). The static contraction test determines the length of time that a submaximal load can be held for on a given exercise. Isokinetic dynamometers may also be used to assess muscular fitness, but requires the use of expensive equipment (34,37).

Body composition is most accurately assessed with CAT, MRI, and dual-energy x-ray absorbance (DXA) scans (34). The additional benefit of the above methods for cancer survivors is that they can be used to determine bone mineral density, which as previously mentioned can have been negatively impacted by a number of cancer treatments (22). Despite being the ideal methods to assess body composition, these techniques require expensive equipment and highly specialized training to be carried out. Less expensive and technically demanding means of assessing body composition carry a greater amount of measurement error and cannot determine bone density (34). These include hydrodensitometry (underwater weighing), air-displacement plethysmography, skinfold analysis, and bioelectrical impedance analysis (34). At a minimum, basic anthropometry, including circumference measures (e.g. waist and hip), and height and weight, which can be used to determine body mass index (BMI), should be completed to assess body composition (34).

General flexibility tests that can be used to assess flexibility include the sit-and-reach test and shoulder elevation tests (33,34). Flexibility and range of motion (ROM) of a specific joint can be assessed using a universal goniometer (33,34). These are likely to be of greater use in cancer survivors who have had specific joints affected resulting from their cancer treatment, usually following surgery or radiation (15).

As stated, the combined fitness component changes experienced by cancer survivors related to their treatments will likely result in a reduction in their overall physical function. It has been suggested that the cancer survivor's physical function can be divided into three components: (*a*) their self-report of "difficulty" in participating in life or role activities, (*b* their self-report of "difficulty" in carrying out physical actions, and (*c*) objective assessment of physical actions by measured performance tests (25). Important in the context of exercise testing is this final suggestion to assess objectively the cancer survivor's ability to perform tasks specific to daily activities and functions. Although many such tests exist, two test batteries that objectively assess a number of dimensions relevant to functional actions include the Senior Fitness Test and Continuous Scale Physical Functional Performance (CS-PFP) Test. The Senior Fitness Test consists of six test items (chair sit-to-stand, arm curls, chair sit-and-reach, back scratch for flexibility, 8-ft up and go, and 6-minute walk test) that measure the underlying physical parameters (i.e., health-related fitness components) associated with functional ability (38). The CS-PFP (16 items) and the 10 item version (PFP-10) of this test include an assortment of tests of increasing difficultly designed to mimic activities of daily living (ADL) and objectively measure upper body strength, lower body strength, flexibility, balance and coordination, and endurance (39). It is important to note that, because these tests have been designed for use in older adults, other tests may be more appropriate when dealing with younger cancer survivors, or when dealing with a group of survivors across a wide age range.

EXERCISE PRESCRIPTION AND PROGRAMMING

Appropriately, early research took a cautious approach to exercise in cancer patients consistent with the physician's rule "First, do no harm." As evidence has emerged in support of the efficacy and safety of exercise, both during and following cancer treatment, there has been an upsurge in the number of research studies and interest in the development of clinical exercise programs for cancer patients and survivors. To date, more than 40 controlled clinical trials have been performed examining exercise interventions for cancer patients and survivors. The optimal form of exercise training for cancer patients and survivors, however, remains undefined (40,41) and further investigation is needed to determine the response to variations in exercise programming in terms of dosage, timing, and type of exercise.

Although physical exercise may be an effective QOL intervention for many cancer patients and survivors, it is important to recognize that mitigating factors may make it unwise or even dangerous for some cancer patients to exercise. Besides the general contraindications that are relevant for any older population (42), additional contraindications apply to cancer patients (15). This cautionary note is not meant to imply that cancer patients

with such conditions could not benefit from an appropriately designed and supervised exercise program, but only that the risk-to-benefit ratio may be higher and close medical supervision may be required.

Prescribing exercise for cancer survivors is complex because the ability to exercise, especially during cancer treatment, may differ, depending on the type of cancer and cancer treatment, and may be limited by factors, such as the survivor's age, overall health and fitness and the presence of a comorbid condition(s). Therefore, the exercise program should be prescribed individually for each survivor using all available clinical data, and should also consider the survivor's needs, goals and abilities. The exercise program may be designed to increase, maintain, or prevent declines in the cancer survivor's overall fitness, and to address specific disease or treatment-related deficits. In general, exercise programs for cancer patients and survivors have closely followed the *American College of Sport Medicine's Guidelines* (43) (Table 15.10).

CARDIORESPIRATORY FITNESS

Traditionally, exercise programs have followed the standard prescription of continuous aerobic exercise in the form of walking or cycle ergometry. The key point when prescribing activity mode in cancer patients and survivors is to take into account any acute or chronic physical impairments that may have resulted from medical treatment. For example, swimming should be avoided by those patients with nephrostomy tubes, non–in-dwelling central venous access catheters, and urinary bladder catheters. Swimming is not contraindicated for patients with continent urinary diversions, uterotomies, or colostomies, but patients should wait 8 weeks post-surgery and avoid open-ended pouch appliances. High-impact exercises or contact sports should be avoided in cancer patients or palliative care patients with primary or metastatic bone cancer. From a clinical perspective, it is probably safest to prescribe walking or cycle ergometry; however, no evidence suggests one type of aerobic exercise is superior to another in the general rehabilitation of cancer patients and survivors.

Most studies have prescribed moderate-intensity exercise performed 3–5 days per week for 20–30 minutes per session. During cancer treatment, however, many patients will not feel like exercising at certain times during their chemotherapy cycles. These so-called "down days" are different for each patient and may even vary from cycle to cycle. The key point is to build flexibility into the exercise prescription so that cancer patients are able to modify the frequency, intensity, or duration of their exercise, depending on how well they tolerate treatment. Results from studies examining aerobic exercise in breast cancer survivors have shown improvements in the range of 10%–20% consistent with improvements reported in the general population (41,43).

TABLE 15.10. EXERCISE PRESCRIPTION CONSIDERATIONS FOR CANCER PATIENTS AND SURVIVORS

	ACSM EXERCISE GUIDELINES	DURING CANCER TREATMENT	POST CANCER TREATMENT	SPECIAL CONSIDERATIONS
Physical activity for health	30 minutes of physical activity, 5 or more days of the week	Remain as active as possible during treatment	Increase volume of exercise through repeated bouts of 10 minute exercise sessions	The disease may limit ability to walk and may necessitate other forms of exercise
Exercise to improve cardiorespiratory fitness	Moderate intensity exercise (e.g. 40%–60% HRR) 20–45 minutes, 3–5 days per week	Symptom limited: modifications to workload to adjust for 'down days'. Consider interval training for those unable to perform continuous exercise.	Slower progression and longer course of treatment for older, sedentary, or more deconditioned survivors.	Assess and monitor for any acute, chronic and long-term side effects of treatment
Exercise to improve muscular strength and endurance	8–10 exercises of major muscle groups of upper and lower extremities and trunk 10–15 repetitions, 1–3 sets, 2–3 days per week	Symptom limited: may have difficulty maintaining exercise volume/progressing through latter stages of treatment. May consider incorporating functional activities in program.	May need to start with low-intensity resistance (e.g. lightest weight on rack or alternatively at 30% of 1 repetition maximum [1-RM]) and progress to standard prescription of 60%–70% of 1-RM.	Avoid exhaustion: monitor symptoms of pain and fatigue, delayed muscle soreness; reduce/adjust workload if worsening of symptoms with exercise
Exercise to improve flexibility	2–4 stretches of each major muscle group Each stretch held for 10–30 seconds, Frequency: 2–3 days per week	May need to prevent/address specific deficits in range of motion or tissue constriction caused by cancer treatment.	May need to increase frequency of stretching to 5–7 days per week to address soft tissue tightness owing to surgery or radiation therapy.	Avoid stretching exercises if acute reaction to radiation therapy (e.g., severe burn/blistering) in region

HRR, heart rate reserve.
(ACSM : American College of Sports Medicine.)

From a duration perspective, it is likely that many cancer patients will not be able to tolerate 30 minutes of continuous exercise at the start of their treatments, especially if they were previously sedentary. Researchers have used intermittent or interval training (i.e., alternating short bouts of exercise and rest) for patients preparing for cancer surgery (44), during chemotherapy treatment (45,46), or immediately following bone marrow transplantation (47,48) as a way of accumulating exercise volume and improving cardiorespiratory fitness. This approach allows for short work periods of higher intensity than would be possible with a continuous exercise protocol and has been shown to improve outcomes, such as body composition and functional capacity, and to reduce days in hospital (40).

After treatment, for the less active and the more deconditioned cancer survivor, the exercise prescription may start by simply encouraging a more active lifestyle (e.g., take the stairs, walk instead of driving) with the goal of increasing daily physical activity to levels advocated by public health guidelines. The potential health benefits of increased physical activity have been long recognized, although minimal changes in cardiorespiratory fitness occur (49). This lower intensity exercise can be easily incorporated into the individual's lifestyle and increases in physical activity can be accomplished through education and behavior change modalities. As an example, Vallance et al. (50) examined the effects of breast-

cancer specific print materials and step pedometers on physical activity and QOL in breast cancer survivors. The authors reported increased physical activity, improvements in QOL, and reductions in fatigue in survivors receiving both the print material and step pedometer when compared with survivors receiving standard physical activity recommendations.

RESISTANCE TRAINING

The evidence for the efficacy of resistance training is only beginning to emerge, with several studies examining resistance exercise alone or in combination with aerobic exercise. Resistance exercise may be prescribed to improve muscular strength and endurance, physical function, and to address changes in peripheral muscle as a result of the cancer or cancer treatment. As many leisure-time activities require lifting, moving or carrying, resistance exercise may prove beneficial in addressing the long-term limitations in physical performance reported among cancer survivors (51).

Standard recommendations for resistance training include a minimum of 1 set of 8–10 exercises that work the major muscle groups. Although these recommendations may be appropriate for many cancer survivors, resistance exercise programs for some survivors may need to focus on specific muscles or muscle groups, or postural correction. For example, Shamley et al. (52) examined muscle cross-sectional area and electromyographic activity of the muscles of the shoulder in 74 women with breast cancer. The authors reported altered muscle activity in upper trapezius, rhomboids, and serratus anterior; reduced muscle size in pectoralis major and minor; and subjective reports of pain with carrying objects and lifting the arm. The results suggest that some breast cancer survivors may need a more focused exercise regimen to address these specific muscles of the upper extremity.

FLEXIBILITY

Stretching and ROM exercises may very likely prove to be important components in the optimal exercise prescription of cancer patients and survivors. Surgery and radiation therapy may result in musculoskeletal problems, such as loss of strength and ROM in the region of the cancer. Moreover, late effects of tissue fibrosis and muscle atrophy can develop in the field of radiation therapy and may limit extensibility of the affected tissue (53). In some cancer patients and survivors, a flexibility training program may need to include a regular set of exercises intended to progressively increase ROM in a joint or to lengthen shortened muscles in a region (e.g., restriction in neck ROM following surgery and radiation therapy for head and neck cancer) or to address the functional needs of the individual (e.g., reaching overhead).

Traditionally, the recommended stretching prescription has consisted of slow, static stretches held for 10–30 seconds. More recently, Lee et al. (54) examined the effect of long duration static stretches to prevent radiation-induced tissue constriction in the ipsilateral pectoral muscles of breast cancer patients undergoing radiation therapy. Although this type of stretching intervention holds promise, in the short term, no significant differences were found between the group performing standard ROM exercises and the group performing long duration static stretching. A number of studies have shown benefit from yoga and Tai Chi movements as alternative exercise methods for the cancer survivor to improve flexibility, as well as balance and agility (55–57).

It is also important to recognize that cancer patients exercise as much for psychological health as for physiologic health (58). Consequently, it is important to take psychological benefits into account when prescribing exercise for cancer patients. As a general guideline, exercise professionals should prescribe exercise that is enjoyable, builds confidence, facilitates perceptions of control, develops new skills, incorporates social interaction, and takes place in an environment that engages the mind and spirit. The overall goal is to encourage and support exercise behavior that results in lifetime physical activity.

EDUCATION AND COUNSELING

Exercise adherence is a major challenge for health professionals, regardless of the demographic profile of the group or the purpose of the exercise. Nevertheless, the significant morbidity caused by cancer and its treatments makes exercise adherence even more difficult for cancer survivors, especially during difficult adjuvant therapies. Not surprisingly, research has documented that a significant decline occurs in the volume of exercise during cancer treatment that is not recovered even years after treatment is completed (58). Research, however, has started to examine the major incentives and barriers to exercise in cancer survivors, which is reviewed by Courneya, et al. (58). Although some general conclusions can be made, the specific incentives and barriers are likely to vary, depending on the type of cancer, extent of disease, type of medical treatment, existence of other comorbid conditions, point along the cancer control continuum, and other personal factors. Table 15.11 lists some of the common incentives and barriers to exercise for several cancer survivor groups.

Overall, studies have indicated that cancer survivors have diverse motives and barriers to exercise, some of

TABLE 15.11. COMMON EXERCISE MOTIVES AND BARRIERS FOR CANCER SURVIVORS

	MOTIVES	BARRIERS
During Treatment	Maintain a normal lifestyle	Feeling sick
	Cope with treatments	Fatigue/tiredness
	Gain control over cancer/life	Nausea/vomiting
	Cope with stress	Lack of time/too busy
	Get mind off cancer/ treatment	Pain/soreness
	Feel better/improve well-being	Chemotherapy day
	Improve immune function	Diarrhea
	Improve energy level	
During Survivorship	Recover from treatments	Lack of time/too busy
	Reduce risk of recurrence	Lack of energy/too tired
	Improve strength and fitness	Deconditioned/too weak
	Increase energy	Poor health/ comorbid Condition(s)
	Relieve stress	Poor weather conditions
	Control/lose weight	Lack of motivation
	Improve self-esteem	Arthritis/bad joints
	Improve cardiovascular health	Lack of facilities/ equipment
	Feel better/improve well-being	Cancer recurrence

which are unique to the cancer experience and some of which are common to other populations. Not surprisingly, motives and barriers vary by treatment status. Barriers to exercise during treatment often reflect the well-known side effects of treatments (e.g., sickness, nausea, diarrhea, fatigue) (59), whereas barriers during survivorship tend to realign with barriers in the general population (e.g., lack of time, too busy). It is also apparent that exercise motives and barriers vary by cancer survivor group, reflecting the unique profile of the particular disease. For example, weight loss is the most common exercise motive in endometrial cancer survivors where obesity rates are high (60) and deconditioning is a major exercise barrier in non-Hodgkin lymphoma survivors where poor physical conditioning is common (61). The key point for fitness professionals is that cancer survivors will have unique incentives and barriers to exercise that need to be understood and addressed. Creative exercise programming and adherence strategies for this population will be required.

SUMMARY AND CONCLUSION

More than 10 million Americans are cancer survivors, and this number is increasing. Moreover, cancer treatments are intensive and cause significant morbidity that results in acute, chronic, and late effects on physical functioning, disease risk, health, and QOL. Good evidence exists for promoting exercise in cancer survivors. Currently, more than 40 studies have addressed this issue using primarily intervention designs. Despite limitations in the studies, the evidence suggests that exercise will improve a broad array of physical and psychosocial functioning parameters, both during and after cancer treatments, and may even reduce the risk of the disease coming back. Exercise testing and prescription in cancer survivors must take into account the morbidity caused by treatments. Guidelines for exercise prescription in this population include moderate-to-vigorous intensity exercise performed 3–5 times per week for 30–60 minutes in an environment that optimizes psychosocial health. Finally, facilitating exercise adherence among cancer survivors requires a good understanding of the unique incentives and barriers in this population and the application of creative behavior change strategies.

REFERENCES

1. American Cancer Society. *Cancer Facts and Figures 2007*. Atlanta, GA: American Cancer Society; 2007.
2. Harvard Report on Cancer Prevention. Volume 1: Causes of human cancer, 1996.
3. Friedenreich CM, Orenstein MR. Physical activity and cancer prevention: Etiologic evidence and biological mechanisms. *J Nutr* 2002;132(11 Suppl):3456S–64S.
4. Samad AK, Taylor RS, Marshall T, et al. A meta-analysis of the association of physical activity with reduced risk of colorectal cancer. *Colorectal Dis* 2005;7(3):204–13.
5. Monninkhof EM, Elias SG, Vlems FA, et al. Physical activity and breast cancer: a systematic review. *Epidemiology* 2007;18(1):137–57.
6. Cust A, Armstrong B, Friedenreich C, et al. Physical activity and endometrial cancer risk: A review of the current evidence, biologic mechanisms and the quality of physical activity assessment methods. *Cancer Causes Control* 2007;18(3):243–58.
7. Oliveria SA, Lee IM. Is exercise beneficial in the prevention of prostate cancer? *Sports Med* 1997;23(5):271–8.
8. Tardon A, Lee WJ, Delgado-Rodriguez M, et al. Leisure-time physical activity and lung cancer: a meta-analysis. *Cancer Causes Control* 2005;16(4):389–97.
9. Patel AV, Rodriguez C, Pavluck AL, et al. Recreational physical activity and sedentary behavior in relation to ovarian cancer risk in a large cohort of US women. *Am J Epidemiol* 2006;163(8):709–16.
10. Pan SY, DesMeules M, Morrison H, et al. Obesity, high energy intake, lack of physical activity, and the risk of kidney cancer. *Cancer Epidemiol Biomarkers Prev* 2006;15(12):2453–60.
11. Lin Y, Kikuchi S, Tamakoshi A, et al. Obesity, physical activity and the risk of pancreatic cancer in a large Japanese cohort. *Int J Cancer* 2007;120(12):2665–71.
12. American Cancer Society. *Cancer Prevention and Early Detection Facts & Figures 2007*. Atlanta, GA: American Cancer Society; 2007.
13. American Joint Committee on Cancer Staging Manual. *AJCC Cancer Staging Manual*, 5th ed. Philadelphia: Lippincott-Raven; 1998.
14. Stanton AL. Psychosocial concerns and interventions for cancer survivors. *J Clin Oncol* 2006;24(32):5132–7.
15. McNeely ML, Peddle CJ, Parliament M, et al. Cancer rehabilitation: Recommendations for integrating exercise programming in the clinical practice setting. *Current Cancer Therapy Reviews* 2006;2(4):351–60.
16. Schmitz KH, Holtzman J, Courneya KS, et al. Controlled physical activity trials in cancer survivors: A systematic review and meta-analysis. *Cancer Epidemiol Biomarkers Prev* 2005; 14(7):1588–95.
17. Spiegel D. Psychosocial aspects of breast cancer treatment. *Semin Oncol* 1997;24(1 Suppl 1):S1-36–S1-47.
18. Aziz NM. Cancer survivorship research: State of knowledge, challenges and opportunities. *Acta Oncol* 2007;46(4):417–32.
19. Rooney M, Wald A. Interventions for the management of weight and body composition changes in women with breast cancer. *Clin J Oncol Nurs* 2007;11(1):41–52.
20. Segal RJ, Reid RD, Courneya KS, et al. Resistance exercise in men receiving androgen deprivation therapy for prostate cancer. *J Clin Oncol* 2003;21(9):1653–9.
21. Ardies CM. Exercise, cachexia, and cancer therapy: a molecular rationale. *Nutr Cancer* 2002;42(2):143–157.
22. Guise TA. Bone loss and fracture risk associated with cancer therapy. *Oncologist* 2006;11(10):1121–31.
23. Blomqvist L, Stark B, Engler N, et al. Evaluation of arm and shoulder mobility and strength after modified radical mastectomy and radiotherapy. *Acta Oncol* 2004;43(3):280–3.
24. McNeely ML, Parliament M, Courneya KS, et al. A pilot study of a randomized controlled trial to evaluate the effects of progressive resistance exercise training on shoulder dysfunction caused by spinal accessory neurapraxia/neurectomy in head and neck cancer survivors. *Head Neck* 2004;26(6):518–30.
25. Bennett JA, Winters-Stone K, Nail L. Conceptualizing and measuring physical functioning in cancer survivorship studies. *Oncol Nurs Forum* 2006;33(1):41–9.
26. Courneya KS, Friedenreich CM. Physical activity and cancer control: An overview and update. *Semin Oncol Nurs*. 2007;23:242–252.
27. Courneya KS, Segal RJ, Mackey JR, et al. Effects of aerobic and resistance exercise in breast cancer patients receiving adjuvant chemotherapy: A multicenter randomized controlled trial. *J Clin Oncol*. 2007;25:4396–4404.
28. Daley AJ, Crank H, Saxton JM, et al. Randomized trial of exercise therapy in women treated for breast cancer. *J Clin Oncol* 2007;25(13):1713–21.

29. Holmes MD, Chen WY, Feskanich D, et al. Physical activity and survival after breast cancer diagnosis. *JAMA* 2005;293(20): 2479–86.

30. Pierce JP, Stefanick ML, Flatt SW, et al. Greater survival after breast cancer in physically active women with high vegetable-fruit intake regardless of obesity. *J Clin Oncol* 2007;25(17):2345–51.

31. Meyerhardt JA, Giovannucci EL, Holmes MD, et al. Physical activity and survival after colorectal cancer diagnosis. *J Clin Oncol* 2006;24(22):3527–34.

32. Meyerhardt JA, Heseltine D, Niedzwiecki D, et al. Impact of physical activity on cancer recurrence and survival in patients with stage III colon cancer: findings from CALGB 89803. *J Clin Oncol* 2006;24(22):3535–41.

33. American College of Sports Medicine. *ACSM's guidelines for exercise testing and prescription*, 7th ed. Baltimore: Lippincott Williams & Wilkins; 2006.

34. American College of Sports Medicine. *ACSM's Resource Manual for Guidelines for Exercise Testing and Prescription*, 5th ed. Baltimore: Lippincott Williams & Wilkins; 2006.

35. ATS/ACCP Statement on cardiopulmonary exercise testing. *Am J Respir Crit Care Med* 2003;167(2):211–277.

36. Palange P, Ward SA, Carlsen KH, et al. Recommendations on the use of exercise testing in clinical practice. *Eur Respir J* 2007;29(1): 185–209.

37. Jaric S. Muscle strength testing: use of normalisation for body size. *Sports Med* 2002;32(10):615–31.

38. Rikli RE, Jones CJ. Development and validation of a functional test for community-residing older adults. *J Aging Phys Act* 1999;7: 129–61.

39. Cress ME, Buchner DM, Questad KA, et al. Continuous-scale physical functional performance in healthy older adults: A validation study. *Arch Phys Med Rehabil.* 1996;77(12):1243–50.

40. Knols R, Aaronson NK, Duebelhart D, et al. Physical exercise in cancer patients during and after medical treatment: A systematic review of randomized and controlled trials. *J Clin Oncol* 2005;23: 3830–41.

41. McNeely ML, Campbell KL, Rowe BH, et al. Effects of exercise on breast cancer patients and survivors: A systematic review and meta-analysis. *CMAJ* 2006;175(1):34–41.

42. Nelson ME, Rejeski WJ, Blair SN, et al. Physical Activity and Public Health in Older Adults: Recommendation from the American College of Sports Medicine and the American Heart Association. *Med Sci Sports Exerc* 2007;39(8):1435–45.

43. Haskell WL, Lee I, Pate RR, et al. Physical Activity and Public Health: Updated Recommendation for Adults from the American College of Sports Medicine and the American Heart Association. *Med Sci Sports Exerc* 2007;39(8):1423–34.

44. Jones LW, Peddle CJ, Eves ND, et al. Effects of presurgical exercise training on cardiorespiratory fitness among patients undergoing thoracic surgery for malignant lung lesions. *Cancer* 2007;110(3): 590–8.

45. MacVicar MG, Winningham ML. Response of cancer patients on chemotherapy to a supervised exercise program. *Cancer Bull* 1986; 13:265–74.

46. Mock V, Burke MB, Sheehan P, et al. A nursing rehabilitation program for women with breast cancer receiving adjuvant chemotherapy. *Oncol Nurs Forum* 1994;21(5):899–907.

47. Dimeo FC, Tilmann MH, Bertz H, et al. Aerobic exercise in the rehabilitation of cancer patients after high dose chemotherapy and autologous peripheral stem cell transplantation. *Cancer.* 1997; 79(9):1717–22.

48. Dimeo FC, Stieglitz RD, Novelli-Fischer U, et al. Effects of physical activity on the fatigue and psychologic status of cancer patients during chemotherapy. *Cancer* 1999;85(10):2273–7.

49. American College of Sports Medicine. Position stand on the recommended quantity and quality of exercise for developing and maintaining cardiorespiratory and muscular fitness, and flexibility in healthy adults [see comment]. *Med Sci Sports Exerc* 1998;30(6):975–991.

50. Vallance JK, Courneya KS, Plotnikoff RC, et al. Randomized controlled trial of the effects of print materials and step pedometers on physical activity and quality of life in breast cancer survivors.[see comment]. *J Clin Oncol* 2007;25(17):2352–9.

51. Ness KK, Wall MM, Oakes JM, et al. Physical performance limitations and participation restrictions among cancer survivors: a population-based study. *Ann Epidemiol* 2006;16(3):197–205.

52. Shamley D, Srinanaganathan R, Weatherall R, et al. Changes in shoulder muscle size and activity following treatment for breast cancer. *Breast Cancer Res Treat* 2007. In press.

53. Stone HB, Coleman CN, Anscher MS, et al. Effects of radiation on normal tissue: consequences and mechanisms. *Lancet Oncol* 2003; 4(9):529–36.

54. Lee TS, Kilbreath SL, Refshauge KM, et al. Pectoral stretching program for women undergoing radiotherapy for breast cancer. *Breast Cancer Res Treat* 2007;102(3):313–21.

55. Culos-Reed SN, Carlson LE, Daroux LM, et al. A pilot study of yoga for breast cancer survivors: physical and psychological benefits. *Psychooncology* 2006;15(10):891–7.

56. Galantino ML, Capito L, Kane RJ, et al. The effects of Tai Chi and walking on fatigue and body mass index in women living with breast cancer: A pilot study. *Rehabil Oncol* 2003;21:17–22.

57. Mustian KM, Katula JA, Zhao H. A pilot study to assess the influence of tai chi chuan on functional capacity among breast cancer survivors. *J Support Oncol* 2006;4(3):139–45.

58. Courneya KS, Karvinen KH, Vallance JKH. Exercise motivation and behavior change. In: Feuersteins M, ed. *Handbook of Cancer Survivorship.* New York: Springer; 2007:113–32.

59. Courneya KS, McKenzie DC, Reid RD, et al. Barriers to supervised exercise training in a randomized controlled trial of breast cancer patients receiving chemotherapy. *Annals of Behavioral Medicine* 2008;35:116–122.

60. Karvinen KH, Courneya KS, Campbell KL, et al. Correlates of exercise motivation and behavior in a population-based sample of endometrial cancer survivors: An application of the theory of planned behavior. *Int J Behav Nutr Phys Act* 2007;4(21).

61. Courneya KS, Vallance JKV, Jones LW, et al. Correlates of exercise intentions in non-Hodgkin's lymphoma survivors: An application of the Theory of Planned Behavior. *J Sport Exerc Psychol* 2005;27: 335–49.

Physical Activity, Diet and the Immune System

Interest in the effects of exercise on immune function arises from several directions (1). First, athletes and coaches believe that athletes experience frequent illness while training intensely. Epidemiologic evidence supports this perception that athletes are susceptible to upper respiratory tract infection (URTI; e.g., common cold, "flu") during prolonged periods of intense training and after major competition. Second, regular physical activity is recommended for the prevention of a number of diseases with significant lifestyle-associated factors, such as cardiovascular disease, osteoporosis, or type 2 diabetes. Interest exists in whether regular exercise may also help prevent other diseases with lifestyle-associated risk factors, such as cancer; epidemiologic evidence suggests that physical activity lowers the risk of some types of cancer, in particular colon cancer, and possibly reproductive system cancers (see Chapter 15). Third, exercise has become an integral part of treatment or management of several diseases with significant immune system involvement, such as human immunodeficiency virus or acquired immunodeficiency syndrome (HIV/AIDS), rheumatoid arthritis, multiple sclerosis, and cancer. Although exercise is often an adjunct therapy to alleviate debilitating symptoms of disease or treatment (e.g., muscle wasting in HIV/AIDS; nausea in cancer patients), it is also useful to understand the immune system response to exercise in healthy individuals and patients. Such information is important to determine whether exercise has any positive or adverse effects on the disease process, and to best tailor exercise prescription for particular patients. Finally, physical and psychological stressors influence immunity to disease, showing the close interaction between the neuroendocrine and immune systems, which share many messenger molecules and hormones. Studying the immune response to a quantifiable physical stress, such as exercise, leads to further understanding of the overall regulation of immune function.

RELEVANCE OF EXERCISE IMMUNOLOGY TO CLINICAL EXERCISE PHYSIOLOGY

The clinical exercise physiologist may encounter persons with diseases or conditions directly affecting immune function or in which treatment may influence the immune system. These persons may range from high-performance athletes to elderly individuals to those with diseases involving the immune system. Athletes may seek advice about avoiding frequent illness during intense training and competition, or when to resume training after viral illness; healthy, active individuals may also seek advice about exercising during mild illness (e.g., common cold or flu). The clinical exercise physiologist may be involved in exercise testing or programming of patients for whom the disease or treatment affect may involve the immune system. For example, in the cancer patient, radiation and chemotherapy can significantly reduce immune cell number and function, as well as blood electrolyte levels (discussed in Chapter 15). Transplant recipients will be taking immunosuppressive drugs to prevent rejection of transplanted tissue; these drugs may influence immune function (Table 16.1). As described in Chapters 17 and 18, HIV infection and chronic fatigue syndrome involve immune system dysfunction. It can be questioned, for example, whether intense exercise is to be recommended for HIV-positive individuals, based on observations that intense exercise may suppress immune function. Individuals with autoimmune diseases, such as myasthenia gravis or multiple sclerosis, may be taking drugs with immunosuppressive activity. Finally, increasing evidence suggests that regular exercise may have 'anti-inflammatory' effects, in that it reduces chronic low-grade inflammation associated with aging, cardiovascular diseases, obesity, and type 2 diabetes. When selecting appropriate exercise test protocols and exercise prescription, the clinical exercise physiologist needs to consider the effects of these diseases and treatments on exercise capacity and, in turn, the effects of exercise on immunity in these patients.

OVERVIEW OF THE IMMUNE SYSTEM

The immune system most likely evolved as a means of self-identification, as a way for the body to distinguish its own cells from those originating outside the body. In theory, the immune system is capable of defending the host against infinite environmental challenges, including foreign cells, proteins, and microorganisms, such as viruses, bacteria, or parasites. To accomplish such a formidable

TABLE 16.1. DISEASES, CONDITIONS, AND MEDICATIONS THAT MAY ALTER IMMUNE FUNCTION

DISEASES	CONDITIONS	MEDICATIONS OR TREATMENT
Some bacterial infections (e.g., staphylococcus)	*Malnutrition*	*Corticosteroids*
Some viral infections (e.g., measles virus, human immunodeficiency virus [HIV])	*Physical stress* (e.g., intense exercise)	*Cytotoxic drugs*
Anemia	*Psychological stress* (e.g., bereavement)	*Radiation therapy*
Inherited *immunodeficiency*	*Trauma, burns*	*Surgery*
Acquired *immunodeficiency* syndrome (AIDS)		Tissue or organ transplantation
Autoimmune diseases (e.g., type 2 diabetes, rheumatoid arthritis)		

(Compiled from Janeway CA, Travers P, Walport M, et al. *Immunobiology: The Immune System in Health and Disease*, 4th ed. New York: Elsevier Science; 1999.)
Items in *italics indicate that immunosuppression may result.*

task, the immune system has evolved as a complex system that incorporates complementary and overlapping functions.

One of the most important functions (although not the only one) of the immune system is to prevent or combat infection by pathogenic microorganisms. The immune system works at several levels to prevent infection: Physical barriers such as the skin and mucous membranes, and chemical barriers provided by substances contained in saliva, tears, and other body fluids, maintain the body's structural integrity to prevent entry by most pathogens. If these defenses are breached, several different cellular mechanisms may be activated to counteract the pathogen: Cells engulf and degrade the pathogen (a process called phagocytosis), other cells directly kill the pathogen or infected cells (cytotoxicity), yet other cells produce antibodies that may neutralize the foreign agent, and many types of cells produce soluble factors that may assist in killing the pathogen. In most instances, this combined effort is sufficient to eventually overcome infection, although at times the body's response is ineffective or inappropriate.

GENERAL SUMMARY OF THE IMMUNE RESPONSE

A simplified scheme of the immune response to a pathogen, such as a virus or bacterium, is depicted in Figure 16.1. The immune response is initiated when a pathogen penetrates the chemical and physical barriers, and is engulfed by phagocytic cells, which degrade the foreign proteins (called antigens). Once degraded, parts of these antigens are displayed on the surface of antigen-presenting cells (e.g., monocytes, macrophages, dendritic cells), along with special self-recognition proteins (termed major histocompatibility complex [MHC] proteins) and costimulatory proteins (CD80/86) that allow communication between different cells of the immune system. Antigen recognition and upregulation of MHC and CD80/86 proteins are coordinated by transmembrane proteins known as toll-like receptors (TLRs). Fragments of the degraded antigen are presented on the MHC proteins to specialized immune cells called T lymphocytes. T lymphocytes are then activated to produce factors that stimulate other

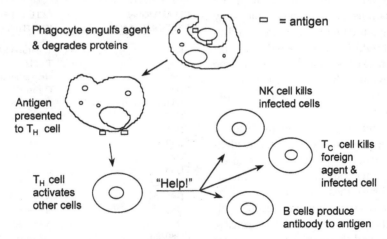

FIGURE 16-1. General scheme of the immune response. T_H, helper (CD4) T lymphocyte; T_C, cytotoxic (CD8) lymphocyte; NK, natural killer cell. (Reproduced with permission from Mackinnon LT. *Advances in Exercise Immunology*. Champaign, IL: Human Kinetics, 1999.)

TABLE 16.2. DESCRIPTION AND NORMAL VALUES FOR MAJOR TYPES OF CIRCULATING LEUKOCYTES

CELL TYPE	PERCENTAGE OF CELLS (%)	REFERENCE NORM	MAJOR FUNCTION(S)
Granulocyte, mainly neutrophil	60–70	3.0–6.0	Phagocytosis, chemotactic factors
Monocyte	10–15	0.15–0.60	Phagocytosis, antigen presentation, cytokine secretion
Lymphocyte	20–25	1.0–2.5	Antigen recognition, antibody production, cytokine secretion, memory
T cell	60–75 of lymphocytes	1.0–2.5	Antibody production, memory
CD4 T cell	60–70 of T cells	0.5–1.6	
CD8 T cell	30–40 of T cells	0.3–0.9	
B cell	5–15 of lymphocytes	0.3	
Natural killer cell	10–20	0.1–0.5	Cytotoxicity, cytokine secretion

Percentage of cells = percentage of total circulating leukocytes unless otherwise stated. Cell concentrations are expressed as number of cells $\times 10^9$/l of blood.
(Compiled from Janeway CA, Travers P, Walport M, et al. *Immunobiology: The Immune System in Health and Disease*, 4th ed. New York: Elsevier Science; 1999.)

immune cells to divide and produce substances to further combat the pathogen. B lymphocytes produce antibody to the foreign proteins, other T lymphocytes may directly kill the foreign cells or infected cells, natural killer (NK) cells may directly kill infected cells, and various cells produce soluble factors that assist in killing or neutralizing the pathogen. During the initial encounter with the pathogen, special "memory" T and B cells are produced, and these respond rapidly to subsequent infection by the same agent (the basis of immunization). Obviously, such a complex response requires close communication between the various effectors of immune function (immune cells and messenger molecules).

Cells of the Immune System

Leukocytes, called white blood cells in the blood, are immune cells produced by several lymphoid tissues. Leukocytes originate from a common stem cell found in the bone marrow and then differentiate into specific immune cells in various lymphoid tissues. Immature and differentiated cells migrate throughout the body through the blood and lymph circulations. At any given time, only about 1%–2% of the body's total leukocytes are found in the blood. This point should be remembered when reviewing the literature on exercise and human immune function; because of obvious ethical limitations in research on humans, cells can be obtained only from the peripheral blood circulation.

Table 16.2 presents a summary of the major types of leukocytes found in the blood. Leukocyte subsets are identified by a unique combination of proteins expressed on the cell surface. Because proteins are antigenic (i.e., an antibody can be raised to them), these cell-surface proteins can be identified and quantified using commercially available monoclonal antibodies. By international consensus, these cell-surface proteins and the cells they identify are now designated by the prefix CD, which stands for clusters of differentiation. For example, helper or inflammatory T lymphocytes are defined as $CD3^+CD4^+$ cells, that is, they

are identified by the CD3 and CD4 antigens expressed on the cell surface. Table 16.3 summarizes the major CD antigens used in the exercise immunology literature.

In the past decade, immunologists have also identified 11 different toll-like receptors, named TLRs 1–11, that are expressed on the surface of monocytes, macrophages, and dendritic cells. As mentioned, these receptors detect and recognize antigens, and form an integral link between the innate and acquired branches of the immune system (2). Increasing attention has also focused on the intracellular expression of heat shock proteins (HSPs) on leukocytes. HSPs are highly conserved proteins that are synthesized in response to a wide variety of environmental, pathologic, and physiologic stimuli. The HSP70 family represents the most conserved and well-known HSPs. The inducible form HSP72 acts as an intracellular

TABLE 16.3. CD ANTIGENS USED TO IDENTIFY LEUKOCYTES IN THE EXERCISE IMMUNOLOGY LITERATURE

CD ANTIGEN PREDOMINANT	CELL TYPE IDENTIFIED
CD2	T, natural killer (NK) cells
CD3	T cells
CD4	Helper, inflammatory T cells
CD8	Cytotoxic T cells
CD11b/CD18 (Mac-1)	Neutrophils, macrophages
CD14	Monocytes
CD16	NK cells, neutrophils
CD19	B cells
CD25	Activated T, B, NK cells
CD45	Leukocytes
CD45RO	Activated T, B cells
CD45RA	Naïve T, B cells
CD56	NK cells
CD69	Activated T, B, NK cells
CD80/86	Activated monocytes, dendritic cells
CD95 (Fas)	Apoptotic lymphocytes
CD122	NK cells, subset of T cells

(Compiled from Janeway CA, Travers P, Walport M, et al. *Immunobiology: The Immune System in Health and Disease*, 4th ed. New York: Elsevier Science; 1999.)

molecular chaperone of naïve, aberrantly folded or mutated proteins, and also exerts cytoprotective effects (3).

Enumeration of leukocyte and various subset concentrations in the blood is important to clinical diagnosis and monitoring of treatment for many conditions. Cell counts may be disturbed by a number of factors, including trauma (e.g., burns, surgery), medication (e.g., corticosteroids), bacterial infection, hematologic disorders (e.g., leukemia, infectious mononucleosis), immune disorders (e.g., HIV infection), treatment (e.g., chemotherapy), inflammation, and allergy (Table 16.1). Monitoring leukocyte and subset numbers may also be useful in assessing the patient's response to treatment (e.g., chemotherapy) or prognosis in immune disorders (e.g., HIV infection). Moreover, acute or chronic stress may also influence circulating immune cell number. As will be discussed later in this chapter, circulating leukocyte number and the ratio of various subsets are dramatically altered during and for up to several hours after intense exercise. Extreme exercise can also induce a systemic inflammatory response syndrome (SIRS) that shares some common characteristics with trauma and infection (5).

Leukocyte Subsets

Polymorphonuclear leukocytes, or granulocytes, are large (10–20 μm) leukocytes containing granules that can be seen with a light microscope. These cells are among the first to react to infection or inflammation. Neutrophils, the most prevalent granulocyte, are phagocytic cells important to early defense against bacterial and viral infection. Neutrophils live only a few days, but are quickly mobilized to sites of infection or inflammation (e.g., damaged tissues). It is thought that neutrophils play a role in degradation and repair of tissues, such as skeletal muscle injured during exercise. Monocytes (in blood) and macrophages (monocytes localized to tissues) are relatively large phagocytic cells crucial to the early response to infection.

Monocyte and macrophage activities include ingesting and killing microorganisms (phagocytosis), presenting antigen to and thus stimulating T cells, and secreting cytokines (regulatory molecules) that further stimulate activity of other immune cells.

Lymphocytes are composed of several subsets with specialized functions. B lymphocytes (or B cells) are small cells (6–10 μm) that produce antibody. Memory B cells rapidly produce antibody in response to previously encountered pathogens. T cells (CD3+) are small (6–10 μm) cells involved in initiating and modulating virtually all aspects of the immune response. T-cell functions include stimulating B cells to differentiate and produce antibody; directly killing some pathogens, tumor cells, and virally infected cells; and secreting cytokines that regulate the activity of many other types of immune cells. The two main subsets of T cells are called helper or inflammatory T cells and cytotoxic T cells (identified by the CD4 and CD8 antigens, respectively). CD4 T cells are

central to regulation of immune function, as shown by the devastating effect on immunity by HIV infection, which destroys these cells. CD4 helper cells stimulate B cells to produce antibody; CD4 inflammatory T cells stimulate monocyte or macrophage antibacterial activity. Both types of CD4 cells produce several types of cytokines. CD8 T cells help combat viral infection by killing infected cells.

Natural killer cells may represent a distinct cell lineage. NK cells are defined as non-T cells (CD3⁻) that express NK-specific markers CD16 and CD56. Because NK cells are capable of recognizing and killing certain tumor and virally infected cells, it is believed that these cells function in the early defense against tumor growth and viral infection. NK cells also release some cytokines.

Soluble Factors

Soluble factors are found in blood and other body fluids, and act as mediators of a wide range of immune functions. These factors may act directly, for example, by killing or neutralizing pathogens, or indirectly, as chemical messengers between different types of immune cells. The major classes of soluble factors relevant to exercise immunology include cytokines, immunoglobulin and antibody, acute-phase proteins, and complement; their major functions are listed in Table 16.4. More recently, immunologicsts have identified extracellular HSP72 as an important soluble factor that mediates innate immunity (3).

Cytokines. Cytokines are polypeptide messenger molecules central to cellular communication and immune regulation. Primarily growth and regulatory factors, cytokines are produced mainly but not exclusively by immune cells. Also, naturally occurring factors exist that inhibit and, thus, help regulate cytokine activity. The major types of cytokines examined in the exercise immunology literature are the interleukins (IL-), interferons (IFN-), and tumor-necrosis factor (TNF). Interleukins, numbered IL-1 through IL-33 (at present) (6), are unrelated cytokines produced primarily by T cells, monocytes, and NK cells, and are involved mainly in the regulation of lymphocyte activation and proliferation. Interferons (α, β, and γ), produced mainly by T and NK cells, exert antiviral activity and stimulate NK cell and macrophage cytotoxicity. TNF-α, produced by macrophages, NK cells, and T cells, is an important mediator of defense against viral infection and tumor growth. Some cytokines are classified as type 1 or type 2 cytokines. Type 1 cytokines (e.g., IFN-γ, TNF-α) are produced by type 1 T helper lymphocytes and activate macrophages and cytotoxic T cells, which protect against viral infections. Type 2 cytokines (e.g., IL-4, IL-5, IL-10, and IL-13) are generated by type 2 helper lymphocytes and stimulate antibody production (humoral immunity) against extracellular pathogens, eosinophil activity, and IgE-mediated allergic reactions.

TABLE 16.4. SOURCES AND MAJOR FUNCTIONS OF SOLUBLE FACTORS

FACTOR	PRODUCED BY	MAJOR FUNCTIONS
Immunoglobulin and antibody	Antigen binding	Resting and mature B lymphocytes Complement activation Inhibition of pathogen entry into the body Neutralization of bacterial toxins Passive immunity in newborn
Cytokines	Various leukocytes and other cells (e.g., fibroblasts, endothelial cells)	Immune system regulation Cellular communication Activation of immune cells to proliferate and differentiate Antiviral activity Cytotoxicity (cell killing) Chemotaxis (attracting cells to sites of inflammation/infection)
Acute Phase Proteins	Liver	Binding to bacteria Binding serum metals, thus limiting bacterial growth Complement activation Stimulation of phagocytosis Chemotaxis
Complement		Direct killing of bacteria Stimulation of phagocytosis Chemotaxis

(Compiled from Janeway CA, Travers P, Walport M, et al. *Immunobiology: The Immune System in Health and Disease*, 4th ed. New York: Elsevier Science; 1999.)

Several cytokines, in particular IL-1, IL-6, and TNF-α, act as mediators of inflammation. Besides involvement in general inflammation, such as in soft-tissue or joint injury, these inflammatory cytokines are also linked to atherosclerosis. It is thought that leukocytes localized to atherosclerotic plaques may release inflammatory cytokines, which act as mediators of damage to the arterial wall. Some anti-inflammatory cytokines, such as IL-4 and IL-10, may be protective against atherosclerosis. As discussed later in this chapter, prolonged weight-bearing exercise induces release of some of these cytokines, which may reflect inflammation within damaged skeletal muscle.

Immunoglobulin and Antibody. Immunoglobulin (Ig) is a class of glycoproteins produced by resting and mature B lymphocytes. Ig is expressed on the B-cell surface and is also found in serum and other body fluids, such as tears and saliva. Because of the unique structure of the Ig molecule, it is able to bind specifically to various foreign proteins or antigens. Antibody is an Ig molecule that binds specifically to a particular antigen; each antibody binds specifically to only one type of antigen. All antibodies are Ig molecules, but not all Igs exhibit antibody activity. Antigen–antibody binding initiates further immune responses by other lymphocytes and cytotoxic cells. Antibody acts in many ways, both directly to inhibit pathogens from entering the body and indirectly by stimulating phagocytosis and cytotoxicity by other immune cells.

There are five classes of Ig—IgA, IgD, IgG, IgE, and IgM—each with different complex structures and functions. IgG is most prevalent in serum, whereas IgA is the major Ig in mucosal fluids, such as saliva and tears. IgA in mucosal secretions plays a major role in preventing infection by viruses that gain entry through mucosal surfaces of the mouth, eye, nose, and respiratory, genitourinary, and gastrointestinal tracts.

Acute Phase Proteins. Acute phase proteins (APPs) are unrelated glycoproteins released from the liver in response to infection or inflammation. Proinflammatory cytokines IL-1, IL-6, and TNF-α stimulate release of APPs. The concentration of APPs increases in the blood following trauma, such as bacterial infection, surgery, and myocardial infarction, and during chronic inflammation. Some APPs stimulate immunity by binding to bacteria and by activating complement and phagocytosis. Others lower serum iron and copper concentrations, inhibiting bacterial growth by limiting availability of these metals. Still other APPs inhibit protein degradation in skeletal muscle and neutralize free radicals.

Complement. Complement represents a complex group of diverse plasma proteins produced in response to infection and inflammation. Complement acts in three main ways: by recruiting immune cells to the site of infection or inflammation; by binding to pathogens and, thus, stimulating phagocytes to kill the pathogens; and by directly killing pathogens, such as bacteria.

Extracellular HSP72. Extracellular HSP72 is a highly conserved protein that is released from many different cell types (including T and B lymphocytes, macrophages and dendritic cells) into the extracellular milieu within exosomes through a nonclassic protein transport pathway that requires intact lipid rafts (3,4). The release of extracellular HSP72 is thought to serve as a "danger signal" to the immune system. It binds to cytotoxic T lymphocytes, NK cells, and antigen-presenting cells to activate intracellular signaling cascades that lead to the expression of co-stimulatory molecules, and the synthesis of proinflammatory cytokines, chemokines, and nitric oxide (3).

METHODS TO ASSESS OR QUANTIFY IMMUNE FUNCTION

Because of the immune system's complexity, there is no single measure of "immune function," and many different types of assays are used to assess particular immune parameters. Only those most commonly used in the exercise immunology literature will be briefly described in this chapter. Assays can be simplistically classified as those quantifying the concentration of a particular factor (e.g., antibody concentration, cell number in the blood) and those measuring the functional status of particular cells (e.g., neutrophil antibacterial activity, lymphocyte proliferation). In humans, most functional assays are performed in vitro because of ethical issues and to specifically measure one parameter independent of the effects of others. Obviously, some limitations exist to applying data from in vitro experiments to in vivo function.

MEASURING CELL COUNT

In the human, leukocytes can be isolated from peripheral blood using density centrifugation. Whole blood is layered over a gradient and centrifuged, which separates the peripheral blood mononuclear cells (PBMCs) from red blood cells and granulocytes. PBMCs include lymphocytes and monocytes. Lymphocytes can be further separated from monocytes by incubating PBMCs in plastic culture dishes; monocytes adhere to the plastic, and the lymphocytes are removed in the culture medium. Cells obtained from peripheral blood may then be used to quantify cell number or function (discussed further below). Leukocytes may also be isolated from sites of inflammation by aspiration (e.g., peritoneal cavity, synovial fluid in rheumatoid arthritis) or, less frequently, by biopsy or surgery. (Animal models are not limited by mode of cell sampling as are humans, and cells may be obtained from various lymphoid tissues.)

Automated electronic cell counters are used to assess blood leukocyte and subset number. In the electronic counter, a stream of blood is passed through a narrow orifice one cell at a time, triggering an electronic signal for each cell. A leukocyte "differential" count gives the number of total leukocytes, as well as neutrophils, lymphocytes, monocytes, basophils, and eosinophils per volume of blood; clinical reference norms for these cell concentrations in blood are given in Table 16.2.

Lymphocyte subsets can be identified and quantified using flow cytometry. In this technique, fluorescently labeled antibodies to specific cell-surface markers (e.g., CD antigens discussed above) are incubated with whole blood or isolated cells, allowing the labeled antibody to bind specifically to the cells through cell surface proteins. Antibodies specific to a variety of cytokines are now available to assess intracellular cytokine production and, therefore, to identify different types of T lymphocytes using flow cytometry. The sample is then passed in front of a special laser that excites the fluorescent dye. The signals are sent to a computer, which calculates a number of variables, cell subset number and proportion relative to other subsets (based on the number of positively stained cells), cell size (based on how cells scatter light), and the density of cell-surface marker per cell (based on the intensity of fluorescent dye bound to the cells). Recent advances allow the detection of up to four different dyes simultaneously; this permits recognition of cell subsets identified by multiple surface markers.

MEASURING THE CONCENTRATION OF SOLUBLE FACTORS

Techniques to quantify the concentration of soluble factors can be broadly divided into those directly assessing concentration and those indirectly assessing concentration by measuring the biological activity of the substance of interest (called a bioassay). Immunoassays are used widely to measure the concentration of immunoglobulin, cytokines, hormones, peptides, and many other proteins. Two commonly used immunoassays are the radioimmunoassay (RIA) and enzyme-linked immunosorbent assay (ELISA). In these assays, the molecule of interest (antigen) is incubated with an antibody directed against it. The antibody binds the antigen in a specific and quantifiable way. In the RIA, a radioactively (^{125}I) labeled antibody is used, and the amount of labeled antibody is detected by counting radioactivity. In the ELISA, an enzyme is attached to the antibody, which develops color when incubated with an appropriate substrate. The amount of radioactivity (RIA) or color developed (ELISA) is directly proportional to the amount of antibody bound to antigen, which in turn is proportional to the concentration of the molecule of interest.

Since the introduction of specific and sensitive immunoassays, bioassays are used less frequently to assess the concentration of soluble factors. In a bioassay, the concentration of the substance of interest is assessed in vitro by incubating that substance with a cell line that requires it for cell growth. Cell growth is then quantified, and the amount or activity of the substance of interest is inferred from the amount of cell growth. The sensitivity of a bioassay may be limited by other growth or inhibitory factors in the sample, which may alternately stimulate or inhibit cell growth.

Cytokine gene expression may be assessed by reverse transcriptase-polymerase chain reaction (RT-PCR). Because cytokines may act only locally and are rapidly removed from the circulation, measuring levels in blood may not give an accurate measure of cytokine production. In RT-PCR, messenger RNA (mRNA) is isolated from cells of interest (e.g., leukocytes, skeletal muscle) and reverse transcription used to make multiple copies of complementary DNA (cDNA) to the mRNA. The cDNA is then amplified chemically and quantified. The amount of cDNA is proportional to the amount of mRNA, which gives a measure of cytokine gene expression. This technique has been applied in studies trying to determine the source of cytokines appearing after exercise (discussed below).

MEASURING LYMPHOCYTE PROLIFERATION

Once activated by an encounter with a pathogen, the lymphocyte proliferates to produce more cells to combat the infection. This process can be simulated in vitro by incubating whole blood or isolated lymphocytes with substances that induce proliferation. These substances are called "mitogens" because of their ability to induce mitosis in lymphocytes. When studying human cells, the most commonly used mitogens include phytohemagglutinin (PHA) and concanavalin A (conA), which stimulate T-cell proliferation, and pokeweed mitogen (PWM), which stimulates T-cell–dependent B cell proliferation. After incubation with the mitogen for a given period of time, DNA synthesis is measured either by quantifying the uptake of radioactively labeled thymidine (used to synthesize DNA) or dyes that bind to newly synthesized DNA, which can be detected using colorimetry or fluorometry.

Because lymphocytes are first activated before proliferating, cell proliferation may also be assessed by expression of activation markers on the cell surface. Monoclonal antibodies to these activation markers are incubated with whole blood or lymphocytes, and flow cytometry is used to quantify the number of cells expressing the activation marker.

MEASURING CELL-MEDIATED CYTOTOXIC ACTIVITY

Both NK cells and cytotoxic T cells can directly kill certain tumor and virally infected cells. Cytotoxic (killing) activity of these cells can be assessed by two general methods. In the standard ^{51}Cr release assay, target cells (those killed by the cytotoxic cells, usually a tumor cell line) are first incubated with radioactively labeled chromium, which is taken up and retained by the target cells. The labeled target cells are then incubated with whole blood or isolated effector cells, during which time the effector cells of interest (either NK or cytotoxic T cells) kill a number of target cells. On death of the target cells, ^{51}Cr is released into the fluid medium. Radioactivity in the fluid medium is proportional to the number of target cells killed, which gives a measure of cytotoxic activity.

Cytotoxicity can also be assessed using flow cytometry. Target and effector cells are incubated together, and dead target cells are identified with a fluorescently labeled dye that distinguishes dead from live target cells.

MEASURING MONOCYTE AND NEUTROPHIL FUNCTION

Monocytes and neutrophils exhibit a wide range of functions, including phagocytosis and killing of pathogens, such as bacteria and viruses. Phagocytosis is a complex process involving several steps, each of which can be assessed independently. The ability of phagocytes to ingest microbes can be assessed in vitro by incubating cells with fluorescently labeled beads (e.g., latex) and then quantifying the amount of internalized beads histologically or with flow cytometry. Once activated or "primed" to kill, phagocytes exhibit an oxidative burst that can be quantified in vitro as production of reactive oxygen or nitrogen species (which are toxic to microbes), or as an increase in respiratory rate. Neutrophil activation can also be assessed by the appearance of proteolytic enzymes, such as elastase released into the incubation medium, the plasma concentrations of myeloperoxidase and calprotectin, or by expression of certain cell-surface markers, such as the complement receptor CD11b.

USING IN VIVO ASSAYS IN HUMANS

In vitro assays are important in studying particular immune parameters. However, methodologic concerns limit the extrapolation of these data to understanding immune competence in the intact body. First, only 1%–2% of all immune cells are in the circulation at any given time. Second, leukocyte function is influenced by hormones, cytokines, and neurotransmitters, and the plasma concentrations of these agents can change in response to exercise. Therefore, measuring the function of isolated leukocytes without these agents present in the incubation medium does not necessarily reflect leukocyte function in vivo. Finally, alterations in blood temperature and pH that may occur during exercise are often also neglected during in vitro studies of isolated leukocyte function. Some of these limitations are overcome when studying immune function in whole blood (7). On the other hand, ethical considerations limit the types of in vivo tests that may be applied in humans. In vivo tests of immune function commonly used in humans involve exposure to a particular antigen and then measuring the response. An antigen can be injected (as in immunization) and the amount of antibody produced to that antigen measured in the blood. Alternatively, the antigen can be applied to the skin (as in the tuberculin test), and the size of the skin reaction gives an indication of T-cell function; this is called delayed-type hypersensitivity.

EXERCISE AND THE IMMUNE SYSTEM

The exercise immunology literature has focused on the effects of exercise on illness, as well as the responses of key components of immunity, such as cell number and function, levels of soluble mediators, and other factors that may influence immunity. As described above, the immune system is very complex, and a physical stress such as exercise can influence immune function at any number of points. Moreover, as will be discussed below, responses can vary between different immune parameters, between acute and chronic exercise, and between trained and untrained individuals.

EFFECTS ON RISK FOR UPPER RESPIRATORY TRACT INFECTION

Athletes and coaches have long perceived an association between intense exercise and increased risk of upper respiratory tract infection (URTI; e.g., common cold, sore throat). This perception is supported by several epidemiologic studies on distance runners, which show increased risk of URTI during the 2 weeks after major competition such as a marathon or ultramarathon (8–10). Of runner, 50%–70% may experience URTI symptoms after a race (8–10). Moreover, the risk of URTI has been related to competition pace (9) and average training distance (8,11).

In contrast to these findings, a recent study reported that the incidence of self-reported URTI in a 3-week period following a marathon race did not differ from the incidence of URTI in the 6 months before the race (12). In addition, the incidence of URTI in the 3 weeks after the race was not related to the training volume before the race. The incidence of URTI after the race was 16% in runners who were free of URTI before the race compared with 33% in runners who experienced URTI before the race. This finding suggests that, in some runners, the stress induced by the race may have reactivated a virus that was responsible for URTI before the race.

A threshold of exercise appears to exist, below which risk of URTI does not increase. For example, the risk of URTI is not elevated in those participating in "fun runs" of 21 km or less (13). Similarly, moderate exercise training (e.g., brisk walking) does not increase, and may even reduce, the incidence of URTI (14–17). Based on these data, a "J-curve" model has been proposed that suggests that the risk of URTI is reduced by regular moderate exercise, but increased by intense exercise. It is not known whether this relationship holds true for other types of athletes, such as sprinters or power athletes, or for the general public. The minimal and optimal amounts of exercise needed to enhance resistance to infectious illness are also currently unknown. From the public health and clinical perspective, however, no evidence suggests that, at least in healthy individuals, resistance to infectious illness is compromised by regular moderate exercise as recommended for long-term health. Recent data also suggest that not all upper respiratory illness in athletes is caused by infectious pathogens. Similar symptoms may result from noninfectious stimuli (e.g., allergies, air-borne pollutants, airway inflammation) (17) or reactivation of a virus (discussed further later in this chapter).

Aerobic exercise capacity and muscular strength decline during febrile viral illness, suggesting that physical performance may be temporarily impaired during illness with fever (18). The athlete is advised not to continue intense exercise training during the active stages of viral infection, because this has been associated with an increased risk of developing viral myocarditis (18) or chronic fatigue syndrome (19). On the other hand, moderate exercise training (e.g., 40 minutes at 70% heart rate reserve, 3 sessions per week) does not influence the severity of mild, experimentally induced URTI (19). Moderate exercise appears to improve survival rates in mice following injection with influenza vaccine (21). An acute bout of cycling 45 minutes before influenza vaccination improves antibody responses to the vaccine in women, but not in men, at 4 and 20 weeks after vaccination (22). An acute bout of eccentric exercise (lengthening muscle contractions) 6 hours before influenza vaccination also improves antibody responses to the vaccine in women at 6 and 20 weeks after vaccination, and enhances cell-mediated immunity in men at 8 weeks after vaccination (23). Another recent study indicated that elderly individuals with high physical fitness ($\dot{V}O_{2max}$ 47 mL $\cdot$ kg^{-1} $\cdot$ min^{-1}) produce more antibodies in response to influenza vaccination than do elderly individuals of low physical fitness ($\dot{V}O_2$max 21 mL $\cdot$ kg^{-1} $\cdot$ min^{-1}) (24). These studies indicate that moderate levels of both acute and chronic exercise enhance immune responses in vivo.

Athletes are advised to follow the "above the neck" rule—if illness is mild, without fever, and affects only the mouth, nose, and throat, as in a common cold, then exercise training is permitted, perhaps with slightly reduced intensity or duration. In contrast, systemic illness (e.g., swollen glands) or illness involving fever should be evaluated by a physician before any intense exercise is performed. All individuals should resume normal physical activity patterns gradually after illness.

EFFECTS ON PERIPHERAL BLOOD LEUKOCYTE NUMBER

Acute exercise causes dramatic changes in the number and relative distribution of circulating leukocyte subsets as reviewed by Mackinnon (1). Changes in cell number are mediated primarily by stress hormones, such as cortisol, epinephrine, and growth hormone, and cytokines, such as IL-6. The magnitude of change is a function of exercise intensity, duration, and mode, and the time of blood sampling after exercise (Table 16.5).

Leukocytes, neutrophils, monocytes, and lymphocytes all increase in concentration during and immediately after exercise. Cell numbers are higher, and remain elevated for longer, after intense or prolonged compared with moderate exercise. Exercise with an eccentric bias (e.g., downhill running) causes greater perturbation of

TABLE 16.5. SUMMARY OF ACUTE AND CHRONIC EXERCISE RESPONSES OF SELECTED IMMUNE PARAMETERS

IMMUNE PARAMETER	ACUTE RESPONSE[a]		CHRONIC RESPONSE[b]
	POSTEXERCISE[c]	1–5 HOURS POSTEXERCISE	
Cell number			
Leukocyte	↑↑	↑↑	− or may ↓
Neutrophil	↑↑	↑↑	−
Lymphocyte	↑	↓	−
NK cell	↑↑	↓	− or may ↑
Cell function			
Neutrophil activity	↑	↑	↓
NK-cell cytotoxic activity	↑	↓	− or may ↑
Lymphocyte proliferation	↓	↓	−

[a]After intense prolonged exercise.
[b]Resting values in athletes compared with nonathletes or clinical norms.
[c]Immediately postexercise.
↑ = increase; ↑↑ = large increase, more than double resting values; ↓ = decrease; − = no change.
(Compiled from various sources.)

cell number compared with level running, even at the same metabolic cost (25), suggesting some form of communication between skeletal muscle and immune cells. The relationship between leukocyte responses and muscle damage may depend on adaptation to previous muscle damage (26).

Leukocyte and neutrophil numbers may increase threefold immediately after prolonged exercise and continue to increase further for several hours. In contrast, brief, intense exercise elicits a biphasic response: Cell number first increases during exercise, returns to resting levels by 1 hour postexercise, and then increases again 1–3 hours after exercise. Lymphocytes also exhibit a biphasic response, but the response follows a different pattern. Lymphocyte numbers increase during and immediately after exercise, but decline and remain below baseline levels between 1 and 5 hours after exercise. T, B, and NK cell counts follow a similar pattern. Normal cell counts are generally restored by 24 hours after exercise.

The postexercise increase in the number of leukocytes does not result from synthesis of new cells, but rather reflects a redistribution of cells between the circulation and other sites (recall that, at any given time, only 1%–2% of all immune cells are in the circulation). Increased cardiac output and release of cells from marginated pools in underperfused tissues (e.g., lungs, bone marrow) and the spleen are all sources of cells appearing in the circulation after exercise. It is not currently known where cells go after leaving the circulation, when normal blood levels are restored during recovery after exercise. The stress of exercise may stimulate the postexercise uptake of lymphocytes into lymphoid tissue and bone marrow (27).

Exercise training appears to have minimal chronic effects on circulating leukocyte number because athletes generally exhibit clinically normal cell counts at rest. Two possible exceptions: Total leukocyte and NK cell numbers may decline during prolonged periods of very intense exercise training. Leukocyte numbers reportedly decreased to clinically low levels after 4 weeks of intensified training in distance runners (28). In a study of elite swimmers, NK cell number declined after 7 months of swim training despite no changes in other cell counts (29). A brief period (6 days) of intense training also attenuates the leukocyte response to acute exercise (30). It is not known whether these changes reflect increased cell turnover or migration of cells out of the circulation, nor whether there are any long-term implications.

Clinicians who treat physically active patients should be aware of both acute and chronic exercise-induced changes in circulating immune cell counts because these data are often used to diagnose or to make decisions about treatment. If an accurate leukocyte differential count is needed for clinical purposes, physically active patients should refrain from exercise for at least 24 hours before blood sampling.

EFFECTS ON LEUKOCYTE FUNCTION

Despite only transient perturbation in circulating leukocyte number, good evidence shows both acute and chronic effects of exercise on immune cell function. Neutrophil and monocyte functions, NK cell cytotoxicity, and lymphocyte proliferation are all affected by intense exercise.

EFFECTS ON NATURAL KILLER CELL FUNCTION

Natural killer cell cytotoxic activity (NKCA) increases during and immediately after moderate and intense exercise; the magnitude of change is directly related to exercise intensity and duration. NKCA returns to resting levels soon after moderate exercise, but declines below baseline values between 1 and 6 hours after intense prolonged exercise. The mechanisms responsible for these changes in NKCA during and after exercise are complex. The increase in NKCA immediately after exercise appears to result from the rise in NK-cell number in the blood. The reasons for the delayed decrease in NKCA have been debated, which is reviewed by Mackinnon (1), and it is beyond the scope of this chapter to discuss this issue fully. Briefly, it appears that this delayed decline in NKCA reflects both decreased number and suppressed killing activity of NK cells in the blood. Given the role of NK cells in defense against viruses, it has been suggested that prolonged suppression of NKCA after intense exercise may provide an "open window," during which the athlete may be susceptible to infection (31).

Despite this apparent suppression of NKCA acutely after intense exercise, NKCA does not appear to be adversely affected by intense exercise training over the long term because resting NKCA is normal in athletes. Moderate exercise training may enhance NKCA. For example, resting NKCA was higher in moderately trained distance runners compared with matched nonrunners (32). In an animal model, exercised mice exhibited higher NKCA and less tumor retention compared with sedentary controls (33).

EFFECTS ON NEUTROPHIL FUNCTION

Acute intense, but not moderate, exercise stimulates several aspects of neutrophil function, including migration, degranulation, phagocytosis, and respiratory burst activity. Stimulation may last for several hours after prolonged exercise, possibly as a result of the recruitment of younger, more active neutrophils into the circulation (34). After exercise, neutrophils infiltrate tissues such as nasal mucosa (35) and skeletal muscle (36), and this has been suggested to cause local inflammation by release of reactive oxygen species and chemotactic factors, which attract inflammatory cells (37).

Although neutrophil function is stimulated by acute exercise, chronic exercise appears to downregulate this response. Athletes undergoing intense training exhibit lower resting and postexercise neutrophil function compared with nonathletes and their own values obtained during moderate training (38,39). This apparent downregulation of neutrophil function may be protective by limiting neutrophil involvement in inflammation associated with daily intense exercise (1,34). Whether such downregulation of neutrophil activity increases susceptibility to illness is not known. One report found no association between depressed neutrophil function and the incidence of URTI in elite swimmers (39). Moderate exercise training appears to have little effect on neutrophil function.

EFFECTS ON LYMPHOCYTE PROLIFERATION

Lymphocyte proliferation is sensitive to exercise intensity and duration. Acute moderate exercise has little or a slight stimulatory effect on proliferation. In contrast, intense exercise appears to suppress proliferation for up to 3 hours after exercise. The mechanism responsible is not fully known and is likely to be complex. Some, but not all, of the suppression can be attributed to increased catecholamine release and fewer lymphocytes in the blood during recovery after exercise (40). A decrease in the number of circulating type 1 T lymphocytes may contribute to lower lymphocyte proliferation after exercise (41). Decreased lymphocyte proliferation following prolonged exercise may also be caused by an increased rate of death of CD4 and CD8 T lymphocytes (42). Exercise training, regardless of intensity, has little effect on resting lymphocyte proliferation, indicating that any effects are transitory and perhaps of limited clinical significance. Exercise training has been associated with increased expression of lymphocyte activation markers, suggesting that chronic exercise may enhance the ability of these cells to respond to immune challenges.

EFFECTS ON SOLUBLE MEDIATORS OF IMMUNE FUNCTION

The exercise immunology literature has explored the effects of exercise on diverse soluble mediators of immune function, focusing mainly on cytokines, immunoglobulin, and antibody, and to a lesser extent on complement and acute phase proteins.

Effects on Cytokines

Intense, prolonged exercise induces release of several cytokines. The plasma concentrations of proinflammatory cytokines (e.g., IL-1 and TNF-α) increase slightly (up to threefold) after exercise (43), whereas those with antiviral activity (e.g., IL-2, IFN-α/β) generally remain unchanged. In contrast, the concentrations of IL-6 increase more than 100 times, anti-inflammatory cytokines (e.g., IL-10, IL-1 receptor antagonist) increase up to 50 times, and chemokines (e.g. granulocyte-colony stimulating factor, monocyte chemotactic protein-1, macrophage inhibitory protein-1β) increase up to 30 times following prolonged, strenuous exercise (43,44).

In response to intense exercise, the percentage of circulating type 1 T lymphocytes decreases, whereas the percentage of circulating type 2 T lymphocytes remains unchanged (30,41). These effects may be mediated by epinephrine and IL-6 (41). This indicates a shift toward type 2 T-lymphocyte responses following intense exercise. Recall that type 1 T lymphocytes regulate cell-mediated immunity and protection against viral infection, whereas type 2 T lymphocytes regulate humoral immunity and IgE-mediated allergic reactions. A shift in favor of type 2 T-lymphocyte responses may increase risk of viral infection in athletes, while also increasing the risk of asthma and allergic reactions.

Initial research suggested that muscle damage is a major stimulus for cytokine production during exercise (45), but more recent research suggests that muscle damage plays a relatively minor role (46). Other factors, such as low blood glucose concentration, muscle glycogen depletion, calcium signaling, and oxidative stress, appear to have a greater influence on the cytokine response to exercise (47–49). The time course of cytokine production in response to exercise differs between cytokines. Early release of inflammatory cytokines, such as IL-1 and TNF-α, after distance running is balanced by later release of other cytokines, such as IL-10 and IL-1 receptor antagonist (IL-1ra) that inhibit the inflammatory cytokines (43). IL-6 is now recognized as an anti-inflammatory cytokine during exercise because it inhibits the production of TNF-α, possibly by stimulating the production of IL-10 and IL-1ra (50).

Cytokine production is not always apparent from blood samples, because cytokines act locally and are rapidly removed from circulation. For example, IL-1β and TNF-α mRNA levels increase to a greater extent in skeletal muscle during exercise (51,52) than does the plasma concentration of these cytokines (53). Skeletal muscle is a major source of IL-6 and accounts for most of the IL-6 circulating during exercise (47,48). IL-8 and IL-10 mRNA are also expressed within skeletal muscle following exercise (52). Because these cytokines are produced in skeletal muscle, they have been termed 'myokines' (47). Whereas some evidence suggests that muscle cells generate IL-6, it is not known whether other myokines are synthesized by muscle cells or other cell types resident in muscle (e.g., leukocytes, fibroblasts, endothelial cells). Recent data suggest that leukocytes present in skeletal muscle may be a source of mRNA for IL-1ra, IL-8, and IL-10 (54). Cytokines are cleared rapidly from the circulation and are detected in urine for up to several days after prolonged exercise (55).

Exercise training may alter the amount and pattern of cytokine release, possibly by downregulating proinflammatory processes and upregulating anti-inflammatory processes (50). This response may have positive implications for individuals with chronic heart failure (56–58), obesity and diabetes (59), and chronic kidney disease (60). Downregulation of TLRs on circulating monocytes may contribute to lower systemic levels of proinflammatory cytokines and C-reactive protein following exercise training (2).

It is not clear whether acute or chronic exercise-induced changes in cytokine levels influence immune function. A shift in the type 1/type 2 cytokine balance toward dominance of type 2 cytokine production may, however, contribute to the overtraining syndrome in athletes (61) and may be one possible mechanism for the higher incidence of URTI symptoms experienced by athletes training intensely or when overtrained, as discussed earlier. The overtraining syndrome is characterized by fatigue, hormonal disturbances, performance decrements, weight loss, and mood changes. Data on changes in resting cytokine levels in response to brief periods of intensified training are equivocal, however. Some research suggests that 1–2 weeks of intensified training increases resting plasma IL-6 concentration (62) and suppresses the number and percentage of T lymphocytes producing IFN-γ (30), whereas other research has reported no change in resting plasma concentrations of IL-6 or TNF-α after a short period of overreaching (63). Alterations in plasma IL-6 concentration during intensified training may depend partly on the degree of muscle damage incurred during exercise (62).

Effects Immunoglobulin (Ig) and Antibody

Serum and mucosal immunoglobulin serve different functions and are regulated independently; exercise appears to affect serum and mucosal immunoglobulin differently (1). Serum immunoglobulin concentration remains relatively unchanged after both acute and chronic exercise, although clinically low concentrations of some IgG subclasses were observed in elite athletes undergoing months of intense training (64). However, the ability to mount a specific antibody response (i.e., to a specific antigenic challenge or immunization) is normal in athletes (65,66); it is not clear whether there are clinical implications of the low levels of serum IgG subclasses in athletes. Recent research indicates that physically fit elderly individuals generate less IgG1 and tend to produce more IgG2 than elderly individuals with low fitness (24).

Mucosal IgA is a major effector of host defense against viruses causing URTI. Low mucosal IgA concentration has been observed in some athletes and low levels may be predictive of risk for URTI (67). Salivary IgA concentration declines after brief or prolonged intense exercise but is unaffected by moderate exercise. Salivary IgA concentrations decrease over long-term training (>6 months), but may not change appreciably over shorter training periods (67). These observations are consistent with the "J-curve" model (discussed above), in which the risk of URTI increases with exercise intensity or volume, and may partially explain the elevated risk of URTI in endurance athletes. Salivary IgA concentration in athletes may depend on fitness level. It is difficult, however, to assess the biological significance of changes in salivary IgA concentration in groups, as interindividual variation tends to obscure trends in individuals (67). The following questions relating to mucosal immunity await further investigation (67): (a) does mucosal immunity reflect overall immune status, (b) does the type of exercise influence acute changes in mucosal immunity, (c) what factors influence responses to long-term training, (d) does moderate exercise enhance mucosal immunity, (e) can markers of mucosal immunity be used to monitor overtraining and (f) what therapeutic and dietary factors influence mucosal immunity?

EFFECTS ON HSP72

Endurance exercise increases intracellular expression of HSP72 in monocytes and granulocytes (68). The intracellular expression of HSP72 is reduced in endurance trained athletes compared with untrained individuals, suggesting an adaptive response to the stress imposed by regular exercise (68). Exercise also increases the extracellular release of HSP72, as indicated by an increase in plasma or serum HSP72 concentration (69–72). Sources of extracellular HSP72 release during exercise include the brain (4) and hepatosplanchnic tissue (69). Extracellular HSP72 is released within exosomes through a nonclassic protein transport pathway (3, 4). The stimuli for the release of extracellular HSP72 may include oxidative stress

(72) and reduced blood glucose availability (70). The biological significance of changes in extracellular HSP72 during exercise is not immediately clear at present, but extracellular HSP72 may serve as a danger signal to activate the innate immune system (3).

EFFECTS ON TOLL-LIKE RECEPTORS

In recent years, increasing attention has focused on changes in the expression of TLRs on circulating monocytes following acute exercise and chronic training. Acute exercise in hot conditions (34°C) suppresses the expression of TLR1, TL2, and TLR4, but not TLR9 on the $CD14^+$ monocytes. Exercise also suppresses the expression of MHC II, co-stimulatory molecules CD80 and CD86 and lipopolysaccharide-stimulated IL-6 on $CD14^+$ monocytes (74). Cross-sectional studies have indicated that TLR4 expression on the surface of $CD14^+$ monocytes is lower in physically active individuals compared with sedentary individuals. These findings have also been confirmed in longitudinal studies of exercise training in previously untrained individuals (2). The biological significance of alterations in the expression of TLRs following strenuous acute exercise and chronic training is unclear at present. Downregulation of TLRs after acute exercise may increase the risk of URTI following strenuous exercise (74). Long-term downregulation of TLRs after training may reduce chronic low grade infection (2). More research is needed to investigate these possibilities.

ARE ATHLETES IMMUNOCOMPROMISED?

As mentioned above, athletes experience high rates of URTI during intense training and after major competition. Viral URTI appears to be the only illness to which athletes are at increased risk, suggesting that, from a clinical perspective, any suppression of immune function is relatively mild. On the other hand, the occurrence of URTI at a particular time in the athlete's training cycle or competition may be critical to the athlete's career.

Thus, although athletes are not considered clinically immune deficient, evidence discussed above suggests that mild suppression of several immune parameters occurs during intense training. It is possible that, in athletes, the combined effects of small changes in several immune parameters may compromise resistance to minor infectious agents or cause reactivation of some viruses. For example, overtrained athletes show some evidence of reactivation of Epstein-Barr virus, a common virus to which most adults are exposed, which causes symptoms of upper respiratory tract infection (75–77). In a double-blind, placebo-controlled study from the same laboratory, an antiviral agent (Valtrex) decreased the Epstein-Barr virus load but did not decrease the incidence of URTI symptoms, when given to elite distance runners over a 4-month period (78). Thus, it is unclear whether the symptoms of URTI associated with overtraining and prolonged

TABLE 16.6. PRACTICAL ADVICE FOR ATHLETES WISHING TO AVOID IMMUNE SUPPRESSION

Avoid Overtraining
- Schedule rest days
- Include periodization and recovery training
- Allow adequate rest after competition
- Avoid too frequent competition

Limit Exposure to Potential Sources of Illness
- Limit exposure to crowds during and after competition
- Avoid extended air travel immediately before and after competition

Ensure Adequate Nutrition
- Total energy, protein, carbohydrates
- Iron, vitamin C
- Avoid rapid weight loss (e.g., wrestlers, lightweight rowers)

Rest or Only Light Exercise During Systemic Viral illness
- Seek medical advice for all but simple head cold
- Avoid exercise when febrile
- Return to training or competition only when asymptomatic

periods of intense training are caused by an infectious agent. It is possible that the localized symptoms of the infection may have an inflammatory rather than an infectious origin (17).

In contrast, moderate exercise training appears to have either no effect, or may slightly enhance, resistance to URTI, possibly by stimulating immune function. Although competitive athletes must train intensely on a regular basis, monitoring athletes' adaptation to training, allowing adequate recovery between sessions and after major competition, and attention to other factors, such as proper nutrition and stress management, may help athletes avoid immune suppression and associated illness (Table 16.6).

EXERCISE AND IMMUNE FUNCTION UNDER ENVIRONMENTAL STRESS

Unaccustomed environmental stress during exercise, such as cold or heat exposure and altitude, places considerable demands on muscle metabolism, in addition to the thermoregulatory, cardiovascular, and pulmonary systems of the body. Such stress also modifies neuroendocrine responses to exercise, which in turn may influence immune function. Exercise in hot conditions increases the concentration of circulating leukocytes and cytokines, whereas the effects of heat on neutrophil, lymphocyte, and NK cell function are variable (79, 80, 81). Immune changes during exercise may contribute in part to exertional heat illness (82). Although current research suggests that exercise in the heat does not significantly impair immune function, most of this research has been performed under tightly controlled laboratory conditions. Strenuous exertion under conditions in the field where ambient temperature is likely to be higher than in the exercise laboratory (e.g., military operations, fire fighting) may pose a greater risk to immune function (79).

Less is known about the effects of exercising in cold conditions and at altitude. During exercise in cold conditions, circulating leukocyte concentrations may be lower (83), whereas NK cell activity (84) and salivary IgA concentration are unaffected by the cold (79). Insufficient evidence currently exists to evaluate whether exercise in the cold increases the risk of URTI (79). Simulated hypoxia during exercise increases circulating NK cell counts but does not influence NK cell activity (85). Tentative evidence suggests that the combination of living in simulated altitude (2,500–3,000 m) while training at lower altitude (1,200 m) tends to reduce salivary IgA concentration (86). The findings of this study (86) should be interpreted cautiously because of limitations in the experimental design and the lack of significant differences in salivary IgA concentration between the experimental and control groups. Symptoms of URTI are often confused with symptoms of acute mountain sickness, which makes it difficult to assess whether exercising at high altitude the increases risk of infection (79).

IMMUNE CHANGES AFTER REPEATED BOUTS OF EXERCISE

Professional athletes often train more than once per day. Repeated bouts of exercise without sufficient recovery can result in fatigue and neuroendocrine disturbances that may influence some immune variables. Shorter recovery time (3 versus 6 hours) between two bouts of endurance exercise is associated with a greater increase in serum catecholamine concentration following the second bout of exercise. In contrast, the length of recovery time does not influence changes in concentrations of serum growth hormone and testosterone, and circulating leukocyte, plasma IL-6, and IL-1ra following a second bout of exercise (87,88). Resting concentrations of plasma IL-6 and IL-1ra, and neutrophils and lymphocytes return to baseline more slowly after exercise when recovery time is shortened (87,88). Therefore, athletes and coaches need to be aware that the recovery time between training sessions influences the sympathetic nervous system and may delay the recovery of some immune variables after exercise. This may have important implications if athletes are exposed to infectious pathogens between training sessions.

DIET, EXERCISE, AND IMMUNE FUNCTION

Proper nutrition is essential to a competent immune system. Malnutrition is the most common cause of immune suppression throughout the world, primarily in less-developed countries (6). In developed countries, where malnutrition is less of an issue, nutrition has relevance to immune function in various groups, including athletes, the elderly, and obese individuals attempting to lose weight.

Optimal immune function depends on adequate intake of a number of factors. Deficiency in immune function can result from inadequate intake of total energy, protein, minerals (e.g., zinc or iron), vitamins (e.g., vitamin C or E), or other antioxidants. On the other hand, it is questionable whether supplementation with any of these substances enhances immune function in the absence of deficiency. It is beyond the scope of this chapter to fully discuss the relationship between diet, exercise, and immune function, and only a brief discussion of some relevant aspects is included.

Physical work capacity may be compromised by inadequate diet. It is well known that athletes may have special dietary needs: Dietary carbohydrate supplementation either before or during prolonged exercise may delay the onset of fatigue, endurance exercise performance is compromised in iron-deficient athletes, and endurance and power athletes require additional protein intake compared with the sedentary population. Athletes are avid consumers of a range of dietary products purported to enhance physical performance or immunity to infection, such as vitamins, minerals, antioxidants, carbohydrate or protein supplements, and glutamine.

DIETARY CARBOHYDRATE

During prolonged exercise, depletion of muscle glycogen and blood glucose contributes to the onset of fatigue. Consumption of a high carbohydrate (CHO) diet in the days before, or CHO-containing fluids (e.g., sports drink) during prolonged exercise helps maintain blood glucose levels and may delay the onset of fatigue. Maintaining blood glucose levels through dietary CHO manipulation also attenuates some of the exercise-induced changes in immune parameters. This is thought to occur by preventing the rise in IL-6 and in stress hormones, such as catecholamines, cortisol, and growth hormone, during exercise.

Ingestion of CHO during prolonged exercise attenuates the changes in blood leukocyte and lymphocyte counts, and cytokines such as IL-6, IL-1ra, and IL-10 (51–53). CHO attenuates plasma IL-6 concentration following exercise by reducing the release of IL-6 from skeletal muscle (89). The effects of CHO on IL-6 gene expression in skeletal muscle depend on the mode of exercise (51,52,89). CHO also reduces IL-8, IL-10, and IL-1ra gene expression in leukocytes (54).

The effects of CHO ingestion on other aspects of immune function vary. Some research has indicated that CHO supplementation during exercise reduces salivary IgA concentration (90), increases NKCA (91), and prevents a decline in T-lymphocyte proliferation (42). Other research has, however, reported different effects or no effects on these immune variables (52,92). Some of this variability may be related to differences in intensity, duration, and mode of exercise; CHO supplementation; and fitness levels of study participants. CHO prevents a decrease in lipolysaccharide-stimulated elastase release from neutrophils following exercise (93). More recent research has demonstrated that CHO prevents the suppression of in vitro production of IFN-γ by CD4$^+$ and CD8$^+$ T lymphocytes (94), and attenuates the release of extracellular HSP72 (70) following exercise. Further research is needed to determine whether there are clinical implications of altering the immune system response to exercise in athletes or other groups.

IRON AND ZINC

Iron and other minerals (e.g., zinc, selenium) are required for normal immune function. Iron deficiency is associated with impaired lymphocyte proliferation, NKCA, and phagocytic function (95,96). Iron is lost from the body during exercise through sweat and the destruction of red blood cells; endurance athletes may have increased iron requirements because of increased turnover of red blood cells. Menstruating female endurance athletes may be especially susceptible to iron deficiency because of additional losses each cycle. The prevalence of iron deficiency among athletes of either sex is not known because the expansion of plasma volume in response to endurance training (a positive adaptive response) can lead to artificially low blood hemoglobin concentration ("pseudoanemia"). This topic is discussed in detail in Chapter 19. Severe zinc deficiency is associated with increased risk of infection, altered cellular immune responses, reduced numbers of blood lymphocytes, and defective neutrophil chemotaxis (97). Similar to iron, zinc is lost from the body during exercise through sweat. Some athletes may also be at risk of low dietary zinc intake because of lower consumption of protein-rich foods coupled with high carbohydrate and fiber intake, which limits zinc absorption.

The relationship between iron and zinc status and immune function has not been studied extensively in athletes. A preliminary report noted lower NKCA in female runners with low compared with normal serum ferritin concentration (98) In this study, 8 weeks' iron supplementation (100 mg elemental iron/day) had no effect on NKCA in the low ferritin runners despite increasing serum ferritin concentration toward normal levels. Eight weeks' supplementation may have been insufficient to alter NKCA. Plasma zinc concentration is lower in endurance runners than in sedentary individuals (97). This lower zinc status does not, however, appear to influence resting leukocyte numbers or lymphocyte proliferation during a moderate increase in training volume (97). Zinc

supplementation does not influence changes in plasma IL-6 concentration following exercise (99), but it attenuates the effects of exercise on neutrophil respiratory burst activity (100).

Various diseases or treatments may influence iron status. For example, cancer therapy can induce anemia and low red blood cell counts (discussed further in Chapters 15 and 19). It is possible that immune suppression may result, although these patients will be taking other medications that may also contribute to impaired immunity (e.g., cytotoxic drugs). Certainly, the clinical exercise physiologist should consider, among other factors, the possible adverse effect of iron status on immune function when prescribing exercise for these patients.

ANTIOXIDANT VITAMINS

A diet rich in antioxidants is thought to protect against cancer, although it is unclear whether such protection directly involves the immune system. Immune cells are susceptible to damage by oxidants, such as free radicals produced in oxidative metabolism, and normal leukocyte function (101). Neutrophils release reactive oxygen and nitrogen species, which are toxic to pathogens but may also cause inflammation and damage within normal cells. Increased oxidative metabolism (as occurs in prolonged exercise) produces reactive oxygen species. This suggests that free-radical–induced damage to leukocytes is one mechanism by which prolonged exercise may impair immune function. Evidence suggests that programmed cell death (apoptosis) occurs in lymphocytes after intense exercise (42). If this hypothesis is correct, then it is possible that antioxidant supplementation prevents or limits exercise-induced immune suppression.

One antioxidant vitamin, vitamin C, has long been purported to be prophylactic against the common cold. Despite years of scrutiny, however, the evidence is still equivocal in normal populations, and it appears that any effect of supplementation can occur by decreasing the duration and severity of symptoms rather than by reducing the incidence (92). On the other hand, evidence does suggest that vitamin C can prevent the common cold in certain conditions, such as physical stress (92). For example, in a double-blind study, 84 distance runners and 73 nonrunners consumed either 600 mg/day of vitamin C or placebo for 3 weeks before a 90-km ultramarathon race (10). In the 2 weeks after the race, the incidence of URTI symptoms was reduced by more than half in runners who took supplements compared with those consuming placebo. In contrast, vitamin C supplementation had no effect on the incidence of symptoms in nonrunners. Vitamins A and E had no effect on URTI incidence after an ultramarathon (103). The mechanisms by which vitamin C protects against URTI are unknown, but it has been suggested that any effects may relate to the vitamin's antioxidant activity and protection against reactive oxygen species produced by activated neutrophils (94). The influence of vitamin C and other antioxidants (e.g., vitamin E, N-acetylcysteine) on exercise-induced changes in other aspects of immune function, such as salivary IgA secretion, lymphocyte production, and cytokine production, is negligible and inconsistent (95,96). One month of daily supplementation with a combination of vitamin C (500 mg), γ-tocopherol (130 IU) and α-tocopherol (290 IU) completely attenuates the release of extracellular HSP72 during exercise (72).

GLUTAMINE

Glutamine is the most abundant amino acid in the body; skeletal muscle provides the largest source of glutamine. Proliferating lymphocytes require glutamine as an energy source and for nucleotide synthesis. A decrease in glutamine levels during physiologic stress, such as surgery, burns, and trauma, has been associated with immunosuppression. Glutamine supplementation helps restore immunity in these conditions (107).

Plasma glutamine concentration declines acutely and remains low for up to several hours after prolonged exercise (108), decreases during intense exercise training, and is lower in overtrained compared with well-trained athletes (107). More recent data indicate no change in plasma glutamine concentration followed a period of intensified training (63). Low plasma glutamine concentration may compromise lymphocyte function and thus impair immunity to infection (107). A brief report suggests the possibility that glutamine supplementation can prevent URTI after endurance competition (distance running) (109). Other data, however, do not support a role of glutamine in preventing immune suppression after exercise. For example, despite significantly lower plasma glutamine concentration in overtrained compared with well-trained swimmers, glutamine concentration did not differ between athletes who developed URTI and those who did not during 4 weeks of intensified training (110). Research findings on the relationship between changes in plasma glutamine concentration and immune changes after exercise are also inconsistent (107,108,111,112). The effects of glutamine may depend on the nature of exericse and may be specific to certain aspects of immune function.

OTHER DIETARY AND PHARMACOLOGIC INTERVENTIONS

One month of supplementation with a probiotic supplement containing *Lactobacillis acidophilus* has been reported to improve the production of interferon-γ in fatigued athletes presenting with reactivation of Epstein-Barr virus (75). Ingestion of nonsteroidal anti-inflammatory drugs before and during an ultramarathon race increases plasma cytokine concentrations after the race (44), whereas anti-inflammatory drugs and analgesics generally do not influence the inflammatory response to exercise-induced muscle damage (46).

DIET, EXERCISE, AND IMMUNE FUNCTION IN THE ELDERLY

Aging is associated with immunosenescence, which refers to dysregulated immune function, rather than impaired immune function. Aging is associated with a number of changes in immune function, including increased mortality rate owing to infection; decreased NK cell number, killing activity, and proliferation; decreased T-cell proliferation, B-cell number, plasma cell differentiation capacity, and the proportion of functional antibody; and an imbalance between type 1 and type 2 cytokines (112). It is unclear, however, whether such changes are inevitable or result from diseases that increase in prevalence with aging, such as cardiovascular disease and cancer, or other factors, such as increased body fat or inactivity. One viewpoint is that, in the absence of disease, age-related changes in immune function are relatively small, as shown in studies of healthy centenarians (people ≥100 years of age). It has been suggested that a "continuous remodeling" of the immune system occurs from birth, during which some immune variables change whereas others are maintained during senescence (114).

The immune response to acute exercise is preserved in the elderly, but it is quantitatively smaller. Cross-sectional studies provide tentative evidence that, compared with sedentary elderly individuals, physically active elderly individuals have slightly higher NKCA (113). In addition, physically active elderly individuals produce more IgG and IgM, generate a stronger lymphocyte proliferative response following vaccination (115), and have a stronger delayed-type hypersensitivity (116). Most prospective studies indicate that a minimum of 6 months of exercise training is necessary to improve immune function in elderly individuals (113). One exception to this trend is that 10 weeks of resistance training in older postmenopausal women does not influence CD4$^+$, CD8$^+$, or NK cell counts, but improves NKCA after an acute bout of resistance exercise (117). Ten months of moderate aerobic exercise training (3 days/week, 25–30 minutes, 65%–75% maximal heart rate) reduces the severity of URTI in elderly individuals (112). Aerobic training increases T-cell activation and CD25 expression (IL-2 receptor-α) in elderly individuals, whereas a combination of resistance and flexibility training is less effective (113). Exercise training also increases salivary IgA concentration and secretion rate (118), increases IL-2 and IL-2 receptor expression (119), downregulates TLR4 expression on CD14$^+$ monocytes, and reduces the plasma concentrations of C-reactive protein and cytokines (113).

The inflammatory response to exercise-induced muscle damage is impaired in elderly compared with young individuals (44,120).

The mechanisms by which exercise training alters immunosenescence require further clarification. Other issues that await further investigation include (113) (a) whether aerobic exercise has different effects than resistance training, (b) the optimal amount of exercise necessary to counter immunosenescence, and (c) whether the benefits of exercise are restricted to certain aging populations.

Whereas the aging process may be responsible for changes in immune function in the elderly, poor nutrition may also play a role; for a number of reasons, including economic, the elderly are often mildly deficient in protein and key vitamins and minerals (121). Daily supplementation of micronutrients may improve immune function in the healthy elderly. For example, 17 weeks of dietary supplements, with or without regular exercise, increases blood indicators of nutritional status (e.g., vitamin, ferritinconcentrations) in elderly subjects (121). The combination of exercise and dietary supplements also induces a greater decrease in serum C-reactive protein concentration than does exercise alone (121).

EFFECTS OF WEIGHT LOSS ON IMMUNE FUNCTION

Obesity is associated with a higher incidence of infection and cancer, suggesting impairment of immune function, although it is not clear whether this results directly from obesity or indirectly from other factors, such as a sedentary lifestyle or nutritional imbalance. Obesity has been linked with high circulating leukocyte concentrations (primarily neutrophils and monocytes) and cytokines, reduced T- and B-lymphocyte proliferation, and lower NKCA (14,56,121). It would seem logical, then, that weight loss may enhance immune function in the obese, although evidence for this view is equivocal. Some studies have shown enhanced immune parameters after weight loss in obese subjects, whereas others have shown the opposite. It appears that the model of weight loss and immune parameters assessed can both influence the results of these studies. For example, in a study of 22 healthy obese women, diet alone (900 kcal/day liquid diet for 8 weeks) resulted in significant declines in NKCA and IL-2 receptor expression by PBMC (122). In contrast, in the same study, a combined diet plus exercise regimem (same diet plus mild aerobic and resistance exercise 3 times/week) prevented the decreases in NKCA and IL-2 receptor expression, despite similar loss of body mass in both regimens (11–12 kg) (122). In another study of 91 obese women, lymphocyte proliferation declined similarly after weight loss regardless of the method (12-week diet alone, exercise alone, or diet plus exercise) compared with controls who did not lose weight (14). Other immune parameters, such as NKCA and phagocytosis, did not change with weight loss, however. Compared with the former study (122), the latter study (14) induced less energy restriction (1200 versus 900 kcal/day), more gradual weight loss (2–8 kg over 12 weeks versus 11–12 kg over 8 weeks), and more exercise (5 versus 3 days/week), which may partially explain the different results. A more recent cross-sectional study reported an inverse relationship between weight loss over a period of 20 years and NKCA in healthy, overweight, sedentary postmenopausal women (123). Another study of middle-aged obese men, with and without type 2 diabetes, indicated that 60 minutes of aerobic exercise five times per week for 12 weeks reduces resting plasma IL-6 concentration without reducing body mass (59). Some evidence suggests that more than 4% loss of body weight in judo athletes over 1 month of training impairs resting lymphocyte function (124).

The mechanisms responsible for changes in immune function after weight loss are unknown at present. It is unclear which factors associated with weight loss influence the immune system: energy deficit, changes in body composition, changes in metabolism, or some combination of factors. At present, it would appear that gradual weight loss induced by moderate dietary restriction and exercise, as generally recommended for good health, may avoid or attenuate any adverse effects on immune function. Certainly, compelling health reasons exist for weight reduction in the obese and overweight (e.g., reduced risk of cardiovascular and metabolic diseases), and any possible mild impairment of immune function does not negate the general recommendation for all individuals to maintain a healthy body weight.

SUMMARY AND CONCLUSIONS

The human immune system is a complex system with overlapping and complementary functions requiring extensive communication and coordination between its various effector cells and messenger molecules. Immune function can be altered by a variety of conditions, including disease, medication, surgery, trauma, dietary imbalance, and physical or psychological stress. Physical stress, such as strenuous exercise, causes an influx of immune cells into the peripheral circulation and may induce changes in immune cell function; most effects are transitory, and normal levels are generally restored within 24 hours. Long-term moderate exercise training appears to have little effect on, and may slightly enhance, immune function. In contrast, prolonged periods of intense exercise training may induce mild suppression of several immune parameters. Although athletes are not considered clinically immune deficient, this mild suppression of immunity may contribute to the high incidence of URTI in endurance athletes. Inadequate nutrition, obesity, and rapid weight loss may also compromise immunity. Dietary supplementation may be of value in some individuals, such as the elderly, or in those with specific deficiencies. Moderate exercise training attenuates adverse effects on immune function resulting from weight loss in obese individuals. The clinical exercise physiologist should be aware of the immune response to exercise in healthy individuals and in those with diseases affecting immune function to safely prescribe exercise for these individuals. Given the suppressive effects of intense exercise on immune function in healthy individuals, it would be prudent to prescribe moderate physical activity for patients with immune system dysfunction, regardless of whether such dysfunction is caused directly by disease or is secondary to treatment.

REFERENCES

1. Mackinnon LT. *Advances in Exercise Immunology*. Champaign, IL: Human Kinetics; 1999.
2. Gleeson M, McFarlin B, Flynn M. Exercise and toll-like receptors. *Exerc Immunol Rev* 2006;12:34–53.
3. Asea A. Stress proteins and initiation of immune response: Chaperokine activity of HSP72. *Exerc Immunol Rev* 2005;11:34–45.
4. Lancaster GI, Febbraio MA. Mechanisms of stress-induced cellular HSP72 release: Implications for exercise-induced increases in extracellular HSP72. *Exerc Immunol Rev* 2005;11:46–52.
5. Fehrenbach E, Schneider ME. Trauma-induced systemic inflammatory response versus exercise-induced immunomodulatory effects. *Sports Med* 2006;36:373–84.
6. Janeway CA, Travers P, Walport M, et al. *Immunobiology: The Immune System in Health and Disease*, 4th ed. New York: Elsevier Science; 693–699.
7. Gleeson M. Immune function in sport and exercise. *J Appl Physiol* 2007. In press.
8. Nieman DC, Johanssen LM, Lee JW, et al. Infectious episodes in runners before and after the Los Angeles Marathon. *J Sports Med Phys Fitness* 1990;30:316–28.
9. Peters EM, Bateman ED. Ultramarathon running and upper respiratory tract infections. *S Afr J Sports Med* 1983;64:582–84.
10. Peters EM, Goetzsche JM, Grobbelaar B, et al. Vitamin C supplementation reduces the incidence of postrace symptoms of upper respiratory tract infection in ultramarathon runners. *Am J Clin Nutr* 1993;57:170–4.
11. Heath GW, Ford ES, Craven TE, et al. Exercise and the incidence of upper respiratory tract infections. *Med Sci Sports Exerc* 1991;23:152–7.
12. Ekblom B, Ekblom O, Malm C. Infectious episodes before and after a marathon race. *Scand J Med Sci Sports* 2006;16:287–93.
13. Nieman DC, Johanssen LM, Lee JW. Infectious episodes in runners before and after a roadrace. *J Sports Med Phys Fitness* 1989;29:289–96.
14. Nieman DC, Nehlsen-Cannarella SL, Henson DA, et al. Immune responses to exercise training and/or energy restriction in obese women. *Med Sci Sports Exerc* 1998;30:679–86.
15. Matthews CE, Ockene IS, Freedson PS, et al. Moderate to vigorous physical activity and the risk of upper-respiratory tract infection. *Med Sci Sports Exerc* 2002;34:1242–8.
16. Chubak J, McTiernan A, Sorensen B, et al. Moderate intensity exercise reduces the incidence of colds among postmenopausal women. *Am J Med* 2006;119:937–42.
17. Spence L, Brown WJ, Pyne DB, et al. Incidence, etiology, and symptomatology of upper respiratory illness in elite athletes. *Med Sci Sports Exerc* 2007;39:557–86.
18. Friman G, Ilback N-G. Acute infection: Metabolic responses, effects on performance, interaction with exercise, and myocarditis. *Int J Sports Med* 1998;19:S172–82.
19. Parker S, Brukner PD, Rosier M. Chronic fatigue syndrome and the athlete. *Sports Med Training Rehab* 1996;6:269–78.
20. Weidner TG, Cranston T, Schurr T, et al. The effect of exercise training on the severity and duration of a viral respiratory illness. *Med Sci Sports Exerc* 1998;30:1578–83.
21. Lowder T, Padgett DA, Woods JA. Moderate exercise protects mice from death due to influenza virus. *Brain Behav Immun* 2005;19:377–80.
22. Edwards KM, Burns VE, Reynolds T. Acute stress exposure prior to influenza vaccine antibody response in women. *Brain Behav Immun* 2006;20:159–68.
23. Edwards KM, Burns VE, Allen LM. Eccentric exercise as an adjuvant to influenza vaccine in humans. *Brain Behav Immun* 2007;21:209–17.
24. Keylock KT, Lowder T, Leifheit KA, et al. Higher antibody, but not cell-mediated responses, to vaccination in high physically fit elderly. *J Appl Physiol* 2007;102:1090–8.
25. Pizza FX, Mitchell JB, Davis BH, et al. Exercise-induced muscle damage: Effect on circulating leukocyte and lymphocyte subsets. *Med Sci Sports Exerc* 1995;27:363–70.
26. Peake JM, Suzuki K, Wilson G, et al. Exercise-induced muscle damage, plasma cytokines and markers of neutrophil activation. *Med Sci Sports Exerc* 2005;37:737–45.
27. Dhabhar FS. Stress-induced enhancement of cell-mediated immunity. *Ann N Y Acad Sci* 1998;840:359–72.
28. Lehmann M, Mann H, Gastmann U, et al. Unaccustomed high-mileage vs intensity training-related changes in performance and serum amino acid levels. *Int J Sports Med* 1996;17:187–92.
29. Gleeson M, McDonald WA, Cripps AW, et al. The effect on immunity of long-term intensive training in elite swimmers. *Clin Exp Immunol* 1995;102:210–6.
30. Lancaster GI, Halson SL, Khan Q, et al. Effects of acute exhaustive exercise and chronic exercise training on type 1 and type 2 T lymphocytes. *Exerc Immunol Rev* 2004;10:91–106.
31. Pedersen BK, Ullum H. NK cell response to physical activity: Possible mechanisms of action. *Med Sci Sports Exerc* 1994;26:140–6.
32. Nieman DC, Buckley KS, Henson DA, et al. Immune function in marathon runners vs sedentary controls. *Med Sci Sports Exerc* 1995;27:986–92.
33. MacNeil B, Hoffman-Goetz L. Chronic exercise enhances in vivo and in vitro cytotoxic mechanisms of natural immunity in mice. *J Appl Physiol* 1993;74:388–95.
34. Suzuki K, Totsuka M, Nakaji S, et al. Endurance exercise causes interaction among stress hormones, cytokines, neutrophil dynamics and muscle damage. *J Appl Physiol* 1999;86:1360–7.
35. Muns G, Rubinstein I, Singer P. Neutrophil chemotactic activity is increased in nasal secretions of long distance runners. *Int J Sports Med* 1996;17:56–9.
36. Raastad T, Risoy BA, Benestad HB, et al. Temporal relation between leukocyte accumulation in muscles and halted recovery 10-20 h after strength exercise. *J Appl Physiol* 2003;95:2503–9.
37. Aoi W, Naito Y, Takanami Y, et al. Oxidative stress and delayed-onset muscle damage after exercise. *Free Radic Biol Med* 2004;37:480–7.
38. Hack B, Strobel G, Weiss M, et al. PMN cell counts and phagocytic activity of highly trained athletes depending on training period. *J Appl Physiol* 1994;77:1731–5.
39. Pyne DB, Baker MS, Fricker PA, et al. Effects of an intensive 12 week training program by elite swimmers on neutrophil oxidative activity. *Med Sci Sports Exerc* 1995;27:536–42.
40. Hinton JR, Rowbottom DG, Keast D, et al. Acute intensive interval training and in vitro T lymphocyte function. *Int J Sports Med* 1997;18:132–7.

41. Steensberg A, Toft AD, Bruunsgaard H, et al. Strenuous exercise decreases the percentage of type 1 T cells in the circulation. *J Appl Physiol* 2001;91:1708–1712.

42. Green K, Croaker SJ, Rowbottom DG. Carbohydrate and exercise-induced changes in T lymphocyte function. *J Appl Physiol* 2003;95:1216–1223.

43. Ostrowski K, Rohde T, Asp S, et al. Pro- and anti-inflammatory cytokine balance in strenuous exercise. *J Physiol* 1999;515:287–91.

44. Nieman DC, Henson DA, Dumke CL, et al. Ibuprofen use, endotoxemia, inflammation, and plasma cytokines during ultramarathon competition. *Brain Behav Immun* 2006;20:578–84.

45. Bruunsgaard H, Galbo H, Halkjaer-Kristensen J, et al. Exercise-induced increase in serum interleukin-6 in humans is related to muscle damage. *J Physiol* 1997;499:833–41.

46. Peake J, Nosaka K, Suzuki K. Characterization of systemic inflammatory responses to eccentric exercise in humans. *Exerc Immunol Rev* 2005;11:64–85.

47. Febbraio MA, Pedersen BK. Contraction-induced myokine production and release: Is skeletal muscle an endocrine organ? *Exerc Sport Sci Rev* 2005;33:114–9.

48. Fischer CP, Hiscock NJ, Penkowa M, et al. Vitamin C and E supplementation inhibits the release of interleukin-6 from contracting human skeletal muscle. *J Physiol* 2004;558:633–45.

49. Steensberg A, Keller C, Hillig T, et al. Nitric oxide production is a proximal signaling event controlling exercise-induced mRNA expression in human skeletal muscle. *FASEB J* 2007;21:2683–2691.

50. Petersen AM, Pedersen BK. The antiinflammatory effect of exercise. *J Appl Physiol* 2005;98:1154–62.

51. Nieman DC, Davis JM, Henson DA, et al. Muscle cytokine mRNA changes after 2.5 h of cycling: Influence of carbohydrate. *Med Sci Sports Exerc* 2005;37:1283–90.

52. Nieman DC, Davis JM, Henson DA, et al. Carbohydrate ingestion influences skeletal muscle cytokine mRNA and plasma cytokine levels after a 3-h run. *J Appl Physiol* 2003;94:1917–25.

53. Nieman DC, Henson DA, Smith LL, et al. Cytokine changes after a marathon race. *J Appl Physiol* 2001;91:109–14.

54. Nieman DC, Henson DA, Davis JM, et al. Blood leukocyte mRNA expression for IL-10, IL-1Ra, and IL-8, but not IL-6, increases after exercise. *J Interferon Cytokine Res* 2006;26:668–74.

55. Sprenger H, Jacobs C, Nain N, et al. Enhanced release of cytokines, interleukin-2 receptors, and neopterin after long-distance running. *Clin Immunol Immunopathol* 1992;53:188–95.

56. Linke A, Adams V, Schulze PC, et al. Antioxidative effects of exercise training in patients with chronic heart failure: Increase in radical scavenger enzyme activity in skeletal muscle. *Circulation* 2005;111:1763–70.

57. Konig D, Deibert P, Winkler K, et al. Association between LDL-cholesterol, statin therapy, physical activity and inflammatory markers in patients with stable coronary heart disease. *Exerc Immunol Rev* 2005;11:97–107.

58. Smith JK, Dykes R, Douglas RE, et al. Long-term exercise and atherogenic activity of blood mononuclear cells in persons at risk of developing ischemic heart disease. *JAMA* 1999;281:1722–7.

59. Dekker MJ, Lee S, Hudson R, et al. An exercise intervention without weight loss decreases circulating interleukin-6 in lean and obese men with and without type 2 diabetes mellitus. *Metabolism* 2007;56:332–8.

60. Castaneda C, Gordon PL, Parker RC, et al. Resistance training to reduce the malnutrition-inflammation complex syndrome of chronic kidney disease. *Am J Kidney Dis* 2004;43:607–16.

61. Lakier Smith L. Overtraining, excessive exercise, and altered immunity: Is this a T helper-1 versus T helper-2 lymphocyte response? *Sports Med* 2003;33:347–64.

62. Robson-Ansley PJ, Blannin A, Gleeson M. Elevated plasma interleukin-6 levels in trained male triathletes following an acute period of intense interval training. *Eur J Appl Physiol* 2006;99:353–60.

63. Halson SL, Lancaster GI, Jeukendrup AE, et al. Immunological responses to overreaching in cyclists. *Med Sci Sports Exerc* 2003;35:854–61.

64. Gleeson M, McDonald WA, Cripps AW, et al. The effect on immunity of long-term intensive training in elite swimmers. *Clin Exp Immunol* 1995;102:210–6.

65. Bruunsgaard H, Hartkopp A, Mohr T, et al. In vivo cell-mediated immunity and vaccination response following prolonged, intense exercise. *Med Sci Sports Exerc* 1997;29:1176–81.

66. Gleeson M, Pyne DB, McDonald WA, et al. Pneumococcal antibody responses in elite swimmers. *Clin Exp Immunol* 1996;105:238–44.

67. Gleeson M, Pyne DB, Callister R. The missing links in exercise effects on mucosal immunity. *Exerc Immunol Rev* 2004;10:107–28.

68. Fehrenbach E, Passek F, Niess AM, et al. HSP expression in human leukocytes is modulated by endurance exercise. *Med Sci Sports Exerc* 2000;32;592–600.

69. Febbraio MA, Ott P, Nielsen HB, et al. Exercise induces hepatosplanchnic release of heat shock protein 72 in humans. *J Physiol* 2002;544:957–62.

70. Febbraio MA, Mesa JL, Chung J, et al. Glucose attenuates the exercise-induced increase in circulating heat shock protein 72 and heat shock protein 60 in humans. *Cell Stress Chaperones* 2004;9:390–6.

71. Fehrenbach E, Niess AM, Voelker K, et al. Exercise intensity and duration affect blood soluble HSP72. *Int J Sports Med* 2005;26:552–7.

72. Fischer CP, Hiscock NJ, Basu S, et al. Vitamin E isoform-specific inhibition of the exercise-induced heat shock protein 72 expression in humans. *J Appl Physiol* 2006;100:1679–87.

73. Fahlman MM, Engels H-J. Mucosal IgA and URTI in American college football players: A year longitudinal study. *Med Sci Sports Exerc* 2005;37:374–80.

74. Lancaster GI, Khan Q, Drysdale P, et al. The physiological regulation of toll-like receptor expression and function in humans. *J Physiol* 2005;563:945–55.

75. Clancy RL, Gleeson M, Cox A, et al. Reversal in fatigued athletes of a defect in interferon gamma secretion after administration of *Lactobacillus acidophilus*. *Br J Sports Med* 2006;40:351–4.

76. Gleeson M, Pyne DB, Austin JP, et al. Epstein–Barr virus reactivation and upper-respiratory illness in elite swimmers. *Med Sci Sports Exerc* 2002;34:411–7.

77. Reid VL, Gleeson M, Williams N, et al. Clinical investigation of athletes with persistent fatigue and/or recurrent infections. *Br J Sports Med* 2004;38:42–5.

78. Cox AJ, Gleeson M, Pyne DB, et al. Valtrex therapy for Epstein–Barr virus reactivation and upper respiratory symptoms in elite runners. *Med Sci Sports Exerc* 2004;36:1104–10.

79. Walsh NP, Whitham M. Exercising in environmental extremes. A greater threat to immune function? *Sports Med* 2006;36:941–76.

80. Severs Y, Brenner I, Shek PN, et al. Effects of heat and intermittent exercise on leukocyte and sub-population cell counts. *Eur J Appl Physiol* 1996;74:234–45.

81. Mitchell JB, Dugas JP, McFarlin BK, et al. Effect of exercise, heat stress, and hydration on immune cell number and function. *Med Sci Sports Exerc* 2002;34:1941–50.

82. Lim C, Mackinnon LT. The roles of exercise-induced immune system disturbances in the pathology of heat stroke: The dual pathway model of heat stroke. *Sports Med* 2006;36:39–64.

83. Rhind SG, Gannon GA, Shek PN, et al. Contribution of exertional hyperthermia to sympathoadrenal-mediated lymphocyte subset redistribution. *J Appl Physiol* 1999;87:1178–85.

84. Brenner I, Castellani JW, Gabaree C, et al. Immune changes in humans during cold exposure: Effects of prior heating and exercise. *J Appl Physiol* 1999;87:699–710.

85. Klokker M, Kjaer M, Secher NH, et al. Natural killer cell response to exercise in humans: Effect of hypoxia and epidural anesthesia. *J Appl Physiol* 1995;78:709–16.

86. Tiollier E, Schmitt L, Burnat P, et al. Living high-training low altitude training: Effects on mucosal immunity. *Eur J Appl Physiol* 2005;94:298–304.

87. Ronsen O, Kjeldsen-Kragh J, Haug E, et al. Recovery time affects immunoendocrine responses to a second bout of endurance exercise. *Am J Physiol Cell Physiol* 2002;283:C1612–20.

88. Ronsen O, Lea T, Bahr R, et al. Enhanced plasma IL-6 and IL-1ra responses to repeated vs. single bouts of prolonged cycling in elite athletes. *J Appl Physiol* 2002;92:2547–53.

89. Febbraio MA, Steensberg A, Keller C, et al. Glucose ingestion attenuates interleukin-6 release from contracting skeletal muscle in humans. *J Physiol* 2003;549:607–12.

90. Bishop NC, Blannin AK, Armstrong E, et al. Carbohydrate and fluid intake affect the saliva flow rate and IgA response to cycling. *Med Sci Sports Exerc* 2000;32:2046–51.

91. McFarlin BK, Flynn MG, Hampton T. Carbohydrate consumption during cycling increases in vitro NK cell responses to IL-2 and IFN-γ. *Brain Behav Immun* 2007;21:202–8.

92. Henson DA, Nieman DC, Blodgett AD, et al. Influence of exercise mode and carbohydrate on the immune response to prolonged exercise. *Int J Sport Nutr* 1999;9:213–8.

93. Bishop NC, Walsh NP, Scanlon GA. Effect of prolonged exercise and carbohydrate on total neutrophil elastase content. *Med Sci Sports Exerc* 2003;35:1326–32.

94. Lancaster GI, Khan Q, Drysdale DT, et al. Effect of prolonged exercise and carbohydrate ingestion on type 1 and type 2 T lymphocyte distribution and intracellular cytokine production in humans. *J Appl Physiol* 2005;98:565–71.

95. Konig D, Weinstock C, Keul J, et al. Zinc, iron, and magnesium status in athletes—Influence on the regulation of exercise-induced stress and immune function. *Exerc Immunol Rev* 1998;4:2–21.

96. Shephard RJ, Shek PN. Immunological hazards from nutritional imbalance in athletes. *Exerc Immunol Rev* 1998;4:48.

97. Peake JM, Gerrard DF, Griffith JFT. Plasma zinc and immune markers in runners in response to a moderate increase in training volume. *Int J Sports Med* 2003;24:212–6.

98. Flynn MG, Mackinnon LT, Gedge V, et al. Iron status and cell-mediated immune function in female distance runners. *Med Sci Sports Exerc* 1996;28:S90.

99. Singh A, Papanicolaou DA, Lawrence LL, et al. Neuroendocrine responses to running in women after zinc and vitamin E supplementation. *Med Sci Sports Exerc* 1999;31:536–42.

100. Singh A, Failla ML, Deuster PA. Exercise-induced changes in immune function: Effects of zinc supplementation. *J Appl Physiol* 1994;76:2298–03.

101. Niess AM, Dickhuth HH, Northoff H, et al. Free radicals and oxidative stress in exercise—Immunological aspects. *Exerc Immunol Rev* 1999;5:22–56.

102. Douglas RM, Hemila H, D'Souza R, et al. Vitamin C for preventing and treating the common cold. *Cochrane Database Syst Rev* 2004; 4:CD000980.

103. Peters EM. Exercise, immunology, and upper respiratory tract infections. *Int J Sports Med* 1997;18:S69–77.

104. Robson PJ, Bouic PJD, Myburgh KH. Antioxidant supplementation enhances neutrophil oxidative burst in trained runners following prolonged exercise. *Int J Sport Nutr Exerc Metab* 2003;13:369–81.

105. Gleeson M, Nieman DC, Pedersen BK. Exercise, nutrition and immune function. *J Sports Sci* 2004;22:115–25.

106. Peake JM, Suzuki K, Coombes JS. The influence of antioxidant supplementation on markers of inflammation and the relationship to oxidative stress after exercise. *J Nutr Biochem* 2007;18:357–71.

107. Rohde T, Kryzwkowski K, Pedersen BK. Glutamine, exercise, and the immune system—Is there a link? *Exerc Immunol Rev* 1998;4: 49–63.

108. Bassit RA, Sawada LA, Bacurau RF, et al. Branched-chain amino acid supplementation and the immune response of long-distance athletes. *Nutrition* 2002;18:376–9.

109. Castell LM, Newsholme EA, Poortmans JR. Does glutamine have a role in reducing infection in athletes? *Eur J Appl Physiol* 1996; 73:488–90.

110. Mackinnon LT, Hooper SL. Plasma glutamine concentration and upper respiratory tract infection during over-training in elite swimmers. *Med Sci Sports Exerc* 1996;28:285–90.

111. Krieger JW, Crowe M, Blank SE. Chronic glutamine supplementation increases nasal but not salivary IgA during 9 days of interval training. *J Appl Physiol* 2004;97:585–91.

112. Hiscock N, Petersen EW, Krzywkoski K, et al. Glutamine supplementation further enhances exercise-induced plasma IL-6. *J Appl Physiol* 2003;95:145–8.

113. Kohut ML, Senchina DS. Reversing age-associated immunosenescence via exercise. *Exerc Immunol Rev* 2005;11:6–41.

114. Franceschi C, Monti D, Sansoni P, et al. The immunology of exceptional individuals: The lesson in centenarians. *Immunol. Today* 1995;16:12–6.

115. Kohut ML, Cooper MM, Nickolaus MS, et al. Exercise and psychosocial factors modulate immunity to influenza vaccine in elderly individuals. *J Gerontol* 2002;57A:M557–62.

116. Smith TP, Kennedy SL, Fleshner M. Influence of age and physical activation the primary in vivo antibody and T-cell mediated responses in men. *J Appl Physiol* 2002;97:491–8.

117. McFarlin BK, Flynn MG, Phillips MD, et al. Chronic resistance exercise training improves natural killer cell activity in older women. *J Gerontol A Biol Sci Med Sci* 2005;60:1315–8.

118. Akimoto T, Kumai Y, Akama E, et al. Effects of 12 months exercise training on salivary secretory IgA levels in elderly subjects. *Br J Sports Med* 2003;37:76–9.

119. Kohut ML, Boehm GW, Moynihan JA. Moderate exercise is associated with enhanced antigen-specific cytokine, but not IgM antibody production in mice. *Mech Ageing Dev* 2001;122:1135–50.

120. Przybyla B, Gurley C, Harvey JF, et al. Aging alters macrophage properties in human skeletal muscle both at rest and in response to acute resistance exercise. *Exp Gerontol* 2006;41:320–7.

121. deJong N, Paw MJ, deGroot LC, et al. Functional biochemical and nutrient indices in frail elderly people are partly affected by dietary supplements but not by exercise. *J Nutr* 1999;129: 2028–36.

122. Scanga CB, Verde TJ, Paolone AM, et al. Effects of weight loss and exercise training on natural killer cell activity in obese women. *Med Sci Sports Exerc* 1998;30:1666–71.

123. Shade ED, Ulrich CM, Wener MH, et al. Frequent intentional weight loss is associated with lower natural killer cell cytotoxicity in postmenopausal women: Possible long-term immune effects. *J Am Diet Assoc* 2004;104:903–12.

124. Imai T, Seki S, Dobashi H,. et al. Effect of weight loss on T-cell receptor-mediated T-cell function in elite athletes. *Med Sci Sports Exerc* 2002;34:245–50.

17

HIV/AIDS: A GLOBAL PANDEMIC

Since the first cases of acquired immunodeficiency syndrome (AIDS) were reported in 1981, infection with human immunodeficiency virus (HIV) has grown to pandemic proportions, resulting in an estimated 65 million infections and 25 million deaths worldwide. In 2005 alone, an estimated 38.6 million people were living with HIV, more than any previous year. An estimated 4.1 million people became newly infected with HIV that year and an estimated 2.8 million died from AIDS (1). Although the pandemic is global in nature, HIV disproportionately affects certain geographic regions. Sub-Saharan Africa is experiencing a generalized epidemic, which is defined as HIV prevalence consistently remaining greater than 1% in pregnant women. Southern Africa, in particular, represents the epicenter of the global pandemic with almost all countries experiencing HIV prevalence rates higher than 10%. Women are disproportionately affected by this generalized epidemic. Other regions, including parts of Asia and eastern Europe, are experiencing concentrated epidemics whereby HIV prevalence is greater than 5% in at least one defined subpopulation. These disproportionately affected subpopulations include injection drug users, sex workers, and men who have sex with men. Yet other regions are experiencing low level epidemics whereby HIV prevalence has not consistently exceeded 5% in any defined subpopulation. In the United States, 1.2 million people were estimated to be living with HIV in 2005, one-quarter of whom were women (1).

Overall, the proportion of people living with HIV in the world (i.e., global prevalence) is leveling off because of decreasing rates of new infections in some countries in combination with rising AIDS mortality rates. The total numbers of people living with HIV has continued to rise, however, because of population growth and, in recent years, the life-extending effects of HIV treatments known as highly active antiretroviral therapy (HAART). First developed in the mid-1990s, HAART is the combination of three or more antiretroviral drugs that together impede different stages of the HIV replication cycle, thus slowing the progression to AIDS. HAART is a treatment as opposed to a cure or vaccine. For those who can access and tolerate these drug regimens, HIV can be transformed, however, from a swiftly fatal disease into a chronic illness characterized by long periods of relative wellness or fluctuating episodes of wellness and illness.

Historically, access to HAART has been grossly inequitable, with high levels of coverage in developed countries (with low level epidemics) and little to no access to treatment in poor countries (with generalized and concentrated epidemics). Since the early 2000s, however, HIV/AIDS has helped drive a global revolution in the delivery of complex treatment in developing countries. Between 2001 and 2005, the number of people on HAART in low- and middle-income countries increased from 240,000 to approximately 1.3 million. Expanded treatment access has been estimated to have averted up to 350,000 AIDS deaths between 2003 and 2005. Globally, however, antiretroviral drugs still reach only one in five in need (1).

WHY EXERCISE MATTERS FOR PEOPLE LIVING WITH HIV

For those who are able to benefit from the life-prolonging effects of HAART as well as those who do not have access to these treatments, exercise may be sought as a tool for minimizing the disablement associated with HIV disease. Goals of exercise may be to restore the body after an HIV-related illness or to combat side effects from HAART. Others may look to exercise as a secondary prevention tool for building up strength, endurance, and body composition to ward off the sequelae of HIV. Exercise might also be pursued for psychological benefits and for body image reasons. This chapter provides a comprehensive overview of the evidence regarding the effects of exercise on the physiology of people living with HIV. We begin by providing a general overview of HIV and AIDS followed by a discussion of exercise physiology in this population. Next, we summarize the research on the effects of aerobic exercise and progressive resistive training in people living with HIV. Finally, we present recommendations for exercise prescription with this population.

CHARACTERISTICS AND CLINICAL MANIFESTATIONS OF HIV/AIDS

OVERVIEW

Human immunodeficiency virus is transmitted through direct contact of a mucous membrane or the bloodstream with a bodily fluid containing HIV. As such, transmission can occur through sexual contact, blood transfusions, contaminated needles, or from mother to baby during pregnancy, delivery, or breastfeeding. HIV is not transmitted through the air, casual contact such as kissing, or contact with sweat, tears, or saliva. After initial HIV infection, people may experience a syndrome typical of an acute viral infection, such as the flu. Symptoms usually resolve quickly, followed by a long asymptomatic phase during which HIV is replicating in lymphoid tissue. Throughout this phase, HIV is slowly destroying CD4 lymphocytes (also known as T-cells), which are required for healthy functioning of the immune system. As the number of CD4 cells declines, individuals are increasingly susceptible to a number of opportunistic infections (e.g., lung or brain infections), malignancies (e.g., Kaposi's sarcoma), or syndromes (e.g., wasting syndrome or AIDS dementia complex), which are all considered to be AIDS-defining conditions. As such, HIV disease can manifest in myriad ways and in almost all body systems. Furthermore, the rate of clinical disease progression varies widely among individuals. As such, exercise prescription depends on the unique presentation and stage of disease for each person living with HIV.

For both HIV and AIDS, disease progression can be estimated through the use of two surrogate markers: CD4 count and viral load. A CD4 count of higher than 500 cells/mm^3 indicates mild or early disease, whereas a CD4 count between 200 and 499 cells/mm^3 represents midstage disease. A CD4 count below 200 cells/mm^3 indicates that an individual's immune system is severely compromised and is considered to be definitive for AIDS. Viral load, measured in number of copies of HIV per milliliter of blood, indicates the amount of virus circulating in the blood. As the virus replicates in the body, the measure of HIV viral load increases. A viral load test can also be reported as undetectable, which gives the optimistic message that the amount of virus in the circulating blood is below the threshold of the test.

METABOLIC AND ANTHROPOMETRIC CHANGES ASSOCIATED WITH HIV/AIDS

Along with the AIDS-defining conditions described above, HIV and the side effects of HAART are associated with a range of metabolic and anthropometric complications that have relevance to exercise, including muscle wasting, adipose tissue redistribution, lipid abnormalities, insulin resistance or glucose intolerance, bone abnormalities, mitochondrial abnormalities, and hyperlactatemia (2,3). Two common syndromes are HIV wasting and lipodystrophy.

An early identifying clinical manifestation of HIV infection is HIV wasting. The traditional definition of AIDS wasting is an involuntary loss of more than 10% of baseline body weight in combination with diarrhea, weakness, or fever (4). Studies have shown, however, that a more subtle decline in weight (e.g., 5%) during a 4-month period can predict poor outcomes in people with AIDS (5). Moreover, the severity of illness in AIDS wasting may relate more to changes in body composition (i.e., proportion of fat and muscle) than to changes in weight (6). Wasting occurred in 10%–20% of people with AIDS in the United States before the advent of HAART and is still a common and serious occurrence despite the benefits of HAART (7). Wasting in people living with HIV is an important predictor of mortality and it is also associated with poor physical functioning, presumably reflecting the loss of skeletal muscle (8,9). The etiology underlying AIDS wasting is complex and may reflect increased energy expenditure, decreased energy intake, impaired absorption of energy substrate, and hormonal factors (10).

Lipodystrophy is the term for a collection of symptoms that have been seen in people living with HIV since the advent of HAART. These symptoms include metabolic changes, such as insulin resistance or glucose intolerance, diabetes, and hyperlipidemia. These symptoms often occur in combination with adipose tissue redistribution characterized by the accumulation of visceral fat in the abdomen, breasts, and neck; a "buffalo hump" on the back of the neck; and a loss of subcutaneous fat in the face and extremities. The pathophysiologic mechanisms underlying lipodystrophy syndrome are unclear and a causal link to certain drugs is uncertain (2,3). Body composition changes can have an impact on quality of life because they can lead to social stigmatization, increased psychological stress, lower self-esteem, and reluctance to initiate antiretroviral therapy (3). The metabolic and fat distribution abnormalities that characterize the lipodystrophy syndrome could also represent a potential health risk (11). A recent study determined the acute myocardial infarction rates and cardiovascular risk factors in 3,851 people living with HIV compared with 1,044,589 HIV-negative people in two tertiary care hospitals (12). Acute myocardial infarction rates per 100 person years were greater in people living with HIV (11.1) versus those who were HIV-negative (6.7), and more so in women than men. In addition, the HIV-positive cohort had significantly higher proportions of hypertension (21.2 versus 15.9%), diabetes (11.5 versus 6.6%), and dyslipidemia (23.3 versus 17.6%) than the HIV-negative cohort.

Given the health risks and potential for decreased self-image with changes in body composition, various strategies attempting to reverse these changes have been tested, including pharmacologic therapies, such as anabolic steroids and growth hormone (13). Because of the side effects associated with pharmacologic therapies, healthcare professionals have turned to changing exercise and dietary habits as a way of combating lipodystrophy syndrome and the associated increased health risk (14).

To date, however, no evidence indicates that exercise can reverse the fat redistribution process associated with this syndrome.

DISABLEMENT IN HIV/AIDS

Along with the medical diagnoses described above, individuals may experience various forms of disablement as a result of HIV/AIDS, their sequelae and the side effects of treatments. The International Classification of Functioning, Disability and Health provides a framework for classifying such health-related consequences of disease according to three concepts: impairments, activity limitations, and participation restrictions. Impairments describe problems of physiologic functioning or anatomic structure, such as muscle wasting or decreased endurance that can occur after HIV infection. Activity limitations are defined as difficulties in executing a task or action, such as climbing stairs or getting dressed. Participation restrictions are challenges relating to life situations, such as may occur during work or parenting (15) (Figure 17.1).

A study of people living with HIV in the province of British Columbia in Canada found that more than 90%, 80%, and 93% of respondents reported experiencing one or more impairments, activity limitations, and participation restrictions in the past month, respectively (16). For example, 40%–50% of respondents reported that they experienced the impairments of weakness, decreased endurance, chronic fatigue, or poor concentration within the previous month. Approximately 40% and 70% reported that they were either "somewhat limited" or "unable to perform" the activities of moderate or vigorous physical activity, respectively (16). These high levels of disablement among people living with HIV highlight the potential importance of incorporating exercise and physical activity as a therapeutic strategy.

EXERCISE PHYSIOLOGY AND HIV/AIDS

The study of exercise physiology and HIV/AIDS is a relatively new field of research. The first published studies of exercise responses in people with HIV during cardiopulmonary exercise testing appeared in the early 1990s (17,18). Also during this period, a number of aerobic or progressive resistive training (PRE) training programs were evaluated in adults living with HIV, primarily to determine their safety, efficacy, and physiologic impacts (19,20). Although the participants in these early studies were primarily men who were having sex with men, more recent research has begun to examine the effects of exercise training in women, people of varied ethnocultural backgrounds, and people who have experienced other mechanisms of HIV transmission (i.e., heterosexual, intravenous drug use) (21,22). In most of these studies, the participants were not reported as being diagnosed with AIDS; only a small number had an AIDS-defining diagnosis or AIDS-related wasting. However, participants' immune status and symptoms varied widely within and between studies. The mean entry CD4 cell counts of participants across studies varied from approximately 40–900 cells/mm^3 (18,22–48) (Figure 17.2). Other more recent developments include the use a greater variety of assessment tools, including cardiopulmonary exercise testing, neuromuscular assessments, muscle biopsies, and imaging technologies to address physiologic limitations to exercise performance and training-induced adaptations in the HIV population (22,30,39,43). These assessments will help to elucidate whether exercise training can minimize the metabolic complications and long-term health risks associated with HIV and HAART.

AEROBIC INSUFFICIENCY IN HIV/AIDS

Cardiopulmonary exercise testing, which includes the direct measurement of oxygen uptake and carbon dioxide production, can be used to determine whether exercise intolerance primarily reflects limitations of the ventilatory, cardiovascular, or muscular systems. In addition, subtle indicators of deconditioning, dyspnea, opportunistic infections, and training-induced adaptations can be deduced from data gathered during cardiopulmonary

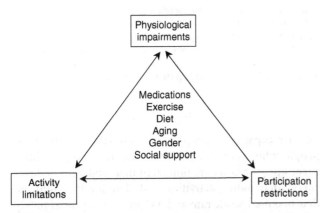

FIGURE 17-1. The relationship between impairments in physiology, activity limitations, and participation restrictions based on the International Classification of Functioning, Disability and Health (15). The *double arrows* indicate the complex interrelationships that exist between each of the three components. For example, the low aerobic capacity and muscle dysfunction (impairments) in people living with human immunodeficiency virus (HIV) likely restrict their ability to perform vigorous activity and this, in turn, could restrict participation in sports and leisure activities. In addition, the relationship among the components can be modified by factors, including medications and lifestyle behaviors such as exercise training, physical activity, and diet. Although highly active antiretroviral therapy (HAART) has extended the lives of many people living with HIV, these medications may exacerbate certain conditions (i.e., lipodystrophy, hyperlactatemia), which can increase the risk of developing cardiovascular and other diseases. Regular exercise training can improve physiologic (i.e., aerobic capacity, strength) and psychological (i.e., mood) outcomes, which may minimize activity limitations, participation restrictions, and disease risks in people living with HIV who are on HAART.

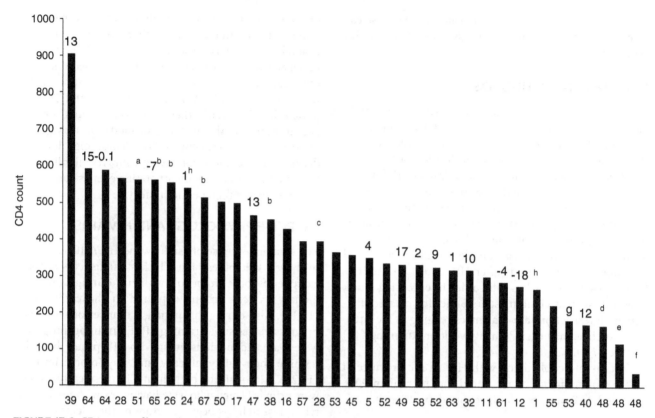

FIGURE 17-2. CD4 counts of human immunodeficiency virus (HIV)-positive adults, with or without metabolic abnormalities, who participated in exercise performance (no training) or exercise training (aerobic or progressive resistive training [PRE]) studies. Each *bar* represents the group mean baseline CD4 count reported in the study indicated on the x-axis. Based on these mean CD4 counts, most participants in exercise-related studies were in midstage disease and relatively few had severely compromised immune function (i.e., CD4 count <200). Numbers above the bars correspond to the percentage increase or decrease in group mean CD4 count after training. None of the changes in CD4 count was significant except for one study (36). Also, only two reports studied women exclusively (23,29). [a]HIV patients with lipodystrophy and/or hyperlactatemia; [b]HIV patients with lipodystrophy and/or dyslipidemia; [c]HIV patients with hyperlactatemia; [d]HIV patients without history of respiratory disease or current lung disease; [e]HIV patients with a previous episode of *Pneumocystis carinii pneumonia* (PCP); [f]HIV patients with current broncopulmonary complications; [g]HIV patients with wasting; [h]women only were tested.

exercise testing (49). Maximal oxygen uptake ($\dot{V}O_2$max), the gold standard measurement of exercise capacity, reflects oxygen delivery by the cardiorespiratory system and oxygen utilization by the exercising muscles (i.e., $\dot{V}O_2$ = heart rate × stroke volume × arterial − venous oxygen content difference. In addition, the ventilatory anaerobic threshold can be determined from gas exchange measurements to provide an indication of the work rate (or $\dot{V}O_2$) at which there is an acceleration of anaerobic metabolism. An individual's health and performance are associated with his or her aerobic capacity and ventilatory anaerobic threshold. Hence, poor exercise performance can be attributed, in part, to a low $\dot{V}O_2$max, low ventilatory anaerobic threshold, or both (50). In addition, the lower the exercise (aerobic) capacity, the higher the risk of developing coronary artery disease (51).

The $\dot{V}O_2$max values reported in people living with HIV and HIV-negative controls are shown in *Figure 17.3*, many of which were determined as part of exercise training studies (24,26,31,35,38,43,44,46–48,52, 53–56). Only a few investigators (17,18,22,39) directly compared the

exercise capacity of people who were HIV-negative with people who were HIV-positive, despite survey findings suggesting the latter are limited in their ability to perform energy-demanding activities (16). The findings indicate that maximal work rate and $\dot{V}O_2$max are approximately 10%–40% lower in HIV-positive adults compared with those who are HIV-negative, although the difference between the groups was significant in only two studies (18,22).

Johnson et al. (17) characterized the cardiorespiratory responses during maximal cycle ergometer exercise in 32 active members of the army who were in the early stages of HIV infection and 22 members who were HIV-negative. Most participants in each group reported engaging in regular aerobic training. Overall, cardiorespiratory differences between the groups during maximal exercise were relatively modest. The group of adults living with HIV had lower values for $\dot{V}O_2$max (2.6 versus 2.8 L/min), although not significantly so ($P > 0.05$), and lower ventilatory anaerobic threshold (49% versus 62% of $\dot{V}O_2$max) compared with the controls. However, a

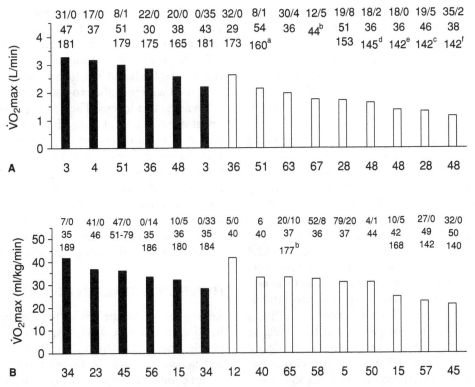

FIGURE 17-3. Directly measured maximal oxygen uptake ($\dot{V}O_2$max) during bicycle ergometer exercise (**A**) or treadmill exercise (**B**) to exhaustion in adults who are HIV-negative (*filled bars*) or HIV-positive (*open bars*). Numbers along the x-axis correspond to the cited references. Values above the bars correspond to the number of men or women in each group (**upper**), mean age or age range of the group (**middle**), and group mean maximal heart rate where provided (**lower**). Values for maximal oxygen uptake and maximal heart rate are generally lower in people living with HIV compared with controls (18,39).

subgroup of adults living with HIV with ventilatory anaerobic thresholds less than 43% of the $\dot{V}O_2$max (the two-tailed 95% confidence interval [CI] for the controls), demonstrated larger deficits in work rate and $\dot{V}O_2$max, and a steeper slope of heart rate–$\dot{V}O_2$ relationship compared with the controls. More of the participants in the subgroup were smokers (8/9) than the remaining participants living with HIV (11/23), but immunologic stage of the disease and prevalence of anemia were similar between the groups. The investigators concluded that large deficits in maximal aerobic power result from a limitation of oxygen delivery to the exercising muscles.

In a subsequent study by this group, nine people living with HIV underwent exercise right-sided heart catheterization to determine presence of cardiac dysfunction (57). Compared with HIV-negative controls, those living with HIV had higher pulmonary capillary wedge pressure and right atrial pressure at similar oxygen consumption, a finding indicative of cardiac disease or dysfunction. One patient underwent endomyocardial biopsy with findings consistent with a cardiomyopathy, including myofiber loss and atrophy. These findings suggest that low ventilatory anaerobic threshold and $\dot{V}O_2$max values may reflect cardiac disease in people living with HIV.

Pothoff et al. (18) compared pulmonary function and exercise capacity in three groups of patients with advanced HIV-infection (CD4 count <200) and HIV-negative controls. Participants living with HIV in group 1 had no history of respiratory disease or current lung disease; group 2 had a previous episode of *Pneumocystis carinii* pneumonia (PCP), but no current lung disease; and group 3 had current bronchopulmonary complications, including PCP. Lung-diffusing capacity, $\dot{V}O_2$max, maximal work rate, and ventilatory anaerobic threshold were all lower in all patient groups compared with the controls, with the largest deficits observed in group 3. No obvious evidence indicated that exercise limitation was related to the decrease in lung diffusing capacity, however, because neither spirometric nor exercise parameters suggested ventilatory limitation or arterial desaturation in any of the patient groups. In addition, the slope of the relationship between oxygen uptake and heart rate during exercise was similar among all groups. In contrast to the conclusion of Johnson et al. (57), this finding suggests that low exercise capacity, at least to the levels tested in these patients, may not result from heart disease. The end exercise maximal heart rates were much lower in the patients (~140 bpm) than the controls (~165 bpm) despite similar ages, a finding reported in those in earlier stages of HIV infection (22,27,39). This observation suggests exercise intolerance in HIV patients may reflect poor effort, neuromuscular fatigue, or a combination of both factors. Most studies, however, did not record the rating of perceived exertion and respiratory exchange ratio, and some did not provide maximal heart rate (HRmax), during exercise testing, making it difficult to assess effort level of the participants.

Cade et al. (27) measured cardiac output (rebreathing method) and estimated the arterial-venous oxygen content difference (indirect Fick method) during a maximal treadmill test among adults living with HIV and a group of HIV-negative controls. The $\dot{V}O_2$max and peak exercise arterial-venous oxygen content difference were lower in the adults living with HIV (25 mL/kg/min and 10.8 vol%) compared with the controls (32 mL/kg/min and 12.4 vol%), whereas stroke volume and cardiac output were similar between the groups. Furthermore, deficits in aerobic capacity and arterial-venous oxygen content difference were more pronounced among participants living with HIV taking HAART compared with HIV-negative participants (58). The authors suggested that the deficit in aerobic capacity in the HIV-positive participants reflected their smaller arterial-venous oxygen content difference, which, in turn, may be owing to limited oxygen extraction and utilization by skeletal muscle. Collectively, the above studies suggest that exercise intolerance with HIV may reflect a combination of poor cardiovascular fitness because of decreased cardiac output and deficits in neuromuscular function. However, the degree to which these limitations can be ascribed to deconditioning owing to a decline in physical activity versus HIV- or HAART-induced pathology remains unclear.

NEUROMUSCULAR DYSFUNCTION IN HIV/AIDS

A number of skeletal muscle abnormalities have been reported in people with HIV/AIDS. HIV, and HAART can cause muscle myopathy that is associated with weakness, elevated creatine phosphokinase, myofibrillar damage, fiber necrosis, and inflammation (59). Several agents, including nucleoside reverse transcriptase inhibitor (NRTI) drugs, have been shown to induce a mitochondrial myopathy and adversely affect cellular bioenergetics (60). The relationship between these muscle abnormalities and exercise performance in vivo is not known, however. For example, no studies have determined whether muscles of individuals with HIV are more fatigable than the muscle of people who are HIV-negative.

In a recent study, Scott et al. (43) measured the cross-sectional area, strength, and neuromuscular (central) activation level of the quadriceps and dorsiflexor muscles in 27 men living with HIV who were taking HAART. Supramaximal tetanic stimulation was applied to the muscle during a maximal voluntary isometric contraction to determine central activation. Of the 27 participants, 11 had an impaired ability to activate the quadriceps as revealed by a mean central activation ratio of 0.72. A greater proportion of these participants had higher viral loads and a history of AIDS-defining illnesses compared with the other 16 participants who could fully activate the quadriceps. The investigators suggested that impairment of central motor function, rather than atrophy, may be a predominant factor compromising muscle performance in the era of HAART. The impaired activation could, however, reflect a lower effort level of these 11 participants during the strength test rather than any real deficit in output from the motor cortex or motor neuron activation. No deficits in activation occurred in the dorsiflexor muscles of these individuals, although this model is less sensitive at detecting activation impairment (61).

HYPERLACTATEMIA IN HIV/AIDS

Resting venous lactate levels are elevated in some adults living with HIV who are taking HAART compared with people who are HIV-negative (62). Higher lactate levels and lipoatrophy may be linked through mitochondrial dysfunction as a result of HAART medications from the NRTI class (31). In theory, elevated blood lactate levels could reflect excessive muscle lactate production via accelerated glycolysis or a defect in mitochondrial oxidative phosphorlyation, a reduction in clearance rate from the blood, or a combination of these factors. The clinical significance and impact on exercise performance of elevated lactate levels in people living with HIV remains unclear, however. At issue is whether elevated lactate levels at rest will lead to early fatigue during exercise (39).

One small study compared eight healthy controls with eight people who were living with HIV, taking HAART, and who had lipodystrophy or elevated lactate (n = 3). All participants exercised until exhaustion on a cycle ergometer (39). Blood lactate and biopsies of the quadriceps were taken before and after exercise. Maximal work rate was lower and $\dot{V}O_2$max tended to be lower ($P = 0.11$) in the people living with HIV (171 W and 2.1 L/min) compared with the controls (235 W and 2.9 L/min). However, the two groups were similar in terms of the slope corresponding to the change in $\dot{V}O_2$ for a given change in work rate, respiratory exchange ratio, maximal lactate and recovery lactate levels, and oxidative enzyme capacity of the biopsy. The investigators concluded that the lower maximal work rate was caused by a decline in physical fitness rather than mitochondrial dysfunction.

Tesiorowski et al. (63) compared the cardiorespiratory responses in 28 HIV-positive adults with hyperlactemia (>2.1 mmol/L) and 8 HIV-positive controls with normal blood lactate levels during symptom-limited maximal cycle ergometer exercise. No difference was seen in maximal work rate, minute ventilation, or $\dot{V}O_2$ between the groups. However, the hyperlactemia patients had a higher respiratory quotient ($V_{CO_2}/\dot{V}O_2$max) and tended to have a lower ventilatory anaerobic threshold (% of $\dot{V}O_2$max; $P = 0.078$).

Furthermore, Duong et al. (31) compared 24 people living with HIV with elevated lactate levels with 27 people living with HIV who had normal lactate levels during cycle ergometer exercise. They found that maximal work rate, peak $\dot{V}O_2$max, and arterial-venous oxygen content difference were all lower in the participants with hyperlactemia than in those with normal lactate levels. In addition, the calculated ratios corresponding to the changes in cardiac output relative to $\dot{V}O_2$ and ventilation relative to $\dot{V}O_2$ were greater in participants with hyperlactemia (8 and 49, respectively) compared with the controls (6 and 42).

Bauer et al. (64) examined the kinetics of lactate metabolism in four groups after submaximal (to a heart rate of 200−age) cycle ergometer exercise: (*a*) people living with HIV who were taking HAART and had normal blood lactate; (*b*) people living with HIV who were taking HAART and had hyperlactemia; (*c*) people living with HIV who were not taking HAART; and (*d*) HIV-negative controls. Maximal lactate levels after exercise were similar in all groups. However, patients with hyperlactemia had the slowest rate of lactate recovery compared to the other three groups. Hence, elevated baseline lactate does not lead to higher end-exercise lactate but is associated with a delayed decline in lactate after exercise, possibly reflecting impaired lactate clearance. The investigators also found that the rate of lactate recovery was slower in the HIV-positive participants taking HAART compared with HIV-negative controls, implying that HIV infection in itself may influence lactate levels.

AEROBIC CAPACITY IN OLDER ADULTS LIVING WITH HIV/AIDS

With the life-prolonging effects of HAART, many people are aging with HIV/AIDS. The proportion of people with AIDS in the United States who are 50 years of age or older has grown from 19% in 2000 to 27% in 2004 (22). Although 50 years of age is not considered old when referring to the general population, current convention in HIV and aging research categorizes this group as older adults (65). Older adults with HIV may have to contend with age-related decrements in physiology and function in addition to the effects of HIV and its treatments. Hence, this population also may benefit from exercise. Only a few studies, however, have examined the physical activity levels or exercise responses in people living with HIV who are older than 50.

Oursler et al. (22) assessed grip strength, the 6-minute walk test, and $\dot{V}O_2$(peak)max during a treadmill test in younger (40–49 years, n =12) and older (50 + years, n = 20) men living with HIV and in 47 age-matched healthy controls. Mean maximal aerobic capacity was lower in the older (19.1 mL/kg/min) versus the younger (25.2 mL/kg/min) men with HIV, but 6-minute walk distance was similar in the two groups. The $\dot{V}O_2$max and 6-minute walk distance were 41% and 8% lower, respectively, in the men living with HIV compared with the age-matched controls. Regression analysis revealed, however, that the rate of decline in aerobic capacity was similar in the two groups, suggesting that primary aging has a comparable effect in both HIV-positive and general populations.

EXERCISE TRAINING AND HIV/AIDS

AEROBIC EXERCISE TRAINING IN PEOPLE LIVING WITH HIV/AIDS

Most HIV and aerobic exercise studies have examined the effects of approximately 12 weeks of thrice weekly aerobic training alone, or in combination with resistance training, on measures such as CD4 count, $\dot{V}O_2$max, endurance time, body composition, and psychological health (19). Aerobic training sessions commonly consisted of 20–40 minutes of continuous or intermittent stationary cycling or walking or running on a treadmill (track). In some cases, stair-climbers, rowing, or cross-country ski machines were used. The intensity of exercise was usually set at 60%–80% of the maximal heart rate.

Results of a recent systematic review suggest that performing aerobic exercise at least three times per week for at least 4 weeks appears to be safe and may lead to significant improvements in cardiopulmonary and psychological outcomes for adults living with HIV (19). Meta-analyses reported statistically significant improvements in $\dot{V}O_2$max of 1.64 mL/kg/min and depression-dejection symptoms of 7.68 points on the Profile of Mood States (POMS) scale among participants engaged in constant or interval exercise compared with nonexercisers. Greater improvements in $\dot{V}O_2$max of 4.3 mL/kg/min were found among participants exercising at heavy intensity compared with those exercising at moderate intensity. No changes in CD4 count or viral load were demonstrated with exercise groups, suggesting that this activity is safe for people living with HIV who are medically stable (*Figure 17.2*).

Other studies that used a cross-sectional design suggested that regular exercise may be associated with improved immunologic and virologic status. For instance, Mustafa et al. (66) conducted an epidemiologic study of exercise behaviors and disease status in 415 men who have sex with men. They found that HIV-infected participants who reported exercising at least three to four times per week had 107.5% higher CD4+ counts compared with HIV-positive men who denied exercise participation. Regular exercisers also displayed slower disease progression to AIDS, less symptomology, and decreased rates of mortality compared with nonexercisers. Bopp et al. (67) examined the relationship between physical activity levels, viral load, and CD4 cell count in 66 HIV-positive participants. They found a significant inverse relationship between physical activity level and viral load; however, no correlation was seen between activity and CD4 counts.

Results from individual studies support findings from the meta-analyses demonstrating improvements in cardiopulmonary, body composition, and psychological outcomes. Specifically, submaximal and maximal exercise performance ($\dot{V}O_2$max) improved posttraining, along with reductions in body fat and an increase in quality of life scores. MacArthur et al. (35) investigated the changes in 25 men living with HIV after 24 weeks of aerobic training. Only six participants were compliant with the exercise program (>80% of the planned sessions attended). Similar to training-induced adaptations in HIV-negative persons, these six participants showed significant increases in $\dot{V}O_2$max and minute ventilation and reductions in heart rate, rate pressure product, and rating of perceived exertion during a submaximal exercise test. A trend was also noted for improved mental health scores (General Health Questionnaire) among the compliant exercisers.

Perna et al. (36) examined the effects of a 12-week aerobic training program on cardiopulmonary function in symptomatic adults living with HIV. They reported that the compliant exercisers (11/18 participants, >50% of the planned sessions attended) increased their $\dot{V}O_2$max, minute ventilation, and maximal work rate. Smith et al. (44) studied 60 men and women living with HIV who were randomized to a thrice weekly aerobic exercise group or control group for 12 weeks. Training intensity was 60%–80% of the $\dot{V}O_2$max for at least 30 minutes. Training improved the $\dot{V}O_2$max by 7.5% ($P = 0.09$) and endurance time on the treadmill by 1 minute (11%). In addition, training-induced reductions in body mass index (BMI), subcutaneous fat (skinfolds), and abdominal girth were found.

Baigis et al. (24) conducted a 15-week home-based aerobic exercise program with adults living with HIV. Results showed no improvement in $\dot{V}O_2$max or health-related quality of life posttraining. The lack of improvement in aerobic capacity may have been owing to their relatively high initial $\dot{V}O_2$max (30 mL/kg/min). Individuals with low levels of fitness usually show the largest gains after training. Other reasons for the lack of aerobic gains may have included the short training sessions and that participants exercised on a ski machine but were tested on a treadmill.

Stringer et al (46) investigated aerobic exercise regimens of varied intensity in 26 men and women living with HIV. The moderate- and high-intensity exercise training groups exercised at work rates that were below and above the ventilatory anaerobic threshold, respectively, three times per week for 6 weeks. The high-intensity group performed a proportionally shorter bout of exercise while maintaining the total work per session

identical to that of the moderate-intensity group. The ventilatory anaerobic threshold increased in both groups, but $\dot{V}O_2$max and maximal power increased only in the high-intensity group, suggesting that intensity of exercise may be more effective in improving aerobic capacity than the amount of exercise in this population. In addition, both groups showed improvements in their quality of life after training based on a self-administered questionnaire.

In another study of aerobic exercise intensity, men and women living with HIV completed a 12-week program of treadmill walking at a moderate intensity (60% of HRmax) or treadmill running at a high intensity (75%–85% of HRmax) (68). The aerobic capacity (maximal treadmill time) increased in both groups, but the improvement was greater in the high-intensity group (190 seconds) than the moderate-intensity (70 seconds) group. Training had no effect on body fat percentage or depression scores.

PROGRESSIVE RESISTIVE EXERCISE IN PEOPLE LIVING WITH HIV/AIDS

Progressive resistive exercise has been used to combat muscle wasting and improve strength in people who are aging and in numerous clinical populations, including patients with renal failure or rheumatoid arthritis (69,70). Given the adverse effect of wasting associated with HIV, investigators have examined the physiologic and psychological effects of PRE alone or in combination with aerobic exercise or androgenic therapy (e.g., testosterone) in people living with HIV (20). For the most part, PRE interventions have consisted of 4–10 isotonic exercises (machines or free weights) of the major muscle groups three times per week for 6–16 weeks. Three sets of 8–12 repetitions were performed for each exercise. The maximal amount of weight that could be lifted once, or the one repetition maximum (1-RM), was determined for each exercise at the start of the program and intermittently throughout the study. The training intensity was set at 50% of the 1-RM during the first few sessions and then increased to 80% of the 1-RM for the remainder of the program.

Results from a systematic review that investigated the effect of PRE in people living with HIV found statistically significant increases in mean body weight of 3.5 kg and mean arm and thigh girth of 7.9 cm among participants engaged in PRE or combined PRE and aerobic exercise compared with nonexercisers (20). Given many of the participants in the individual studies included in this review were diagnosed with AIDS-related wasting syndrome, these increases in weight and body composition were interpreted as favorable outcomes. Despite statistical nonsignificance, results showed a trend toward improvements in cardiopulmonary fitness (HR submax). Similar to the aerobic exercise review (19), no significant changes in CD4 count were reported. Individual study results support findings from the above meta-analyses. In an early randomized control trial (RCT), 24 men living with HIV who had recovered from PCP and were on zidovudine therapy were evenly divided into a PRE group and a nonexercise control group for 6 weeks (71). Body weight and upper and lower body strength increased in the PRE group but not the control group after 6 weeks.

Roubenoff et al. (40,41) implemented an 8-week PRE program in a group of 25 men living with HIV, 6 of whom had AIDS-related wasting. Significant increases were seen in strength and lean body mass after training. Moreover, increases in weight, strength, and lean body mass were greatest in people who demonstrated features of AIDS wasting. Also, self-reported physical function only increased among the participants with wasting and was positively correlated to improvements in strength and lean body mass. In one of the few studies focusing on women living with HIV, Agin et al. (23) examined the separate and combined effects of 14 weeks of PRE and protein supplementation on body composition, strength, and quality of life in 30 women. PRE increased body cell mass, muscle mass, strength, and quality of life, but protein supplementation provided no additional benefit.

Testosterone levels are generally lower in men living with HIV, and even more so in people with wasting. Low testosterone levels correlate with deficits in muscle mass and disease progression. Of the various therapies being considered for the treatment of HIV-associated weight loss, testosterone and exercise are attractive because they are relatively inexpensive and safe. In a 12-week trial, Sattler et al. (42) examined the effects of the anabolic steroid, nandrolone, alone or in combination with PRE in men living with HIV without wasting. Both groups showed increases in body weight, body cell mass, thigh muscle area, and strength. The steroid plus PRE group showed greater increases than the steroid-only group in lean body mass and strength. Although this study did not employ placebo or PRE-only control groups, it suggested that exercise combined with steroids might be a more effective treatment for increasing mass and strength than steroids alone.

The effects of 8 weeks of thrice weekly PRE, with or without an anabolic steroid (oxandrolone), were compared in a group of HIV-positive men who had experienced at least a 5% weight loss over the preceding 2 years (45). They found that PRE increased weight, nitrogen retention, lean body mass, and strength, and that these improvements were greater in those who took the steroid. High-density lipoprotein (HDL) cholesterol declined in the steroid group, however, which suggests a detrimental effect of this treatment on blood lipid profile. Bhasin et al. (25) examined the separate and combined effects of 16 weeks of PRE and testosterone supplementation on strength and body composition in a group of men living with HIV who also had wasting and low serum testosterone levels. Both testosterone and PRE individually

produced significant increases in body weight, strength, and thigh muscle volume, but no added benefit was found with the treatments in combination. Grinspoon et al. (32) compared the effects of 12 weeks of thrice weekly exercise (20 minutes of aerobic training and PRE) and testosterone supplementation in men with wasting. Testosterone or exercise alone increased arm and leg muscle area and muscle mass, but the two treatments combined did not enhance these gains. Levels of HDL cholesterol increased in response to training, but decreased in response to testosterone therapy.

Collectively, the evidence suggests that PRE can result in increases in strength, body weight, lean body mass, HDL cholesterol, and improvements in quality of life measures, whereas nonexercising controls showed little change in these measures. Hence, in addition to increasing lean body mass, PRE is also associated with a potential cardioprotective effect. When androgenic therapy is added to PRE, minimal improvements were noted in strength and body composition over those achieved with PRE alone, but HDL cholesterol did not increase (25,32,42).

EXERCISE TRAINING EFFECTS ON METABOLIC COMPLICATIONS ASSOCIATED WITH HIV AND HAART

Exercise training and physical activity are well-known to reduce central adiposity, blood lipids, and carbohydrate disorders in people who are HIV-negative. It remains inconclusive whether exercise and physical activity have similar benefits for people with HIV and lipodystrophy. Gavrila et al. (72) examined 117 men and 13 women with HIV infection on HAART, in which the patients self-reported habitual exercise and diet. They found that the total exercise index (equal to exercise intensity × duration of exercise × number of exercise sessions per week) was inversely correlated with triglycerides and insulin resistance.

Intervention studies that determined the effects of exercise training on metabolic outcomes in people with HIV and lipodystrophy are in their infancy (13). These studies have a number of methodologic limitations, including the lack of a nonexercising control group, small sample sizes, short training durations, and variable criteria used to define lipodystrophy. Hence, positive outcomes that are noted below should be interpreted cautiously until more rigorous controlled studies are completed. Yarasheski et al. (73) examined whether 16 weeks of PRE reduced hypertriglyceridemia in HIV-positive men on HAART. PRE increased lean body mass (1.4 kg) and thigh muscle area, but did not reduce adipose tissue mass. However, serum triglycerides were decreased at the end of training. Similarly, Jones et al. (33) found that 10 weeks of aerobic and PRE training decreased the waist-to-hip ratio, body fat percentage, total cholesterol (18%), and triglycerides (25%) and increased body mass and arm and leg girths in six participants (one women) with HIV lipodystrophy.

In another study, Thoni et al. (48) reported improvements in body composition and blood lipids after a 4-month program of aerobic cycling exercise in lipodystrophic adults. They found that total abdominal fat (13%), visceral abdominal fat (12%), total cholesterol (23%) and triglycerides (43%) all decreased, and HDL (6%) increased. More recently, Driscoll et al. (30,74) conducted a prospective randomized controlled trial on the effects of receiving the diabetic drug metformin alone or in combination with 12 weeks of exercise training (aerobic and PRE) in 25 HIV-infected patients with fat redistribution and insulin resistance. They found that exercise plus metformin resulted in greater reductions in waist-to-hip ratio, thigh adiposity, blood pressure, and fasting insulin, and larger increases in muscle area and exercise time compared with subjects receiving metformin alone. Moreover, reductions in trunk fat and thigh adiposity were associated with lower insulin levels. Neither intervention, however, altered blood lipid levels (triglycerides, total cholesterol, low-density lipoprotein [LDL] and HDL), a finding also reported by others (26,47). The authors concluded that exercise may improve glucose and insulin metabolism in addition to improving cardiovascular disease indices and body composition in people with HIV lipodystrophy. The absence of an effect on blood lipids may relate to the unique pathophysiology of lipid abnormalities in HIV infection or an ongoing effect of antiretroviral treatment that may prevent positive training-induced adaptations of lipid metabolism in some individuals.

RECOMMENDATIONS FOR EXERCISE PRESCRIPTION AND PROGRAMS

No specific guidelines exist for exercise prescription in people living with HIV. However, the aerobic and PRE programs prescribed in previous exercise intervention studies appear to be safe among adults with HIV who are medically stable. These programs were in accordance with guidelines developed by the American College of Sports Medicine (ACSM) for apparently healthy people (75). It should be noted, however, a number of limitations in the existing HIV and exercise literature should be taken into account. Studies were often fraught with large drop-out rates of exercise participants and adverse effects were not reported in some studies. The excessive drop-out rate highlights the importance of focusing on strategies to promote exercise adherence. One such strategy is to recommend a qualified personal trainer, particularly for those who have little experience with exercise. Another approach that may improve exercise adherence is to promote exercising in groups or with a partner. Research results should also be interpreted cautiously for women

living with HIV because women comprised such a small proportion of the participants in the studies reviewed.

Despite the limitations, the most prudent exercise prescription strategy for people living with HIV to follow is the general ACSM guidelines developed for apparently healthy people. However, these guidelines should be catered to each person's overall health and fitness, specific medical conditions, goals, and practical concerns. In addition, special exercise programming considerations developed by ACSM for people who have conditions such as type 2 diabetes, dyslipidemia, metabolic syndrome, or osteoporosis may need to be consulted when those with HIV have these or related conditions. The exercise professional should have at least a rudimentary knowledge of HIV infection and an understanding of the person's medications and their potential effects on exercise performance. In addition, he or she may need to work closely with or consult other members of the patient's healthcare team to discuss potential adverse effects of exercise and to clarify treatment issues that may have an impact on exercise tolerance.

Two examples illustrate potential approaches for exercise prescription with this population. Client A, who is HIV-positive with lipodystrophy and is new to exercise, may want to become more active to improve her health and reduce the level of truncal adipose tissue. A program for this person ought to focus more on health-related fitness; an "active living" program that emphasizes more daily activity, such as walking or climbing stairs, could be promoted. One goal would be to accumulate a certain amount of activity per week to improve insulin sensitivity and reduce blood lipids. A simple home-based PRE program could be included once the client has completed several weeks of increased physical activity. One of the goals of an exercise intervention for patients with lipodystrophy is to optimize body composition and offset the potential deleterious health effects associated with central adiposity. Hence, a combination of PRE and aerobic exercise can be recommended for persons with lipodystrophy.

Client B is HIV-positive but does not have lipodystrophy. He is active in sports and is interested in a general conditioning program. In this case, a program centered on improving performance-related fitness may be appropriate. Hence, depending on the client's initial fitness, aerobic training for 3–5 days per week lasting for 30–60 minutes at an intensity of 70%–85% of the HRmax may be suitable for this individual. PRE for this client could be incorporated two times per week using free weights and machines to focus on the major muscle groups for 2–3 sets of 8–10 repetitions.

SUMMARY

For people who can access and tolerate HAART, HIV has evolved from a fatal disease to a chronic condition with associated metabolic abnormalities. Studies indicate that people living with HIV have lower aerobic capacity and ventilatory (or blood lactate) anaerobic threshold compared with noninfected controls. These deficits in aerobic fitness may reflect the direct effects of HIV and HAART on body cells (i.e., dysfunctional muscle mitochondria) as well deconditioning of the cardiovascular and neuromuscular systems. These physiologic deficits provide some explanation for impairments, such as weakness and decreased endurance, commonly experienced by people living with HIV, and highlight the need for exercise training in this population. Further studies in the HIV population should determine both exercise physiology and functional measures in the same individual before and after exercise training to more fully understand their interdependence.

Exercise training in adults living with HIV has demonstrated positive outcomes similar to those observed in the HIV-negative population. For example, aerobic exercise training increased maximal aerobic capacity, reduced body fat (i.e., waist-to-hip ratio, skinfolds) and showed improvements in anxiety, depression, and life satisfaction. Moreover, PRE alone or in combination with aerobic training increased strength and lean body mass, particularly in those with wasting, and provided an additional potential cardioprotective effect as reflected by increased HDL levels. The addition of androgen therapy to exercise training may not add much benefit over exercise training alone and may prevent the exercise-induced increase in HDL. Exercise training studies in adults with HIV and lipodystrophy also showed increases in strength, lean body mass (muscle area), and reduced trunk fat, but inconsistent effects on blood lipids after training, possibly reflecting the effects of HAART. The cardioprotective effects of increased aerobic fitness, reduced trunk fat, and lower blood lipids may be particularly important to counteract the increased risk of heart disease in people living with HIV who are on HAART.

Aerobic training, PRE, or a combination of both, appears to be safe for adults living with HIV who are medically stable, as demonstrated by the lack of change in immunologic or virologic status with the exercise interventions. In many studies, however, participants who withdrew from exercise programs were not included in the final analysis of the data. This raises concerns about the safety and effectiveness of exercise among participants who stopped exercising. Future studies should make an effort to include all participants in an intention-to-treat analysis, which involves reporting findings for all subjects who withdraw from exercise programs.

Most studies assessed groups of individuals with widely ranging stages of HIV disease progression. Few investigators grouped participants according to disease stage. Hence, the impact of illness stage on the acute or chronic responses to exercise are not well understood. Most participants in studies of HIV/AIDS and exercise have been men between 30 and 40 years of age. Relatively few women, older adults, or children have been studied, despite gender- and age-related differences in exercise responses in the HIV-negative population. In addition, when both men and women living with HIV were included as study participants, the results were presented as one group without examining gender differences in exercise responses. Additional studies should attempt to study more homogenous subject groups, particularly those who are more severely immunocompromised and older adults. These individuals may demonstrate the lowest fitness reserves and, thus, may benefit most from exercise training. As well, greater numbers of women should be studied and findings should be presented by gender in samples that are sufficiently large to power appropriate analyses.

Despite the limitations of previous studies, sufficient evidence supports the advice that people living with HIV should be encouraged to increase their daily physical activity and participate in a formal aerobic, PRE exercise program, or both, if interested. Exercise should be tailored to meet the particular needs of individuals and should follow ACSM guidelines. Hence, the exercise professional should consider the stage of the disease, symptoms, drug side effects, functional ability, and the frequency, intensity, duration, and the exercise mode.

REFERENCES

1. UNAIDS. Joint United Nations Programme on HIV/AIDS. *2006 Report on the Global AIDS Epidemic.* Geneva, Switzerland: UNAIDS; July 2006.
2. Jacobson DL, Tang AM, Spiegelman D, et al. Incidence of metabolic syndrome in a cohort of HIV-infected adults and prevalence relative to the US population (National Health and Nutrition Examination Survey). *J Acquir Immune Defic Syndr* 2006;43(4):458–66.
3. Monier PL, Wilcox R. Metabolic complications associated with the use of highly active antiretroviral therapy in HIV-1-infected adults. *Am J Med Sci* 2004;328(1):48–56.
4. Centers for Disease Control and Prevention. Revision of the CDC surveillance case definition for acquired immunodeficiency syndrome. *MMWR* 1987;36(2S):3S–15S.
5. Wheeler DA, Gibert CL, Launer CA, et al. Weight loss as a predictor of survival and disease progression in HIV infection. Terry Beirn Community Programs for Clinical Research on AIDS. *J Acquir Immune Defic Syndr Hum Retrovirol* 1998;18(1):80–5.
6. Dudgeon WD, Phillips KD, Carson JA, et al. Counteracting muscle wasting in HIV-infected individuals. *HIV Med* 2006;7(5):299–310.
7. Wanke CA, Silva M, Knox TA, et al. Weight loss and wasting remain common complications in individuals infected with human immunodeficiency virus in the era of highly active antiretroviral therapy. *Clin Infect Dis* 2000; 31(3):803–5.
8. Palenicek JP, Graham NM, He YD, et al. Weight loss prior to clinical AIDS as a predictor of survival. Multicenter AIDS Cohort Study Investigators. *J Acquir Immune Defic Syndr Hum Retrovirol* 1995; 10(3):366–73.
9. Wilson IB, Jacobson DL, Roubenoff R, et al. Changes in lean body mass and total body weight are weakly associated with physical functioning in patients with HIV infection. *HIV Med* 2002;3(4):263–70.

10. Corcoran C, Grinspoon S. Treatments for wasting in patients with the acquired immunodeficiency syndrome. *N Engl J Med* 1999; 340(22):1740–50.

11. Balasubramanyam A, Sekhar RV, Jahoor F, et al. Pathophysiology of dyslipidemia and increased cardiovascular risk in HIV lipodystrophy: A model of 'systemic steatosis'. *Curr Opin Lipidol* 2004; 15(1):59–67.

12. Triant VA, Lee H, Hadigan C, et al. Increased acute myocardial infarction rates and cardiovascular risk factors among patients with human immunodeficiency virus disease. *J Clin Endocrinol Metab* 2007;92(7):2506–12.

13. Yarasheski KE, Roubenoff R. Exercise treatment for HIV-associated metabolic and anthropomorphic complications. *Exerc Sport Sci Rev* 2001;29(4):170–4.

14. Ciccolo JT, Jowers EM, Bartholomew JB. The benefits of exercise training for quality of life in HIV/AIDS in the post-HAART era. *Sports Med* 2004;34(8):487–99.

15. World Health Organization. *The International Classification of Functioning, Disability and Health-ICF*. Geneva: World Health Organization; 200.

16. Rusch M, Nixon S, Schilder A, et al. Impairments, activity limitations and participation restrictions: Prevalence and associations among persons living with HIV/AIDS in British Columbia. *Health Qual Life Outcomes* [Internet]. 2004 [cited 2007 June 10];2:46. Available from:http: //www. hqlo.com/ content /2/1/46. doi:10. 1186/1477-7525-2-46

17. Johnson JE, Anders GT, Blanton HM, et al. Exercise dysfunction in patients seropositive for the human immunodeficiency virus. *Am Rev Respir Dis* 1990;141(3):618–22.

18. Pothoff G, Wassermann K, Ostmann H. Impairment of exercise capacity in various groups of HIV-infected patients. *Respiration* 1994;61(2):80–5.

19. O'Brien K, Nixon S, Tynan AM, et al. Aerobic exercise interventions for people living with HIV/AIDS: Implications for practice, education, and research. *Physiotherapy Canada* 2006; 58(2): 114–29.

20. O'Brien K, Nixon S, Glazier RH, et al. Progressive resistive exercise interventions for adults living with HIV/AIDS. *Cochrane Database Syst Rev* 2004;(4):CD004248.

21. Fitch KV, Anderson EJ, Hubbard JL, et al. Effects of a lifestyle modification program in HIV-infected patients with the metabolic syndrome. *AIDS* 2006;20(14):1843–50.

22. Oursler KK, Sorkin JD, Smith BA, et al. Reduced aerobic capacity and physical functioning in older HIV-infected men. *AIDS Res Hum Retroviruses* 2006;22(11):1113–21.

23. Agin D, Gallagher D, Wang J, et al. Effects of whey protein and resistance exercise on body cell mass, muscle strength, and quality of life in women with HIV. *AIDS* 2001;15(18):2431–40.

24. Baigis J, Korniewicz DM, Chase G, et al. Effectiveness of a home-based exercise intervention for HIV-infected adults: A randomized trial. *J Assoc Nurses AIDS Care* 2002; 13(2):33–45.

25. Bhasin S, Storer TW, Javanbakht M, et al. Testosterone replacement and resistance exercise in HIV-infected men with weight loss and low testosterone levels. *JAMA* 2000;283(6):763–70.

26. Birk TJ, MacArthur RD, Lipton LM, et al. Aerobic exercise training fails to lower hypertriglyceridemia levels in persons with advanced HIV-1 infection. *J Assoc Nurses AIDS Care* 2002; 13(6): 20–4.

27. Cade WT, Fantry LE, Nabar SR, et al. Decreased peak arteriovenous oxygen difference during treadmill exercise testing in individuals infected with the human immunodeficiency virus. *Arch Phys Med Rehabil* 2003;84(11):1595–603.

28. Cade WT, Peralta L, Keyser RE. Aerobic capacity in late adolescents infected with HIV and controls. *Pediatr Rehabil* 2002; 5(3): 161–9.

29. Dolan SE, Frontera W, Librizzi J, et al. Effects of a supervised home-based aerobic and progressive resistance training regimen in women infected with human immunodeficiency virus: A randomized trial. *Arch Intern Med* 2006;166(11):1225–31.

30. Driscoll SD, Meininger GE, Ljungquist K, et al. Differential effects of metformin and exercise on muscle adiposity and metabolic indices in human immunodeficiency virus-infected patients. *J Clin Endocrinol Metab* 2004;89(5):2171–8.

31. Duong M, Dumas JP, Buisson M, et al. Limitation of exercise capacity in nucleoside-treated HIV-infected patients with hyperlactataemia. *HIV Med* 2007;8(2):105–11.

32. Grinspoon S, Corcoran C, Parlman K, et al. Effects of testosterone and progressive resistance training in eugonadal men with AIDS wasting. A randomized, controlled trial. *Ann Intern Med* 2000; 133(5):348–55.

33. Jones SP, Doran DA, Leatt PB, et al. Short-term exercise training improves body composition and hyperlipidemia in HIV-positive individuals with lipodystrophy. *AIDS* 2001;15(15):2049–51.

34. LaPerriere A, Klimas N, Fletcher MA, et al. Change in CD4+ cell enumeration following aerobic exercise training in HIV-1 disease: Possible mechanisms and practical applications. *Int J Sports Med* 1997;18(Suppl 1):S56–61.

35. MacArthur RD, Levine SD, Birk TJ. Supervised exercise training improves cardiopulmonary fitness in HIV-infected persons. *Med Sci Sports Exerc* 1993;25(6):684–8.

36. Perna FM, LaPerriere A, Klimas N, et al. Cardiopulmonary and CD4 cell changes in response to exercise training in early symptomatic HIV infection. *Med Sci Sports Exerc* 1999;31(7): 973–9.

37. Rigsby LW, Dishman RK, Jackson AW, et al. Effects of exercise training on men seropositive for the human immunodeficiency virus-1. *Med Sci Sports Exerc* 1992;24(1):6–12.

38. Robinson FP, Quinn LT, Rimmer JH. Effects of high-intensity endurance and resistance exercise on HIV metabolic abnormalities: A pilot study. *Biol Res Nurs* 2007;8(3):177–85.

39. Roge BT, Calbet JA, Moller K, et al. Skeletal muscle mitochondrial function and exercise capacity in HIV-infected patients with lipodystrophy and elevated p-lactate levels. *AIDS* 2002; 16(7): 973–82.

40. Roubenoff R, Weiss L, McDermott A, et al. A pilot study of exercise training to reduce trunk fat in adults with HIV-associated fat redistribution. *AIDS* 1999;13(11):1373–5.

41. Roubenoff R. Wilson IB. Effect of resistance training on self-reported physical functioning in HIV infection. *Med Sci Sports Exerc* 2001;33(11):1811–7.

42. Sattler FR, Jaque SV, Schroeder ET, et al. Effects of pharmacological doses of nandrolone decanoate and progressive resistance training in immunodeficient patients infected with human immunodeficiency virus. *J Clin Endocrinol Metab* 1999; 84(4):1268–76.

43. Scott WB, Oursler KK, Katzel LI, et al. Central activation, muscle performance, and physical function in men infected with human immunodeficiency virus. *Muscle Nerve* 2007; 36(3):374–83.

44. Smith BA, Neidig JL, Nickel JT, et al. Aerobic exercise: Effects on parameters related to fatigue, dyspnea, weight and body composition in HIV-infected adults. *AIDS* 2001;15(6):693–701.

45. Strawford A, Barbieri T, Van Loan M, et al. Resistance exercise and supraphysiologic androgen therapy in eugonadal men with HIV-related weight loss: A randomized controlled trial. *JAMA* 1999; 281(14):1282–90.

46. Stringer WW, Berezovskaya M, O'Brien WA, et al. The effect of exercise training on aerobic fitness, immune indices, and quality of life in HIV+ patients. *Med Sci Sports Exerc* 1998;30(1):11–6.

47. Terry L, Sprinz E, Stein R, et al. Exercise training in HIV-1-infected individuals with dyslipidemia and lipodystrophy. *Med Sci Sports Exerc* 2006;38(3):411–7.

48. Thoni GJ, Fedou C, Brun JF, et al. Reduction of fat accumulation and lipid disorders by individualized light aerobic training in human immunodeficiency virus infected patients with lipodystrophy and/or dyslipidemia. *Diabetes Metab* 2002;28(5):397–404.

49. Stringer WW. Mechanisms of exercise limitation in HIV+ individuals. *Med Sci Sports Exerc* 2000;32(7 Suppl):S412–21.

50. Bassett DR Jr, Howley ET. Limiting factors for maximum oxygen uptake and determinants of endurance performance. *Med Sci Sports Exerc* 2000;32(1):70–84.

51. Finley CE, LaMonte MJ, Waslien CI, et al. Cardiorespiratory fitness, macronutrient intake, and the metabolic syndrome: The Aerobics Center Longitudinal Study. *J Am Diet Assoc* 2006;106(5): 673–9.

52. Astrand I, Astrand PO, Hallback I, et al. Reduction in maximal oxygen uptake with age. *J Appl Physiol* 1973;35(5):649–54.

53. Babcock MA, Paterson DH, Cunningham DA. Effects of aerobic endurance training on gas exchange kinetics of older men. *Med Sci Sports Exerc* 1994;26(4):447–52.

54. Dehn MM, Bruce RA. Longitudinal variations in maximal oxygen intake with age and activity. *J Appl Physiol* 1972;33(6):805–7.

55. Hossack KF, Bruce RA. Maximal cardiac function in sedentary normal men and women: Comparison of age-related changes. *J Appl Physiol* 1982;53(4):799–804.

56. Schiller BC, Casas YG, Desouza CA, et al. Maximal aerobic capacity across age in healthy Hispanic and Caucasian women. *J Appl Physiol* 2001;91(3):1048–54.

57. Johnson JE, Slife DM, Anders GT, et al. Cardiac dysfunction in patients seropositive for the human immunodeficiency virus. *West J Med* 1991;155(4):373–9.

58. Cade WT, Fantry LE, Nabar SR, et al. A comparison of Qt and a-$\dot{V}O_2$ in individuals with HIV taking and not taking HAART. *Med Sci Sports Exerc* 2003;35(7):1108–17.

59. Bailey RO, Turok DI, Jaufmann BP, et al. Myositis and acquired immunodeficiency syndrome. *Hum Pathol* 1987; 18(7):749–51.

60. Chapplain JM, Beillot J, Begue JM, et al. Mitochondrial abnormalities in HIV-infected lipoatrophic patients treated with antiretroviral agents. *J Acquir Immune Defic Syndr* 2004;37(4):1477–88.

61. Belanger AY, McComas AJ. Extent of motor unit activation during effort. *J Appl Physiol* 1981;51(5):1131–5.

62. Boubaker K, Flepp M, Sudre P, et al. Hyperlactatemia and antiretroviral therapy: The Swiss HIV Cohort Study. *Clin Infect Dis* 2001;33(11):1931–7.

63. Tesiorowski AM, Harris M, Chan KJ, et al. Anaerobic threshold and random venous lactate levels among HIV-positive patients on antiretroviral therapy. *J Acquir Immune Defic Syndr* 2002;31(2): 250–1.

64. Bauer AM, Sternfeld T, Horster S, et al. Kinetics of lactate metabolism after submaximal ergometric exercise in HIV-infected patients. *HIV Med* 2004;5(5): 371–6.

65. Stoff DM, Khalsa JH, Monjan A, et al. Introduction: HIV/AIDS and Aging. *AIDS* 2004;18(Suppl 1):S1–2.

66. Mustafa T, Sy FS, Macera CA, et al. Association between exercise and HIV disease progression in a cohort of homosexual men. *Ann Epidemiol* 1999;9(2):127–31.

67. Bopp CM, Phillips KD, Fulk LJ, et al. Physical activity and immunity in HIV-infected individuals. *AIDS Care* 2004;16(3):387–93.

68. Terry L, Sprinz E, Ribeiro JP. Moderate and high intensity exercise training in HIV-1 seropositive individuals: A randomized trial. *Int J Sports Med* 1999;20(2):142–6.

69. Castaneda C, Gordon PL, Uhlin KL, et al. Resistance training to counteract the catabolism of a low-protein diet in patients with chronic renal insufficiency. A randomized, controlled trial. *Ann Intern Med* 2001;135(11):965–76.

70. Hakkinen A, Sokka T, Kotaniemi A, et al. A randomized two-year study of the effects of dynamic strength training on muscle strength, disease activity, functional capacity, and bone mineral density in early rheumatoid arthritis. *Arthritis Rheum* 2001;44(3): 515–22.

71. Spence DW, Galantino ML, Mossberg KA, et al. Progressive resistance exercise: Effect on muscle function and anthropometry of a select AIDS population. *Arch Phys Med Rehabil* 1990; 71(9):644–8.

72. Gavrila A, Tsiodras S, Doweiko J, et al. Exercise and vitamin E intake are independently associated with metabolic abnormalities in human immunodeficiency virus-positive subjects: A cross-sectional study. *Clin Infect Dis* 2003;36(12):1593–601.

73. Yarasheski KE, Tebas P, Stanerson B, et al. Resistance exercise training reduces hypertriglyceridemia in HIV-infected men treated with antiviral therapy. *J Appl Physiol* 2001;90(1):133–8.

74. Driscoll SD, Meininger GE, Lareau MT, et al. Effects of exercise training and metformin on body composition and cardiovascular indices in HIV-infected patients. *AIDS* 2004;18(3):465–73.

75. American College of Sports Medicine. *ACSM's Guidelines For Exercise Testing and Prescription*, 7th ed. Philadelphia: Lippincott Williams & Wilkins; 2006.

Chronic Fatigue Syndrome

EPIDEMIOLOGY AND PATHOPHYSIOLOGY

A cluster of symptoms and signs of abnormal functioning that have no discernible medical cause define chronic fatigue syndrome (CFS). The major patient-reported symptom is a prolonged and debilitating feeling of fatigue that is not improved with rest and is often worsened after even minimal mental or physical stress.

The term CFS arose out of four reports in the first half of the 1980s concerning patients suffering from a chronic and recurring complex of symptoms of unknown origin that included severe fatigue, fever, tender lymph nodes, sore throat, decreased memory, confusion, and depression (1–4). Preliminary clinical serologic investigation revealed that many patients exhibited antibody profiles consistent with mononucleosis-associated Epstein-Barr virus (EBV) infection. This illness came to be called the *chronic EBV syndrome* or the *chronic mononucleosislike syndrome*. Data from two subsequent scientific investigations cast doubt on EBV as the syndrome's etiology by indicating that these patients would be just as likely to have serologic profiles consistent with infections by cytomegalovirus, herpes simplex virus types 1 and 2, or the measles virus (5,6).

CASE DEFINITION

In 1988, the U.S. Centers for Disease Control and Prevention (CDC) formulated a working case definition for the syndrome discussed above and named it CFS. This was done in an attempt to help identify the illness, prevent association with a specific unproved etiology, and provide guidelines for investigators concerned with ascertaining its true etiology and pathology. This working definition states that a diagnosis of CFS can be made if a patient exhibits a new onset of severe fatigue that has persisted or relapsed for at least 6 months, caused at least a 50% reduction in premorbid activity, and cannot be attributed to known medical conditions. The patient must also exhibit eight or more of the following symptoms: mild fever, sore throat, painful lymph nodes, muscle weakness, myalgia, severe fatigue after mild exercise, headaches, migratory arthralgia, neuropsychological complaints, sleep disturbance, and sudden onset of symptoms. Diagnosis is

to be excluded with any presence or history of psychiatric disease or personality disorder (7).

Additional case definitions were also developed (8,9). The Oxford or British definition accounts for the fact that in many patients, psychological symptoms, such as depression, anxiety, and loss of interest, cannot explain the severe fatigue reported and may actually have developed as a result of the chronic illness. Therefore, this definition does not exclude for many psychological conditions (9).

In 1991, the National Institutes of Health (NIH) recommended that revisions be made in the CDC guidelines for diagnosing CFS to accommodate for the premorbid and comorbid presence of certain psychiatric disorders, diseases, or syndromes. Also, the NIH recommended specific laboratory and psychological tests to help rule out a diagnosis of CFS in the presence of known causes of fatigue (10).

An international working group, including representatives from the CDC, NIH, United States, Britain, and Australia, convened in 1994 to amend the CDC case definition and research guidelines. The result was the most widely accepted case definition (11). Here, a diagnosis of CFS is established

" . . . by the presence of the following: 1) clinically evaluated, unexplained, persistent or relapsing chronic fatigue that is of new or definite onset (has not been lifelong); is not the result of ongoing exertion; is not substantially alleviated by rest; and results in substantial reduction in previous levels of occupational, educational, social, or personal activities; and 2) the concurrent occurrence of four or more of the following symptoms, all of which must have persisted or recurred during 6 or more consecutive months of illness and must not have predated the fatigue: self-reported impairment in short-term memory or concentration severe enough to cause substantial reduction in previous levels of occupational, educational, social, or personal activities; sore throat; tender cervical or axially lymph nodes; muscle pain, multi joint pain without joint swelling or redness; headaches of a new type, pattern, or severity; unrefreshing sleep; and postexertional malaise lasting more than 24 hours" (11; p 956).

This definition has gone a long way in providing research guidance and clarity in the identification process of patients with CFS. Many ambiguities remain, however, as evidenced by the existence of groups of patients that meet the criteria for CFS but have different degrees of fatigue and heterogeneity of symptoms. An international group of experts has published specific recommendations to address these problems. They provide a clarification of the inclusion and exclusion criteria and a descriptive list of questionnaires and medical diagnostic techniques that have been shown to be valid for use with patients with CFS (12).

THEORIES OF ETIOLOGY AND PATHOPHYSIOLOGY

Volumes of data from research studies investigating possible causes of CFS have been published, but a definitive cause or marker has not been identified. Therefore, it is somewhat difficult to separate the etiology and pathophysiology of this illness.

The first suspected etiology of CFS was a viral or bacterial infection, which originated from patients reporting that fatigue symptoms started suddenly after a "flulike" illness. Many viruses have been suspected, such as human herpesvirus-6 (HHV-6), which often becomes latent after early infection, can be reactivated, and affects a number of body systems. In one study, CFS patients (57%) were found to have higher HHV-6 blood antibody levels when compared with healthy controls (16%) (13). In a study of 22 pairs of twins where one twin was diagnosed as having CFS while the other remained healthy, no significant differences were found in assays for several viruses, including HHV-6 (14). A multitude of viruses and bacteria have been investigated, but to date, no single infectious organism has consistently been found in patients with CFS such that it would be considered a marker for the illness. Data have been presented indicating that a variety of viruses may precipitate the development of CFS in a significant number of postinfective patients (15).

Because so many different viral agents have been implicated and patients seem to have an exaggerated response to infections, many theorize that an abnormal immune system may be the origin of CFS. Data exist to support a possible chronic immune activation (16) or an insufficient immune response in patients with CFS (17). Often reported are abnormal CD8+ cytotoxic T-cell activation (16) and a depression of natural killer (NK) cell activity (17). Others, however, have reported no abnormal blood concentration or activation of lymphocyte cell surface markers in CFS (18). Several authors have reported immune activation associated with interleukins (i.e., IL-1, IL-2, IL-4, and IL-6) and tumor-necrosis factor (TNF), as well as other cytokines (19). However, others have not found a difference in the cytokine levels in patients with CFS when compared with healthy control subjects (20). In an attempt to clarify these inconsistencies, a systematic review of the CFS immunologic literature was conducted. This review rated the various studies on the quality of the reported methodology. No consistent pattern of immuno-

logic abnormalities in CFS was identified as a result of this review process. However, immune dysfunction, particularly T cell changes, could not be definitively ruled out as a potential factor in the etiology of CFS (21).

Neuroendocrine abnormalities have also been implicated in the etiology of CFS. The research here has centered primarily on the hypothalamic-pituitary-adrenal axis (HPA). The HPA is considered the primary axis in response to both physical and psychologic stress. Deficiency of glucocorticoids released by the adrenal gland can result in fatigue, and evidence of low glucocorticoid levels in patients with CFS has been presented, which may be caused to a blunted release of corticotropin (22). The adrenal glands in patients with CFS have also been shown to have a low secretory reserve when stimulated and to be reduced in size (23). Many reports, however, have not found HPA hypoactivity in patients with CFS (24). Some investigators have concluded that, although no specific dysfunction of the HPA axis causes the onset of CFS, the illness may perpetuate an abnormally functioning HPA axis, which in turn, may be one of many factors contributing to the exacerbation of symptoms during the progression of the disease (25).

Because the symptoms of CFS are so heterogeneous and the illness seems to affect numerous body functions, many speculate that the nervous system must be involved, either as a primary or secondary cause. Neurologic studies have shown that, when compared with controls, patients with CFS had significantly more abnormalities in the cerebral white matter (26), brainstem hypoperfusion (27), decreased regional cerebral blood flow (27), decreased serotonin activity (28), and alterations in the processing of motor activities (29,30). Others have reported, however, no neurologic abnormalities in patients with CFS. For example, no difference was found in resting regional brain blood flow in twins with CFS when compared with their healthy co-twins (31).

Investigations of the autonomic nervous system have revealed both parasympathetic and sympathetic abnormalities in patients with CFS, whereas others have found normal autonomic activity. Some reports have indicated a high percentage (90%) of patients with CFS who exhibit neurally mediated hypotension (NMH) during tilt-table testing (32). Conversely, data have shown no difference in the percentage of patients with CFS with orthostatic intolerance when compared with healthy sedentary controls (33). Furthermore, when NMH was successfully treated in patients with CFS no significant improvement was seen in their fatigue (34).

Psychological factors are significantly involved in many CFS cases. Some physicians feel that patients with CFS are suffering from primary psychiatric disorders or psychophysiologic reactions. Suggested psychological causes of chronic fatigue include depression, anxiety disorder, somatization disorder, and dysthymia and grief (35). High premorbid and comorbid incidences of these disorders are associated with CFS. For example, comorbid major depression has been indicated in 50% of patients with CFS (35). In some investigations, 66% have been found to have a history of major depression at sometime during their lives (35). This may not be unexpected owing to significant lifestyle disruption. Arguably, comorbid presence of symptoms of depression does not necessarily indicate a cause for fatigue, because these symptoms may result from being chronically ill and physically compromised. Also, it has been pointed out that the biological abnormalities found in depression differ from those found in CFS. Furthermore, a significant number of patients with CFS have no indication of psychopathology (36).

The proposed causes and pathologies discussed above are just a sample of those reported in the medical and scientific literature concerned with CFS. Also, several unifying theories of the origins of CFS have been suggested, but to date, none are supported by sufficient clinical evidence to be validated as the true etiology.

PREVALENCE AND INCIDENCE

Estimates of the incidence of CFS in the general population are difficult to make because no definitive marker exists and, therefore, estimates must be approached with caution. A population-based study conducted in Wichita, Kansas found the prevalence of adult CFS to be approximately 0.24% (37). In San Francisco it was found that 0.2% of adults satisfied criteria for CFS (38). In a randomly selected sample of the general population of Chicago, Illinois, the prevalence rate for CFS was higher (0.42%), with the highest rates found among women, minority groups, and the less educated (39).

In a rigorously controlled population study of the prevalence of CFS in metropolitan, urban, and rural Georgia, investigators estimated that 2.54% of the adult population experiences CFS. No differences were found in the prevalence rates in the three population stratifications for the women, but men in the rural areas had a significantly higher rate (2.89%) when compared with men in the metropolitan area (0.42%). Metropolitan women had a rate that was 11.2 times that of metropolitan men. No significant differences were found for prevalence rates for white and black persons. The researchers attributed the increased prevalence rates found in their study to different screening criteria and the use of more sensitive and specific measures of CFS (40).

RISK FACTORS

No health organization, such as the NIH or CDC, has published or endorsed a list of risk factors for CFS. One risk factor that seems to be consistently reported, however, is being female, for which the relative risk has been estimated to be between 1.3 to 1.7 per 100,000 (41). Childhood trauma and psychopathology have also been shown to be important predisposing factors (42). Other risk factors which have been indicated in the CFS scientific literature include genetics, neuroticism, introversion, childhood inactivity, and inactivity after mononucleosis (43).

FUNCTIONAL CONSEQUENCES

Data concerned with the degree of disability in CFS are biased by the fact that one primary criterion for diagnosis is a substantial reduction in daily activity. However, on the Medical Outcomes Study Short-Form General Health Survey (SF-36) (44) when comparing individuals with chronic fatigue, major depression, acute infectious mononucleosis, and healthy controls, patients with CFS scored lowest on physical functioning, role functioning, social functioning, general health, and body pain subscales (45). In a population-based study, patients diagnosed with CFS and patients with severe fatigue associated with comorbid conditions had similar reductions in energy and time spent on hobbies, schooling, or volunteer work when compared with nonfatigued controls (46). Electronic activity monitors have indicated that daily activity levels of patients with CFS were approximately 15% less when compared with healthy sedentary control (47).

In the U.S. population of patients with CFS, it is estimated that there is an overall reduction in employment of 27%, with a 37% decline in household productivity, and a 54% reduction in labor force productivity. This lost productivity is projected to cost the U.S. economy $9.1 billion per year representing about $20,000 per person with CFS (48).

The functional limitations reduce the individuals' social and vocational opportunities and result in varying degrees of isolation (9). When the illness is severe, the functional impairments can cause school and work absenteeism, social isolation, and an eventual breakdown of a normal family life (43). Additionally, data from community-based studies suggest that women, minorities, and those nonworking individuals who have CFS experience greater functional disability and severity of symptoms than men, whites, and working individuals (49).

PROGNOSIS

Nothing indicates that untreated CFS is a fatal condition, but the prognosis for patients is not very promising in terms of complete recovery (50,51). However, during the progression of the illness, patients with CFS will often have periods where symptoms will get better and then relapse. A systematic review of studies concerned with CFS prognosis indicated that the median full recovery rate was 5% (range: 0–31%), at follow-up the median proportion with improved symptoms was 39.5% (range: 8%–63%), and the return to work was 8%–30% (50). Factors related to a poor prognosis have been reported to be older age, chronic illness before diagnosis of CFS, comorbid psychiatric disorders, and patients holding on to the belief of a physical cause for their illness (51).

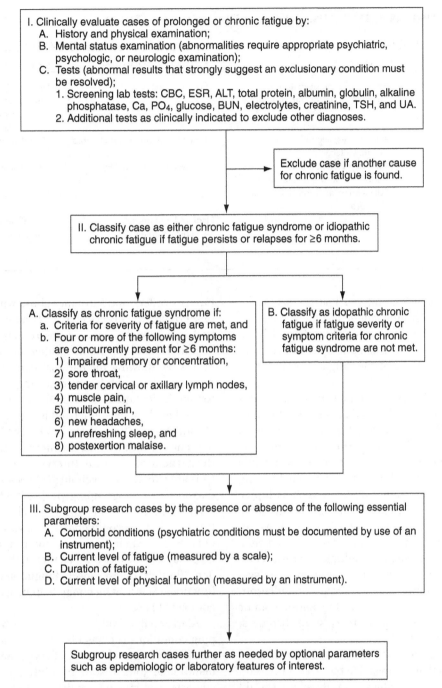

I. Clinically evaluate cases of prolonged or chronic fatigue by:
   A. History and physical examination;
   B. Mental status examination (abnormalities require appropriate psychiatric, psychologic, or neurologic examination);
   C. Tests (abnormal results that strongly suggest an exclusionary condition must be resolved);
      1. Screening lab tests: CBC, ESR, ALT, total protein, albumin, globulin, alkaline phosphatase, Ca, PO₄, glucose, BUN, electrolytes, creatinine, TSH, and UA.
      2. Additional tests as clinically indicated to exclude other diagnoses.

Exclude case if another cause for chronic fatigue is found.

II. Classify case as either chronic fatigue syndrome or idiopathic chronic fatigue if fatigue persists or relapses for ≥6 months.

A. Classify as chronic fatigue syndrome if:
   a. Criteria for severity of fatigue are met, and
   b. Four or more of the following symptoms are concurrently present for ≥6 months:
      1) impaired memory or concentration,
      2) sore throat,
      3) tender cervical or axillary lymph nodes,
      4) muscle pain,
      5) multijoint pain,
      6) new headaches,
      7) unrefreshing sleep, and
      8) postexertion malaise.

B. Classify as idopathic chronic fatigue if fatigue severity or symptom criteria for chronic fatigue syndrome are not met.

III. Subgroup research cases by the presence or absence of the following essential parameters:
   A. Comorbid conditions (psychiatric conditions must be documented by use of an instrument);
   B. Current level of fatigue (measured by a scale);
   C. Duration of fatigue;
   D. Current level of physical function (measured by an instrument).

Subgroup research cases further as needed by optional parameters such as epidemiologic or laboratory features of interest.

FIGURE 18.1. Evaluation and classification of unexplained chronic fatigue. ALT, alanine aminotransferase; BUN, blood urea nitrogen; CBC, complete blood count; ESR, erythrocyte sedimentation rate; PO4, phosphorus; TSH, thyroid-stimulating hormone; UA, urinalysis. (Reprinted with permission from Fukuda et al. The chronic fatigue syndrome: A comprehensive approach to its definition and study. *Ann Intern Med* 1994;121:953–959, the American College of Physicians—American Society of Internal Medicine.)

DIAGNOSTIC TECHNIQUES

To date, no diagnostic tests definitively establish the presence of CFS. Therefore, establishing if the 1994 CDC case definition, described earlier, applies to an individual patient ruling out any definable medical cause of the fatigue must be done to make a diagnosis of CFS. A flow chart of the suggested diagnostic steps to take when evaluating a patient and further subgrouping for research purposes is presented in Figure 18.1 (11).

Because many patients presenting themselves to a clinic express fatigue as a symptom, the first diagnostic step is to

TABLE 18.1. EXCLUSIONS AND INCLUSIONS FOR A DIAGNOSIS OF CHRONIC FATIGUE SYNDROME (CFS)

EXCLUSIVE		INCLUSIVE	
MEDICAL CONDITION	**EXAMPLES**	**MEDICAL CONDITION**	**EXAMPLES**
Active or untreated	Hypothyroidism, sleep apnea, narcolepsy, iatrogenic conditions	Symptom defined	Fibromyalgia, anxiety disorders, somatoform disorders, mild depression, neurasthenia, multiple chemical sensitivity
Unresolved premorbid CFS	Malignancies, hepatitis B or C virus infection	Treated and symptoms elevated	Hypothyroidism, asthma
Major psychological	Major depression, bipolar affective disorders, schizophrenia, delusional, dementias, anorexia or bulimia nervosa	Resolved premorbid CFS	Lyme disease, syphilis
Alcohol and substance abuse		Isolated and unexplained clinical finding	Insignificant elevated antinuclear antibody titer
Severe obesity (body mass index [BMI] ≥45)			

make a distinction between prolonged fatigue lasting for at least 1 month and chronic fatigue lasting or relapsing for at least 6 months. Next, specific clinical and laboratory tests are recommended when attempting to rule out medically definable causes of the fatigue (Figure 18.1) (11).

A diagnosis of CFS is excluded if a patient has a clinically defined and treatable illness that is known to cause fatigue (Table 18.1). Reeves et al. (12) describe the need to clarify further the exclusionary criteria to improve the uniformity of diagnosis. Their recommendations include (*a*) organ failure, including lung, cardiac, or renal failure; (*b*) rheumatic or inflammatory diseases, such as lupus, Sjögren's syndrome, rheumatoid arthritis, or irritable bowel syndrome; (52) chronic infections, such as acquired immunodeficiency syndrome (AIDS) or hepatitis; (*d*) neurologic diseases, such as multiple sclerosis, cerebrovascular accidents, or traumatic brain injury; (*e*) systemic treatments, such as chemotherapy or radiation; (*f*) major endocrine diseases, such as hypopituitarism or adrenal insufficiency; and (*g*) primary sleep disorders, such as apnea or narcolepsy.

Reeves et al. (12) also describe several temporary medical conditions that are treatable but over time could contribute to the fatiguing illness and, therefore, should be monitored. These conditions may include medication effects, sleep deprivation, untreated hypothyroidism, diabetes, or active infection. These temporary medical conditions might also include those that resolve, such as pregnancy including the postpartum period, the 6-month period following major surgery and 3 months following minor surgery, restless leg disorders, 5 years following major conditions such as myocardial infarction or heart failure, and finally, morbid obesity (body mass index [BMI] >40).

Permanent psychiatric conditions are exclusionary, including a lifetime diagnosis of bipolar affective disorders, schizophrenia, delusional disorders, dementias, organic

brain disorders, and substance abuse within 2 years of the onset of fatigue. Reeves et al. (12) note that the Composite International Diagnostic Instrument (CIDI) (53) can be a useful tool for the determination of psychiatric disorders by allowing for national comparisons of psychiatric prevalence while not requiring neuropsychologists for implementation. The CIDI can be administered by general medical personnel and is supported by the World Health Organization (WHO) (54). The National Institute of Mental Health Diagnostic Interview Schedule (55) and the Structured Clinical Interview for DSM-IV (SCID) (56) are two of the psychological tests recommended for diagnostic or subgrouping purposes (11). Instruments, such as the SF-36 (44) and the Sickness Impact Profile (SIP) (57), are recommended to assess functional status (11). For research purposes, subgrouping patients with CFS may also be based on factors such as gradual or sudden "flulike" illness onset, fatigue severity ratings, or functional status, which may help in ascertaining disease etiology (11).

Afari and Buchwald (58) also describe several overlapping conditions such as fibromyalgia, multiple chemical sensitivities, irritable bowel syndrome and tempromandibular joint disorders. Fibromyalgia syndrome is characterized by tender points and chronic, diffuse pain (59). Several authors report the relationship of CFS and fibromyalgia, with estimates of 20%–70% of patients having overlying symptoms (60–62).

PHYSICAL EXAMINATION

A crucial part of the evaluation of a patient with CFS is the medical and psychosocial history, given the chronicity of the illness. Qualitative research indicates problematic relationships between patients with CFS and healthcare practitioners, where patients often report feeling unaccepted, marginalized, and not prioritized (23). Doctors and healthcare practitioners also feel helpless and skeptical when dealing with this syndrome owing to its uncertain etiology (23). Thus, it is the professional's responsibility to acknowledge the patient's subjective experiences, despite the lack of objective signs (63).

When beginning the physical examination, the professional must realize that the clinical presentation of fatigue is the hallmark of CFS. Defining symptoms and ruling out medical conditions play such major roles in diagnosing this illness that physical examinations of the patient are often uneventful. Several scales have been adopted to measure fatigue. These include the Chalder Fatigue Scale (64) or the Krupp Fatigue Severity Scale (16). Along with severe fatigue, the patient with CFS may express any number of symptoms. The most frequent complaints cited from the symptoms listed in the case definition, secondary to fatigue, are sleep disturbances, impaired memory or concentration, and postexertional fatigue (38). Sleep disturbances can be measured using instruments such as the Pittsburgh Sleep Quality Index (65) or the Sleep Assessment Questionnaire (66). Psychological testing can be done using the CIDI, whereas neurocognitive function can be measured with instruments such as the Cambridge Neuropsychological Test Automated Battery (12,67). It is important to document postexertional fatigue. Many patients report excellent preillness fitness and energy (26) before an abrupt onset of fatigue after a flulike illness (27,30). Following the flulike illness, minimal physical exertion appears to be required to exacerbate fatigue. Recording those activities that tend to worsen fatigue, identifying other symptoms, noting how long they persist and what resolves these symptoms is key. Attention should also be given to whether a stressful event has recently occurred because this may have an impact on symptoms. Many individuals complain of frequent fevers; however, an increase in body temperature greater than 100.4°F may be a sign of acute infection. In these cases, the recommendation is to limit physical activity and prescribe rest until the infection is treated and the fever is resolved (68).

Many of these chronically ill patients are extremely inactive and tend to rest for long periods of time. This inactivity can result in extreme muscle weakness, muscle wasting, orthostatic intolerance, and loss of balance. It is suggested that the patient with CFS should be tested for these conditions and perhaps be prescribed physical rehabilitation (68). Significant functional limitations exist, depending on illness severity. Several scales measure functional limitations. The Medical Outcomes Short Form-36 measures the effect of symptoms experienced by persons on their health perception (44). The Sickness Impact Profile questionnaire measures disability in different areas of functioning such as home management, leisure activities, and sleep (57). Objective information can be obtained utilizing diaries where patients record their physical activity and by monitoring individuals using an activity monitor (actigraphy) (47).

The Chronic Fatigue Syndrome/Myalgic Encephalomyelitis (CFS/ME) working group from London (69) proposed a four-stage functional classification system that ranges from mild to very severe. A mild rating denotes a person who is mobile and able to carry out basic daily activities. A moderate rating identifies a person with reduced mobility and a limited ability to carry out activities of every day life. A severe rating describes the patient who uses a wheelchair and is restricted to very simple activities such as face washing. Very severe, on this scale, describes the patient who is bedridden and unable to care for self in any way. Incidentally, the individuals rated as severe are unable to participate in research activities or even seek clinical care. Many patients with CFS have become unemployed and have withdrawn socially, thus it is important to identify realistic vocational goals and socialization activities, which should become an early part of the recovery prescription.

PHARMACOLOGY

No universal pharmacologic regimen is prescribed or recommended for CFS. However, patients with CFS use various over-the-counter and prescribed drugs to help relieve specific symptoms. Many pharmacologic therapies that are based on the different theories of the etiology of CFS have been investigated, but the results have been inconclusive or have shown no significant effect (70). These include antidepressants (e.g., fluoxetine and pheneizine), corticosteroids (e.g., hydrocortisone and fludrocortisones), immunologic therapy (e.g., intravenous immunoglobulin G and interferon-alpha), and nutritional supplements (e.g., ginseng and essential fatty acids) (70).

When compared with nonfatigued controls, patients with CFS take a significantly larger amount of pain relievers, supplements and vitamins, hormones, antidepressants, gastrointestinal agents, central nervous system drugs, and benzodiazepines (71). The CDC recommends the use of as few drugs as possible, careful monitoring of drug side effects, and individualization of pharmacologic therapy. Furthermore, because many patients with CFS are very sensitive to medications, especially to those that affect the central nervous system, medication regimens should begin by using below standard doses and be titrated up to an effective level (72).

Over-the-counter drugs, such as antihistamines or sleep products, can be used to treat sleep disturbances after nonpharmacologic therapies have failed. If these do not help, sleep-initiating and sleep-sustaining drugs may be prescribed. Pain drug therapy can range from analgesics, aspirin, or nonsteroidal anti-inflammatory drugs to narcotics, depending on specific patient complaints. Because depression is a common comorbid condition in CFS, various antidepressant drugs may be prescribed. Stimulants may also be prescribed for cognitive problems in some patients with CFS (72).

Because of the heterogeneity of CFS complaints and that pharmacologic treatment of CFS is based on relieving specific symptoms expressed by the patient, a thorough medication list should be obtained before exercise testing or prescription. In most cases, the dose of antidepressants prescribed for patients with CFS is small and may have no effect on exercise performance. In therapeutic doses, however, some antidepressants, especially tricyclic antidepressants, can increase heart rate, decrease blood pressure, and cause electrocardiographic (ECG) changes (52). Most patients with CFS with suspected or demonstrated orthostatic intolerance are prescribed fludrocortisone or increased salt intake for treatment. A smaller number of these patients, however, may be given β-blockers that can affect exercise by decreasing heart rate and blood pressure, reducing exercise capacity in patients without angina (52).

MEDICAL AND SURGICAL TREATMENTS

No medical treatments for CFS have been found to be universally effective, and no therapy can be endorsed on the basis of sound clinical research. Many pharmacologic, immunologic, and nutritional therapies have been studied, but have demonstrated limited results. Also, survey data indicate that a significant number of patients with CFS turn to complementary and alternative medical therapy, such as massage therapy, homeopathic remedies, and osteopathy (73). However, these therapies have been shown to be of little or no benefit in the treatment of CFS (70). Other treatments investigated have included prolonged rest, cognitive behavioral therapy, and graded exercise training. Prolonged rest has not been shown to be an effective treatment. Some evidence suggests that prolonged rest after a viral infection may perpetuate or worsen fatigue and CFS symptoms (74).

The CDC recommends that treatment of CFS should be directed toward relief of the most disabling symptoms after the possible underlying causes of these symptoms have been ruled out. For example, with unrefreshing sleep they recommend good sleep hygiene techniques as the initial treatment strategy. The use of drug therapy is only suggested if the implementation of good sleep hygiene techniques does not alleviate the sleep problems. When cognitive problems are present, the CDC suggests encouraging activities that stimulate the mind, such as puzzles and games. Other symptoms commonly treated include pain, depression, and orthostatic instability (72).

The CDC also suggests counseling to assist with anxiety and other psychosocial factors. Cognitive behavioral therapy can help individuals manage their condition and form effective coping mechanisms. Nutritional guidance can be important, not only to assure that patients are getting a well balanced diet, but also to make sure they are not using supplements that can worsen symptoms or adversely interact with other medications. Exercise therapy and guidance is recommended to prevent too little or too much physical activity, both of which can exacerbate fatigue (72).

CLINICAL EXERCISE PHYSIOLOGY

PHYSIOLOGIC RESPONSES TO ACTIVITY AND EXERCISE

A number of studies have investigated the aerobic capacity and cardiopulmonary functioning of patients with CFS during a graded exercise test to exhaustion. Most have found patients with CFS to have low normal [overdotV]O_2 peak values with comparatively normal cardiopulmonary responses (75–77). Mullis et al. (78) found, however, that the patients with CFS they tested only achieved 77% of age-related predicted maximal heart rate. On close inspection, the data do not seem to indicate heart chronotropic problems in patients with CFS as much as they indicate an early voluntary termination of the maximal test, because the average respiratory exchange ratio was only 0.95, with no one achieving greater than 0.97 (78). Other researchers have found significantly reduced aerobic power in patients with CFS when compared with controls, which they have attributed to low maximal heart rates (79). In contrast, other researchers found that during an incremental exercise test to exhaustion, 80% of patients with CFS achieved higher than 90% of age-related predicted maximal heart rate with no evidence of an abnormal heart rate to [overdotV]O_2 relationship in these patients (80).

Some of the variability in these data may be explained by different testing methods, the inclusion of both men and women in some of the comparison groups, or control groups not being properly matched to CFS according to activity levels. Additionally, the heterogeneity of symptoms found within the CFS patient population may be a confounding factor. Vanness et al. (81) found that stratifying patients with CFS according to aerobic capacity may help in the interpretation of responses to exercise. Furthermore, Cook et al. (75) found that patients with CFS who had concurrent symptoms of fibromyalgia had significantly lower aerobic capacity and different physiologic responses during the test when compared with controls. These differences were not seen when comparing patients with only CFS symptoms with control participants (75).

Many studies of aerobic capacity report a significantly higher rating of perceived exertion (RPE) at every workload by patients with CFS when compared with healthy controls (82,83). The conclusion is that the limiting factors in the exercise capacity of patients with CFS may be central in origin as opposed to peripheral. Reported, however, is that when an RPE at a relative percentage of peak oxygen uptake is compared, patients with CFS and sedentary healthy controls do not indicate a difference in perception of effort (77,84).

Limitations in muscle strength and endurance for patients with CFS were not observed in earlier studies (85,86). In contrast, using twitch interpolated voluntary isometric contractions investigators found that patients with CFS had significantly weaker quadriceps muscle when compared with controls. These differences were attributed to deconditioning (87).

Some studies have reported limitations in muscle endurance (88); however, many of these studies did not normalize exercise levels to maximal strength. Kent-Braun et al. (89) found increased fatigue in muscles with superimposed electrical twitches and explained this phenomenon as a drop in neural activation rather than a change in muscle function. Magnetic resonance spectroscopy (MRS) studies suggest that a subpopulation of patients with CFS have muscle metabolic abnormalities, such as abnormally high or low adenosine diphosphate (ADP) levels during steady exercise, which represents the degree of mitochondrial activation (90). Additional MRS studies have shown that some patients with CFS have abnormal phosphocreatine (PCr) recovery rates after exercise, which are related to increased muscle acidification (91). One study utilizing both MRS and near-infrared spectroscopy revealed a reduced muscle oxygen delivery capacity in patients with CFS (92). In a follow-up investigation, which added Doppler ultrasound measurements, the data showed evidence of decreased control of muscle blood flow but no deficiencies in muscle metabolism (93). The lack of blood flow control could be a result of decreased autonomic function; however, many of these abnormalities have been associated with deconditioning in healthy volunteers, which suggests that many of the deficiencies seen in the muscle functioning of patients with CFS could be the result of deconditioning.

Much of the earlier data indicated that the occurrence of muscle pathology is rare (94) and, therefore, was thought not to play a significant role in CFS. More recent reports indicate, however, that DNA damage, lipid oxidative damage, and increased activity of the antioxidant enzymes have been seen in the muscles of patients with CFS (95,96). Additionally, these same researchers presented evidence that the fluidity of the muscle membrane is adversely affected by CFS. These data suggest that oxidative damage may be a potential organic origin of CFS (95,96).

During a 12-week graded aerobic exercise program which increased gradually until patients were working for 30 minutes per day at 60% $\dot{V}O_2$max 5 days per week, self-reported symptoms of fatigue and functional well-being scores improved in persons with CFS (97). At least two additional studies have indicated beneficial effects of graded aerobic training on CFS symptoms and work capacity (98,99). Furthermore, graded exercise training was not associated with a worsening of CFS symptoms (98).

SUPERVISION AND MONITORING

A heart rate monitor allows for independent monitoring of the prescribed target heart rate range during exercise sessions. Also, it is important to monitor heart rate during recovery from exercise. The typical response of a slow return to resting heart rate owing to deconditioning is not always the case. Some individuals with CFS demonstrate an abnormally rapid decline in heart rate during the postexercise period and should be instructed to continue low-level exercise to lower the heart rate more gradually. Blood pressure monitoring can be used for those individuals who demonstrate postural hypotension. In this case, blood pressure monitoring provides the practitioner and the patient with feedback about those postures producing undesirable responses. For example, exercises may have to be done supine, progressing to semireclining, sitting, standing, and finally walking while monitoring blood pressure. Blood pressure responses help to determine whether or not exercises can be progressed or if the patient needs to return to a reclined position.

Early on during exercise intervention, monitoring should occur every other day or twice a week, but as patients begin to learn the management of their symptoms, exercise supervision may be more protracted. If individuals with CFS demonstrate serious cognitive difficulties, more frequent supervision may be needed to correct exercise errors. Providing written and pictorial exercise reminders is extremely important in these situations.

EXERCISE/FITNESS/ FUNCTIONAL TESTING

As a group, patients with CFS tolerate standard cardiopulmonary and strength testing fairly well and without signs of muscle damage (91), compromised immune system (86), or severe signs of a worsened disease state (78). Patient complaints of fatigue are increased for several days after testing (77), however, and there are some signs of decreased cognitive abilities. It is recommended that patients adjust their daily affairs so that they do very little physical activity before testing and have time to rest afterward. Also, it would be helpful for a patient to be accompanied by someone to provide assistance after the exercise testing.

Because of the heterogeneity of symptoms, the variety of prescribed medications, and the fluctuation of illness severity, the history and physical examination before testing are very important. Cardiopulmonary testing with metabolic measurements is often used to help rule out known causes of the fatigue. However, one should not assume that heart disease has been specifically ruled out, and the *American College of Sports Medicine (ACSM) Guidelines for Exercise Testing and Prescription* (52) should be applied. Despite that many physicians doubt the existence of chronic fatigue as a distinct illness and that the syndrome's etiology is unknown, these patients are ill and do present symptoms. Medical clearance and clinical exercise tests are recommended for these individuals before they participate in an exercise program.

Standard protocols may be utilized when measuring aerobic power on either a cycle ergometer or a treadmill. Workload increments are typically 20–25 W or 1–2 metabolic equivalents (METS). A ramping protocol may be appropriate. Interpretation of gas exchange data and measurement of aerobic power can reveal signs of possible underlying vascular, metabolic, or muscle disease. Additional specialized diagnostic testing may then be recommended. Because one of the primary goals of an exercise program used in the treatment of CFS would be to increase the patient's functional capacity, tests of daily activities, such as the continuous-scale physical functional performance test (100), could be used to evaluate a patient's progress. Also, questionnaires, such as the SF-36 (44), can be used to evaluate the subjective effects of the prescribed exercise program. Reeves et al. (12) have suggested several valid instruments that can be used to evaluate such variables as fatigue, accompanying symptoms of the illness, functional capacity, and activity levels in patients with CFS.

EXERCISE PRESCRIPTION AND PROGRAMMING

Various treatments for CFS have been subjected to randomized, controlled trials. To date only two classifications of treatments, cognitive behavioral therapy or graded exercise therapy, have been scientifically proved to benefit people with CFS (101,102). Both interventions address a paced approach so that the patient may acquire control over their symptoms. Cognitive behavioral therapy addresses the fatigue-related cognitions, along with a gradual increase in physical activity, and the graded exercise therapy exposes the patient to individually adjusted structured exercise (43,97,99). When patients experience exercise that is too strenuous, compliance falls; therefore, a graded approach appears to be most beneficial. One recent research clinical trial found that a graded exercise program improved measures of fatigue, physical functioning, and depression compared with relaxation and flexibility (98). It is important to note that follow-up studies reveal that the improvements seen with cognitive behavioral therapy appear to be sustained at least 8 months after the intervention (103).

MULTIDISCIPLINARY TREATMENT INTERVENTION

The management strategy for individuals with CFS should be individualized. The first principle that must be applied to most patients with CFS is that exercise training must be very light to light and progress extremely gradually. Probably the greatest error that occurs when providing an exercise regimen for individuals with CFS is to approach the exercise regimen as if it is a case of simple deconditioning. This conclusion leads to the erroneous approach that a standard strengthening and conditioning program will return the patient to healthy functioning. This is most definitely not the case.

Individuals with the diagnosis of CFS have been chronically ill for at least 6 months and often longer. They have most likely attempted to return to their previous level of exercise either on their own or with assistance from healthcare professionals or personal trainers. These efforts have often met with little success and sometimes with detrimental results. The term "kinesophobia" or fear of movement has been described in a group of Dutch patients with CFS (104). This study utilized kinesophobia and activity questionnaires and maximal graded exercise testing. A significant association was seen between kinesophobia and decreased activity but not with maximal exercise capacity. Therefore, the possible negative effects associated with approaching patients with CFS with a standard strengthening and reconditioning program include an exacerbation of flulike symptoms, severe fatigue for days to weeks, and cognitive dysfunction, leading to a fear of movement or exercise.

This is not to imply that exercise of any form is unbeneficial to the patient with CFS. Fulcher and White (97) evaluated aerobic exercise versus flexibility and relaxation exercise. Nearly twice as many patients reported feeling better as a result of the aerobic exercise than from the flexibility and relaxation exercises. These authors acknowledge the benefits of graded aerobic exercise in the management of CFS. Gradual and careful pacing of an exercise program can be a key to its success. Wallman et al. (98) suggest that patients with CFS reduce exercise on days that symptoms are worse and not increase exercise beyond the prescribed amount on their good days which could make them more susceptible to relapse. It is important to recognize that CFS is a multifactorial illness, and consequently, the treatment intervention should be multidisciplinary. Patients with CFS may have anxiety or affective disorders, sleep disorders, pharmacologic management requirements, difficulties in pacing activity, and family difficulties as a result of the illness. Therefore, exercise alone will not usually help the patient manage the overall illness. Communication with other professionals, such as psychologists, physical and occupational therapists, vocational counselors, and physicians, is essential. Marlin et al. (105) reported that a significant number of patients returned to work or functioned at a level equivalent to gainful employment when a multidisciplinary intervention was applied. This intervention entailed optimal medical management; pharmacologic treatment of the affective, anxiety, or sleep disorder; activity management; and "coping" techniques.

PROGRAM GUIDELINES AND INITIAL EXERCISE PRESCRIPTION

Establishing Goals

Goals should be patient-focused in the areas of self-care, whether it is in-house or not; productivity for either school or work, and leisure activity. Basic self-care goals might include activities of daily living (e.g., morning hygiene, walking within the house, and meal preparation). Intermediate self-care goals might include activities such as stair climbing, walking longer distances, and activities that involve leaving the home environment. It is advisable for the patient to make a regular weekly commitment to exercise as soon as possible. This might include social activity, such as visiting a friend; educational activity, such as attending a lecture; or other leisure activities that demand only a very low intensity of physical activity. To avoid a relapse, care should be taken when attempting to integrate more intense leisure activity, such as golfing or dancing with the exercise program.

Breathing and Relaxation Exercises

Patients with CFS often have an apical breathing pattern and are susceptible to hyperventilation (94,106). Therefore, proper diaphragmatic breathing exercises, coupled with relaxation techniques, may help to reduce these problems. Some individuals with CFS also have a concomitant history of panic attacks. Teaching proper breathing and relaxation exercises is extremely successful in reducing panic attacks and giving the individual a sense of control over his or her condition. Breathing and relaxation exercises are recommended during any time of stress, even during challenging exercises. In particular, these exercises should be recommended at night to promote sleep.

Stretching and Flexibility Exercises

Individuals with CFS are typically sedentary and often experience significant muscle aches and pains lasting several months to years. Posture is usually faulty and cannot be corrected without incorporating a stretching routine into their daily activity. Stretching exercises should focus on the anterior chest wall and neck region. Gentle stretching of the anterior and posterior neck region can provide great relief for common headache complaints. Stretching exercises should be done daily. Stretching performed on waking allows for an improved sense of mobility and vitality when the day begins.

Strengthening Exercises

During the initial stages, strengthening exercises should address active motion with gravity-only resistance. When adding weight training to the exercise routine, exercises should first focus on trunk stability, followed by extremity-strengthening exercises. It is recommended that weight be added only when the individual can perform three sets of 15 repetitions. Sometimes, individuals fatigue and relapse if the entire exercise routine is done in one bout, in which case they should be encouraged to split the tasks between the morning and afternoon. Depending on the patient's response to exercise, it is recommended to alternate days of strengthening with submaximal aerobic exercise. Particular attention should be paid to pacing with the patient, first beginning with just a couple of exercises which are added every week or two as they adapt (98,107). Again it is recommended (98) that on days when symptoms are worse, reduce the workout, and on days when symptoms are less do not do any more than the prescribed program to avoid relapse.

Submaximal Aerobic Exercise

Aerobic exercises should begin at a low level and increase in duration before increasing the intensity. The decision to increase exercise intensity or duration is often based on the individual's current level of activity. For example, if an individual is bedridden or extremely sedentary, walking on a treadmill may, at the start, be limited to 1 minute or less. Conversely, if daily activities are more frequent, treadmill walking may initially be prescribed for 5 or 10 minutes. It is important for individuals to monitor their heart rate and stay within the prescribed range. If individuals are extremely ill and fatigued most of the time, working at 50% of the age-predicted maximal heart rate is not unreasonable. Exercise intensity is usually increased to 55%, 60%, and 65% of maximal heart rate. Higher-functioning patients may be able to progress to 70%–85% of maximal heart rate. A rating of perceived exertion scale where patients should keep their intensity at a level they feel is very light to moderate can be useful (107). Patients should be reminded to breathe properly during all exercises. They should also be advised to avoid exercise if other significant duties are to be conducted that day.

Exercise Progression

Once an initial level of exercise intensity is determined to be tolerated, better results are more often achieved if there is no additional increase in intensity within a 1-week period. This time allows for an adjustment period during which unexpected exacerbations of the patient's condition may occur. If this does occur, a decrease of exercise intensity is recommended. If an exercise program is progressed every session, it becomes unclear whether it was the exercise intensity that was too extreme for the patient or whether the exacerbation was caused by the cumulative effect of the exercise program. During this initial period, it is important to point out to patients that their other daily activities should not be significantly altered. Altering several activities simultaneously makes it difficult to determine the impact of the increased intensity of the exercise regimen apart from that of an increase in home or social activity. After submaximal aerobic exercise reaches 30 minutes, patients are usually ready for an increase in exercise intensity. Again, the use of ratings of perceived exertion can be important indicators of how well patients are coping with the current protocol and when they are ready to progress the exercise intensity (107). Initially, supervised exercise is best administered approximately twice per week. Clapp et al. (108) determined that approximately 15 minutes of discontinuous low level treadmill exercise was the upper limit before patients with CFS indicated a significant increase in their acute fatigue level. Their data also indicated, however, that these patients could complete a 30-minute aerobic exercise session, where the protocol was 10 minutes of exercise followed by 3 minutes of rest, and their CFS symptoms were not exacerbated immediately following or up to 7 days after exercise. This allows for exercise adaptation to the volume of work.

EXERCISE CONSIDERATIONS AND SYMPTOM RELAPSE

Patients with CFS must understand that they will continue to have periods of worsening symptoms, but should be informed that with graded exercise, which includes pacing techniques, as well as energy-conservation techniques, these symptoms should occur less frequently and be less severe. Smith (109) described the course of recovery for patients with CFS: The symptom severity decreases and periods of symptom exacerbation become more predictable. This information provides a psychological benefit to the patient by demonstrating the practitioner's understanding of the recovery trajectory and increasing the patient's hope of eventual recovery to an improved state. It is very important that patients with CFS learn how to manage their activity during a period of relapse, recognizing that rest is needed and excess mental or physical exertion can cause further deterioration. Some simple exercises can be performed based on the individual's symptoms. These can include breathing, relaxation, and stretching exercises. If symptoms are worsening, simple strengthening exercises that the patient is already familiar with should be done but with less intensity, frequency, or duration than usual.

STRATEGIES FOR PROMOTING ADHERENCE

Patient education about the need to interrupt the continuous downward cycle of inactivity, relapse, rest, and deconditioning is usually sufficient to promote exercise adherence, provided the patient is given a manageable program that does not result in frequent relapses. Most patients with CFS want to feel better and welcome guidance on how to enhance recovery. It is important for the patient to learn self-management of symptoms to avoid frustration. For example, if severe headaches limit activity, teaching relaxation, breathing, and neck-stretching exercises to reduce pain will lead to a sense of control over the illness. This improvement in control reinforces the use of treatments prescribed, and patients are often quite willing to proceed with exercise maintenance and progression. It is advisable to remind patients that as they begin to feel better, it is common to overdo other activities, because they may not be viewed as exercise. In fact, all daily activities must be taken into account when determining how strenuous the exercise should be. When daily activities are significant, exercise might be skipped altogether for that day. Patients should be encouraged to take control of their activity planning and be given permission for lapses in their planned exercise regimen owing to other required activities or responsibilities.

PRECAUTIONS

Patients with CFS often report a relapse of severe symptoms following acute and even mild exercise for hours (82,110) to days (47,77). Furthermore, there appears to be no clear warning of the point at which too much exercise will trigger a relapse (106). In other words, by the time the individual reports that he or she feels tired enough to stop exercising, it is likely to be too late to avoid exacerbation of symptoms. Using only the patient's response as an end limit to exercise bouts is likely to prove unsuccessful. Setting exercise intensity thresholds using a rating of perceived exertion scale can serve as a safety mechanism to prevent over-exertion (107). Therefore, a structured mild and gradually progressed exercise regimen usually helps to avoid most severe relapsing.

EDUCATION AND COUNSELING

Patients with CFS should be instructed about fitness as a lifetime goal as well as the detrimental effects of deconditioning, and informed that increases in the fitness regimen should be taken on gradually. Patients should stay on track and avoid the tendency to overdo the workout because of the immediate sense of well-being. This is a common problem that results in significant frustration. Patients should be instructed not to increase the intensity and duration of fitness exercises more than once a week. To avoid relapse in very patients with severe CFS, sometimes a 2-week period of exercise adaptation is needed. Also, the frequency of exercise should always allow for a rest day in between sessions. For example, an individual could begin an independent outdoor exercise program by walking one block every other day and monitoring the time needed to complete the walk. This walking may be increased to include longer distances and consequently requiring a longer time to complete. Generally, when 30 minutes of continuous exercise is achieved, then patients can be instructed to modify their walking pace to a faster speed, thereby covering a greater distance in the same amount of time. Patients should be instructed to increase their program as tolerated, but energy should be saved for leisure, social, and work activities.

Patients should be counseled to self-manage symptoms while continually but gradually raising the level of exercise intensity. These management instructions can be in the form of home exercise programs. The home exercise program should include relaxation, stretching, strengthening, and aerobic exercises. When designing these exercise programs for the home, it is important to keep the directions simple and concise, while graphics should be used to demonstrate stretching and exercise techniques.

Patients with CFS may experience barriers to exercise. Sometimes, these individuals may demonstrate avoidance of exercise because of somatic complaint (111). This is often learned behavior resulting from those times when exercise attempts have failed and serious exacerbation has occurred. Cognitive limitations may also preclude patients with CFS from completing

tasks according to the exercise guidelines recommended. For example, individuals may not comply owing to their inability to recall and follow instructions. When patients are limited by serious exacerbation, they should be encouraged to rest and be reminded that in time, the exacerbation will become less severe and shorter in duration. Many patients also require a significant number of medical visits that consumes their energy and may result in an inability to comply with an exercise regimen. Patients should be reminded to set aside a few minutes for gentle exercises on these days to avoid getting out of the habit of regular exercise.

Finally, patients with CFS must advocate for themselves. As a group they are, and should continue to be, well-informed and generally have a strong community network. Self-help and support groups can provide patients with information and a sense of community. Care should be taken to be sure that the information obtained from these sources is consistent with evidence-based medicine (112). Patient advocacy groups also promote research on CFS as well as addressing the social and medical and treatment implications of labeling CFS as a medical or psychiatric disorder.

CASE STUDIES

The examples illustrate the management of a severe and a moderate-to-mild case of CFS. The cases do not represent the only mechanism for management of CFS but are an attempt to illustrate the complexity and uniqueness of exercise prescription.

CASE 1

A 35-year-old woman complains of severe fatigue for 2 years. The onset occurred after she had suffered a week-long bout with the flu. The fatigue from the flu only partially subsided. Fatigue and cognitive problems are her primary complaints. She reports a history of seeing a variety of doctors and psychologists who were unable to make an affirmative diagnosis until 6 months ago, when she received the diagnosis of chronic fatigue syndrome by an immunologist.

Since her initial illness, she has become extremely weak and unable to sustain everyday activities for longer than 15 minutes at a time, less if there is a significant cognitive demand. Her strength tests are within the normal range; however, she complains of a lack of vigor and inability to complete more than one repetition of antigravity limb exercises. She complains that her greatest difficulty is carrying heavy objects, especially up a flight of stairs.

She is able to walk within her house for short intervals and avoids out-of-house activities altogether. She

requires the assistance of friends and relatives to do her shopping and errands. She has become depressed because of an inability to participate in even minimal activities socially.

Before her illness, she was a competitive jogger, and she has attempted exercising on her own several times since. Each time she exerted herself even at a minimal intensity, she would suffer from worsening fatigue a day or two later. This was true although she did not experience any deleterious effects during the exercise. This exacerbation of fatigue would often last several days, during which most of the time was spent in bed. Because of her long bouts of rest during the day, her dietary and hydration habits were poor. Medications caused significant weight gain and resulted in dry mouth and eyes.

S: Easy fatigability with minimal exertion

O: Range of motion and strength when tested statically were within normal limits. Unable to repeat antigravity limb exercises more than once. Heart rate was 80 bpm at rest and increased to 100 during standing activities. Able to walk on a treadmill at 1 mph for 5 minutes, however, this resulted in worsening fatigue reported at the next visit. Peak $\dot{V}O_2$ is 20 mL/kg/min. Blood pressure was 120/80 mm Hg in sitting and lying but dropped to 100/60 initially on standing. Medications include Florinef to improve postural hypotension and Paxil to reduce anxiety. Occasionally, Halcyon was taken at bedtime if sleep was difficult.

A: Low endurance and conditioning; hypotension upon standing

P: 1. Gentle antigravity exercise strengthening and conditioning

2. Gentle aerobic conditioning

EXERCISE PROGRAM

Goal: Increase antigravity exercise endurance repetitions for trunk and limbs.

Mode: Antigravity exercise without weights, treadmill, and sitting or supine cycle ergometry; calf strengthening, and/or elastic stockings to promote venous return during standing activities; may have to exercise initially in sitting or lying.

Intensity: Active exercise without weights with arms, legs, and trunk to tolerance to establish initial repetition level (i.e., 3–5 repetitions for each muscle group; treadmill at 0.5 to 1 mph or leg cycle ergometry at 20 to 25 W).

Frequency: Every other day; reevaluate weekly to determine if repetitions should be decreased or increased.

Duration: 10–20 minutes of active exercise; 5 minutes on treadmill or cycle ergometry on alternate days from active exercise days, monitoring exercise and recovery heart rate.

Time course of supervised exercise: 3 months

Note: Exercise intensity should be evaluated weekly to determine any exacerbation of symptoms of fatigue or flulike symptoms. If symptoms are present, intensity should be reduced or exercise bouts should be more spaced. With no symptoms, exercise intensity should be increased slightly and reevaluated again each week.

CASE 2

A 30-year-old woman complains of severe fatigue for 2 years. The onset was after suffering a week-long bout with the flu. The fatigue from the flu only partially subsided. Her primary complaints are fatigue and cognitive problems. She claims that she has seen a variety of doctors who were unable to make an affirmative diagnosis until 6 months ago when she received the diagnosis of chronic fatigue syndrome by a neurologist. She was previously a regular exerciser and jogged three times per week to total approximately 15 miles per week.

She is able to work her full-time job, but when she comes home and on weekends, she is unable to do anything but sleep until the next morning. Her strength tests are within the normal range; however, she complains of lack of vigor and inability to concentrate on mental tasks during complex multisequencing tasks. She complains of

difficulty carrying heavy objects. She requires the assistance of friends and relatives to do her shopping and errands. She has become depressed owing to inability to participate in even minimal activities socially outside of work.

She has attempted exercising on her own several times since, before her illness, she was a competitive jogger. Each time she exerted herself at what she considered a minimal amount, she would still suffer from worsening fatigue a day or two later, although she did not experience any deleterious effects during that exercise. This exacerbation of fatigue would often last several hours.

S: Easy fatigability with minimal exertion

O: Range of motion and strength when tested statically were within normal limits. She was unable to repeat antigravity limb exercises more than 10 times. Heart rate was 70 bpm at rest, and she was able to walk on a treadmill at 2.5 mph for 15 minutes; however, this resulted in worsening fatigue reported at the next visit. Her peak $\dot{V}O_2$ is 33 mL/kg/min. Blood pressure was 120/80 mm Hg in sitting and standing. Medications include Paxil to reduce anxiety and Flexeril for muscle pain.

A: Low endurance and conditioning

P: 1. Gentle strengthening and conditioning

2. Gentle aerobic conditioning

EXERCISE PROGRAM

Goal: Increase antigravity exercise endurance repetitions for trunk and limbs

Mode: Antigravity exercise without weights, treadmill, and sitting or supine cycle ergometry

Intensity: Active exercise without weights with arms, legs, and trunk to tolerance to establish initial repetition level (i.e., 10–15 repetitions for each muscle; treadmill or cycle ergometry at an intensity of 2.5 to 3 METS).

Frequency: Every other day; reevaluate weekly to determine if repetitions should be decreased or increased.

Duration: 20 minutes of active exercise; 5–10 minutes on treadmill or cycle ergometry on alternate days from active exercise days, monitoring exercise and recovery heart rate.

Time course of supervised exercise: 1–5 months

Note: Exercise intensity should be evaluated weekly to determine any exacerbation of symptoms of fatigue or flulike symptoms. If symptoms are present, intensity should be reduced and/or exercise bouts should be more spaced. With no symptoms, exercise intensity should be increased slightly and reevaluated again each week.

S, subjective data; O, objective data; A, assessment; P, plan of action.

REFERENCES

1. DuBois RE, Seeley JK, Brus I, et al. Chronic mononucleosis syndrome. *South Med J* 1984;77(11):1376–82.

2. Jones JF, Ray CG, Minnich LL, et al. Evidence for active Epstein-Barr virus infection in patients with persistent, unexplained illnesses: Elevated anti-early antigen antibodies. *Ann Intern Med* 1985;102(1):1–7.

3. Straus SE, Tosato G, Armstrong G, et al. Persisting illness and fatigue in adults with evidence of Epstein-Barr virus infection. *Ann Intern Med* 1985;102(1):7–16.

4. Tobi M, Morag A, Ravid Z, et al. Prolonged atypical illness associated with serological evidence of persistent Epstein-Barr virus infection. *Lancet* 1982;1(8263):61–4.

5. Buchwald D, Sullivan JL, Komaroff AL. Frequency of 'chronic active Epstein-Barr virus infection' in a general medical practice. *JAMA* 1987;257(17):2303–7.

6. Holmes GP, Kaplan JE, Stewart JA, et al. A cluster of patients with a chronic mononucleosis-like syndrome. Is Epstein-Barr virus the cause? *JAMA* 1987;257(17): 2297–302.

7. Holmes GP, Kaplan JE, Gantz NM, et al. Chronic fatigue syndrome: A working case definition. *Ann Intern Med* 1988;108(3): 387–9.

8. Lloyd AR, Hickie I, Boughton CR, et al. Prevalence of chronic fatigue syndrome in an Australian population. *Med J Aust* 1990; 153(9):522–8.

9. Sharpe MC, Archard LC, Banatvala JE, et al. A report—Chronic fatigue syndrome: Guidelines for research. *J R Soc Med* 1991;84(2): 118–21.

10. Schluederberg A, Straus SE, Peterson P, et al. NIH conference. Chronic fatigue syndrome research. Definition and medical outcome assessment. *Ann Intern Med* 1992;117(4):325–31.

11. Fukuda K, Straus SE, Hickie I, et al. The chronic fatigue syndrome: A comprehensive approach to its definition and study. International Chronic Fatigue Syndrome Study Group. *Ann Intern Med* 1994;121(12):953–9.

12. Reeves WC, Lloyd A, Vernon SD, et al. International Chronic Fatigue Syndrome Study Group: Identification of ambiguities in the 1994 chronic fatigue syndrome research case definition and recommendations for resolution. *BMC Health Serv Res* [Internet]. 2003 [cited 2003 Dec 31]; 3(1):25. Available from: http://www.biomedcentral.com/1472-6963/3/25

13. Ablashi DV, Eastman HB, Owen CB, et al. Frequent HHV-6 reactivation in multiple sclerosis (MS) and chronic fatigue syndrome (CFS) patients. *J Clin Virol* 2000;16(3):179–91.

14. Koelle DM, Barcy S, Huang ML, et al. Markers of viral infection in monozygotic twins discordant for chronic fatigue syndrome. *Clin Infect Dis* 2002;35(5):518–25.

15. Hickie I, Davenport T, Wakefield D, et al. Dubbo Infection Outcomes Study Group. Post-infective and chronic fatigue syndromes precipitated by viral and non-viral pathogens: Prospective cohort study. *BMJ* 2006;333:575–80.

16. Landay AL, Jessop C, Lennette ET, et al. Chronic fatigue syndrome: Clinical condition associated with immune activation. *Lancet* 1991;338(8769):707–12.

17. Barker E, Fujimura SF, Fadem MB, et al. Immunologic abnormalities associated with chronic fatigue syndrome. *Clin Infect Dis* 1994;18(Suppl 1):S136–41.

18. Natelson BH, LaManca JJ, Denny TN, et al. Immunologic parameters in chronic fatigue syndrome, major depression, and multiple sclerosis. *Am J Med* 1998;105(3A):43S–9S.

19. Evengard B, Schacterle RS, Komaroff AL. Chronic fatigue syndrome: New insights and old ignorance. *J Intern Med* 1999;246(5): 455–69.

20. Dickinson CJ. Chronic fatigue syndrome—Aetiological aspects. *Eur J Clin Invest* 1997;27(4):257–67.

21. Lyall M, Peakman M, Wessely S. A systematic review and critical evaluation of the immunology of chronic fatigue syndrome. *J Psychosom Res* 2003;55(2):79–90.

22. Demitrack MA, Dale JK, Straus SE, et al. Evidence for impaired activation of the hypothalamic-pituitary-adrenal axis in patients with chronic fatigue syndrome. *J Clin Endocrinol Metab* 1991; 73(6):1224–34.

23. Scott LV, Teh J, Reznek R, et al. Small adrenal glands in chronic fatigue syndrome: A preliminary computer tomography study. *Psychoneuroendocrinology* 1999;24(7):759–68.

24. Hudson M, Cleare AJ. The 1microg short Synacthen test in chronic fatigue syndrome. *Clin Endocrinol* (Oxf) 1999;51(5):625–30.

25. Cleare AJ. The HPA axis and the genesis of chronic fatigue syndrome. *Trends Endocrinol Metab* 2004;15(2):55–9.

26. Natelson BH, Cohen JM, Brassloff I, et al. A controlled study of brain magnetic resonance imaging in patients with the chronic fatigue syndrome. *J Neurol Sci* 1993;120(2):213–7.

27. Costa DC, Tannock C, Brostoff J. Brainstem perfusion is impaired in chronic fatigue syndrome. *QJM* 1995;88(11):767–73.

28. Cleare AJ, Messa C, Rabiner EA, et al. Brain 5-HT1A receptor binding in chronic fatigue syndrome measured using positron emission tomography and [11C]WAY-100635. *Psychiatry* 2005;57: 239–46.

29. Boda WL, Natelson BH, Sisto SA, et al. Gait abnormalities in chronic fatigue syndrome. *J Neurol Sci* 1995;131(2):156–61.

30. Samii A, Wassermann EM, Ikoma K, et al. Decreased postexercise facilitation of motor evoked potentials in patients with chronic fatigue syndrome or depression. *Neurology* 1996;47(6):1410–4.

31. Lewis DH, Mayberg HS, Fischer ME et al. Monozygotic twins discordant for chronic fatigue syndrome: Regional cerebral blood flow SPECT. *Radiology* 2001;219:766–73.

32. Bou-Holaigah I, Rowe PC, Kan J, et al. The relationship between neurally mediated hypotension and the chronic fatigue syndrome. *JAMA* 1995;274(12):961–7.

33. LaManca JJ, Peckerman A, Walker J, et al. Cardiovascular response during head-up tilt in chronic fatigue syndrome. *Clin Physiol* 1999;19(2):111–20.

34. Rowe PC, Calkins H, DeBusk K, et al. Fludrocortisone acetate to treat neurally mediated hypotension in chronic fatigue syndrome: A randomized controlled trial. *JAMA* 2001;285(1):52–9.

35. Buchwald D. Fibromyalgia and chronic fatigue syndrome: Similarities and differences. *Rheum Dis Clin North Am* 1996;22(2): 219–43.

36. Johnson SK, DeLuca J, Natelson BH. Chronic fatigue syndrome: Reviewing the research findings. *Ann Behav Med* 1999;21(3): 258–71.

37. Reyes M, Nisenbaum R, Hoaglin DC, et al. Prevalence and incidence of chronic fatigue syndrome in Wichita, Kansas. *Arch Intern Med* 2003;163(13):1530–1536.

38. Steele L, Dobbins JG, Fukuda K, et al. The epidemiology of chronic fatigue in San Francisco. *Am J Med* 1998;105(3A): 83S–90S.

39. Jason LA, Richman JA, Rademaker AW, et al. A community-based study of chronic fatigue syndrome. *Arch Intern Med* 1999;159(18): 2129–37.

40. Reeves WC, Jones JF, Maloney E, et al. Prevalence of chronic fatigue syndrome in metropolitan, urban, and rural Georgia. *Popul Health Metr* [Internet]. 2007 [cited 2007 Jun 8];5:5. Available from: http://www.pophealthmetrics.com/content/5/1/5. Accessed June 15, 2007.

41. Wessely S. The epidemiology of chronic fatigue syndrome. *Epidemiol Rev* 1995;17(1):139–51.

42. Heim C, Wagner D, Maloney E, et al. Early adverse experience and risk for chronic fatigue syndrome: Results from a population-based study. *Arch Gen Psychiatry* 2006;63(11):1258–66.

43. Prins JB, van der Meer JW, Bleijenberg G. Chronic fatigue syndrome. *Lancet* 2006;367(9507):346–55.

44. Ware JE Jr, Sherbourne CD. The MOS 36-item short-form health survey (SF-36). I. Conceptual framework and item selection. *Med Care* 1992;30(6):473–83.

45. Buchwald D, Pearlman T, Umali J, et al. Functional status in patients with chronic fatigue syndrome, other fatiguing illnesses, and healthy individuals. *Am J Med* 1996;101(4): 364–70.

46. Solomon L, Nisenbaum R, Reyes M, et al. Functional status of persons with chronic fatigue syndrome in the Wichita, Kansas, population. *Health Qual Life Outcomes* [Internet]. 2003 [cited 2003 Oct 3];1(1):48. Available from: http:// www.hqlo.com/content/1/1/48

47. Sisto SA, Tapp WN, LaManca JJ, et al. Physical activity before and after exercise in women with chronic fatigue syndrome. *QJM* 1998; 91(7):465–73.

48. Reynolds KJ, Vernon SD, Bouchery E, et al. The economic impact of chronic fatigue syndrome. *Cost Eff Resour Alloc* [Internet]. 2004 [cited 2003 Jun 21];2(1):4. Available from http://www. resource-allocation.com/content/2/1/4

49. Jason LA, Taylor RR, Kennedy CL, et al. Chronic fatigue syndrome: Sociodemographic subtypes in a community-based sample. *Eval Health Prof* 2000;23(3):243–63.

50. Cairns R, Hotopf M. A systematic review describing the prognosis of chronic fatigue syndrome. *Occup Med* (Lond) 2005;55(1):20–31.

51. Joyce J, Hotopf M, Wessely S. The prognosis of chronic fatigue and chronic fatigue syndrome: A systematic review. *QJM* 1997;90(3): 223–33.

52. American College of Sports Medicine. *ACSM's Guidelines for Exercise Testing and Prescription*, 7th ed. Baltimore: Lippincott Williams & Wilkins; 2006.

53. Robins LN, Wing J, Wittchen HU, et al. The Composite International Diagnostic Interview. An epidemiologic Instrument suitable for use in conjunction with different diagnostic systems and in different cultures. *Arch Gen Psychiatry* 1988;45(12):1069–77.

54. Andrews G, Peters L. The psychometric properties of the Composite International Diagnostic Interview. *Soc Psychiatry Psychiatr Epidemiol* 1998;33(2):80–8.

55. Robins LN, Helzer JE, Croughan J, et al. National Institute of Mental Health Diagnostic Interview Schedule. Its history, characteristics, and validity. *Arch Gen Psychiatry* 1981;38(4):381–9.

56. Spitzer RL, Williams JB, Gibbon M, et al. The Structured Clinical Interview for DSM-III-R (SCID). I: History, rationale, and description. *Arch Gen Psychiatry* 1992;49(8):624–9.

57. Bergner M, Bobbitt RA, Carter WB, et al. The Sickness Impact Profile: Development and final revision of a health status measure. *Med Care* 1981;19(8):787–805.

58. Afari N, Buchwald D. Chronic fatigue syndrome: A review. *Am J Psychiatry* 2003;160(2):221–36.

59. Wolfe F, Smythe HA, Yunus MB, et al. The American College of Rheumatology 1990 Criteria for the Classification of Fibromyalgia. Report of the Multicenter Criteria Committee. *Arthritis Rheum* 1990;33(2):160–72.

60. Buchwald D, Garrity D. Comparison of patients with chronic fatigue syndrome, fibromyalgia, and multiple chemical sensitivities. *Arch Intern Med* 1994;154(18):2049–53.

61. Hudson JI, Goldenberg DL, Pope HG Jr, et al. Comorbidity of fibromyalgia with medical and psychiatric disorders. *Am J Med* 1992;92(4):363–7.

62. White KP, Speechley M, Harth M, et al. Co-existence of chronic fatigue syndrome with fibromyalgia syndrome in the general population. A controlled study. *Scand J Rheumatol* 2000;29(1): 44–51.

63. Wyller VB. The chronic fatigue syndrome—An update. *Acta Neurol Scand Suppl* 2007;187:7–14.

64. Mawle AC, Reyes M, Schmid DS. Is chronic fatigue syndrome an infectious disease? *Infect Agents Dis* 1993;2(5):333–41.

65. Smyth C. The Pittsburgh Sleep Quality Index (PSQI). *J Gerontol Nurs* 1999;25(12):10–1.

66. Cesta A, Moldofsky H, Sammut C: The University of Toronto Sleep Assessment Questionnaire (SAQ). *Sleep Res* 1996;25:486.

67. Sahakian BJ, Owen AM. Computerized assessment in neuropsychiatry using CANTAB: Discussion paper. *J R Soc Med* 1992;85(7): 399–402.

68. Sharpe M, Chalder T, Palmer I, et al. Chronic fatigue syndrome. A practical guide to assessment and management. *Gen Hosp Psychiatry* 1997;19(3):185–99.

69. U. K. Department of Health. *A Report of the CFS/ME Working Group: A Report to the Chief Medical Officer of an Independent Working Group*. London: Department of Health; 2002:82. Available from DH Publications Orderline, London.

70. Rimes KA, Chalder T. Treatments for chronic fatigue syndrome. *Occup Med* (Lond) 2005;55(1):32–9.

71. Jones JF, Nisenbaum R, Reeves WC. Medication use by persons with chronic fatigue syndrome: Results of a randomized telephone survey in Wichita, Kansas. *Health Qual Life Outcomes* [Internet]. 2003 [cited 2003 Dec 2];1(1):74. Available from: http://www. hqlo.com/content/1/1/74. Accessed June 14, 2007.

72. Center for Disease Control and Prevention Web site [Internet]. Atlanta (GA): Center for Disease Control and Prevention; [cited 2006 May 26]. Available from: http://www.cdc.gov/cfs/cfstreatmentHCP.htm. Accessed June 20, 2007.

73. Jones JF, Maloney EM, Boneva RS, et al. Complementary and alternative medical therapy utilization by people with chronic fatiguing illnesses in the United States. BMC Complement Altern Med [Internet]. 2007 [cited 2007 Apr 25];7:12. Available from: http://www.biomedcentral.com/1472–6882/7/12

74. Reid S, Chalder T, Cleare A, et al. Chronic fatigue syndrome. *Clinical Evidence* 2005;(14):1366–78.

75. Cook DB, Nagelkirk PR, Poluri A, et al. The influence of aerobic fitness and fibromyalgia on cardiorespiratory and perceptual responses to exercise in patients with chronic fatigue syndrome. *Arthritis Rheum* 2006;54(10):3351–62.

76. Sargent C, Scroop GC, Nemeth PM, et al. Maximal oxygen uptake and lactate metabolism are normal in chronic fatigue syndrome. *Med Sci Sports Exerc* 2002;34(1):51–6.

77. Sisto SA, LaManca J, Cordero DL, et al. Metabolic and cardiovascular effects of a progressive exercise test in patients with chronic fatigue syndrome. *Am J Med* 1996;100(6):634–40.

78. Mullis R, Campbell IT, Wearden AJ, et al. Prediction of peak oxygen uptake in chronic fatigue syndrome. *Br J Sports Med* 1999; 33(5):352–6.

79. De Becker P, Roeykens J, Reynders M, et al. Exercise capacity in chronic fatigue syndrome. *Arch Intern Med* 2000;160(21):3270–7.

80. LaManca JJ, Sisto SA, Zhou XD, et al. Immunological response in chronic fatigue syndrome following a graded exercise test to exhaustion. *J Clin Immunol* 1999;19(2):135–42.

81. Vanness JM, Snell CR, Strayer DR, et al. Subclassifying chronic fatigue syndrome through exercise testing. *Med Sci Sports Exerc* 2003;35(6):908–13.

82. Gibson H, Carroll N, Clague JE, et al. Exercise performance and fatiguability in patients with chronic fatigue syndrome. *J Neurol Neurosurg Psychiatry* 1993;56(9):993–8.

83. Riley MS, O'Brien CJ, McCluskey DR, et al. Aerobic work capacity in patients with chronic fatigue syndrome. *BMJ* 1990;301(6758):953–6.

84. Cook DB, Nagelkirk PR, Peckerman A, et al. Perceived exertion in fatiguing illness: Civilians with chronic fatigue syndrome. *Med Sci Sports Exerc* 2003;35(4):563–8.

85. Lloyd AR, Gandevia SC, Hales JP. Muscle performance, voluntary activation, twitch properties and perceived effort in normal subjects and patients with the chronic fatigue syndrome. *Brain* 1991; 114 (Pt 1A):85–98.

86. Stokes MJ, Cooper RG, Edwards RH. Normal muscle strength and fatigability in patients with effort syndromes. *BMJ* 1988;297(6655): 1014–7.

87. Fulcher KY, White PD. Strength and physiological response to exercise in patients with chronic fatigue syndrome. *J Neurol Neurosurg Psychiatry* 2000;69(3):302–7.

88. Wong R, Lopaschuk G, Zhu G, et al. Skeletal muscle metabolism in the chronic fatigue syndrome. In vivo assessment by 31P nuclear magnetic resonance spectroscopy. *Chest* 1992;102(6):1716–22.

89. Kent-Braun JA, Sharma KR, Weiner MW, et al. Central basis of muscle fatigue in chronic fatigue syndrome. *Neurology* 1993;43(1):125–31.

90. Barnes PR, Taylor DJ, Kemp GJ, et al. Skeletal muscle bioenergetics in the chronic fatigue syndrome. *J Neurol Neurosurg Psychiatry* 1993;56(6):679–83.

91. McCully KK, Natelson BH, Iotti S, et al. Reduced oxidative muscle metabolism in chronic fatigue syndrome. *Muscle Nerve* 1996;19(5):621–5.

92. McCully KK, Natelson BH. Impaired oxygen delivery to muscle in chronic fatigue syndrome. *Clin Sci (Lond)* 1999;97(5):603–8.

93. McCully KK, Smith S, Rajaei S, et al. Muscle metabolism with blood flow restriction in chronic fatigue syndrome. *J Appl Physiol* 2004;96(3):871–8.

94. Edwards RH, Gibson H, Clague JE, et al. Muscle histopathology and physiology in chronic fatigue syndrome. *Ciba Foundation Symposium* 1993;173:102–17.

95. Fulle S, Belia S, Vecchiet J, et al. Modification of the functional capacity of sarcoplasmic reticulum membranes in patients suffering from chronic fatigue syndrome. *Neuromuscul Disord* 2003;13(6): 479–84.

96. Fulle S, Mecocci P, Fano G, et al. Specific oxidative alterations in vastus lateralis muscle of patients with the diagnosis of chronic fatigue syndrome. *Free Radic Biol Med* 2000;29(12):1252–9.

97. Fulcher KY, White PD. Randomised controlled trial of graded exercise in patients with the chronic fatigue syndrome. *BMJ* 1997;314(7095):1647–52.

98. Wallman KE, Morton AR, Goodman C, et al. Randomised controlled trial of graded exercise in chronic fatigue syndrome. *Med J Aust* 2004;180(9):444–8.

99. Wearden AJ, Morriss RK, Mullis R, et al. Randomised, double-blind, placebo-controlled treatment trial of fluoxetine and graded exercise for chronic fatigue syndrome. *Br J Psychiatry* 1998;172: 485–90.

100. Cress ME, Petrella JK, Moore TL, et al. Continuous-scale physical functional performance test: Validity, reliability, and sensitivity of data for the short version. *Phys Ther* 2005;85(4): 323–35.

101. Edmonds M, McGuire H, Price J. Exercise therapy for chronic fatigue syndrome. Cochrane Database of Systematic Reviews [Internet]. 2004 [cited 2004 May 8]; 3 (CD003200). Available from: http://mrw.interscience.wiley.com/cochrane/clsysrev/articles/CD0 03200/frame.html. Accessed June 14, 2007.

102. Prins JB, Bleijenberg G, Bazelmans E, et al. Cognitive behaviour therapy for chronic fatigue syndrome: A multicentre randomised controlled trial. *Lancet* 2001;357(9259):841–7.

103. Sharpe M. Chronic fatigue syndrome. *Psychiatr Clin North Am* 1996;19(3):549–73.

104. Nijs J, De Meirleir K, Duquet W. Kinesiophobia in chronic fatigue syndrome: Assessment and associations with disability. *Arch Phys Med Rehabil* 2004;85(10):1586–92.

105. Marlin RG, Anchel H, Gibson JC, et al. An evaluation of multidisciplinary intervention for chronic fatigue syndrome with long-term follow-up, and a comparison with untreated controls. *Am J Med* 1998;105(3A):110S–4S.

106. Sisto SA. Chronic fatigue syndrome: An overview and intervention guidelines. *Neurol Rep* 1993;17:30–4.

107. Wallman Ke, Morton AR, Goodman C, et al. Exercise prescription for individuals with chronic fatigue syndrome. *Med J Aust* 2005;183(3):142–3.

108. Clapp LL, Richardson MT, Smith JF, et al. Acute effects of thirty minutes of light-intensity, intermittent exercise on patients with chronic fatigue syndrome. *Phys Ther* 1999;79(8):749–56.

109. Smith DG. The management of postviral fatigue syndrome in general practice. In: Jenkins R, Mowbray J, eds. *Postviral Fatigue Syndrome*. New York: John Wiley & Sons; 1991.

110. Komaroff AL. Clinical presentation of chronic fatigue syndrome. *Ciba Foundation Symposium* 1993;173:43–54; discussion 54–61.

111. Fischler B, Dendale P, Michiels V, et al. Physical fatigability and exercise capacity in chronic fatigue syndrome: Association with disability, somatization and psychopathology. *J Psychosom Res* 1997;42(4):369–78.

112. Kisely SR. Treatments for chronic fatigue syndrome and the Internet: A systematic survey of what your patients are reading. *Aust N Z J Psychiatry* 2002;36(2):240–5.

IRON DEFICIENCY

EPIDEMIOLOGY AND PATHOPHYSIOLOGY

At a global level, iron-deficiency anemia is the most commonly occurring nutritional deficiency. In developing countries or among high-risk groups, iron deficiency can affect 30%–40% of the population, whereas the prevalence of iron-deficiency anemia in the general community is typically 1%–3%. Recently, athletes have come under scrutiny as one such high-risk group. During the 1970s, exercise scientists commented on some interesting differences in the hematologic characteristics of long-distance runners. Endurance athletes were seen to have reduced plasma hemoglobin concentrations, a characteristic that seemed unfavorable for the performance of events reliant on the delivery of oxygen to working muscles (1). After study, this phenomenon was found to be a dilutional anemia, resulting from the increase in plasma volume that accompanies aerobic training (2). It is not considered to be a pathologic state and is not disadvantageous to performance, does not limit the production of red blood cells, and does not respond to iron-supplementation therapy (3).

THE ROLE OF IRON

About 3–5 g of iron is found in the body in three main pools: *storage iron* (ferritin and hemosiderin) found predominantly in the spleen, liver, and bone marrow; *transport iron* (transported through the plasma and extravascular fluids by the carrier, transferrin); and *oxygen-transport iron* (within the active centers of hemoglobin in the erythrocyte and myoglobin in the muscle). Most iron in the body is recycled, with iron from senecent erythrocytes being salvaged for storage or reincorporation into new reticulocytes. Iron status is a result of the balance between the small amounts of dietary iron that are absorbed each day and small iron losses from skin, sweat, and the gastrointestinal and urinary tracts. It should be noted that, apart from blood loss, no mechanism exists to remove excess iron from the body. Important functions of iron and iron-related compounds in the body are as follows:

- Transport of oxygen in the blood (hemoglobin) and muscle (myoglobin)
- As a component of enzyme systems, such as the electron transport chain, ribonucleotide reductase (required for the production of DNA), catalase, and succinate dehydrogenase
- As a catalyst in the production of free oxygen radicals

Whereas a small percentage of the population (usually male) suffers from the clinical effects of hemochromatosis, or iron-overload disease, whereby excessive amounts of iron are absorbed and deposited in major organs, the more common problem related to iron status is iron depletion. (For further reviews of iron metabolism, see references 16, 19, and 49.)

Reduction in iron stores is thought to progress through a number of stages with different functional and diagnostic criteria. These stages are summarized in Table 19.1. The end stage of iron-deficiency anemia is detected by a hemoglobin level below the reference range in association hypochromic, microcytic red cells, and iron-related parameters consistent with iron deficiency. At this stage, inadequate iron is available in the bone marrow for the normal manufacture of hemoglobin and erythrocytes. Interference with oxygen transport and enzyme function leads to clinical symptoms associated with the impairment of muscle metabolism, brain metabolism, immunity, and temperature control.

CAUSES OF IRON DEFICIENCY

Iron deficiency occurs in athletes and people who exercise for the same overall reason that it occurs in sedentary populations: iron requirements or losses exceed iron intake over a sufficient period of time. Iron requirements are increased during periods of growth, reflected by the higher recommended daily allowances for iron during adolescence and during pregnancy (Table 19.2). Iron needs are higher in females of reproductive age than in males because of the monthly menstrual blood losses (Table 19.2).

Increased iron losses can also occur through conditions or problems that cause substantial or prolonged blood loss, such as tumors, gastrointestinal ulcers, surgery, or severe bruising. Given the individual characteristics of athletes, it

TABLE 19.1. DIAGNOSTIC VALUES OF IRON-RELATED PARAMETERS FOR FOUR LEVELS OF IRON STATUS

IRON STATUS	NORMAL	STORAGE IRON DEPLETION	IRON DEFICIENT ERYTHROPIOESIS	IRON DEFICIENCY ANEMIA
Hemoglobin	Normal	Normal	Normal	Reduced
Ferritin	Normal (>22 µg/L)	<22 µg/L	<22 µg/L	<22 µg/L
sTfR	Normal (1.15–2.75 mg/L)	Normal	>2.75 mg/L	>3.6 mg/L
TfR-ferritin Index	Normal (<1.8)	>1.8	>2.2	>2.8

sTfR, soluble transferrin receptors.
Reproduced from reference 18.

is not possible to make general recommendations for iron requirements of people who exercise; however, generally, an increase occurs in iron requirements and iron turnover in those who undertake prolonged and heavy training. It is believed that iron losses are greater in athletes because of increased iron losses through sweating (4), gastrointestinal blood loss (5), and mechanical trauma to red blood cells (6). Although these losses might seem small and inconsequential, over a prolonged period they can lead to iron depletion unless a compensatory increase in iron intake occurs. Although undetected blood losses are generally the cause of iron deficiency in older populations, at a global level, inadequate intake of iron is the major cause of iron deficiency. This is probably also true in the sports world.

Iron is found in a range of plant and animal food sources, with the iron density of a mixed diet being 5–6 mg/1,000 kcal. Dietary iron is found in two forms: as *heme iron*, found only in flesh or blood containing animal foods, and *organic iron*, which is found in both animal foods and plant foods (Table 19.3). Whereas heme iron is relatively well absorbed from single foods and mixed meals (15%–35% bioavailability), the absorption of nonheme iron from single plant sources is low and variable (2%–8%) (7). The bioavailability of nonheme iron is affected by the presence of enhancing or inhibiting factors in foods eaten during the same meal. Enhancing factors include vitamin C (found in citrus, tropical, and berry fruits, and some vegetables), peptides from meat, fish, or chicken (often called the meat-enhancement factor),

alcohol, and some foods with a low pH owing to fermentation or the presence of citric or tartaric acids (3). Inhibiting factors include phytate (found in whole-grain cereals and soy protein), polyphenol (found in tea and red wine), calcium (found in milk and cheese), and peptides such as soy protein (found in plants) (3). Until recently, the absorption of heme iron was considered to be relatively unaffected by other dietary compounds; however, updated study techniques have shown that other meal components, such as calcium and plant peptides, may reduce heme iron bioavailability (8). The absorption of both heme and nonheme iron is increased as an adaptive response in people who are iron deficient or who have increased iron requirements. It should be noted that iron bioavailability studies from which these observations have been made have not been undertaken in special groups, such as athletes. However, it is generally assumed that the results can be applied across populations of healthy people.

TABLE 19.2. RECOMMENDED DIETARY ALLOWANCES FOR IRON FOR INFANTS (7–12 MONTHS), CHILDREN, AND ADULTS

AGE	MALES (mg/day)	FEMALES (mg/day)	PREGNANCY (mg/day)	LACTATION (mg/day)
7–12 months	11	11	N/A	N/A
1–3 years	7	7	N/A	N/A
4–8 years	10	10	N/A	N/A
9–13 years	8	8	N/A	N/A
14–18 years	11	15	27	10
19–50 years	8	18	27	9
51+ years	8	8	N/A	N/A

Adapted from reference 63.

TABLE 19.3. DIETARY SOURCES OF IRON

FOOD	SERVING	IRON (MG)
ANIMAL SOURCES: Containing Both Heme and Nonheme Iron		
Liver (beef, cooked)	3.5 oz (100 g)	8.8
Liver pâté	1 oz (30 g)	1.6
Lean cooked beef steak	3.5 oz (100 g)	4.0
Lean cooked roast lamb	3.5 oz (100 g)	3.2
Lean cooked chicken breast	3.5 oz (100 g)	1.1
Lean cooked chicken drumstick	(50 g)	1.4
Oysters	1/2 doz (100 g)	5.5
Canned tuna	6.5 oz (185 g)	2.1
Fish, white flesh	3.5 oz (100 g)	0.9
Sliced ham (lean)	1 oz (30 g)	0.3
PLANT SOURCES: Containing Nonheme Iron		
Fortified oat flakes cereal	2/3 cup (30 g)	8.1
Nonfortified cornflakes	1 cup (30 g)	0.8
Porridge	3/4 cup (170 g)	1.2
Whole wheat bread	1 slice (24 g)	0.8
White bread	1 slice (24 g)	0.6
Baked beans in sauce	8 oz (225 g)	3.6
Lentils	2/3 cup (100 g)	2.1
Raisins	2/3 cup (100 g)	1.8
Almonds	1 oz (30 g)	1.4
Spinach (cooked)	1/2 cup (90 g)	2.0
Apple	small (140 g)	0.3

Adapted from reference 64.

In a mixed diet where lean meats are consumed regularly, heme iron may provide about half of the absorbable iron. In many western countries, such as the United States and Australia, cereal products such as bread and breakfast cereals are the single greatest source of total dietary iron because of the fortification of these products with additional iron and the frequency with which they are consumed (3). Assessment of total dietary iron intake is not necessarily a good predictor of iron status; the mixing and matching of foods at meals plays an important role in determining the bioavailability of dietary iron intake. For example, in two groups of female runners who reported similar intakes of total dietary iron, the group who reported regular intake of meat was estimated to have a greater intake of absorbable iron and showed higher iron status than a matched group of runners who were semivegetarian (9).

PREVALENCE OF IRON DEFICIENCY IN ATHLETES

Finding the true prevalence of problematic iron deficiency in people who exercise is dependent on answering the following questions:

1. Can the reference standards for biochemical and hematologic parameters used to diagnose the stages of iron deficiency in normal populations be applied to athletes?
2. At what stage of iron depletion are impairments to exercise performance observed?
3. What is optimal iron status for an athlete, particularly an endurance athlete?

Changes in iron status associated with exercise are shown in Table 19.4. Our current understanding of these issues will be discussed later in this chapter. When examining the literature related to iron deficiency in athletes, it should be noted, however, that the prevalence was overstated in earlier times because of different interpretations of this information. In fact, there are a number of ways in which acute or chronic exercise itself alters iron status parameters independently of true iron status. According to the review by Haymes (10), the prevalence of anemia reported among groups of athletes ranges from 0 to 12.5%, whereas low ferritin levels might be expected in 0–44% of

an athletic group. Because many studies lack control groups for comparison and use different cut-off values to designate low or suboptimal levels, it is hard, however, to gain an overview of the true problem. Fogelholm (11) has also undertaken a sophisticated summary of the literature, in which only those studies that included control groups were evaluated. He concluded that the reported prevalence of iron-deficiency anemia is quite low (~3%) and similar between athletes and untrained individuals. Meanwhile, the pooled mean prevalence of low serum ferritin was 37% (range: 13%–50%) in male and female athletes and 23% (range: 10%–46%) in controls. The highest prevalence of low ferritin levels was seen in endurance sports, and among female and adolescent athletes, irrespective of the type of sport and intensity of training (11).

CLINICAL EXERCISE PHYSIOLOGY

EFFECT OF ANEMIA ON EXERCISE PERFORMANCE

The effects of iron deficiency anemia on aerobic capacity and exercise performance have been frequently demonstrated and have been summarized in a recent review (12). In cases of severely reduced hemoglobin levels, individuals may be unable to carry out everyday activities and work tasks and may report a noticeable breathlessness on even the mildest exertion. This results from impairment of oxygen transport in blood and muscle and impaired functioning of iron-related enzymes; however, reductions in cognition, temperature control, and immunity may also exacerbate the impaired exercise tolerance.

Although the effects of gradually reduced hemoglobin on performance have not been systematically studied, it is believed that even a small decline in hemoglobin levels (e.g., 1–2 mg/100 mL) will reduce the competition performance of athletes (13). Because the range of "normal" hemoglobin levels is reasonably wide, it is possible that an athlete may show a level that is within reference standards, but is below the level that is "usual" for him or her, and below that required for his or her optimal performance. If this were to occur, however, a specific clinical reason should exist for it and this could be detected by recourse, initially, to the characteristics of the red cells and

TABLE 19.4. REPORTED CHANGES IN IRON STATUS PARAMETERS IN CONDITIONS ENCOUNTERED BY EXERCISE

	HEMOGLOBIN	TRANSFERRIN SATURATION	SERUM IRON	FERRITIN
Plasma volume expansion in response to aerobic training	↓	↓	↓	↓
Dehydration at the time of testing	↑	↑	↑	↑
Infection (URTI, flu, virus) or inflammation	↓	↓	↓	↓
After acute strenuous exercise (after 24 hours)	↓	↓	↓	↓

(Adapted from Deakin V. Iron depletion in athletes. In: Burke L, Deakin V, eds. *Clinical Sports Nutrition*, 3rd ed. Sydney: McGraw Hill; 2006:263–312.)

the presence of a reticulocytosis and later to the results of other investigations, such as iron studies. Although a low hemoglobin level may be relatively easy to detect, it is difficult to confirm optimal iron status from a single blood test. Great value is seen in establishing a history of iron status results from individual athletes to establish a feel for what is normal for them, and how parameters may vary even when steps are taken to prevent or interpret these fluctuations (see below).

Athletes often believe that the "more is better" principle applies to hemoglobin levels per se. In the absence of hemoconcentration owing to dehydration, very high hemoglobin levels are usually explained by genetic individuality or drug use (e.g., erythropoietin [EPO]) and are not possible for most athletes to achieve.

EFFECT OF REDUCED IRON STATUS WITHOUT ANEMIA ON EXERCISE PERFORMANCE

Serum ferritin is almost universally used to assess iron storage status in both athletes and the general population (14,15). Generally, in healthy individuals, serum ferritin is the most sensitive test of iron deficiency (16) with values of <12 µg/L indicating absence of iron stores (17). Serum ferritin, however, does not accurately reflect tissue iron deficiency when stores are nearly or completely exhausted and, in this situation, soluble transferrin receptor is a more accurate indicator of iron status (18).

The transferrin receptor is a transmembrane glycoprotein expressed on the surface of erythroid and other cells, with about 80% of the total number of receptors present on cells of the erythron (19). It binds transferrin and is endocytosed releasing inorganic iron into the cytoplasm for use in erythropoiesis (20). The number of transferrin receptors on the cell surface reflects the intracellular iron requirement and iron deprivation rapidly induces transferrin receptor synthesis by interaction between iron responsive elements and iron regulatory proteins (21,22). Control of transferrin receptor synthesis appears to be mainly posttranscriptional, mediated by the iron responsive element in the messenger RNA (mRNA) for the receptor (23).

Concentrations of plasma or soluble transferrin receptors (sTfR) have a constant relationship to tissue receptors (24) and have been correlated with increases in reticulocytes (25). Increases in sTfR occur in conditions of increased red cell production and in iron deficiency (26), with increases in the concentration of this protein being suggested as a sensitive measure of tissue iron deficiency (27,28). sTfR is not an acute phase reactant and this has relevance in assessment of iron status in patients with conditions in which this might be a consideration and in the assessment in those involved in exercise.

Of recent interest and some controversy has been the effect of iron depletion in nonanemic persons on performance. Iron supplementation studies, based on reduced levels of serum ferritin (generally less than 20 µg/L) as markers for iron depletion, generally failed to show increases in aerobic capacity after supplementation (29–33). Friedmann et al. (34) demonstrated, however, a significant increase in $\dot{V}O_2$ max in young, nonanemic athletes with serum ferritin concentration <20 µg/L after 12 weeks of supplementation with 200 mg of ferrous iron per day. Endurance capacity was found to be increased in the studies by Rowland et al. (32) and Hinton et al. (35), but not in those of Klingshirn et al. (29) and Zhu and Haas (33). It should be noted, that in the study by Hinton et al. (35), multiple regression analysis suggested that increases in both iron stores and hemoglobin were associated with the improvement in performance.

More recently, three randomized, placebo-controlled trials of iron supplementation in iron-depleted, nonanemic women using soluble transferrin receptor as an indicator of iron depletion have been published (36–38). Brownlie et al. (36) studied 41 iron depleted (serum ferritin <16 µg/L) nonanemic women before and after receiving either 100 mg iron sulphate or placebo for 6 weeks. Supplementation for 6 weeks led to an increase in $\dot{V}O_2$ max and serum ferritin in the iron group but no change in sTfR (36). After stratification by baseline sTfR (>8.0 mg/L vs. ≤ 8.0 mg/L), it was shown that the improvement in fitness was owing to changes in iron status in the subjects with poor baseline iron status. A separate report from the same study noted that all subjects trained on a cycle ergometer for 5 days per week for the last 4 weeks of the supplementation (37). Endurance capacity was assessed by a 15-km time trial on a cycle ergometer. Significant treatment effects were found for time to complete the time trial, work rate, and percentage of maximal oxygen uptake in subjects with a serum transferrin receptor concentration of more than 8.0 mg/L. Finally, Brutsaert et al (38) studied 20 iron-depleted (serum ferritin <20 µg/L) women performing static, maximal, voluntary contractions (MVC) in the quadriceps and dynamic knee extensions to fatigue, before and after iron supplementation. After treatment, the rate of decrease in MVC was attenuated in the iron group but not in the placebo group. The improvement was not related to changes in iron status indices or tissue iron stores.

The main conclusion to be drawn from these studies is that, in women in the absence of anemia, decrements in performance may be caused by tissue iron deficiency sufficient to cause an elevation in sTfR greater than 8.0 mg/L. This has implications for iron supplementation to avoid decrements in performance. As iron stores in athletes are generally measured by assessment of serum ferritin, knowledge of the level of this parameter at which sTfR is greater than 8.0 using this method of analysis is important.

The normal range for the Ramco Laboratories method for determination of sTfR used in the studies by Brownlie et al. (39) is 3–8.2 mg/L. This suggests that the athletes who are not anemic and who benefit from iron supplementation are those who are at the verge of, or who have, iron deficient erythropoiesis. Although the serum ferritin concentration at the upper limit of normal of sTfR has not been specifically determined using the method used by Brownlie, other studies, using other analytic methods, suggest that the upper limit of normality for sTfR lies at a serum ferritin concentration of approximately 22 μg/L (18,40).

RECOMMENDATIONS FOR SUPPLEMENTATION

Despite much having been published on iron deficiency in athletes, recommendations relating to a cut-off value for iron supplementation in athletes are remarkably hard to find and are generally related to serum ferritin concentrations. The exact basis on which some of these recommendations have been made is unclear.

Neilsen and Nachtigall (41) reported on a survey of 26 sport centers in Germany and found that, for females, 50% recommended supplementation at a serum ferritin concentration less than 25 μg/L and 71% at less than 35 μg/L and for males, 21% recommended supplementation at 20 μg/L and 57% at less than 30 μg/L. Their recommendation was for "supplementation for all athletes with serum ferritin <35 μg/L." Chatard et al. (42) suggested that "in normal training conditions, with no infection or inflammatory syndrome, as long as ferritin levels are above 20–30 μg/L, and the degree of saturation of the transferrin above 16%, iron supplements are not necessary." Other more recent reviews of hematologic issues in sport have not offered a recommendation (43,44).

Based on published research, an athlete with iron deficiency anemia would clearly be treated. It would also be unwise to wait until iron stores were fully depleted, a condition correlated with a serum ferritin concentration of less than 12 μg/L. Despite the controversy over some of the studies of supplementation of nonanemic, iron-depleted female athletes, it would be prudent to avoid levels in the range of 16–20 μg/L.

Iron deficient erythropoiesis should also be avoided and, based on the work of Suominen (18), using the Orion test method, this occurs at a serum ferritin level of less than approximately 22 μg/L. Although this level was derived in a nonathletic population, it was exactly the level above which sTfR was not elevated, using the Roche method in the elite athlete sample studied by Pitsis et al. (40).

Some margin for error is appropriate as the day-to-day total variability of venous serum ferritin has been demonstrated to be 27.4% in young women and 14% in young males (45). In a group of female athletes, the average day-to-day error for ferritin concentration was found to be 46%, compared with 21.6 % in a control group (46). Indeed, this degree of variability suggests that more than one assessment should occur before a clinical decision is made. In addition, a conservative approach is prudent, particularly when screening new athletes, when considering the 25% reduction of serum ferritin found to be associated with the onset of rigorous daily training in an elite program in both weight-bearing and non–weight-bearing sports (47).

Taking all of the above into account, it would seem reasonable to suggest that at least assessment and correction of dietary iron intake, exclusion of medical disorders which might lead to iron loss and, generally, oral iron supplementation should occur in all athletes with serum ferritin concentrations less than 30 μg/L. Again, in relation to the avoidance of iron deficient erythropoiesis, athletes with an increase in sTfR beyond the upper limit of normal should be placed on iron supplementation.

Based on sensitivity and specificity data from Pitsis et al. (40) and the conclusion of Mast (48) that "measurement of sTfR does not provide sufficient additional information to ferritin to warrant routine use," it appears that serum ferritin will remain the standard method of assessment of iron status in athletes. Measurement of the soluble transferrin receptor will, however, be useful in situations in which assessment of iron status is undertaken in the presence of an acute phase response, such as in athletes with intercurrent infections, disorders associated with inflammation, or close in time to the types of exercise which have been shown to induce this response.

In addition, a number of athletes, usually female, appear habitually to have low levels of serum ferritin, some returning relatively rapidly to these levels following a course of supplementation. Clearly, these athletes have normally low levels of serum ferritin. Demonstration of normal levels of soluble transferrin receptor in these athletes will lead to reassurance for both the athlete and coach and avoidance of repeated, unnecessary course of supplementation and blood testing.

PRESENCE OF OTHER RISK FACTORS

Support for an assessment of low iron status and, in particular, a substantial reduction in blood parameters of iron status, can often be found by looking for the presence of risk factors for iron drain or negative iron balance. Important risk factors are listed in Table 19.5.

PHARMACOLOGY

Iron Injections

A rapid reversal of iron depletion and an increase in iron stores can be achieved via intramuscular injections of

TABLE 19.5. RISK FACTORS FOR IRON DRAIN OR NEGATIVE IRON BALANCE

Predictors of Increased Iron Requirements
- Recent growth spurt in adolescents
- Pregnancy (current or within the past year)

Predictors of Increased Iron Losses or Iron Malabsorption
- Sudden increase in heavy training load, particularly involving running on hard surfaces
- Gastrointestinal malabsorption problems (e.g., Crohn's disease, ulcerative colitis, parasite infestation)
- Gastrointestinal bleeding caused by chronic use of some anti-inflammatory drugs, ulcers, or other problems
- Heavy menstrual blood losses
- Excessive blood losses, such as frequent nose bleeds, recent surgery, substantial contact injuries
- Frequent blood donation

Predictors of Inadequate Intake of Bioavailable Iron
- Chronic low energy intake (<2,000 kcal/day)
- Vegetarian eating—especially poorly constructed diets in which alternative food sources of iron are ignored (e.g., legumes, nuts, seeds)
- Fad diets or erratic eating patterns
- Restricted variety of foods in diet and failure to promote mixing and matching of foods at meals (especially vitamin-C–containing fruit and vegetables)
- Heavy reliance on convenience foods and micronutrient-poor sports foods (high carbohydrate [CHO] powders, bars, and gels)
- Very high carbohydrate diet with high fiber content and infrequent intake of meats/fish/chicken
- Natural food diets: failure to consume iron-fortified cereal foods, such as commercial breakfast cereals and bread

iron. This is sometimes provided in cases of extreme iron depletion, which carry a significant penalty to the individual involved, or where oral iron intake is not tolerated. In some athletic circles, however, it has become popular as a more "high-tech" method of supplementation and is even known to be used in cases where iron deficiency has not been characterized. Iron injection does not provide a superior technique of iron repletion *per se*, particularly as a significant proportion of the iron remains in the buttock, unabsorbed. Because it carries a risk of anaphylactic shock as well as iron overload, it should not be regarded as the first choice of treatment or a benign therapy. Iron injections will not increase hemoglobin levels or other iron parameters in people who are not otherwise suboptimal in iron status (49).

IRON SUPPLEMENTS

Oral iron supplements provide part of the usual therapy recommended to treat iron deficiency and anemia. Most authorities recommend that such therapy should be prescribed on a case-by-case basis, as part of a treatment plan involving strategies to reduce or prevent unusual iron losses, and dietary counseling to maximize the intake of bioavailable iron (3,50). The recognized therapy is a daily dose of 100 mg elemental iron (which may be equal to 500 mg of ferrous sulphate), taken on an empty stomach.

Many people take a vitamin C supplement or juice with their supplement to enhance the absorption of this organic iron. A 3-month period of supplementation is needed to restore depleted iron stores (50). In some cases, when it is not possible to enhance dietary iron intake sufficiently, it may be necessary to continue iron supplementation at a lower dose, or as a 1–2 times per week intake to prevent ongoing iron drain.

Although iron supplements are available as over-the-counter medications, there are dangers in self-prescription as a "tonic," or long-term supplementation in the absence of medical follow-up. Iron supplementation is not a replacement for medical and dietary assessment and therapy, because it fails to correct underlying problems that have caused iron drain. In many cases, a diet that is inadequate in iron will also fail to meet other sports nutrition goals. Chronic supplementation with high doses of iron carries a risk of iron overload, especially in males in whom clinical expression of hemochromatosis is more frequent. Iron supplements can also interfere with the absorption of other minerals, such as zinc and copper. Some individuals experience gastrointestinal side effects arising from the use of iron supplements.

DIETARY PRESCRIPTION AND COUNSELING

The major goal of dietary counseling is to increase the person's intake of bioavailable iron, with eating patterns that are compatible with his or her other nutritional goals (e.g., achieving fuel requirements for sport, achieving desired physique). This is often a specialized task, requiring the expertise of a dietitian. Key dietary goals are summarized below:

- Consume sufficient energy to allow nutritional goals to be met. Avoid chronic periods of energy restriction and severe weight loss.
- Include small amounts of lean red meats in meals at least 3–4 times each week. Meat can be added to a high-carbohydrate meal to achieve overall sports nutrition goals (e.g., sandwich with roast beef, pasta with meat sauce, lamb kabobs with rice, beef stir fry with vegetables and noodles). The presence of meat enhances iron absorption from other foods at the meal.
- Add chicken and pork at other meals to provide a reasonable source of iron and to enhance iron absorption at the meal.
- Consider shellfish or liver (e.g., pâté) as an alternative to red meat.
- Make use of cereals that are iron fortified (e.g., many commercial breakfast cereals).
- Include iron-rich foods, such as whole grains, dried fruit, legumes, eggs, nuts, and seeds, in meals, and use with an iron-absorbing food (meat or vitamin-C–containing food) to enhance the bioavailability of

iron. For example, combine parsley with an omelet, or tomato sauce with rice and lentils.

- Combine vitamin-C–containing foods at meals where whole-grain cereals are eaten (to counteract the iron-inhibiting phytate). For example, drink a glass of juice with breakfast cereal, or have fruit or salad vegetables with a whole-meal sandwich.
- If you are at risk of iron drain, drink tea and coffee between meals rather than at meals.

EXERCISE PRESCRIPTION

Exercise prescription for people with iron deficiency depends on the degree to which reduced iron status interferes with exercise capacity and the possibility that exercise is increasing the iron depletion. Because fatigue is one of the principal symptoms of anemia and possibly also iron deficiency without anemia, it may reduce the ability to undertake or enjoy exercise. Therefore, it is prudent not to commence or increase an exercise regimen for an iron-deficient person. Rather, exercise prescription should achieve a level that is comfortable for the individual and his or her symptoms of fatigue. Depending on the individual, the duration, frequency, and intensity of exercise sessions should be considered. These factors may need to be reduced or modified until iron-replacement therapy has progressed sufficiently to abate the feelings of fatigue or poor recovery between sessions. This may be simple for the recreational exerciser but is likely to require careful planning in the case of the serious athlete, so that long-term fitness and competition goals are minimally compromised.

Exercise prescription should also consider the possibility that activity patterns can cause iron losses that are adding to the iron drain. In this case, it may be prudent to modify exercise patterns or associated activities to provide an opportunity for iron status to be improved. A sudden increase in exercise load, particularly involving foot strike damage, blood loss, or contact injuries, may exacerbate iron drain in individuals with low iron intake and precarious iron balance. Although iron-replacement treatment and improved iron intake are the cornerstones of therapy, it also makes sense to monitor exercise patterns to avoid excessive iron losses. Tactics may include choosing a slower rate of introducing or increasing a training program, finding softer surfaces to run on, replacing worn shoes with footwear that offers better cushioning, and avoiding activities with a high risk of blood loss or substantial bruising. Some activities associated with exercise, such as the use of certain nonsteroidal anti-inflammatory drugs to manage pain or overuse injuries, may need to be examined for their possible role in causing gastrointestinal blood losses. Again, the modification of an exercise program may be simple in the case of the recreational exerciser, but compromise and creativity are often needed for the care of the serious or elite athlete.

CASE STUDIES

CASE 1

A female crosscountry skier presented with moderate anemia. Ferritin and other parameters were normal, eliminating chronic iron-deficiency anemia, but suggestive of acute blood loss. She began iron therapy, and her hemoglobin increased from 10.2 to 12.5 g/100 mL in 3 weeks. Symptoms of fatigue abated, leaving her ready to compete. It was subsequently found that she had suffered from gastric bleeding as a result of self-directed use of a nonsteroidal anti-inflammatory drug to treat an injury.

CASE 2

A female basketball player presented for a routine blood screen. Hemoglobin level was just below the normal range. On questioning, she revealed symptoms of lethargy and poor recovery between training sessions. She reported that she had been following a strict weight-loss diet over the previous 3 months and was avoiding the intake of all meats, which were considered to be "too fatty." Further blood tests were taken on the suspicion of low iron status, which was confirmed by a low ferritin level. She was referred for dietary counseling to allow her to achieve body fat goals, while increasing her intake of well-absorbed iron.

Simultaneously, she was started on a 3-month course of oral iron supplements. Review after 3 months showed an increase in ferritin levels from 8 to 42 ng/mL and improvement in well-being. After assessment of high iron eating patterns, iron supplementation was ceased, and a further blood and dietary review was organized for 6 months.

CASE 3

A female swimmer was reviewed by a new doctor in the sports medicine clinic after her routine blood tests revealed a ferritin concentration of 28 ng/mL. She reported training well and performing well. She had been eating all her meals in an athlete dining hall for the previous year and reported eating a varied menu, including meat-containing meals at least 3 times a week. All other hematologic and biochemical tests were normal. Her medical history showed that ferritin test results from the previous 2 years, during similar periods of training, were 29, 32, 27, and 35 ng/mL; soluble transferrin receptor concentrations were also within the normal range. It was concluded that the present results represented normal iron status for this swimmer, and no therapy was needed.

CASE 4

A male triathlete presented with tiredness and a history of mild to moderate diarrhea persisting over the previous month. The triathlete reported being under the care of a sports dietitian and was following a high-carbohydrate diet, with attention to a good intake of bioavailable iron. History revealed that the gastrointestinal problems had begun after completing a triathlon swim in a dam in an area where *Giardia lamblia* infestation was common. Cultures confirmed this problem, and a course of treatment was commenced. A blood screen also showed, however, a ferritin level of 23 ng/mL, in comparison to his previous test results of 85 ng/mL. Hemoglobin levels were within the normal range. Iron supplementation was prescribed to replete iron stores, and a 3-month follow-up check was organized.

SICKLE-CELL ANEMIA

EPIDEMIOLOGY AND PATHOPHYSIOLOGY

The most common structural hemoglobinopathy, sickle-cell anemia, was first recorded by James Herrich of Chicago in 1910 (51). He described crescent-shaped "sickle cells" in a young black student from the West Indies. The greatest prevalence of sickle-cell anemia is in Africa; however, the gene is also common in northern Mediterranean countries; North, Central, and South America; the Middle East; and India. The heterozygous form (sickle-cell trait-HbAS) is found in up to 8%–10% of blacks and, in some regions of Africa, may reach as high as 40% (52). The prevalence of HbS in professional football players (53) and high school athletes (54) has been shown to be nearly identical to the prevalence in the corresponding general population. In a study conducted in the Ivory Coast, the incidence of the gene was 12% (55). The homozygous form (HbSS) has an incidence of up to 1.3% (52). It is of interest that the gene occurs most frequently in areas where malarial infection caused by the parasite *Plasmodium falciparum* is common. This suggests a selective advantage, and immunity to this form of malaria may exist in these individuals; consequently, the gene frequency has built up over time.

HbSS usually presents as a moderate to severe anemia and, consequently, affected individuals cannot perform at a level consistent with elite competition because of the low total Hb mass. Conversely, heterozygous sickle-cell anemia (sickle-cell trait) with normal hemoglobin levels allows affected individuals to compete at the elite level. Evidence collected since the early 1970s suggests, however, that individuals with sickle-cell trait are at increased risk of exertional rhabdomyolysis and sudden death, after exercise (51,56–58). This is a significant issue, given the prevalence of the gene in the black population.

Hemoglobin S (HbS) is the mutant hemoglobin produced when nonpolar valine is substituted for polar glutamic acid in the β-chain. The solubility of HbS in the deoxygenated state (sickled cells) is markedly reduced, producing a tendency for deoxyhemoglobin S molecules to polymerize into rigid aggregates, causing occlusions in the capillaries. Exercise, which can substantially influence temperature, hypoxia, acidosis, and dehydration, can potentially trigger changes in hemoglobin of individuals with HbS, by promoting deoxygenation and the formation of HbS polymers. The hypoxic, acidotic, and hypertonic microenvironments of the kidney, spleen, and retina also promote HbS polymerization and sickling, and intense exercise may exacerbate this (52).

The concentration of hemoglobin also influences sickling. The more concentrated the HbS within the red blood cell, the greater the potential for HbS aggregates to form. Some have speculated that hydrating the cells can prevent sickling (52).

Polymerization of deoxyhemoglobin S begins when the oxygen saturation of hemoglobin falls below 85% and is complete at about 38% oxygen saturation. Altitude exposures for training or acclimatization purposes are important issues to consider in individuals with HbS (52).

The oxygen affinity of HbS may result in important physiologic changes in vivo. HbS has reduced oxygen affinity. The 2,3-diphosphoglycerate levels of homozygote HbS are increased, and hence, the right shift in the oxygen dissociation curves means more oxygen is released to the tissues. This results in an increase in the concentration of deoxyhemoglobin S, promoting the formation of sickle cells. This may occur in the heterozygous state; however, the presence of HbA ensures that any polymers formed are weak (52).

CLINICAL EXERCISE PHYSIOLOGY

Ample evidence suggests that individuals with HbS (sickle cell trait) can perform at levels normal or near normal in relation to exercise capacity and maximal oxygen uptake when compared with appropriate control individuals (58). In a half-marathon held in the Ivory Coast, no significant differences were seen in the rankings of

HbS individuals and healthy individuals (59). One HbS individual finished second; however, it was later determined that he was a double heterozygote HbS/alpha thalassemia. The authors noted that of all the internationally ranked runners in the race, none had HbS, and that this may indicate that HbS is a limiting factor in endurance performance. They also made the point that presence of double heterozygoticity may be a performance-enhancing factor.

PHARMACOLOGY

HbS, because it is generally a benign condition, no agents or drugs are used to treat it. There are, however, pharmacologic agents that can reduce intracellular sickling in patients homozygous for HbS. Hydroxyurea and butyrate are drugs currently used to prevent sickling. These agents elevate fetal hemoglobin (HbF) levels, causing a decrease in intracellular polymerization of HbS.

MEDICAL TREATMENT

Aside from sudden collapse during exercise, other signs of exertional rhabdomyolysis include muscular weakness, muscle swelling, or cramping with darkened urine. In advanced cases of exertional rhabdomyolysis and sickling, appropriate emergency medical care is required to alleviate symptoms and prevent renal and other organ failure.

In acute cases of sickling, which can lead to significant morbidity and mortality, the most effective treatment regimen to minimize organ damage is to remove the stimulus precipitating sickling, such as dehydration or altitude exposure.

PHYSICAL EXAMINATION

In homozygous HbSS individuals, a physical examination may reveal findings associated with sickling, such as anemia, splenomegaly, and dyspnea. In heterozygous HbS, the physical findings are not so obvious, and only an adequate history and appropriate blood tests would identify such individuals. Diagnostic tests include hemoglobin electrophoresis, where up to 35%–45% of the total hemoglobin is made up of HbS; a sickling test, where red blood cells are induced to sickle in the presence of a reducing agent, such as sodium metabisulphite; and a solubility test, in which HbS is deoxygenated with dithionite.

EXERCISE PRESCRIPTION

Between 1977 and 1981, the sudden, unexplained exercise-induced deaths of 62 recruits involved in basic training revealed that individuals with HbS (sickle cell trait) were at 28–40 times greater risk (57). These sudden deaths could, however, have been related to other causes such as acute cardiac arrest of undefined mechanism, exertional heat stroke, or heat stress.

Exertional rhabdomyolysis, a syndrome characterized by skeletal muscle degeneration and muscle enzyme leakage (58), has been linked to at least 17 cases of sudden collapse and deaths in persons with HbS (51,56–58). There are also links to numerous cases of nonfatal exertional collapse (60). The mechanisms leading to sudden death in this condition are not known. Renal tubule damage can be caused, however, when myoglobin is released from working muscles during extreme physical exertion. A metabolite of myoglobin breakdown, ferriheme, has been shown to be toxic to renal tubule epithelium in vitro (61). Another possible mechanism for such catastrophic events is the "sickling" of red blood cells. This sickling may occur for a number of reasons, and the end result is organ failure caused by the polymerization of HbS, causing vaso-occlusion in the capillaries (52).

It is unlikely that the risks will deter athletes with HbS from competing. Any coach or athlete associated with, or afflicted by, HbS should at all times practice caution during training and competition. Primary risk factors, such as extreme heat and humidity, high altitude, illness, and fatigue, should be evaluated and addressed before each session of intense exercise. Attention to hydration status is particularly important, and strict compliance should be observed with fluid replacements in all athletes and not just those with HbS.

Ignoring such simple strategies could lead to fatal outcomes, which emphasizes the importance of HbS in the sporting context. Table 19.6 lists recommended measures for preventing exertional rhabdomyolysis in athletes with HbS (56).

TABLE 19.6. SUGGESTED STRATEGIES FOR THE PREVENTION OF EXERTIONAL RHABDOMYOLYSIS IN ATHLETES WITH HbS (SICKLE CELL TRAIT)

1. Develop and implement conditioning programs before resuming intense training or competition.
2. Develop and implement aggressive hydration policies before, during, and after all activity.
3. Avoid the use of beverages that have diuretic effects (e.g., caffeine, alcohol).
4. Avoid strenuous exercise in hot, humid conditions, and at altitudes of 2,500 feet or higher.
5. Modify activities during or following viral illness, particularly when vomiting and diarrhea has occurred.
6. Modify activities during periods of poor sleep or general fatigue.
7. Avoid stressful exercise routines, such as time trials or repeated high-intensity interval sessions with brief recovery periods.

Reproduced from reference 56.

CASE STUDIES

CASE 5

In 1991, a 22-year-old football player suddenly collapsed after completing an 800-m run. The athlete had been training intensively for 4 weeks and had passed a preevent physical. Despite aggressive and immediate treatment for exertional rhabdomyolysis, the athlete died 46 hours after his collapse. It was subsequently found that the athlete had HbS (62).

CASE 6

In a 20-year-old black football player with HbS, bilateral pain in the lower back, hamstrings, and calves after completing a timed 1–1.5-mile run resulted in his hospitalization. The diagnosis was exercise-induced asthma and rhabdomyolysis. Blood chemistries, excluding creatine kinase, were normal, and he was allowed to return to supervised training and within 2 weeks had returned to full practice except distance runs. He was "aggressively" hydrated before, during, and after all activity. He completed the season with no other adverse health effects (60).

CASE 7

A black crosscountry runner with HbS collapsed suddenly on two separate occasions. After the first incident, the athlete vomited and complained of shortness of breath, abdominal pain, nausea, and leg cramps. He also reported that he had taken a decongestant the previous evening. Although recovering without complications, he was advised to discontinue competitive running. He continued running until a second incident a year later. He collapsed and required mouth-to-mouth resuscitation and was transported to the local emergency facility. He was diagnosed with rhabdomyolysis and renal insufficiency. After regaining consciousness, he was disorientated and complained of severe leg cramps. He was discharged 1 month later with some residual renal damage, and he no longer runs competitively (56).

REFERENCES

1. Brotherhood J, Brozovic B, Pugh LG. Haematological status of middle- and long-distance runners. *Clin Sci Mol Med* 1975; 48: 139–45.
2. Dill DB, Braithwaite K, Adams WC. Blood volume of middle-distance runners: Effect of 2,300 m altitude and comparison with nonathletes. *Med Sci Sports Exerc* 1974;6:1–7.
3. Deakin V. Iron depletion in athletes. In: Burke L, Deakin V, eds. *Clinical Sports Nutrition*, 3rd ed. Sydney: McGraw Hill; 2006: 263–312.
4. Lamanca JJ, Haymes EM, Daly JA, et al. Sweat iron loss of male and female runners during exercise. *Int J Sports Med* 1988;9:52–5.
5. Rudzki SJ, Hazard H, Collinson D. Gastrointestinal blood loss in triathletes: Its etiology and relationship to sports anemia. *Aust J Science Med* 1995;27:3–8.
6. Miller BJ, Pate RR, Burgess W. Foot impact force and intravascular hemolysis during distance running. *Int J Sports Med* 1988;9:56–60.
7. Monsen ER, Hallberg L, Layrisse M, et al. Estimation of available dietary iron. *Am J Clin Nutr* 1978;31:134–41.
8. Hallberg L, Hultén L, Gramatkovski E. Iron absorption from the whole diet in men: How effective is the regulation of iron absorption? *Am J Clin Nutr* 1978;66:347–56.
9. Snyder AC, Dvorak LL, Roepke JB. Influence of dietary iron source on measures of iron status among female runners. *Med Sci Sports Exerc* 1989;21:7–10.
10. Haymes EM. Trace minerals and exercise. In: Wolinsky I, ed. *Nutrition in Exercise and Sport*, 3rd ed. Boca Raton: CRC Press; 1998, 77–107
11. Fogelholm M. Indicators of vitamin and mineral status in athletes' blood: a review. *Int J Sports Nutr* 1995;5:267–84.
12. Haas JD, Brownlie T. Iron deficiency and reduced work capacity: A critical review of the research to determine a causal relationship. *J Nutr* 2001;131:676S–90S.
13. Eichner ER. Minerals: iron. In: Maughan R, ed. *Nutrition in Sport.* London: Blackwell Science; 2000.
14. Garza D, Shrier I, Kohl 111 HW, et al. The clinical value of serum ferritin tests in endurance athletes. *Clin J Sport Med* 1997;7: 46–53.
15. Malczezewska J, Raczynski G, Siwinska D, et al. Ferritin—A diagnostic index of iron status in athletes. *Biol Sport* 1996;13:21–30.
16. Ahluwalia N. Diagnostic utility of serum transferrin receptors measurement in assessing iron status. *Nutr Rev* 1998;56:133–41.
17. Ali MAM, Luxton AW, Walker WHC. Serum ferritin concentration and marrow iron stores: a prospective study. *Can Med Assoc J* 1978; 118:945–6.
18. Souminen P, Punnonen K, Rajamaki A, et al. Serum transferrin receptor and transferrin receptor-ferritin index identify healthy subjects with sub-clinical iron deficits. *Blood* 1998;92: 2934–9.
19. Beguin Y. The soluble transferrin receptor: Biological aspects and clinical usefulness as quantitative measure of erythropoiesis. *Haematologica* 1992;11:1–10.
20. Cook JD. Iron-deficiency anaemia in clinical disorders of iron metabolism. *Bailliere's Clinical Haematology* 1994;7:787–804.
21. Eisenstein RS, Blemings KP. Iron regulatory proteins, iron responsive elements and iron homeostasis. *J Nutr* 1998;128: 2295–8.
22. Rao KK, Shapiro D, Mattia E, et al. Effects of alterations in cellular iron on biosynthesis of the transferrin receptor in K562 cells. *Mol Cell Biol* 1983;5:595–9.
23. Baynes RD, Skikne BS, Cook JD. Circulating transferrin receptors and assessment of iron status. *J Nutr Biochem* 1994;5:322–30.
24. Huebers HA, Beguin Y, Pootrakal P, et al. Intact transferrin receptors in human plasma and their relation to erythropoiesis. *Blood* 1990; 75:102–7.
25. Kohgo Y, Niitsu Y, Kondo H, et al. Serum transferrin receptor as a new index of erythropoiesis. *Blood* 1987;70:1955–8.
26. Punnonen K, Irjala K, Rajamaki A. Iron deficiency anemia is associated with high concentrations of transferrin receptor in serum. *Clin Chem* 1994;40:774–6.

27. Cook JD, Skikne BS, Baynes RD. Serum transferrin receptor. *Ann Rev Med* 1993;44:63–74.

28. Skikne BS, Flowers C, Cook J. Serum transferrin receptor: A quantitative measure of tissue iron deficiency. *Blood* 1990;75:1870–6.

29. Klingshirn LA, Pate RR, Bourque SP, et al. Effect of iron supplementation on endurance capacity in iron-depleted female runners. *Med Sci Sports Exerc* 1992;24:819–24.

30. Newhouse IJ, Clement DB, Taunton JE, et al. The effects of prelatent/latent iron deficiency on physical work capacity. *Med Sci Sports Exerc* 1989;21:263–68.

31. Peeling P, Blee T, Goodman C, et al. Effect of iron injections on aerobic exercise performance of iron depleted female athletes. *Int J Sport Nutr Ex Metab* 2007;17:221–31.

32. Rowland TW, Deisroth MB, Green GM, et al. The effect of iron therapy on the exercise capacity of non-anemic iron-deficient adolescent runners. *Am J Dis Child* 1988;142:165–9.

33. Zhu YI, Haas JD. Altered metabolic response of iron-depleted, non-anemic women during a 15-km time trial. *J Appl Physiol* 1998;84:1768–75.

34. Friedmann B, Weller E, Mairbaurl H, et al. Effects of iron repletion on blood volume and performance capacity in young athletes. *Med Sci Sports Exerc* 2001;33:741–6.

35. Hinton PS, Giordano C, Brownlie T, et al. Iron supplementation improves endurance after training in iron-depleted, non-anaemic women. *J Appl Physiol* 2000;88:1103–11.

36. Brownlie IV T, Utermohlen V, Hinton PS, et al. Marginal iron deficiency without anemia impairs aerobic adaptation among previously untrained women. *Am J Clin Nutr* 2002;75:734–42.

37. Brownlie IV T, Utermohlen V, Hinton PS, et al. Tissue iron deficiency without anemia impairs adaptation in endurance capacity after aerobic training in previously untrained women. *Am J Clin Nutr* 2004;79:437–43.

38. Brutsaert TD, Hernandez-Cordero S, Rivera J, et al. Iron supplementation improves progressive fatigue resistance during dynamic knee extensor exercise in iron-depleted, non-anemic women. *Am J Clin Nutr* 2003;77:441–8.

39. Van den Bosch G, Van den Bosche J, Wagner C, et al. Determination of iron metabolism related reference values in a healthy adult population. *Clin Chem* 2001;47:1465–7.

40. Pitsis GC, Fallon KE, Fallon SK, et al. Response of soluble transferrin receptor and iron-related parameters to iron supplementation in elite, iron-depleted, nonanemic female athletes. *Clin J Sports Med* 2004;14:300–4.

41. Neilsen P, Nachtigall D. Iron supplementation in athletes—Current recommendations. *Sports Med* 1998;26:207–16.

42. Chatard J-C, Mujika I, Guy C, et al. Anemia and iron deficiency in athletes. Practical recommendations for treatment. *Sports Med* 1999;27:229–40.

43. Mercer KW, Densmore JJ. Hematologic disorders in the athlete. *Clin Sports Med* 2005;24:599–621.

44. Shaskey DG, Green GA. Sports hematology. *Sports Med* 2000;29:27–38.

45. Cooper MJ, Zlotkin SH. Day to day variation of transferrin receptor and ferritin in healthy men and women. *Am J Clin Nutr* 1996;64:738–42.

46. Stupnicki R, Malczewska, Ilde K. Hackney AC. Day to day variability in the transferrin receptor/ferritin index in female athletes. *Br J Sports Med* 2003; 37: 267–9.

47. Ashenden MJ, Martin DT, Dobson GP, et al. Serum ferritin and anaemia in trained female athletes. *Int J Sport Nutr* 1998:8:223–9.

48. Mast AE, Blinder MA, Gronowski AM, et al. Clinical utility of the soluble transferrin receptor and comparison with serum ferritin in several populations. *Clin Chem* 1998; 44: 45–51.

49. Ashenden MJ, Fricker PA, Ryan RK, et al. The haematological response to an iron injection amongst female athletes. *Int J Sports Med* 1998;19:474–8.

50. Nielsen P, Nachtigall D. Iron supplementation in athletes: current recommendations. *Sports Med* 1998;26:207–16.

51. Eichner ER. Sickle cell trait, heroic exercise, and fatal collapse. *Phys Sports Med* 1993;21(7):51–64.

52. McKenzie SB. *Textbook of Hematology.* Baltimore: Williams & Wilkins; 1996.

53. Murphy JR. Sickle cell hemoglobin (HbAS) in black football players. *JAMA* 1973;225:981–2.

54. Ferguson BJ, Skikne BS, Simpson KM, et al. Serum transferrin receptor distinguishes the anemia of chronic disease from iron deficiency anemia. *J Lab Clin Med* 1992;19:385–90.

55. Diggs L, Flowers E. High school students with sickle cell trait (HbA/S). *J Natl Med Assoc* 1976;68:492–3.

56. Harrelson G, Fincher L, Robinson J. Acute exertional rhabdomyolysis and its relationship to sickle cell trait. *J Athl Training* 1995; 30(4):309–12.

57. Kark JA, Posey DM, Schumacher HR, et al. Sickle cell trait as a risk factor for sudden death in physical training. *N Eng J Med* 1987; 317:781–7.

58. Kark JA, Ward FT. Exercise and hemoglobin S. *Semin Hematol* 1994; 31:181–225.

59. Le Gallais D, Prefaut C, Mercier J, et al. Sickle cell trait as a limiting factor for high level performance in a semi-marathon. *Int J Sports Med* 1994;15:309–402.

60. Browne RJ, Gillespie CA. Sickle cell trait: a risk factor for life-threatening rhabdomyolysis? *Phys Sports Med* 1993;21(6):80–8.

61. Milne CJ. Rhabdomyolysis, myoglobinuria, and exercise. *Sports Med* 1988;6:93–106.

62. Rosenthal MA, Parker DJ. Collapse of a young athlete. *Ann Emerg Med* 1992;21:1493–8.

63. Institute of Medicine. Food and Nutrition Board. *Dietary Reference Intakes for Vitamin A, Vitamin K, Arsenic, Boron, Chromium, Copper, Iodine, Iron, Manganese, Molybdenum, Nickel, Silicon, Vanadium and Zinc.* Washington, DC: National Academy Press; 2001.

64. Pennington JA, Church HN. *Bowes and Church's Food Values of Portions Commonly Used,* 14th ed. Philadelphia: JB Lippincott; 1985.

IV

Clinical Practice Issues for the RCEP

WILLIAM HERBERT AND ANTHONY KALETH, *Section Editors*

Evolution of the Clinical Exercise Physiologist

THE ORIGINS OF CLINICAL EXERCISE PHYSIOLOGY

Their names ring through the corridors of exercise science departments and exercise physiology laboratories throughout the world—Borg, Astrand, Saltin, Buskirk, Faulkner, Costill, Naughton, Robinson, Kasch, Wilmore, Brooks, Bruce, Balke, Fox, Haskell, and Pollock. These are just some of the many pioneers who helped originate and shape the field of exercise physiology, within which clinical exercise physiology now serves as a subspecialty. They came from many professions, as physicians, academicians, scientists, epidemiologists, kinesiologists, physical educators, physiologists, and biologists, all with a common interest in exercise. Their research and passion to teach and train others were central to the development of the knowledge base that led to the creation of the guidelines, protocols, and materials that resulted in the clinical certifications now offered through the American College of Sports Medicine (ACSM). Specifically, the Clinical Exercise Specialist (CES) and Registered Clinical Exercise Physiologist (RCEP) certifications.

In the 1950s and 1960s, exercise physiology was, for the most part, an academic discipline and not a profession (1). Exercise physiologists during those early years were more focused on developing proper exercise training programs for healthy adults and athletes than applying their trade to patients with a clinically manifest disease (2). At that same time, however, the use of exercise as an adjunctive treatment in medicine began to emerge, along with academic training programs such as those found at the University of Wisconsin at La Crosse, the University of South Carolina, Wake Forest University, Penn State University, and San Diego State University. Many of the academicians working in these programs, and others, integrated their teaching into what quickly became (and remains to this day) a gold standard reference source for the field: *Guidelines for Graded Exercise Testing and Prescription,* first published in 1975 (3).

WHAT IS A CLINICAL EXERCISE PHYSIOLOGIST?

In the 1970s, the question of "What is an exercise physiologist?" surfaced and was subsequently defined by the ACSM

as a "doctoral-level research scientist" who studied mechanisms of biological function in relation to the exercise state (2). Throughout the 1980s and 1990s, some confusion remained regarding the nature of the required training and the practice areas that are unique to those who apply exercise physiology in the clincial setting. Specifically, was it necessary for this emerging allied health professional to be doctorally prepared or was the ACSM Exercise Specialist certification sufficient, regardless of academic degree?

In the mid-1990s the ACSM undertook the arduous task of defining the scope of practice for the clinical exercise physiologist (CEP), which quickly led to the development of the RCEP certification. With a clear delineation of the knowledge, skills, and abilities (KSAs) for the CEP now in hand, including the required amount of practical experience and emergency skills, the foundation was set up similar to what physical therapists, respiratory therapists, nurses, dietitians, and occupational therapists experienced in the evolution of their professions.

Although the CEP now has standardized academic and examination requirements (Box 20.1) as provided by the Clinical Exercise Physiology Association (CEPA), some questions persist regarding the job duties of this professional. Fortunately, owing to the hard work and coordinating efforts of numerous individuals and much research demonstrating the favorable effects of exercise therapy in patients with various chronic diseases, the CEP has become well-integrated into the healthcare team.

JOB DUTIES OF THE CEP

The skills and duties unique to the training of the CEP include: (*a*) prescribing safe and effective cardiorespiratory and musculoskeletal exercise in patients with a chronic disease; (*b*) evaluating and interpreting the acute cardiorespiratory and metabolic adaptations of patients to a single bout of submaximal or maximal exercise; and (*c*) establishing and evaluating behavioral, functional, clinical, and physiologic outcomes that result from participating in a chronic exercise training regimen. Some of the roles that a CEP undertakes in the practice of these skills include the following:

• Supervise noninvasive exercise testing laboratory personnel (e.g., manage the clinical exercise and cardio-

BOX 20.1 Definition of the Clinical Exercise Physiologist by the Clinical Exercise Physiology Association

A clinical exercise physiologist (CEP) is a healthcare professional who is trained to work with patients with chronic diseases where exercise training has been shown to be of therapeutic benefit, including but not limited to cardiovascular disease, pulmonary disease, and metabolic disorders. CEPs work primarily in a medically supervised environment that provides a program or service that is directed by a licensed physician. A CEP holds a minimum of a master's degree* in exercise physiology, exercise or movement science, or kinesiology AND is either licensed under state law or holds a

professional certification from a national organization that is functionally equivalent to either the ACSM's Certified Clinical Exercise Specialist or ACSM's Registered Clinical Exercise Physiologist credentials. An individual with a bachelor's degree in exercise physiology, exercise or movement science, or kinesiology and certified as an ACSM Certified Clinical Exercise Specialist is also considered qualified to perform exercise physiology services. All individuals providing exercise physiology services are trained in basic and advanced cardiac life support.

*Individuals with bachelors degrees in exercise science *and* who hold the ACSM CES or RCEP certification or equivalent before July 1, 2010 are considered Clinical Exercise Physiologists.

vascular technologists who perform ultrasound studies, nuclear imaging studies, Holter monitor scanning, pacemaker analysis, and graded exercise testing)
- Supervise and perform all forms of graded exercise testing in the clinical setting, including nuclear exercise tests, exercise echocardiographic studies, metabolic studies using measured gas analysis, and pharmacologic nuclear imaging studies;
- Develop, implement, and supervise the exercise components of cardiac and pulmonary rehabilitation programs, exercise oncology programs, and similar programs developed for patients with obesity, diabetes, chronic kidney disease and peripheral arterial disease;
- Serve as personal trainers for both healthy participants and those with a chronic disease or comorbid conditions;
- Work in the corporate fitness setting, screening employees for clinically covert disease and developing individualized exercise programs for employee health and wellness; and
- Work in the work-hardening setting, helping to train individuals with medical limitations or those who have been injured to regain their work skills in a particular active job setting.

WHAT FALLS WITHIN AND BEYOND THE SCOPE OF THE CEP?

To better appreciate the duties of the CEP, we encourage the reader to review closely the 2008 scope of practice for the RCEP as outlined by the ACSM (Box 20.2). Note that, as discussed in Boxes 20.1 and 20.2, the duties performed by a CEP are linked closely to treating patients with a chronic disease in which exercise has been shown to provide therapeutic benefit. This duty, among others, rests at the core of what we as CEPs do every day. Relative to what tasks should be avoided, we encourage the CEP to research and review the scopes of practice for registered dietitians, physical therapists, nurses, respiratory therapists, and athletic trainers. Just as with the CEP, each of these allied health professionals are academically prepared to provide KSAs that are unique to their field of study (4).

KSA 1.3.2-RCEP: Conduct a brief physical examination, including evaluation of peripheral edema; measuring blood pressure, peripheral pulses, and respiratory rate; and auscultate heart and lung sounds.

BOX 20.2 Scope of Practice for the Registered Clinical Exercise Physiologist by the American College of Sports Medicine

The Registered Clinical Exercise Physiologist is an allied health professional who works in the application of exercise and physical activity for those clinical and pathological situations where it has been shown to provide therapeutic or functional benefit. Persons for whom RCEP services are appropriate may include, but are not limited to those individuals with cardiovascular, pulmonary, metabolic, orthopedic, musculoskeletal, neuromuscular, neoplastic, immunologic, or hematologic disease. The RCEP performs exercise screening,

exercise and fitness testing, exercise prescription, exercise and physical activity counseling, exercise supervision, exercise and health education/promotion, and measurement and evaluation of exercise and physical activity related outcomes. The RCEP works individually or as part of an interdisciplinary team in a clinical, community, or public setting. The practice and supervision of the RCEP is guided by published professional guidelines, standards, and applicable state and federal regulations.

KSA 1.3.21-RCEP: Discuss patient test results with other healthcare professionals.

KSA 3.3.4-RCEP: Recognize and respond to abnormal signs and symptoms to exercise in individuals with pulmonary diseases.

SUPERVISION OF GRADED EXERCISE AND METABOLIC TESTING

As mentioned above, one of the duties that the CEP is trained to perform is the supervision of noninvasive graded exercise testing. Clinical internships and sufficient on-the-job training can well prepare CEPs to supervise graded exercise tests performed on both apparently healthy people and patients with clinically manifest disease. Thus, the job of safely performing or supervising graded exercise tests is a common occurrence in the United States. Concerning safety, CEPs routinely perform or supervise graded exercise tests on low-, intermediate-, and even high-risk populations with stable disease (5,6). Although it has also been shown that other nonphysician health professionals can safely supervise graded exercise tests (7,8), utilization of CEPs does offer one important advantage—much of the graduate course work that a CEP undertakes specifically addresses normal and abnormal cardiorespiratory responses to graded exercise.

Therefore, one opportunity for a career in exercise physiology is that of manager of a cardiac noninvasive laboratory, or supervisor of graded exercise or nuclear pharmacological testing. For the latter, the CEP usually performs the test with adjunct staff who are responsible to acquire the initial history and prepare the patient for testing (e.g., attach electrocardiographic [ECG] electrodes, measure resting vital signs). The CEP supervises the test and, once completed, he or she makes the initial written interpretation of the test and then consults with the supervising physician who makes the final clinical interpretation and follow-up recommendations for the patient (9).

THE DEVELOPMENT OF THE ACSM CERTIFICATIONS

Certifications offered through the ACSM continue to represent a "gold standard" for exercise professionals—one that many hospitals and medical fitness facilities often inquire about when they interview an employee candidate. In fact, many organizations now require ACSM certification for employment, or at the least, require an employee to gain ACSM certification within the first year of employment.

The ACSM certification process began in the mid 1970s, coinciding with the publication of the first *ACSM Guidelines for Graded Exercise Testing and Prescription* in

1975 (3). In the late 1970s and throughout the 1980s, the ACSM developed what was then referred to as the *Clinical Track* and the *Health Fitness Track* certifications. Included in the *Clinical Track* certifications were the Exercise Test Technologist (ETT), the Exercise Specialist (ES, now titled Clinical Exercise Specialist) and the Program Director (PD). Included in the *Health Fitness Track* certifications were the Exercise Leader (EL), the Health Fitness Instructor (HFI) and the Health Fitness Director (HFD) certifications.

Clinical Track certifications were designed for exercise professionals who worked with individuals with cardiac, pulmonary and metabolic diseases (e.g., diabetes), typically cared for in a cardiac or pulmonary rehabilitation program. A certification through the *Health Fitness Track* was designed for exercise professionals working in the fitness fields, such as personal trainers, exercise leaders in health fitness facilities and directors of YMCAs or corporate fitness programs. The goal of each certification is to assess the cognitive and practical proficiencies and skills of the aspiring exercise professional.

During this period, the ACSM also developed certification workshops at various colleges and universities around the country (10). These workshops were not designed to provide test materials for the candidate, but rather were structured to educate the applicant in most areas of the particular certification that he or she was going to take. For example, the ES workshop provided a number of courses taught by Master's- and Doctorate-prepared exercise professionals that covered areas such as pharmacology, exercise testing, injury prevention, pathophysiology, kinesiology and exercise prescription for special populations—all topics that were included on the ES written and practical examinations.

In the late 1980s and early 1990s, the ACSM tied each certification examination to a set of learner objectives or KSAs, which to this day, still provide the framework on which each certification is based. Questions on each examination are prevalidated, with each one testing a specific KSA. Every 3 years the KSAs are revalidated or revised, using a survey technique called a Job Task Analysis (JTA). The JTA is completed by a representative sample of professionals currently working in the field to ensure all KSAs are contemporary and important.

In response to market forces, in the late 1990s the ACSM consolidated its certifications. As a result, several of the examinations and their related credentials were eliminated (i.e., ETT, PD, EL, and HFD). Those who hold these certifications still must complete continuing education credits to maintain these certifications and each continues to be recognized and valued in the health profession.

The certification process for the exercise professional residing in the United States still represents a dynamic journey that continues to this day. Two relatively recent and important milestones for the ACSM along the way were the elimination of the practical component from the certification examination and use of computer-based testing in place of the traditional paper-and-pencil format. The latter modification in the process is consistent with the certification examinations given to other professionals throughout the United States. A primary reason for the above changes was a realization that assessing the practical skills of each candidate could not easily be made uniform nationwide. To correct this, practical skills are now incorporated into the computer-based examination using case studies, vinettes, and video loops that require the applicant to identify the correct and incorrect method for completing a task. This approach was an important step that allowed the entire ACSM certification program to become certified by the National Commission of Credentialing Agencies (NCCA). The use of the computer-based examinations also gives applicants the opportunity to have immediate feedback on whether they passed or failed the examination, as well as the ability to sit for the examination at any one of thousands of testing locations throughout the world.

THE DEVELOPMENT OF THE ACSM RCEP EXAMINATION

The development of the ACSM RCEP certification was a long and arduous process, with a remarkable amount of dialog and debate along the way. On one side were those who were opposed to this certification, seeing it as a certification that might conflict with the ES (retitled Clinical Exercise Specialist in 2008) and PD certifications. On the other side were those who felt that a new certification was needed to accommodate the expanding role and use of exercise in the care and treatment of patients with other chronic diseases (e.g., neuromuscular, musculoskeletal, immunologic, oncologic). Today, the RCEP certification is now available exclusively to Master's-prepared individuals trained in exercise physiology. At the same time, it was agreed that the CES examination would continue to be made available to a wide range of professionals, including nurses, physical therapists, and Bachelor's-prepared exercise professionals.

Highlighted below is a brief summary of the time line depicting the development of the RCEP.

- May 1996: The CEP scope of practice is adopted by the ACSM.
- October 1997: *ACSM's Exercise Management for Persons with Chronic Diseases and Disabilities* is first published, providing a strong impetus for the development of a certification for an exercise professional proficient in prescribing safe exercise for patients with a multitude of medical conditions.
- May 1998: The ACSM Fellows vote to establish an RCEP Registry Board.

- November 1998: The RCEP KSAs are completed for the pilot year (1998) by expert panels for each practice domain and are approved by the Registry Board.
- June–September 1999: The first RCEP written pilot examinations are given, totaling 87 participants.
- June 2000: The first official written RCEP examination is given at the national ACSM meeting in Indianapolis, IN with 33 participants.
- February 2002: *ACSM's Resources for Clinical Exercise Physiology: Musculoskeletal, Neuromuscular, Neoplastic, Immunologic, and Hematologic Conditions* is first published (Myers, Herbert, and Humphrey senior editors; Figoni, Neiman, and Pitetti section editors)
- January 2006: The inaugural RCEP workshop is offered at Henry Ford Hospital in Detroit, MI. Two other workshops are held that year, one at Henry Ford and the other at the University of Louisiana at Monroe, Monroe, LA.
- May 2006: The first on-line, computer-based RCEP examination is offered at multiple sites across the United States.

The RCEP examination is unique in that it covers areas not included in the CES examination. The six clinical practice areas of the RCEP include the cardiovascular (30% of test questions), pulmonary (10%), metabolic (20%), orthopedic/musculoskeletal (20%), neuromuscular (10%), and oncologic, immunologic and hematologic (10%) domains. Currently, to be eligible to take the RCEP examination applicants must have: (*a*) a Master's degree in an approved clinical exercise science field, (*b*) ACSM CES certification (current or expired) or 600 hours of broad-based clinical experience involving diseases germane to the RCEP examination, (*c*) submission of Master's degree transcripts, and (*d*) verification of current Basic Cardiac Life Support (BLS) certification. The RCEP certification continues to gain popularity and is now required for CEPs due to the broad range of disease states encountered in daily practice.

ACADEMIC STANDARDIZATION AND CURRICULUM ACCREDITATION

For years, healthcare professionals and hospital administrators relied heavily on anecdotal comments from other practitioners and individual academic centers to discern the quality of the many exercise science academic programs around the country (11,12). In 2002, the ACSM introduced the University Connection (UC) program, which served for several years as an endorsement program for undergraduate and graduate studies that prepared individuals for the ACSM credentials. Although initially quite popular, this program was ultimately superceded by the Committee on Accreditation for the Exercise Sciences (CoAES; www.coaes.org). Working under the auspices of the Commission on Accreditation of Allied Health

Education Programs (CAAHEP), the CoAES is composed of nine sponsoring organizations, all charged with the task of initially establishing and now maintaining the standards and guidelines for academic curriculum in the exercise sciences. Presently, the nine professional organizations that co-sponsor the CoAES are as follows:

- American College of Sports Medicine
- American Alliance for Health, Physical Education, Recreation, and Dance
- American Association of Cardiovascular and Pulmonary Rehabilitation
- American Council on Exercise
- American Kinesiotherapy Association
- Medical Fitness Association
- National Academy of Sports Medicine
- National Strength and Conditioning Association
- The Cooper Institute (Institute for Aerobics Research)

Although not exclusive to ACSM credentials, the CoAES offers standards and guidelines that are consistent with the KSAs for the ACSM CES, RCEP and other ACSM certifications relevant to the health-fitness field. The CoAES recognizes four professional categories specific to the exercise practitioner (12):

- **Graduate programs for the CEP**—practitioners who work under the direction of a physician in the application of physical activity and behavioral interventions in clinical situations where they have been scientifically proven to provide therapeutic or functional benefit.
- **Graduate programs for the applied exercise physiologist**—practitioners who manage programs to assess, design, and implement individual and group exercise and fitness programs for apparently healthy individuals and individuals with controlled diseases.
- **Undergraduate programs in exercise science**—practitioners of undergraduate exercise science programs who are trained to assess, design, and implement individual and group exercise and fitness programs for individuals who are apparently healthy, as well as those with controlled diseases. These individuals are skilled in evaluating health behaviors and risk factors, conducting fitness assessments, writing appropriate exercise prescriptions and motivating individuals to modify negative health behaviors and to maintain positive lifestyle behaviors for overall health promotion.
- **Certificate and Associate degree programs for the personal fitness trainer**—practitioners who work with a wide variety of client demographics in one-on-one and small group environments. Certified personal trainers are familiar with a wide variety of exercise interventions to improve and maintain overall health. They are also proficient in leading and demonstrating safe and effective methods of exercise and motivating individuals to begin and continue with healthy behaviors.

They consult with appropriate health and medical professionals when the client's physical condition exceeds the expertise of the personal trainer's level of education, training and experience.

Over the next several years, as more and more graduate programs become accredited through CAAHEP, the graduates from these programs will bring into the profession a uniform level of training and preparation that will do much to further standardize the role and use of the CEP within healthcare. Moreover, graduating from a CAAHEP accredited program will help define for human resource personnel working in healthcare, the specific nature of the training completed by those who apply for exercise-related job openings.

THE PROFESSION TAKES SHAPE

Although it has taken some 30 years to reach the point of professionalization that the CEP enjoys today, many of the key elements are now in place. A standardized curriculum exists at the Master's level for universities to adopt through CAAHEP; a professional organization (CEPA) is in place to address relevant policy issues and to advocate on behalf of the profession; a standardized examination (RCEP) exists to evaluate proficiencies on completion of graduate studies; and several textbooks (bodies of knowledge) are published that apply the practice of clinical exercise physiology across a broad array of patients with chronic diseases and disabilities.

Of all of these, perhaps the greatest ongoing force in the continued shaping of the profession rests with CEPA (www.ACSM-CEPA.org). This professional organization is now responsible for continuing to address the issues important to the field, advocating on behalf of the profession, providing its members with continuing education and training, and working with other organizations and public policy makers to ensure that CEPs are fully integrated into the healthcare delivery team.

LICENSURE ISSUES FOR THE CLINICAL EXERCISE PHYSIOLOGIST

Another important issue that deserves to be discussed addresses the question: "Should the CEP be licensed to practice their profession?" (9,11,13–27). In a 1993 survey of ACSM members, 94% were in favor of licensure for practicing exercise professionals. In a 2007 survey of North Carolina exercise physiologists, an almost identical percentage of practitioners favored pursuing licensure. Currently, in the United States only Louisiana requires licensure for exercise physiologists (signed into law on June 20, 1995). Other states such as West Virginia, Massachusetts, and California have tried unsuccessfully to develop state licensure for CEPs. The major hurdle in California was that no quantitative studies could be cited demonstrating, as scientifically as possible, that licensure was needed to safeguard the consumer (22). States such as North Carolina are still in the early stages of investigating licensure issues.

Within any discussion of licensure, it is first necessary to distinguish the differences between licensure, accreditation, and professional certification (13,14,27). *Licensure* is granted by a political or governmental body in a particular state to individuals applying for licensure (not programs) and provides a legal basis to engage in or practice a profession. In turn, the practice is usually defined with very specific and delimited authorizations. A license is the minimal qualification required to practice in a regulated area and, conversely, if a CEP wishes to practice in a state then licensure is required. Because statutory requirements for licensure vary from state to state, when a licensed professional moves from one state to another, he or she must first become licensed in that state before practicing in the field. *Accreditation* refers to a special recognition or status granted to academic programs (not individuals) offered at schools, colleges, institutes, or universities by an association, organization, or commission (e.g., CAAHEP) that has developed and established eligibility and performance standards. *Certification*, or in the case of the ACSM a registry examination, is granted by an association to an individual who meets predetermined qualifications and competency standards established by the granting agency (e.g., the RCEP). Accreditation, certification and registry are voluntary processes that do not necessarily advantage or restrict an individual's employment.

The language in the Louisiana bill was simple and clearly defined the CEP, their qualifications for licensure, and the "grandfathering" of current practitioners. The process took approximately 14 months (April 1994 to June 1995) and was made possible by a core group of practicing CEPs in Louisiana. Their licensure requirements now include the following (24):

1. Have a Master of science or Master of education degree in an exercise studies curriculum from an accredited school.
2. Be certified as an ACSM CES.
3. Successfully complete an internship of 300 hours in a cardiopulmonary program under the supervision of a CEP.

The bill also includes provisions for those exempt from licensing requirements, such as those employed or supervised by a physician to perform graded exercise testing, exercise science students performing an internship under the supervision of a licensed CEP, and CEPs employed by federal or state agencies.

Although this was a landmark step for the profession, much work remains both within that state and elsewhere. Salaries for CEPs continue to remain low when compared with other allied health practitioners and state health officials and hospital administrators rarely look to this qualification in matters related to provision of exercise

services in healthcare. Given that Louisiana licensure has been in existence for less than 15 years, it is possible that more time is required before the CEP achieves the level of recognition that is commensurate to that of other allied health professionals.

In addition to Louisiana, another template for state licensure is underway in Massachusetts through the Massachusetts Association of Clinical Exercise Physiologists (MACEP). This model uses the RCEP examination as the state licensure examination. The process began in 2001 and in 2009, a fifth attempt will be made.

Four important license-related issues that needed to be addressed became evident through the CEP licensure initiative in Massachusetts (26):

1. Is there a technical basis for practice?
2. Is there a distinct scope of practice?
3. Is there a link between the practice, skills, and standards of training?
4. Is there public acceptance of the profession?

A key point of importance regarding CEP licensure in Massachusetts pertained to restricting the practice of clinical exercise physiology to persons meeting a minimal standard of practice. In this respect, the issue came down to a case of public safety, with the Council of State Governments indicating that four additional points needed to be addressed relative to securing licensure (28):

1. Whether the unregulated practice of an occupation would endanger or harm the health, safety, or welfare of citizens and whether the potential harm is recognizable and not remote;
2. Whether the practice of an occupation requires specialized skill or training and whether the public needs assurance of initial and continuing occupational abilities;
3. Whether the public is, or could be, effectively protected by other means; and
4. Whether the cost and economic effectiveness of regulation outweighs any anti-competitive or detrimental effects to the public.

Given the experiences of the MACEP, CEPs in other states must carefully evaluate their needs, including the potential cost of regulation and possible resistance from other health professional groups. Additionally, another possible disadvantage of state licensure is that licensing may mean some loss of professional autonomy and possible regulation and restriction of practice. There may also be an increased risk of exposure to malpractice claims and litigation, making malpractice insurance essentially mandatory for the CEP (25).

For example, in the proposed licensing bill in Massachusetts, licensed CEPs would be required to work under the authority of a physician, seeing only those clients with a physician's referral. How this applies to the CEP who also wishes to provide and be compensated for personal trainer services he or she renders is unsure. A major advantage of state licensure is that it restricts those people who are not qualified or who call themselves CEPs without proper academic training from incorrectly dispensing exercise recommendations or advice, thereby lessening the chance of harming the client or patient.

SALARIES FOR CLINICAL EXERCISE PHYSIOLOGISTS

The annual starting salaries for CEPs in the United States vary widely by area of the country. In general, this level of compensation is less than that paid to other allied health professionals (e.g., physical therapists, nurses, and respiratory therapists.) Part of the discrepancy is owing to the fairly recent origin of the profession and the prior absence of a well-shaped and defined profession. In this respect, registration and licensure efforts, as well as the work of the CEPA, have greatly added to the credibility of the profession, providing a far more defined scope of practice than previously. Nevertheless, the "base pay" for the CEP during his or her first year of full-time employment has yet to catch up with what is paid to other allied health professionals.

The most comprehensive survey of salaries for exercise physiologists to date was published by Porcari in 1996 in the AACVPR *News and Views* (29). In this three-page document, he summarized the compensation of 242 exercise physiologists, based on degree of education, years of work experience, ACSM certifications and region of the country. Salaries for exercise physiologists who served as a director of a cardiac rehabilitation program ranged from $28,421 with a Bachelor's degree and less than 3 years experience to $59,112 for those with an EdD/PhD and more than 10 years experience. Exercise professionals with ACSM certification made approximately $2,000–$3,000 more per year than those who did not have ACSM certification. Among the general staff, exercise physiologists with a Master's degree made approximately $5,000–$6,000 more per year than those with a Bachelor's degree, varying by region of the country.

THE FUTURE OF CLINICAL EXERCISE PHYSIOLOGY

Despite wide-spread public health efforts to the contrary, many Americans experience and remain at increased risk for the development of chronic lifestyle-related diseases or disorders. Specifically, heart disease, hypertension, certain cancers, diabetes, arthritis, peripheral arterial disease, and obesity remain important health concerns that have all been shown to benefit from regular, safe exercise. As unfortunate as these disease trends may be, they do suggest that the future for the CEP remains optimistic— one that is full of growth potential for the professional properly trained to use exercise to improve clinical out-

comes and reduce future risk. This need is magnified by the fact that the baby boomer generation continues to expand, increasing the number and percentage of people age 60 years and older.

Moreover, while Americans are now living longer, we are also currently in obesity and diabetes "epidemics" resulting from sedentary living, poor dietary habits, high stress lifestyles, and overall lack of physical activity in our daily lifestyles. The need for the expertise of the CEP is now greater than ever before! With the passage of the Pulmonary and Cardiac Rehabilitation Act of 2008, the CEP will now be valued and treated as an equal with all other allied health professionals who work in cardiopulmonary rehabilitation and health/wellness programs. Clearly, a favorable work-force environment awaits the practicing CEP.

REFERENCES

1. Brown SP. Profession or discipline: The role of exercise physiology in allied health. *Clinical Exercise Physiology* 2000;2:168.
2. Foster C. ACSM and the emergence of the profession of exercise physiologist. *Med Sci Sports Exerc* 2003;35(8):101.
3. American College of Sports Medicine. *Guidelines for Graded Exercise Testing and Prescription.* Philadelphia: Lippincott Williams & Wilkins, 1975.
4. Sass C, Eickhoff-Shemek JM, Manore M, et al. Crossing the line: Understanding the scope of practice between registered dietitians and health/fitness professionals. *ACSM's Health & Fitness Journal* 2007;11(3):12–19.
5. Knight JA, Laubach CA, Butcher RJ, et al. Supervision of clinical exercise testing by exercise physiologists. *Am J Cardiol* 1995;75:390–1.
6. Franklin BA, Gordon S, Timmis GC, et al. Is direct supervision of exercise stress testing routinely necessary? *Chest* 1997;111: 262–5.
7. Zecchin RP, Chai YY, Roach KA, et al. Is nurse-supervised exercise stress testing a safe practice? *Heart Lung* 1999;28(3):175–85.
8. Cahalin LP, Blessey RL, Kummer D, et al. The safety of exercise testing performed independently by physical therapists. *J Cardiopulm Rehabil* 1987;7:269–76.
9. Gillespie WJ. A model for licensure of exercise professionals. *Exercise Standards and Malpractice Reporter* 1993;7(6):81–7.
10. Otto RM, Wygand J. American College of Sports Medicine Exercise Specialist workshop/certification—A modality for career preparation. *J Cardiopulm Rehabil* 1996;16:353–5.
11. Foster C, Roitman J, Harnett C. Profession or discipline: Asking the right questions or turf protection? *Clinical Exercise Physiology* 2000;2:168.
12. Costanzo D. Recognizing academic excellence. *ACSM's Health & Fitness Journal* 2007;11(2):31–2.
13. Baechle TR. National guidelines for certification programs. *Exercise Standards and Malpractice Reporter* 1993;7(6):91–4.
14. Gillespie WJ, Protas EJ. A pro/con debate about registration, licensure of exercise practitioners. *American College of Sports Medicine Certified News* 1995;4(2):4–7.
15. Pescatello LS, Lynch EA. Health care reform and the exercise professional. *American College of Sports Medicine Certified News* 1994;4(2):1–3.
16. Herbert WG. The clinical exercise physiologist: a viewpoint on current status. *Exercise Standards and Malpractice Reporter* 1992;9(3):33–7.
17. Ribisl P. Certification or licensure for health/fitness professionals. *Exercise Standards and Malpractice Reporter* 1991;5(2):22–4.
18. Herbert WG. Is fitness instruction legislation necessary? *Exercise Standards and Malpractice Reporter* 1994;8(3):38–40.
19. Sol N. Certification or licensure of fitness professionals: the debate begins. *Exercise Standards and Malpractice Reporter* 1990;4(5):65–9.

20. Editorial: Licensure or certification of fitness professionals. *Exercise Standards and Malpractice Reporter* 1990;4(4):59.

21. Herbert DL. Association responses to proposed licensure requirements for fitness professionals. *Exercise Standards and Malpractice Reporter* 1994;8(4):49–53.

22. Herbert DL. Is licensure "the future" for CEPs? *Exercise Standards and Malpractice Reporter* 1992;5(2):91–4.

23. Herbert WG. The clinical exercise physiologist: brief speculation on the future. *Exercise Standards and Malpractice Reporter* 1995;9(4):53–5.

24. Boulet BM. Licensure of clinical exercise physiologists in Louisiana—A retrospective look at the process. *Exercise Standards and Malpractice Reporter* 1995;9(6):81–5.

25. Herbert WG. Licensure of clinical exercise physiologists: impressions concerning the new law in Louisiana. *Exercise Standards and Malpractice Reporter* 1995;9(5):65:68–70.

26. Garber CE. Should clinical exercise physiologists be regulated in Massachusetts? A case for support of HB 3950. Publication presented to the Massachusetts Board of Licensure, October 2005, pp.1–16.

27. Eickhoff-Shemek JM, Herbert DL. Is licensure in your future? Issues to consider—Part I. *ACSM's Health and Fitness Journal* 2007;11(5):35–7.

28. The Council of State Government. Occupational Licensing Legislation in states. Chicago, 1952.

29. Porcari JP. Exercise physiologists salary survey results. *AACVPR News & Views* 1996;10(1):5–7.

Client Referral and Consulting Relations with Allied Professions

APPROPRIATE SCREENING METHODOLOGIES, TESTS, AND OBSERVATIONS TO GUIDE THE NECESSITY OF A REFERRAL

FIRST DO NO HARM

The American College of Sports Medicine (ACSM) defines the scope of care for a Clinical Exercise Physiologist (CEP) as follows:

> The CEP works in the application of exercise and physical activity for those clinical and pathological situations where it has been shown to provide therapeutic or functional benefit. Patients for whom services are appropriate may include, but not be limited to those with cardiovascular, pulmonary, metabolic, musculoskeletal, neuromuscular, neoplastic, immunologic, and hematologic diseases and conditions. The CEP applies exercise principles to groups such as geriatric, pediatric, or obstetric populations, and to society as a whole in preventive activities. The CEP performs exercise evaluation, exercise prescription, exercise supervision, exercise education, and exercise outcome evaluation. The practice of CEPs should be restricted to clients who are referred by and are under the continued care of a licensed physician (1).

Anytime the results from an assessment indicate that a needed treatment falls outside the CEP's scope of care, a referral should be initiated. Failure to practice within one's scope of care can lead to allegations of malpractice and potentially serious legal ramifications (2). A careful, well-planned assessment of a patient's medical history and current health status, as well as a thorough discussion with that person will reveal a wealth of information including the presence of cardiovascular disease risk factors, orthopedic limitations, medication use and drug allergies, and exercise and physical activity history. Obtaining a complete history is extremely important for the appropriate and safe planning of an individual's exercise program, as well as to guide decisions about the need for a possible medical referral.

Problem-focused client assessment should always precede any treatment. The plan for any exercise treatment recommendations should be, to a large extent, the result of a thorough assessment that includes, but may not be limited to, functional capacity, musculoskeletal strength and endurance, balance and gait, and body composition. Depending on the person's age, medical history, and present health status, additional tests may be requested from either the referring physician or the primary care physician. For those above the age of 45 years for men and 55 years for women, a graded exercise test may be recommended to determine the cardiovascular risk associated with increasing physical activity. Additionally, a measure of fasting blood glucose may reveal the need for diabetic counseling and will help to identify individual who have the metabolic syndrome.

If an abnormal finding is observed, either during the course of taking a client's history or other fitness assessment, it may become necessary to request additional information from the referring physician or, possibly, refer the client back to the referring physician. Signs or symptoms suggesting the need for physician referral include, but may not be limited to, persistent muscle or joint pain, claudication, and chest, jaw, back, or arm pain associated with exertion. The use of an appropriate screening tool, such as the Physical Activity Readiness Questionnaire (PAR-Q) (3) or modified American Heart Association (AHA)/ACSM Health/Fitness Facility Preparticipation Screening Questionnaire (4), may help determine global risk and possible need for exercise testing or exercise therapy.

REFERRAL FOR PHYSICAL THERAPY

Physical therapists provide services to persons who have physical impairments, functional limitations, disabilities, or changes in physical function and health status resulting from injury, disease, or other causes (5). During the assessment of an individual by a CEP, a test may reveal the need for specific skills related to the practice of physical therapy. For example, an initial assessment of gait and balance may have revealed that the person has balance issues that place him or her at higher risk for falls. A more advanced assessment of gait, balance, and fall risk may require the skills of a physical therapist. Persistent musculoskeletal complaints, such as knee pain with mild to moderate exertion, may require a physical therapy evaluation. Additionally, the need for advanced treatment for musculoskeletal injuries and inflammation generally requires the skills of a physical therapist.

REFERRAL FOR NUTRITIONAL COUNSELING

The typical western diet is associated with increased risk for chronic diseases, such as coronary artery disease (CAD) and certain types of cancer and stroke. According to the Centers for Disease Control and Prevention (CDC), 14% of all deaths in the United States can be attributed to poor diets, sedentary lifestyle, or both 20% from CAD and stroke, and 30% of cancers may be prevented by eating an appropriate diet. Additionally, the CDC estimates that 30% of type 2 diabetes cases can be prevented through dietary intervention and obesity control. Hypertension can be reduced with added consumption of fruits and vegetables and bodyweight reduction. The United States Department of Agriculture (USDA) Economic Research Service estimates that improved dietary patterns could save upwards of $43 billion in medical care costs and lost productivity resulting from disability associated with CAD, cancer, stroke and diabetes in the United States each year (6).

An assessment of dietary status, blood lipids, and fasting blood glucose can assist the CEP with the decision regarding the need for a referral. Dietary assessment tools, such as the Diet Habit Survey (7) or Medfcts (8), can guide the decision-making process by providing information on the adequacy of the present eating pattern and the need for a referral.

All persons who present with a diagnosis of diabetes (type 1 or type 2), renal disease, CAD, or pulmonary disease should be referred to a registered, licensed dietitian for assessment and dietary intervention. The cornerstone of treatment for all of the above-mentioned conditions is dietary in nature. Commitment to appropriate dietary modifications or treatments is often difficult because of the many social situations that revolve around food consumption, which may require the additional services of a behaviorist in addition to a dietitian.

REFERRAL FOR STRESS MANAGEMENT AND PSYCHOSOCIAL COUNSELING

Psychosocial distress is now well documented as a major risk factor for death, nonfatal myocardial infarction, ischemia, angina, and noncompliance to therapeutic lifestyle changes, such as exercise training, smoking cessation, and diabetic treatment regimens (9). Depression alone is responsible for more than $44 billion in lost productivity and absenteeism each year, and is the number one cause for disability claims. The average annual cost of medical treatment per depressed patient is $8,600 (6).

The ability to adhere to any lifestyle modification, including exercise training, often depends on an individual's psychosocial status at the time of treatment. In particular, depression, anxiety, and hostility have been shown to dramatically affect the ability to comprehend and act on recommended lifestyle changes, such as exercise training. An assessment of psychosocial status such as the Beck Depression Inventory (10) or the Anger Inventory section of the Minnesota Multiphasic Personality Inventory-2 (MMPI-2) (11) may assist the CEP on the need for referral to a mental health specialist.

REFERRAL FOR WEIGHT MANAGEMENT

During the past 20 years, Americans have become increasingly overweight and obese. The CDC now estimates that 127 million Americans more than 20 years of age are considered overweight (body mass index, [BMI] >25 kg/m^2) (6). The assessment of weight-related risk should be a part of all initial evaluations related to beginning an exercise program and increasing a person's habitual level of physical activity. Relatively simple strategies that should be part of all initial assessments include the calculation of BMI, abdominal adiposity (circumference measures), and percent body fat estimates. Although limitations exist to the use of BMI, it remains an essential first tool for the risk stratification of weight-related issues.

Risk stratification by BMI category allows the CEP to grossly determine if a person is obese (BMI >30 kg/m^2) and determine the necessity for referral to other disciplines, including, but not necessarily limited to, a registered or licensed dietitian and behaviorist. Abdominal adiposity has been shown to increase the risk of developing CAD and diabetes and accelerates the risk of progression of those diseases. For screening purposes, abdominal adiposity can be estimated by obtaining the "waist" girth. Accurate use of the "waist" girth as a surrogate measure of abdominal adiposity depends on the location and measurement of that girth. The National Cholesterol Education Program (NCEP) in the Adult Treatment Panel (ATP) III guideline (12) recommends that the girth be measured at the iliac crest. Use of this waist girth to estimate abdominal adiposity and to assess for the risk of the metabolic syndrome requires an accurate site determination and an accurate measurement using an appropriate tape measure with a known constant tension. Determination of the percentage body fat is somewhat more difficult to estimate accurately and requires the use of skinfold calipers in the hands of a well-trained technician, water or air displacement technologies, or the use of radiologic tests such as the dual-energy x-ray absorptiometry (DXA) scan.

REFERRAL TO HOME OR COMMUNITY-BASED PROGRAMS

The goal of the exercise intervention is long-term health enhancement. The major consideration for home or community-based referral is safety of the individual with secondary concerns around that person's ability to achieve and or maintain the evidence-based medicine goals that will lead to overall risk reduction and health enhancement. Home programs can be effective if they are appropriately designed to match an individual's physiologic status and psychological make-up. The CEP will probably find it easier to prescribe the mode, intensity, duration, and frequency of the exercise intervention than to determine the likelihood of long-term adherence and success. Because the goal is long-term health enhancement, however, factors such as motivation and self-efficacy must be carefully considered and may require the assistance of a behavioral specialist.

When determining to refer an individual to a home program, multiple factors need to be taken into consideration, including the patient's ability to self monitor, activity preferences, time constraints, equipment needs, and preferences as related to an individual or group environment. Generally, home programs should be restricted to low- or moderate-risk individuals. Both low- and moderate-risk patients should be able to verbalize a complete understanding of their exercise prescription and monitor heart rate and perceived exertion, recognize signs and symptoms of exercise intolerance, and have a plan in place should an adverse event occur. Moderate risk patients also should have an exercise partner who is trained in cardiopulmonary resuscitation (CPR) and a heart rate monitor to assist with exercise intensity control. Additionally, an informed consent for home exercise that clearly explains the risks and responsibilities of the client should be carefully reviewed and signed by the client.

Home and community based programs with little or no trained supervision should be limited to persons with a low to moderate level of risk for the development of adverse events, particularly cardiovascular events. The ACSM has developed a simple tool for the assessment of cardiovascular risk that stratifies patients' risk into low, moderate, and high and should be used to risk stratify a client before entrance into any exercise program (4). Additionally, those with moderate to high risk who chose a community-based program should discuss their risk status, the level of training of the supervising staff, and the emergency plan for that facility with the staff of the community program. They should plan with the supervising staff to wear some mutually agreed on type of distinguishing clothing, such as a red hat or arm band, to allow for quick identification in case of an adverse event.

Certain types of psychosocial issues, such as depression, may determine the recommended level of supervision necessary to maximize the likelihood of success of a home or community-based exercise program. Persons with even mild to moderate depression or health-related anxiety may benefit from a more structured environment and at least a moderate level of supervision. It is also important to determine the type of facility and equipment needed to match the client's health status and preferences. For example, clients with no muscular or orthopedic issues may be able to achieve their goals with a relatively simple program of walking with a minimal amount of equipment needed for strength and flexibility training. The only facility and equipment needs would be a suitable place to walk, a heart rate monitor, a pedometer, and some resistance bands for strength training. On the other hand, a patient with significant orthopedic limitations may need to be referred to a community-based aquatic program to minimize weight-bearing musculoskeletal stress.

Program affordability and travel requirements also are important issues that need to be considered when recommending a community-based exercise program. Even relatively low cost programs may place considerable strain on an individual's financial resources. Therefore, it is important to discuss financial limitations with the client before designing or recommending a home or community-based program.

Typically, persons are willing to travel up to 30 minutes one way to participate in a community-based program. A travel time of greater than 30 minutes may be time and cost prohibitive and may adversely affect adherence. An individual's ability to drive must also be considered. If the person does not drive, the availability and cost of public transportation must also be taken into consideration.

REFERENCES

1. Myers J, Herbert W, Humphrey R, eds. *ACSM'S Resources for Clinical Exercise Physiology: Musculoskeletal, Neuromuscular, Neoplastic, Immunologic, and Hematologic Conditions.* Philadelphia: Lippincott Williams & Wilkins; 2002:243.
2. Herbert DL, Herbert WG. *Legal Aspects of Preventive and Rehabilitative Exercise Programs,* 2nd ed. Canton, Ohio: Professional Reports Corporation; 1989:74–9.
3. *Canadian Society for Exercise Physiology. PAR-Q and You.* Gloucester, Ontario: Canadian Society for Exercise Physiology; 1994:1–2.
4. *ACSM's Guidelines for Exercise Testing and Prescription,* 7th ed. Baltimore: Lippincott Williams & Wilkins, 2006.
5. Guide to physical therapy practice, 2nd ed. *Phys Ther* 2001;81: 9–744.
6. United States Department of Agriculture Economic Research Service: Diet Quality and Nutrition. www.ERS.USDA.GOV/BROWSE/Diethealthsafety/dietquality/nutrition.htm
7. Connor SL, Gustafson JR, Sexton G, et al. The Oregon Diet Habit Survey: A new method of dietary assessment that relates to plasma cholesterol changes. *J Am Diet Assoc* 1992;92:41–7.
8. Kris-Etherton P, Eissenstat B, Jaxx S, et al. Validation for MEDFICTS, a dietary assessment instrument for evaluating adherence to total and saturated fat recommendations of the National Cholesterol Education Program Step 1 and Step 2 diets. *J Am Diet Assoc* 2001;101:81–6.
9. Ketterer MW, Mahr G, Goldberg AD. Psychological factors affecting a medical condition: Ischemic coronary heart disease. *J Psychosomatic Res* 2000;48 (4/5):357–68.
10. Beck AT, Steer, RA. *Beck Depression Inventory Manual.* Oronto, Canada: Psychological Corp. Harcourt, Brace, Jovanovich; 1987.

11. Butcher JN, Dahlstrom WG, Graham JR, et al. *MMPI-2: Minnesota Multiphasic Personality Inventory-2. Manual for Administration and Scoring.* Minneapolis, Minn: University of Minnesota Press; 1989.

12. National Cholesterol Education Program (NCEP) Expert Panel on Detection, Evaluation, and Treatment of High Blood Cholesterol in Adults (Adult Treatment Panel III), Final Report. *Circulation* 2002;106(25):3143–421.

The Clinical Exercise Physiologist (CEP) provides professional service and advice to a variety of individuals with a broad range of chronic diseases and disabling conditions. These services, which include health screenings, fitness assessments, exercise testing, exercise prescriptions, and physical activity counseling, are increasingly being performed outside of hospital-based facilities. In this regard, the ability to accurately assess and document pre- and postexercise functional outcomes is particularly important in the long-term clinical and exercise management of these patients. This chapter briefly addresses important skills for assessing and reporting functional outcomes that can be used for a variety of clinical conditions and chronic health problems.

WHAT IS FUNCTIONAL OUTCOMES REPORTING

Documentation is a familiar term to anyone working in the healthcare industry. With the increasing complexity of interventional medical practices, third-party reimbursement, and federal privacy laws (Health Insurance Portability and Accountability Act of 1996, HIPAA) (46), the need for careful, focused documentation and reporting of clinical and functional outcomes has received increased attention. *Functional outcomes reporting* is a method of documentation that emphasizes the patient's medical condition relative to his or her ability to perform activities of daily living (ADLs). Adapted from the SOAP format of note writing (**S**–Subjective; **O**–Objective; **A**–Assessment; **P**–Plan) (49), functional outcomes reporting is increasingly being used by various health professionals to improve the quality and continuity of patient care and improve communication between the medical community and third-party payers. These outcomes provide important information regarding a person's ability to perform basic ADLs considered essential for daily self-care. In addition, healthcare providers and third-party payers are interested in a person's ability to perform activities that are considered *instrumental* to maintaining functional independence within their homes, workplace, and other social environments. See Table 22.1 for examples of basic and instrumental ADLs.

CONSIDERATIONS FOR REPORTING FUNCTIONAL OUTCOMES

To ensure high-quality patient care, the CEP must consider the target audience for whom the report is being written (patient versus physician versus third-party provider). Accurate and concise documentation is essential to bridge the gap between services provided, medical management, and third-party reimbursement. Several factors, including prior and current levels of function, description of current impairments (and how they affect function), goals and expected outcomes, and the exercise plan (frequency, intensity, duration, modes), should be included in the initial documentation (Fig. 22.1). Follow-up documentation, or progress reports, should summarize the exercise intervention provided, describe any changes in functional status, and update patient goals and exercise recommendations. Therefore, the CEP should consider several objective (O) and subjective (S) areas when reporting functional outcomes:

- Physical examination findings and test results (O)
- Past and current medical history (O)
- Patient complaints and symptoms (S)
- Goals and expected outcomes (S)
- Prior and current levels of physical function (S)

PHYSICAL EXAMINATION FINDINGS AND MEDICAL HISTORY REVIEW

Although the details of the clinical evaluation lie beyond the scope of this text, several key components are particularly important for the CEP working in preventive and rehabilitative settings. The physical examination is typically performed by a licensed physician or other qualified licensed healthcare provider. CEPs working in clinical settings should, however, understand the importance of the physical examination for identifying abnormal findings and evaluating the severity of patient symptoms or complaints during any exercise assessment or intervention they may plan, implement, and supervise for their client. When used in conjunction with appropriate exercise and functional assessments, these findings may provide valuable information concerning the beneficial outcomes of various treatments, including exercise.

TABLE 22.1. EXAMPLES OF BASIC AND INSTRUMENTAL ACTIVITIES OF DAILY LIVING (ADLs)

Basic ADLs
Bathing
Dressing and undressing
Feeding
Using the bathroom
Grooming
Transfer from bed to chair, and back

Instrumental ADLs
Driving
Household cleaning
Laundry
Preparing meals
Taking medications
Shopping
Managing household finances
Taking garbage out
Climbing one or more flights of stairs
Care of pets
Use of telephone or other communication device

In addition to reviewing the findings from the physical examination, the CEP should integrate some form of standardized Health History Questionnaire (HHQ) to evaluate the patient's past medical history and current health status, including cardiovascular disease (CVD) risk factors, symptom history, medication use and drug allergies, orthopedic problems, and exercise or physical activity history. Many standardized screening questionnaires are available, including the Physical Activity Readiness Questionnaire (PAR-Q) (7) and modified American Heart Association (AHA)/American College of Sports Medicine (ACSM) Health/Fitness Facility Participation Screening Questionnaire (2). Both screening tools are helpful in identifying individuals who would benefit from medical consultation before beginning an exercise program; however the AHA/ACSM questionnaire provides greater detail regarding CVD risk factors, symptoms, and other important diagnoses the patient may have. Because no single form for preparticipation health screening can cover all conditions or situations,

Personal Information

Client Name: _____   Date of Birth: _____   Date: _____

Gender: M   F   Height: _____ in.   Weight: _____ lb.

Referring Physician: _____   Phone: _____

Medical diagnosis and reason for referral:
Medication, drug/supplement use; allergies:

Subjective Information
Prior medical history
Family history
Previous physical exam findings
Symptom history and pain assessment
Recent illness, hospitalizations, surgeries
Exercise and work history

Objective Information
Anthropometric measures
Blood pressure
Pulse rate and rhythm
Auscultation of heart and lungs
Cardiorespiratory fitness (VO_2)
Muscle strength/endurance
Flexibility/ROM
Skin inspection (edema)
Balance
Gait
Posture
General observations/comments

Summary of Findings/Goals/Expected Functional Outcomes

Exercise Plan
Aerobic modes
Resistance exercise
Flexibility exercise
Balance exercise
Adaptations to exercise equipment

FIGURE 22.1. Functional outcome documentation format.

TABLE 22.2. KEY COMPONENTS OF THE MEDICAL HISTORY AND PHYSICAL EXAMINATION

MEDICAL HISTORY	PHYSICAL EXAMINATION
Medical Diagnosis and Reason for Referral Cardiovascular, pulmonary, metabolic, musculoskeletal, neuromuscular, immunologic, neoplastic, hematologic	**Anthropometric Measures** Height, weight, body fat distribution, girth measures
Family History of Disease or Early Death	**Blood Pressure** Including postural changes
Previous Physical Examination Findings Abnormal heart or lung sounds, blood lipids, blood glucose, hypertension, edema, or other significant laboratory abnormalities	**Pulse Rate and Rhythm** Peripheral pulses (carotid, abdominal, femoral, popliteal, pedal)
Symptom History and Pain Assessment Discomfort in the chest, neck, jaw, back, or arms; shortness of breath, dizziness or syncope; rapid heart rate or palpitations; transient numbness, tingling, or weakness	**Auscultation of Heart and Lungs** Breath sounds (presence of rales, wheezes, other breathing sounds) Heart sounds (presence of murmurs, gallops, clicks, rubs)
Orthopedic Problems Arthritis, joint swelling	**Examination and Palpation of the Abdomen** Bowel sounds, masses, visceromegaly, tenderness
Recent Illness, Hospitalizations, Surgeries Including depression/other mental health issues	**Orthopedic Evaluation** Musculoskeletal strength, endurance, flexibility, balance, gait, posture
Medication, Drug and Supplement Use; Allergies Cardiovascular, non-cardiovascular, illicit drug use, vitamins, herbs, other supplements	**Neurologic Evaluation** Reflexes and cognition
Exercise and Work History Habitual level of activity, current or expected physical demands, stress	**Skin Inspection** Peripheral or central edema, skin ulcers, lesions

Cardiovascular: cardiac, peripheral vascular, or cerebrovascular disease; *Pulmonary*: chronic obstructive pulmonary disease, asthma, interstitial lung disease, or cystic fibrosis; *Metabolic*: diabetes (types 1 and 2), thyroid disorders, renal or liver disease; *Hematologic*: relating to the study of blood and blood disorders; *Neoplastic*: relating to abnormal and uncontrollable cell growth; *Visceromegaly*: enlargement of the internal organs in the abdomen.

the CEP must pay careful attention to the patient's symptoms and chief complaints because these may provide important information regarding the patient's current health status, need for further diagnostic evaluation, treatment modifications, or the need for referral to other health professionals. (See Chapter 21 for additional information on referral to other allied health professionals.) In addition, this information will aid in establishing appropriate goals and may reveal important barriers or contraindications to exercise testing or training that may affect patient safety or impede adherence to the overall treatment program.

PATIENT COMPLAINTS AND SYMPTOMS

The evaluation of perceptual responses (e.g., pain, discomfort, fatigue, dyspnea) can provide valuable clinical information. These responses are, however, inherently subjective experiences that are often difficult to quantify, let alone compare among other individuals. They can be acute or chronic and vary in terms of frequency, intensity, affect, and location. Unalleviated, these symptoms can have significant functional, cognitive, emotional, and psychosocial consequences. For example, pain that is associated with physical activity, whether somatic or psychosomatic, may exacerbate an already sedentary lifestyle that leads to further cardiorespiratory or musculoskeletal deconditioning, poor flexibility, gait disturbances, injuries from falls, and reduced quality of life. Pre-exercise

assessments of individual's suffering from acute or chronic symptoms therefore should include a thorough review of the patient's medical background, symptom history, and physical examination findings (Table 22.2). Because symptoms are highly individualized and subjective, self-report measures are the preferred form of assessment. Therefore, treatments that include medical management or exercise intervention require that symptoms be quantified in order to report successful functional outcomes.

Several validated self-report scales, such as the visual analogue scale (VAS) (24), body maps (39), and the McGill Pain Questionnaire (31), are commonly used by licensed healthcare professionals to assist in quantifying pain. Similar scales are used by CEPs and other medical professionals to quantify chest pain, chest discomfort, and breathing difficulty (2), and perceived exertion while performing various activities (6). The CEP should periodically assess the patient's level of discomfort (or difficulty) during exercise and select functional or occupational tasks relative to the beginning of care to support documentation of progress. For example, after completing 12 weeks of supervised pulmonary rehabilitation, the client reports a dyspnea rating of "1" while walking at 2.5 miles per hour compared with a rating of "3" at baseline. Specific attention should be paid to the precipitating and relieving factors (especially during exercise and performance on functional tasks) to gain a more thorough description of the discomfort. Results from these assessments will provide valuable information about the need for further medical evaluation and in decision-making regarding implementation of an exercise plan, relative to intensity, frequency, duration, and modes.

GOALS AND EXPECTED OUTCOMES

Information obtained from the medical history review, physical examination, and other baseline evaluations will assist in understanding the patient's functional limitations and allow the CEP to theorize on the relationship between these limitations and findings from other objective (functional) assessments. Furthermore, this information will help establish appropriate and attainable goals, which will be useful in structuring an exercise program that is specific to the needs of each patient. When evaluating patient complaints related to daily functional tasks, it is helpful to consider the various components required to complete each task. The CEP should break down the functional task in terms of individual and related components to identify areas of deficiency that could be related to the objective findings or to client complaints and related symptoms. For example, when climbing stairs, cardiorespiratory fitness, muscular strength, muscular endurance, and balance are all required components of the functional task. Therefore, aerobic activities (stair stepping), strength training (lower extremity exercises), and proprioceptive activities (one-leg standing drills) would be appropriate modes to include in the exercise program.

Depending on the patient's diagnosis, prognosis, and length of involvement with the CEP, both short- and long-term goals should be established. In many cases, the short-term goals are steps toward achieving the long-term goals. In particular, the long-term goals should identify the functional level the patient is expected to reach by the time he or she is discharged from services. In this regard, each goal should be reasonable and measurable within a specified time period, and expressed in functional terms, when possible. For example, if a person's main functional complaint is the need to take at least two rest breaks when walking up a flight of stairs, an appropriate goal (and successful functional outcome) would be walking up three flights of stairs, without a single rest break. At regular intervals, the CEP should determine if the functional outcomes have been achieved, need to be revised or upgraded, or if the current exercise plan needs to be discontinued or altered based on the achievement of previously stated functional outcomes.

REPORTING OUTCOMES RELATED TO PHYSICAL FUNCTION

Aerobic Capacity

The assessment of aerobic exercise capacity ($\dot{V}O_{2pk}$) using open-circuit spirometry is generally accepted as the gold standard for assessing cardiorespiratory fitness. Objective and subjective data obtained from maximal exercise testing provide important diagnostic and prognostic information in a wide variety of clinical settings and can effectively aid physician decisions regarding medical and surgical management in a broad range of patients. For the CEP, exercise testing provides valuable information for activity counseling, exercise prescription, return to work evaluations, disability assessment, and the evaluation of exercise training outcomes (2). When performed appropriately, the $\dot{V}O_{2pk}$ test is a valid tool for assessing all-cause mortality and prognosis relative to CVD events. Therefore, the CEP should consider several factors when performing exercise tests (and interpreting results), including type and extent of disease, exercise test procedures (e.g., maximal versus submaximal, estimated versus measured $\dot{V}O_{2pk}$, test end-points, exercise modes), and other clinical and demographic factors (e.g., age, physical activity status, presence of comorbid conditions, smoking history, medications).

Despite the numerous benefits, maximal cardiorespiratory exercise testing is underutilized in the evaluation of patients with chronic disease. Explanations for this include additional cost, patient discomfort, perceived risk-to-benefit ratio, and resource availability. When direct measurement of maximal oxygen uptake is not possible or indicated based on clinical evaluation, $\dot{V}O_{2pk}$ can be predicted from steady-state or graded submaximal exercise tests (walking, running, stepping, arm/cycle ergometry) (2). These equations have limited precision, however, owing to factors such as subject habituation, fitness level, presence of heart disease, patient motivation or anxiety, handrail holding, and choice of protocol. This error is amplified in individuals with reduced exercise capacities. Submaximal exercise testing, however, remains useful clinically for patients with a high probability of serious dysrhythmias, as well as for making appropriate physical activity recommendations, modifying the medical treatment regimen, and for identifying the need for further interventions in the early post-myocardial infarction or postsurgery period (9,33). Individualized, low-level protocols (no more than one metabolic equivalent [1-MET] increment per stage) should be used to optimize information obtained from submaximal exercise testing. Test endpoints for submaximal testing have traditionally been arbitrary, but should always be based on clinical judgment. A heart rate limit of 140 beats/minute and a functional capacity greater than 7 METs are often used for patients younger than 40 years of age; limits of 130 beats/minute and MET level of 5 are frequently used for patients older than 40 years. For patients taking beta-blockers, a perceived exertion level of 7–8 (Borg 1–10 scale) or 15–16 (Borg 6–20 scale) are appropriate endpoints (16). Additional information on maximal and submaximal exercise testing, including common tests and protocols, measurements, and contraindications to exercise testing can be found in Chapters 4 and 5 of *ACSM's Guidelines for Exercise Testing and Prescription (GETP)*, 7th edition (2).

Muscular Strength and Endurance

Musculoskeletal disorders are among the leading causes of disability in the United States. Arthritis and rheumatism, back and spine problems, and extremity and limb weakness account for 38.2% of all disabilities (8). Poor muscular strength and flexibility can result in considerable pain and discomfort, loss of income, increased disability, and premature retirement. As such, several professional health organizations consider resistance training a key component of an overall physical fitness program for both apparently healthy and many patients with chronic disease (1,22,36,44). When performed properly (and regularly), resistance training is a safe and effective method for the development of muscular strength and endurance, which may help preserve bone mass and fat-free mass, improve glucose tolerance and musculotendinous integrity, and enhance a person's ability to live a functionally independent lifestyle (1,15,17).

Before exercise testing or training, the CEP should identify any major areas of patient discomfort and self-reported limitations related to muscular movement. Several factors, including orthopedic conditions, presence (and severity) of neuromuscular disease, inadequate muscular strength and endurance, muscle imbalances, reduced flexibility, or abnormalities in gait, balance, or posture could partially explain patient complaints and physical restrictions of movement. Performing muscular strength and endurance tests before exercise training will provide important information about the patient's muscular fitness level and help the CEP identify areas of muscle weakness or imbalance. Combined with information obtained from the HHQ, results from baseline muscular fitness assessments can serve as a basis for designing individualized exercise training programs and a means to monitor patient improvements as a result of the training program.

Several muscle function tests are available to evaluate muscular strength and endurance; however, these tests are specific to the muscle group tested, the type of contraction, velocity of muscle movement, type of equipment, and joint range of motion (ROM). Furthermore, the results obtained from any one test are specific to the procedures used and no single test exists to evaluate total body muscular strength and endurance (2). Muscular strength can be assessed statically or dynamically and is often expressed as the amount of resistance lifted. Isometric or static strength can be measured using cable tensiometers or handgrip dynamometers that record the maximal voluntary contraction (MVC) of a muscle group at a specific joint angle. Special computer-controlled iso-

kinetic testing equipment can assess strength of a muscle throughout a joint's ROM at a specific angular velocity (e.g., 30 degrees/second). In addition, these devices can be used to measure muscular power (the ability of the muscle to work at a certain rate). Muscular power can be particularly important to assess, because research has demonstrated that leg muscle power is more important than strength for older adults performing daily activities, such as walking, rising from a chair, and stair climbing (3,4) and could aid in the prevention of falls and fractures in older adults (13).

The equipment required to perform specialized muscle function testing is expensive compared to other methods (19), however and it is often unavailable to many medical professionals, including physicians and therapists. In clinical settings, manual muscle testing (MMT) frequently is used to evaluate and grade muscular strength (30). Because MMT is subjective, practice and appropriate training is essential for obtaining accurate and reliable measures (27). For CEPs (and other health or fitness professionals), the one repetition maximum (1-RM), the greatest resistance that can be moved through a complete ROM, remains a popular and commonly used test for evaluating dynamic muscular strength. When administered properly, reports of cardiovascular events and injuries from maximal strength testing in older adults are no more frequent than those experienced by younger individuals (14,23). However, the CEP should pay particular attention to medical contraindications that may preclude vigorous exercise, including high blood pressure, musculoskeletal injury, neuromuscular disorders, and heart disease. Multiple repetitions of submaximal loads, such as the 6-RM or 10-RM to momentary muscle fatigue, can be used with individuals where maximal strength testing is less appropriate and may provide a safer index of strength changes over time. Procedures for administering the 1-RM (or multiple RM) test are provided in *ACSM's GETP*, 7th edition (2).

Muscular endurance refers to the ability of muscles to perform repeated contractions over a period of time sufficient to cause muscular fatigue. Most of the devices for measuring strength also can be used for assessing muscular endurance. As with muscular strength, no single test, however, exists to evaluate total body muscular endurance. Relative muscular endurance can be assessed using a percentage of the patient's RM capability before and after testing (e.g., 50% of 1-RM), whereas absolute muscular endurance is determined using the same resistance before and after testing. For example, the YMCA bench press test (18), which uses an absolute weight (35-pound barbell for women; 80 pounds for men), is considered highly reliable because it controls for repetition duration and posture. Other simple and easy to administer field tests can be used to evaluate static or dynamic muscular endurance. The curl-up (crunch) test and the maximum number of push-ups to fatigue are commonly used to evaluate endurance of the abdominal and upper body muscles, respectively. Normative data and procedures for performing these tests are provided in *ACSM's GETP*, 7th edition (2).

Flexibility

Flexibility is joint specific and is defined as the ability to move a joint through its complete ROM. Inadequate flexibility can hinder ROM, contribute to poor posture and alignment, and impede a person's ability to perform common daily tasks. Limitations can be caused by ligament or tendon restrictions or the distensibility of the joint capsule itself. Common tools used to measure flexibility or joint ROM include goniometers, inclinometers, tape measures, or visual estimation of ROM. Directly measured ROM is preferred to visual estimates of ROM; measures can include flexibility of neck and trunk, hip, lower extremity, and shoulder, and postural assessment. Precise measurement of joint ROM can be assessed with the proper use of a goniometer and strict adherence to guidelines for its use (10,34). Experience, proper training, and an extensive knowledge of anatomy are essential to improve the accuracy of measurements obtained (2).

During the initial evaluation, the CEP should consider how an individual's limitations in ROM or flexibility affect function. Can the patient reach overhead to retrieve items on a top shelf or get a serving platter out of a high cabinet (shoulder flexibility)? Can the person reach down and tie his or her shoes, or pick up an object from the floor (low back or hip-joint flexibility)? The sit-and-reach test is frequently performed in the health and fitness industry to evaluate low back and hip-joint flexibility. However, its ability to measure low back flexibility or predict the incidence of low back pain is questionable (25,26). Regardless, it likely will remain a component of flexibility assessment until a more valid measurement tool of low back flexibility is available. The CEP should use this test cautiously, particularly in persons with limb-length discrepancies, arthritis, or a history of low back pain. When reporting improvements in flexibility and ROM, it is important to provide functional examples in the notation. For example, after completing the exercise program, the patient now exhibits hamstring flexibility "within normal limits," and reports less low back discomfort while walking.

Gait and Balance

In many older adults and patients with neuromuscular disorders, altered balance and gait abnormalities increase the risk for falls and significant injuries, such as bone fractures, hematomas, and head injuries. At a minimum, these injuries can result in a diminished ability to carry out common daily activities, such as dressing or bathing. Severe injuries resulting in significant disability are associated with high morbidity and mortality, and can result in expensive medical intervention. The initial interview should include a review of patient complaints related to difficulties performing daily activities. For example, does the patient require the assistance of a walking device for any (or all) activities? Can the patient balance sufficiently well to safely step into or out of the bath tub without aid? For the CEP, this information is particularly important when making decisions for exercise testing (protocols and modes) as well as exercise programming. During visual observation of the patient, look for noticeable difficulties performing common tasks (e.g., standing up from a chair, walking around the room, stepping over objects). Any obvious abnormalities in gait (or balance) should be evaluated by a qualified licensed professional.

Several simple, inexpensive, and easy-to-administer global or practical tests of musculoskeletal function are available to evaluate the extent of impairment and functional limitations (5,11,29,45,47). The Timed Up and Go test (TUG) (29) is a reliable assessment tool that correlates well with other validated measures of gait and functional status (50) and is able to distinguish between recurrent fallers and nonfallers (43). For the TUG test, the time to rise from a chair, walk 3 m, turn around, walk back to the chair, and sit down is measured. A total time of 16 seconds has been found to be predictive of future falls in older adults (32). The Functional Reach test (11) evaluates forward balance by measuring the maximal distance a person can reach forward while standing upright and bending forward with the shoulder flexed 90 degrees. The inability to reach 6 inches beyond arm reach is associated with an increased risk for recurrent falls (adjusted odds ratio, 4.0) (12). The Berg Balance Scale (5) and Tinetti Balance Assessment tool (45) provide a quantifiable index of balance and gait by evaluating specific functional tasks (sitting–standing balance, rising from a chair, sitting down, turning 360 degrees) with the patient receiving a score based on criteria met within each task. Both are easy to administer and require minimal equipment and space. The CEP should pay particular attention to procedures and safety considerations when performing balance assessment tests because of the increased risk for falls, particularly in older adults and patients with neuromuscular disorders.

Functional Task and Return to Work Evaluations

Increased aerobic capacity, muscular strength, endurance, and flexibility can greatly affect overall health and performance in persons with chronic health conditions. When reporting functional outcomes, the CEP should pay particular attention to the motivating factors that prompted the healthcare provider to make the referral and the third-party payer to support the intervention. A primary goal for physicians and CEPs is the patient's safe return to an optimal functional status and not necessarily to normal strength, ROM, or exercise capacity. For some, this involves the ability to perform routine work-related lifting, climb several flights of stairs, or simply walk for extended periods without rest. For most patients, the traditional $\dot{V}O_{2pk}$ test provides sufficient information necessary to assess functional tolerance for resumption of normal work activities. When maximal exercise testing is not indicated (or available), however, or if the job demands are substantially different from that evaluated with the traditional exercise test, the CEP should consider other tests in the exercise evaluation that provide sufficient information regarding the patient's ability to return to work safely and perform routine activities important to daily living. For example, can the patient carry two bags of groceries to upstairs to his or her apartment without needing to rest? Can the person lift a 50-pound crate at work and carry across a distance of 40 feet, 6 times in 1 hour without low back pain? Tasks that simulate work (or daily living) requirements can be administered when additional information is needed regarding a patient's ability to resume physically demanding activities safely. Certain tasks require activities, such as lifting, pulling, pushing, or carrying, that elicit disproportionate myocardial stress compared with the traditional graded exercise test (GXT). Additionally, some tasks require intermittent heavy work or are performed under stressful environmental conditions (extreme temperatures, altitude, air pollution). Inclusion of additional functional assessments may benefit patients with lower aerobic exercise capacities (relative to job or activity demands), ischemia at submaximal levels, left ventricular dysfunction, complex dysrhythmias, or those hesitant about returning to work (21,42,48). Work simulator tests are available (51), as well as other simple, inexpensive tests that can be modified to evaluate work activities not evaluated with traditional exercise testing. Weight carrying and repetitive weight-lifting protocols that combine static and dynamic work activities have been published and can be individualized to evaluate specific job activities (42). Additional information on occupation and functional task assessments can be found in Chapter 18 of the *ACSM's Resource Manual for GETP*, 5th edition (41).

Walking tests, such as the 6-minute walk test (total distance walked in 6 minutes) are useful for patients incapable of performing maximal exercise tests. In addition to being well accepted by patients, they are inexpensive, require minimal training, are highly reproducible, and are relevant to many daily activities and functional abilities. Previous research has demonstrated that walking tests may be a better indicator of a patient's ability to perform challenging physical ADLs compared with traditional tests performed by cycle ergometry (20). In this regard, choosing the appropriate exercise test mode (principle of specificity) is important in the evaluation of clinical populations. When indicated, similar tests could be implemented for stair climbing, cycle- or arm-ergometry, and wheelchair ergometry. Reductions in submaximal cardiopulmonary measures (heart rate, blood pressure, ventilation, oxygen uptake) and perceived exertion (RPE) can provide further evidence to suggest improvements in functional capacity.

The Senior Fitness Test (SFT) (38) and Physical Performance Test (PPT) (37) were developed in response to a need for improved functional assessment tools in older adults. The SFT has been shown to correlate well with other muscular fitness tests such as the 1-RM; the PPT has been shown to be a reliable and valid instrument for use in other clinical populations (28,35,40). Each of these tests incorporates a series of simple functional task tests designed to evaluate important physiologic measures (strength, endurance, balance, and agility) associated with common everyday functional tasks. For example, two tests in the SFT, the 30-second chair stand and the single arm curl, can be used by CEPs safely and effectively to assess muscular strength and muscular endurance. When evaluated concurrently, results from maximal exercise testing and other functional tests may provide important information about a patient's physical capacity for performing daily living and work activities that would be particularly important to referring physicians and third-party providers.

SUMMARY

The changing healthcare system requires that all health professionals exhibit proficient documentation and outcome reporting skills. Accurate and concise documentation can strengthen the quality of patient care by providing a link between services provided, healthcare, and third-party providers. Properly stated goals (and expected outcomes) should be established from evaluating the patient's current abilities and limitations from performance on both standardized tests and functional task evaluations. Results from these tests can assist other healthcare professionals in making decisions about the need for further diagnostic evaluation or modifications to the treatment plan. When reporting functional outcomes, the CEP should relate the patient's medical history, symptoms and complaints, physical examination findings, and results from other objective and subjective assessments to the limitations that affect functional tasks. In addition to providing evidence of improvement from standardized tests, supplementing the documentation with functional examples offers helpful insight to the referring physician regarding the safe return to daily activities.

REFERENCES

1. American Association of Cardiovascular and Pulmonary Rehabilitation. *Guidelines for Cardiac Rehabilitation and Secondary Prevention Programs.* Champaign, IL: Human Kinetics; 2004:288.

2. American College of Sports Medicine. *ACSM's Guidelines for Exercise Testing and Prescription.* Baltimore: Lippincott Williams & Wilkins, 2006:366.

3. Bassey EJ, Fiatarone MA, O'Neill EF, et al. Leg extensor power and functional performance in very old men and women. *Clin Sci (Lond).* 1992;82:321–327.

4. Bean JF, Kiely DK, Herman S, et al. The relationship between leg power and physical performance in mobility-limited older people. *J Am Geriatr Soc* 2002;50:461–467.

5. Berg KO, Wood-Dauphinee SL, Williams JI, et al. Measuring balance in the elderly: validation of an instrument. *Can J Public Health.* 1992;83 (Suppl 2):S7–S11.

6. Borg G. Perceived exertion as an indicator of somatic stress. *Scand J Rehabil Med.* 1970;2:92–98.

7. Canadian Society for Exercise Physiology Web site. *PAR-Q and You.* Canadian Society for Exercise Physiology. 2002. Available from: http://www.csep.ca.

8. Centers for Disease Control and Prevention. Prevalence of disabilities and associated health conditions among adults—United States, 1999. *MMWR.* 2001;50:120–125.

9. Chang JA, Froelicher VF. Clinical and exercise test markers of prognosis in patients with stable coronary artery disease. *Curr Probl Cardiol.* 1994;19:533–587.

10. Clarkson HM. *Musculoskeletal Assessment: Joint Range of Motion and Manual Muscle Strength.* Philadelphia: Lippincott Williams & Wilkins, 2000.

11. Duncan PW, Weiner DK, Chandler J, et al. Functional reach: a new clinical measure of balance. *J Gerontol.* 1990;45:M192–M197.

12. Duncan PW, Studenski S, Chandler J, et al. Functional reach: predictive validity in a sample of elderly male veterans. *J Gerontol.* 1992;47:M93–M98.

13. Evans WJ. Exercise strategies should be designed to increase muscle power. *J Gerontol A Biol Sci Med Sci* 2000;55:M309–M310.

14. Faigenbaum AD, Milliken LA, Westcott WL. Maximal strength testing in healthy children. *J Strength Cond Res* 2003;17:162–166.

15. Fiatarone MA, Marks EC, Ryan ND, et al. High-intensity strength training in nonagenarians. Effects on skeletal muscle. *JAMA.* 1990; 263:3029–3034.

16. Froelicher VF, Myers J. *Exercise and the heart.* Philadelphia: WB Saunders; 2006.

17. Frontera WR, Meredith CN, O'Reilly KP, et al. Strength conditioning in older men: skeletal muscle hypertrophy and improved function. *J Appl Physiol.* 1988;64:1038–1044.

18. Golding LA. *YMCA Fitness Testing and Assessment Manual.* Champaign, IL: Human Kinetics, 1989.

19. Graves JE, Pollock ML, Bryant CX. Assessment of muscular strength and endurance. In: Roitman JL, ed. *ACSM's Resource Manual for Guidelines for Exercise Testing and Prescription.* Philadelphia: Lippincott Williams & Wilkins; 2001: 376–380.

20. Guyatt GH, Thompson PJ, Berman LB, et al. How should we measure function in patients with chronic heart and lung disease? *J Chronic Dis.* 1985;38:517–524.

21. Haskell WL, Brachfeld N, Bruce RA, et al. Task Force II: Determination of occupational working capacity in patients with ischemic heart disease. *J Am Coll Cardiol* 1989;14:1025–1034.

22. Haskell WL, Lee IM, Pate RR, et al. Physical activity and public health: updated recommendation for adults from the American College of Sports Medicine and the American Heart Association. *Med Sci Sports Exerc* 2007;39:1423–1434.

23. Humphries B, Newton RU, Bronks R, et al. Effect of exercise intensity on bone density, strength, and calcium turnover in older women. *Med Sci Sports Exerc* 2000;32:1043–1050.

24. Huskisson EC. Measurement of pain. *Lancet.* 1974;2:1127–1131.

25. Jackson AW, Baker AA. The relationship of the sit and reach test to criterion measures of hamstring and back flexibility in young females. *Res Q Exerc Sport.* 1986;57:183–186.

26. Jackson AW, Morrow JR Jr., Brill PA, et al. Relations of sit-up and sit-and-reach tests to low back pain in adults. *J Orthop Sports Phys Ther.* 1998;27:22–26.

27. Kendall FP, Mcreary EK, Provance PG, et al. *Muscles: Testing and Function with Posture and Pain.* Baltimore: Lippincott Williams & Wilkins, 2005:480.

28. King JT Jr., Tsevat J, Roberts MS. The physical performance test and the evaluation of functional status in patients with cerebral aneurysms. *J Neurosurg* 2006;104:525–530.

29. Mathias S, Nayak US, Isaacs B. Balance in elderly patients: The "get-up and go" test. *Arch Phys Med Rehabil* 1986;67:387–389.

30. McPeak LA. Physiatric history and examination. In: Branddom RL, et al., eds. *Physical Medicine and Rehabilitation.* Philadelphia: WB Saunders, 1996:3–42.

31. Melzack R. The McGill pain questionnaire. In: *Pain Measurement and Assessment.* Melzack R. ed. New York: Raven Press; 1983: 41–47.

32. Okumiya K, Matsubayashi K, Nakamura T, et al. The timed "up & go" test is a useful predictor of falls in community-dwelling older people. *J Am Geriatr Soc* 1998;46:928–930.

33. Olona M, Candell-Riera J, Permanyer-Miralda G, et al. Strategies for prognostic assessment of uncomplicated first myocardial infarction: 5-year follow-up study. *J Am Coll Cardiol* 1995;25: 815–822.

34. Palmer ML, Epler MF. *Fundamentals of Musculoskeletal Assessment Technique.* Philadelphia: JB Lippincott; 1998.

35. Paschal K, Oswald A, Siegmund R, et al. Test-retest reliability of the physical performance test for persons with Parkinson disease. *J Geriatr Phys Ther* 2006; 29:82–86.

36. Pescatello LS, Franklin BA, Fagard R, et al. American College of Sports Medicine position stand. Exercise and hypertension. *Med Sci Sports Exerc* 2004;36:533–553.

37. Reuben DB, Siu AL. An objective measure of physical function of elderly outpatients. The Physical Performance Test. *J Am Geriatr Soc* 1990; 38:1105–1112.

38. Rikli RE, Jones CJ. *Senior Fitness Test Manual.* Champaign, IL: Human Kinetics; 2001.

39. Ryden O, Lindal E, Uden A, et al. Differentiation of back pain patients using a pain questionnaire. *Scand J Rehabil Med* 1985;17: 155–161.

40. Sato D, Kaneko F, Okamura H. Reliability and validity of the Japanese-language version of the physical performance test (PPT) battery in chronic pain patients. *Disabil Rehabil* 2006;28: 397–405.

41. Sheldahl LM. Occupational and functional assessments. In: Kaminsky LA, ed. *ACSM's Resource Manual for Guidelines for Exercise Testing and Prescription.* Baltimore: Lippincott Williams & Wilkins; 2006:266–276.

42. Sheldahl LM, Wilke NA, Tristani FE. Evaluation and training for resumption of occupational and leisure-time physical activities in patients after a major cardiac event. *Med Exerc Nutr Health* 1995;4: 273–289.

43. Shumway-Cook A, Brauer S, Woollacott M. Predicting the probability for falls in community-dwelling older adults using the Timed Up & Go Test. *Phys Ther* 2000;80:896–903.

44. Sigal RJ, Kenny GP, Wasserman DH, et al. Physical activity/exercise and type 2 diabetes. *Diabetes Care.* 2004;27:2518–2539.

45. Tinetti ME, Williams TF, Mayewski R. Fall risk index for elderly patients based on number of chronic disabilities. *Am J Med.* 1986;80: 429–434.

46. United States Department of Health and Human Services Web site. Medical Privacy-National Standards to Protect the Privacy of Personal Health Information. 1996. Available from: http://www.hhs.gov/ocr/hipaa/.

47. Vellas BJ, Wayne SJ, Romero L, et al. One-leg balance is an important predictor of injurious falls in older persons. *J Am Geriatr Soc* 1997;45:735–738.

48. Vona M, Capodaglio P, Iannessa A, et al. The role of work simulation tests in a comprehensive cardiac rehabilitation program. *Monaldi Arch Chest Dis* 2002;58:26–34.

49. Weed LL. Medical Records, Patient Care, and Medical Education. *Ir J Med Sci* 1964;17:271–282.

50. Whitney SL, Poole JL, Cass SP. A review of balance instruments for older adults. *Am J Occup Ther* 1998;52:666–671.

51. Wilke NA, Sheldahl LM, Dougherty SM, et al. Baltimore Therapeutic Equipment work simulator: Energy expenditure of work activities in cardiac patients. *Arch Phys Med Rehab* 1993;74: 419–424.

Legal and Ethical Considerations

A variety of legal and ethical considerations, as well as a number of practical concerns, have an impact on the delivery of client services by Clinical Exercise Physiologists (CEPs). CEPs have been providing service for many years in a number of settings, including fitness, healthcare, and clinical venues. Unlike other healthcare professionals, such as physicians, nurses, physical therapists, dietitians and others, CEPs are currently licensed only in the state of Louisiana; however, efforts are underway in other states to license CEPs (e.g., Massachusetts HB 2252, an act relative to the licensure of exercise physiologists) (1). Perhaps because of the lack of licensure or other substantive governmental regulation, most health insurance carriers do not pay for services rendered by CEPs unless payment is made through otherwise permissible means, such as billing through physician provider billing authorizations on a delegation of service basis. As a consequence of all of the aforementioned, the legal "rules" and "regulations" surrounding the delivery of service by CEPs can be somewhat broad.

HEALTHCARE PRACTICE REGULATION

In the United States, the more established healthcare professions are typically governed by the statutes and regulations of each respective state or region. These statutes define "scopes of practice," which specify the types of service each respective profession is authorized to provide. Although each of these professions has defined scopes of practice, situations arise where particular scopes of practice overlap with other healthcare provider statutes and regulations so that who can do what is sometimes called into question. Typically, each professional community or organization "guards" its own scopes of practice to protect the interests of their membership.

Physicians are at the top of the healthcare provider practice list and typically have very broad legislative and administrative authority to provide service to patients. All other providers have narrower practice authorizations and function in more specific roles. Almost all CEPs and some others within the fitness and wellness compendium have no statutory or administratively defined scope of practice to examine by reference to governmental action. Therefore, any analysis related to the delivery of service

by CEPs must look to general legal principles and statutes and regulations pertaining to other healthcare providers to see what CEPs may lawfully do in their delivery of certain services. If healthcare services are rendered, then the authority of CEPs to engage in such practices must depend on whether the care they provide is properly delegated.

PROVIDER OVERSIGHT AND DELEGATION OF DUTIES

Typically, healthcare providers, especially physicians, have the ability to delegate lawfully the delivery of service rendered to patients by other licensed and even nonlicensed providers. Although such service delegation may occur, providers are always responsible for the delivery of delegated services and must exercise supervision and oversight in accordance with statutory authorization or rules and regulations promulgated under those statutes.

In some states, such as Texas for example, physicians are provided with legislative authorization related to the delegation of services provided to patients. The related physician practice statute in Texas providing this right is the following:

§157.001.General Authority of Physician to Delegate
(a) A physician may delegate to a qualified and properly trained person acting under the physician's supervision any medical act that a reasonable and prudent physician would find within the scope of sound medical judgment to delegate if, in the opinion of the delegating physician:
   (2) the act:
      (A) can be properly and safely performed by the person to whom the medical act is delegated;
      (B) is performed in its customary manner; and
      (C) is not in violation of any other statute; and
   (3) the person to whom the delegation is made does not represent to the public that the person is authorized to practice medicine.
(b) The delegating physician remains responsible for the medical acts of the person performing the delegated medical acts.

Statutes such as the foregoing one in Texas and in Ohio (Box 23.1) are often subject to determinations made by

BOX 23.1 Administrative Rules for Physician's Delegation of Medical Task (Ohio Revised Code Section 4731.053)

(A) As used in this section, "physician" means an individual authorized by this chapter to practice medicine and surgery, osteopathic medicine and surgery, or podiatric medicine and surgery.

(B) The state medical board shall adopt rules that establish standards to be met and procedures to be followed by a physician with respect to the physician's delegation of the performance of a medical task to a person who is not licensed or otherwise specifically authorized by the Revised Code to perform the task. The rules shall be adopted in accordance with Chapter 119 of the Revised Code and shall include a coroner's investigator among the individuals who are competent to recite the facts of a deceased person's medical condition to a physician so that the physician may pronounce the person dead without personally examining the body.

(C) To the extent that delegation applies to the administration of drugs, the rules adopted under this section shall provide for all of the following:

(1) On-site supervision when the delegation occurs in an institution or other facility that is used primarily for the purpose of providing healthcare, unless the board establishes a specific exception to the on-site supervision requirement with respect to routine administration of a topical drug, such as the use of a medicated shampoo;

(2) Evaluation of whether delegation is appropriate according to the acuity of the patient involved;

(3) Training and competency requirements that must be met by the person administering the drugs;

(4) Other standards and procedures the board considers relevant.

(D) The board shall not adopt rules that do any of the following:

(1) Authorize a physician to transfer the physician's responsibility for supervising a person who is performing a delegated medical task to a health professional other than another physician;

(2) Authorize an individual to whom a medical task is delegated to delegate the performance of that task to another individual;

(3) Except as provided in divisions (D)(7) to (11) of this section, authorize a physician to delegate the administration of anesthesia, controlled substances, drugs administered intravenously, or any other drug or category of drug the board considers to be inappropriate for delegation;

(4) Prevent an individual from engaging in an activity performed for a handicapped child as a service needed to meet the educational needs of the child, as identified in the individualized education program developed for the child under Chapter 3323. of the Revised Code;

(5) Conflict with any provision of the Revised Code that specifically authorizes an individual to perform a particular task;

(6) Conflict with any rule adopted pursuant to the Revised Code that is in effect on April 10, 2001, as long as the rule remains in effect, specifically authorizing an individual to perform a particular task;

(7) Prohibit a perfusionist from administering drugs intravenously while practicing as a perfusionist;

(8) Authorize a physician assistant, anesthesiologist assistant, or any other professional regulated by the board to delegate tasks pursuant to this section.

state medical boards to whether particular services may be properly delegated. Consequently, because of variations in state regulation pertaining to the delegation of service delivery to, among others, CEPs, particular state statutes and regulations where CEPs provide service must be consulted to determine what can be permissibly done by them in the referring physician's recommendation of healthcare services. If services are provided that are not healthcare, then such laws and/ regulations do not apply.

UNAUTHORIZED PRACTICE AND LIMITATIONS ON PRACTICE

Even in those states where the provision of service may be properly delegated by licensed healthcare providers to CEPs, CEPs must be cognizant of their potential liability for engaging in practices that might violate particular laws or applicable regulations. Virtually all jurisdictions have statutes that prohibit the unauthorized practice of medicine, physical therapy, nursing, and so forth by those

---

BOX 23.2 Unauthorized Practice (Ohio Revised Code Section 4731.34)

(A) A person shall be regarded as practicing medicine and surgery, osteopathic medicine and surgery, or podiatric medicine and surgery, within the meaning of this chapter, who does any of the following:
 (1) Uses the words or letters, "Dr.," "Doctor," "M.D.," "physician," "D.O.," "D.P.M.," or any other title in connection with the person's name in any way that represents the person as engaged in the practice of medicine and surgery, osteopathic medicine and surgery, or podiatric medicine and surgery, in any of its branches;
 (2) Advertises, solicits, or represents in any way that the person is practicing medicine and surgery, osteopathic medicine and surgery, or podiatric medicine and surgery, in any of its branches;
 (3) In person or, regardless of the person's location, through the use of any communication, including oral, written, or electronic communication, does any of the following:
  (a) Examines or diagnoses for compensation of any kind, direct or indirect;
  (b) Prescribes, advises, recommends, administers, or dispenses for compensation of any

kind, direct or indirect, a drug or medicine, appliance, mold or cast, application, operation, or treatment, of whatever nature, for the cure or relief of a wound, fracture or bodily injury, infirmity, or disease.

(B) The treatment of human ills through prayer alone by a practitioner of the Christian Science church, in accordance with the tenets and creed of such church, shall not be regarded as the practice of medicine, provided that sanitary and public health laws shall be complied with, no practices shall be used that may be dangerous or detrimental to life or health, and no person shall be denied the benefits of accepted medical and surgical practices.

(C) The use of words, letters, or titles in any connection or under any circumstances as to induce the belief that the person who uses them is engaged in the practice of medicine and surgery, osteopathic medicine and surgery, or podiatric medicine and surgery, in any of its branches, is prima-facie evidence of the intent of such person to represent the person as engaged in the practice of medicine and surgery, osteopathic medicine and surgery, or podiatric medicine and surgery, in any of its branches.

---

who are not licensed in that particular practice domain. For example, in the state of Ohio, the unauthorized provision of such service is defined in Box 23.2. Although the unauthorized practice of medicine may *generally* be enjoined by an injunction action, the unauthorized practice of medicine is also a crime. As of mid-2007, a violation of Ohio practice act 4731.41 (Box 23.3) is a felony of

the fifth degree on a first offense and one of the fourth degree on a subsequent offense. The penalties applicable in Ohio to a fifth-degree felony include a prison term of up to 1 year, whereas a fourth-degree felony can be up to 1.5 years (Ohio Revised Code Section 2929.14); in addition, fines of up to $5,000.00 may be imposed for a felony of the fourth-degree offense and of up to $2,500.00 for a

---

BOX 23.3 Practicing Medicine without Certificate (Ohio Revised Code Section 4731.41)

No person shall practice medicine and surgery, or any of its branches, without the appropriate certificate from the state medical board to engage in the practice. No person shall advertise or claim to the public to be a practitioner of medicine and surgery, or any of its branches, without a certificate from the board. No person shall open or conduct an office or other place for such practice without a certificate from the board. No person shall conduct an office in the name of some person who has a certificate to practice medicine and surgery, or any of its branches. No person shall practice medicine and surgery, or any of its branches, after the person's certificate has been

revoked, or, if suspended, during the time of such suspension.

A certificate signed by the secretary of the board to which is affixed the official seal of the board to the effect that it appears from the records of the board that no such certificate to practice medicine and surgery, or any of its branches, in this state has been issued to the person specified therein, or that a certificate to practice, if issued, has been revoked or suspended, shall be received as prima-facie evidence of the record of the board in any court or before any officer of the state. (16)

felony of the fifth-degree offense (Ohio Revised Code Section 2929.18). Similar penalties exist in other jurisdictions for violations of like statutes. Much more serious charges could be leveled against a service provider who is found to have caused harm or death to another owing to some unauthorized practice. In such situations, assault or even homicide charges could be instituted against those found to have violated such statutes in the event of injury or death resulting therefrom.

Although instances have occurred wherein certain practitioners have been charged with violations of unauthorized practice acts and even more serious criminal offenses, given the multitiered combination of healthcare services delivered by healthcare providers and a plethora of others, sometimes under cost containment restrictions and in efforts to speed the delivery of reasonably available care, such concerns should be minimal for CEPs. Providers, including CEPs, need to remember, however, that if their conduct should be judged to be limited to provision by a healthcare provider and they are not so licensed, that care may well be judged in a civil personal injury or wrongful death litigation by reference to the presumed care expected of a licensed provider—a situation which an unlicensed provider could never meet.

The American College of Sports Medicine's (ACSM's) knowledge, skills and abilities (KSAs) applicable to, and expected of, CEPs do not include the examination, diagnosis, treatment, or administration of healthcare for conditions limited for provision by licensed healthcare providers. For example, although KSA 1.3.2 provides that a CEP be able to "Conduct a brief physical examination including evaluation of peripheral edema, measuring blood pressure, peripheral pulses, respiratory rate and auscultating heart and lung sounds," the process is to be used to present and discuss these matters with other healthcare professionals. This type of examination provides a screening mechanism wherein the CEP is acting as a "suspectitian" and not a "diagnostician." Moreover, although KSA 1.3.1 and 1.3.21 provide for CEPs "to evaluate functional capacity, strength, and flexibility in patients with (specific conditions)" the CEP is not called on in the KSA to diagnose or treat. Indeed, as properly interpreted and applied, all of the ACSM's KSAs are written and drafted to enable CEPs to "work in cooperation" with "physicians and physician assistants" and other healthcare providers to meet the specific needs of "patient populations (4)." So long as CEPS do not inadvertently attempt to render services limited to provision by licensed healthcare providers, unauthorized practice of medicine problems and other similar concerns should not be of significant concern to these professionals.

INFORMED CONSENT

One of the most fundamental and valued rights that all patients have in the United States is the right to exercise informed consent to what particular healthcare procedures will be done to them. This cherished right involves a process, not just the provision, of a written document authorizing the performance of a particular procedure. Every patient who is to undergo a medical procedure has the right to receive information about that procedure, the risks and benefits associated with that procedure, and then on the basis of that information to make a decision—to exercise free will and choose whether or not to undergo that procedure. If sufficient information has been conveyed to enable a reasonable person to make such a choice on the basis of that information, then the process has been completed. If the process is flawed in some respect, a legal action based on a failure to secure such an informed consent can be filed. Such actions are usually based on negligence principles rather than on breach of contract type claims.

All CEPs have the obligation legally and in accordance with ACSM's KSAs to participate in the informed consent process associated with the provision of service. From a legal and risk management perspective, pertinent issues associated with informed consent typically arise in the exercise testing process often used with patients or even with healthy individuals who participate in functional evaluations.

Legal cases dealing with informed consent in the exercise testing area have focused on alleged failures to disclose the risk of untoward cardiovascular incidents during exercise testing, such as with a Veteran's Administration patient (1) and an alleged failure to disclose the risk of death during the performance of a diagnostic exercise stress test (5).

Although the performance of the informed consent process is not limited to the execution of a document, the use of written informed consents can greatly assist in not only ensuring that the process is regularly and consistently followed, but also in providing tangible evidence of compliance with the process in the event that later complaints are made. Patient chart records should also be complete as to the process to provide notations as to completion of the process and to document the question and answer opportunity associated with the process, all of which can provide evidence of legal compliance with the process.

NEGLIGENCE AND MALPRACTICE

In law, a cause of action based on negligence is predicated on the proof of certain elements. These elements of proof are (*a*) duty; (*b*) breach of duty; (*c*) proximate cause; and, (*d*) damage. These basic requirements for negligence actions are the same in relatively all jurisdictions and for all kinds of actions, such as personal injury actions in automobile accident cases, or slip and fall cases, to actions against physicians and other professionals, which are referred to as *malpractice cases*. Although proof of duty and breach thereof in automobile accident type negligence cases may be predicated on proof of the violation of particular traffic laws, negligence cases against professionals, such as physicians and others similarly situated, including probably, CEPs, are almost always predicated on testimony provided by other experts who offer their opinions on the standard of care and breach of that standard in these cases. Standard of care opinions are generally based on a reference to what other providers would do in like circumstances.

When expert opinion is provided on standard of care issues in these cases, professionals almost always refer to published evidence related to the appropriate delivery of service. These opinions may be based on practice statements promulgated and published by professional associations or similar groups which have developed and distributed information about particular parameters of practice relating to the provision of professional service.

For CEPs, standards of practice have been developed primarily by the American College of Sports Medicine (ACSM) (6,7), the American Association of Cardiovascular and Pulmonary Rehabilitation (AACVPR) (3), the American College of Cardiology (ACC), and the American Heart Association (AHA) (2). A number of these standards statements have been used in litigation to evaluate, through expert witness testimony, the actual care rendered to particular patients who claimed to have been the victims of malpractice, or in other words, substandard care. These claims have dealt not only with alleged deficiencies in the aforementioned consent process as previously reviewed, but with alleged failures, properly and timely, to terminate exercise stress testing (8), mishaps occurring during treadmill procedures (9), and deficiencies in a variety of emergency response cases (10).

Sometimes issues also arise to which professionals should be allowed to provide expert testimony in malpractice cases against other professionals. The issue of whether or not exercise physiologists should be permitted to testify as experts in particular cases has even been judicially determined at least in that jurisdiction (11).

Although published standards and guidelines were originally developed to minimize the importance of individual expert testimony in negligence and malpractice cases, the lack of truly uniform and singularly authoritative guidelines has precluded the abrogation of at least some individualized expert opinions in some cases. More truly uniform guidelines might assist in the application of more relatively constant determinations in particular cases.

RISK MANAGEMENT PRACTICES AND INSURANCE

Although a number of potential legal concerns are related to the provision of various services by CEPs, also a number of techniques and strategies can be utilized as tools to reduce the applicable risks through the proper prospec-

tive application of risk management techniques. Risk management is a consistently applied, forward looking process, modified by time and experience used to:

1. Identify applicable legal risks
2. Reduce legal risks so identified
3. Eliminate those risks which are possible to eliminate
4. Minimize applicable risks which cannot be eliminated
5. Transfer relevant risks which cannot be eliminated or minimized

The risk management process is really designed to reduce and curtail the occurrence of untoward events that can lead to patient or participant injury and legal claim and lawsuit. Perhaps the foremost risk management tool for all CEPs is the recommendation to adhere to the best standard of care toward those served by consistent application of care in accordance with ACSM's KSAs and authoritative standards from prominent, professional associations, such as ACSM, AHA, ACC and the AACVPR. Secondary measures to apply in this risk management process would seem to include the use of program documentation for required and necessary components of service delivery, such as written informed consent documents, express assumption of risk forms, and where permissible, the use of prospectively executed waivers of liability—so called releases, the provision of appropriate liability insurance coverage to transfer risks that cannot be eliminated to third parties, and adherence to proper emergency response protocols where needed. The provision of care within legally permissible statutes and regulatory frameworks in the particular state where service is provided would also seem to be a necessary risk management step to avoid relevant concerns.

The use of prospectively executed waivers, or so-called releases, those exculpatory documents signed by participants in advance of the potential occurrence of an untoward event whereby the participant releases the provider from legal responsibility for such events and from provider negligence, are recognized in a number of states. There are a few states where such documents are not recognized either by statute in particular situations, as in New York State, or where such documents are deemed to be against public policy, as in Virginia (12). As a nearly universal rule, however, release documents executed prospectively in advance of the occurrence of untoward events are almost never recognized nor given legal effect in healthcare settings. The judicial system has determined that the use of these documents in such a setting where anyone should be entitled to unrestricted medical care, which should be provided in accordance with acceptable standards of care, should not "encourage" substandard care by allowing those who provide substandard service to escape the legal consequences of their own misdeeds through the use of such documents. As a consequence, where CEPs are providing service within a healthcare or medical setting, prospectively executed release documents will probably not be effective as a risk management tool to avoid the legal consequences of untoward events. In other settings, however, where medical care is not involved, such documents may well be effective in transferring the legal consequences of untoward events, including those which arise out of negligent acts or omissions.

Any risk management plan must also include the provision of liability insurance to cover those risks which can not be eliminated, minimized, or transferred through other means. It is important that such insurance meet the potential claims that may be involved with the provision of service and provide both a defense (insurance paid legal counsel) and indemnification (payment of any claim or judgment) arising out of any potential lawsuit. The services of attorneys and insurance professionals may be necessary to ensure that appropriate coverage is secured and provided for particular CEP practices.

ETHICAL CONCERNS

All CEPs have the benefit of, and are subject to, a Code of Ethics established by the Clinical Exercise Physiology Practice Board/ACSM. Others, including the Clinical Exercise Physiology Association (CEPA), an affiliate society of ACSM, also have established Codes of Ethics for exercise physiologists (13,14) and other similar exercise professionals (15). The State of Louisiana has also passed legislation to provide for a Code of Ethics for the CEPs licensed in that state. Presumably, a violation of any applicable Ethical Code may lead to disciplinary action and even loss of certification or licensure where applicable.

SUMMARY

Whether licensed, certified, or otherwise providing service in the healthcare or fitness fields, CEPs are presented with a variety of opportunities to provide diverse services. From a legal perspective, some of these opportunities have not yet been clearly defined. As a consequence, any analysis of the practice provided by CEPs depends on both the setting within which services are rendered and certain delivery concerns, such as whether services are provided through a permissible licensed healthcare provider delegation.

Services rendered by CEPs are subject to provision in accordance with the so-called standard of care which is usually set in the legal arena by reference to state statutes and regulations. As a consequence, healthcare-related service as delivered by CEPs will be evaluated from a legal perspective by reference to state statutes and regulations to determine if services are permissibly rendered by nonlicensed persons and in case of an untoward event by reference to malpractice and negligence principles evaluated by standard of care statements. Therefore, CEPs need to ensure that their services are properly rendered in accordance with state laws and regulations and standard of care statements. CEPs who render service within a healthcare model need to conform to healthcare provider type requirements, such as informed consent. Codes of Ethics must also be followed to maintain professional standing as well as licensure or certification, whichever the case may be.

REFERENCES

1. Hedgecorth v. United States. 618 F.Supp. 627 (Dist. Ct., E.D. Mo.), 1985.
2. ACC/AHA Clinical Competence statement on stress testing: A report of the American College of Cardiology/American Heart Association/American College of Physicians–American Society of Internal Medicine Task Force on Clinical Competence. *J Am Coll Cardiol* 2000;36:1441–53.
3. American Association of Cardiovascular & Pulmonary Rehabilitation. *Guidelines for Cardiac Rehabilitation and Secondary Prevention Programs.* Champaign, IL: Human Kinetics; 2004.
4. American College of Sports Medicine. *ACSM's Resources for Clinical Exercise Physiology: Musculoskeletal, Neuromuscular, Neoplastic, Immunologic, and Hematologic Conditions.* Philadelphia: Lippincott Williams & Wilkins; 2002.
5. Smogor v. Enke. 874 F.2d 295 (5ᵗʰ Cir 1989), 1971.
6. American College of Sports Medicine. *ACSM's Guidelines for Exercise Testing and Prescription,* 7th ed. Philadelphia: Lippincott Williams & Wilkins; 2006.
7. American College of Sports Medicine. *ACSM's Health/fitness Facility Standards and Guidelines,* 3rd ed. Champaign, IL: Human Kinetics; 2007.
8. Tart v. McGann. 697 F.2d 75, (2d Cir), 1982.
9. Darling v. Fairfield Medical Center. Ohio App. LEXIS 3268, 2001.
10. DL Herbert. Large Verdict Against AED Deficient Health and Fitness Facility. *The Exercise Standards and Malpractice Reporter* 2006;20(4):49;52–4.
11. Chadderton v. Bongivonni, Inc. 647 A.2d 137 (Ct.Spec, Appeals, Maryland), 1993.
12. DL Herbert & WG Herbert. *Legal Aspects of Preventive, Rehabilitative and Recreational Exercise Programs,* 4th ed. Canton, Ohio: PRC Publishing; 2002.
13. American Society of Exercise Physiologists (ASEP). Standards of Professional Practice. Available at http://www.asep.org/services/standards. Accessed November 20, 2007.
14. Clinical Exercise Physiology Association (CEPA). Code of Ethics. Available at http://www.acsm-cepa.org. Accessed October 23, 2008.
15. National Board of Fitness Examiners (NBFE), http://www.nbfe.org. Accessed July 2, 2007.
16. DL Herbert. Massachusetts Considering Bill to License Clinical Exercise Physiologists (CEPs). *The Exercise Standards and Malpractice Reporter* 2007;21(2):17;20–2.

American College of Sports Medicine Certifications

This appendix details information about American College of Sports Medicine (ACSM) Certification and Registry Programs, as well as a complete listing of the current knowledge, skills, and abilities (KSAs) that comprise the foundations of these certification and registry examinations. The mission of the ACSM Committee on Certification and Registry Boards is to develop and provide high-quality, accessible, and affordable credentials and continuing education programs for health and exercise professionals who are responsible for preventive and rehabilitative programs that influence the health and well-being of all individuals.

ACSM CERTIFICATIONS AND THE PUBLIC

The first ACSM clinical certification was initiated over 30 years ago in conjunction with publication of the first edition of the *Guidelines for Exercise Testing and Prescription*. That era was marked by rapid development of exercise programs for patients with stable coronary artery disease (CAD). ACSM sought a means to disseminate accurate information on this health care initiative through expression of consensus from its members in basic science, clinical practice, and education. Thus, these early clinical certifications were viewed as an aid to the establishment of safe and scientifically based exercise services within the framework of cardiac rehabilitation.

Over the past 30 years, exercise has gained widespread favor as an important component in programs of rehabilitative care or health maintenance for an expanding list of chronic diseases and disabling conditions. The growth of public interest in the role of exercise in health promotion has been equally impressive. In addition, federal government policy makers have revisited questions of medical efficacy and financing for exercise services in rehabilitative care of selected patients. Over the past several years, recommendations from the U.S. Public Health Service and the U.S. Surgeon General have acknowledged the central role for regular physical activity in the prevention of disease and promotion of health.

The development of the health/fitness certifications in the 1980s reflected ACSM's intent to increase the availability of qualified professionals to provide scientifically sound advice and supervision regarding appropriate physical activities for health maintenance in the apparently healthy adult population. Since 1975, more than

35,000 certificates have been awarded. With this consistent growth, ACSM has taken steps to ensure that its competency-based certifications will continue to be regarded as the premier program in the exercise field.

The ACSM Committee on Certification and Registry Boards (CCRB) Publications Sub-Committee publishes *ACSM's Certified News*, a periodical addressing professional practice issues whose target audience is those who are certified. The CCRB Continuing Professional Education Sub-Committee has oversight of the continuing education requirements for maintenance of certification and auditing renewal candidates. Continuing education credits can be accrued through ACSM-sponsored educational programs, such as ACSM workshops (ACSM Certified Personal Trainer, ACSM Health/Fitness Instructor, ACSM Exercise Specialist, ACSM Registered Clinical Exercise Physiologist), regional chapter and annual meetings, and other educational programs approved by the ACSM Professional Education Committee. These enhancements are intended to support the continued professional growth of those who have made a commitment to service in this rapidly growing health and fitness field.

In 2004, ACSM was as a founding member of the multiorganizational Committee on Accreditation for the Exercise Sciences (CoAES), and assisted with the development of Standards and Guidelines for educational programs seeking accreditation under the auspices of the Commission on Accreditation of Allied Health Education Programs (CAAHEP). Additional information on outcomes-based, programmatic accreditation can be obtained by visiting www.caahep.org, and specific information regarding the Standards and Guidelines can be obtained by visiting www.coaes.org. Because the standards and guidelines refer to the KSAs that follow, reference to specific KSAs as they relate to given sets of standards and guidelines will be noted when appropriate.

The ACSM also acknowledges the expectation from successful candidates that the public will be informed of the high standards, values, and professionalism implicit in meeting these certification requirements. The College has formally organized its volunteer committee structure and national office staff to give added emphasis to informing the public, professionals, and government agencies about issues of critical importance to ACSM. Informing these constituencies about the meaning and value of

ACSM certification is one important priority that will be given attention in this initiative.

ACSM CERTIFICATION PROGRAMS

The ACSM Certified Personal Trainer is a fitness professional involved in developing and implementing an individualized approach to exercise leadership in healthy populations and in those individuals with medical clearance to exercise. Using a variety of teaching techniques, the ACSM Certified Personal Trainer is proficient in leading and demonstrating safe and effective methods of exercise by applying the fundamental principles of exercise science. The ACSM Certified Personal Trainer is familiar with forms of exercise used to improve, maintain, and optimize health-related components of physical fitness and performance. The ACSM Certified Personal Trainer is proficient in writing appropriate exercise recommendations, leading and demonstrating safe and effective methods of exercise, and motivating individuals to begin and to continue with their healthy behaviors.

The ACSM Health/Fitness Instructor (HFI) is a degreed health and fitness professional qualified for career pursuits in the university, corporate, commercial, hospital, and community settings. The HFI has knowledge and skills in management, administration, training, and supervising entry-level personnel. The HFI is skilled in conducting risk stratification and physical fitness assessments, and in interpreting results; and in constructing appropriate exercise prescriptions and motivating apparently healthy individuals and individuals with medically controlled diseases to adopt and maintain healthy lifestyle behaviors.

The ACSM Exercise Specialist (ES) is a health care professional certified by ACSM to deliver a variety of exercise assessment, training, rehabilitation, risk factor identification, and lifestyle management services to individuals with or at risk for cardiovascular, pulmonary, and metabolic disease(s). These services are typically delivered in cardiovascular or pulmonary rehabilitation programs, physicians' offices, or medical fitness centers. The ACSM Exercise Specialist is also competent to provide exercise-related consulting for research, public health, and other clinical and nonclinical services and programs.

The ACSM Registered Clinical Exercise Physiologist (RCEP) is an allied health professional who works in the application of physical activity and behavioral interventions for those clinical conditions where they have been shown to provide therapeutic and functional benefit. Persons for whom RCEP services are appropriate may include, but are not limited to, those individuals with cardiovascular, pulmonary, metabolic, orthopedic, musculoskeletal, neuromuscular, neoplastic, immunologic, or hematologic disease. The RCEP provides primary and secondary prevention strategies designed to improve fitness and health in populations ranging from children to older adults. The RCEP performs exercise screening, exercise and fitness testing, exercise prescription, exercise and physical activity counseling, exercise supervision, exercise and health education and promotion, and measurement and evaluation of exercise and physical activity related outcome measures. The RCEP works individually or as part of an interdisciplinary team in a clinical, community or public health setting. The practice and supervision of the RCEP is guided by published professional guidelines, standards, and applicable state and federal regulations.

Certification at a given level requires the candidate to have a knowledge and skills base commensurate with that specific level of certification. In addition, the HFI level of certification incorporates the KSAs associated with the ACSM Certified Personal Trainer certification, the ES level of certification incorporates the KSAs associated with the CPT and HFI certification, and the RCEP level of certification incorporates the KSAs associated with the CPT, HFI, and ES levels of certification, as shown in Table 1.

TABLE 1. REQUIREMENTS AND RECOMMENDED COMPETENCIES FOR THE ACSM REGISTERED CLINICAL EXERCISE PHYSIOLOGIST

LEVEL	REQUIREMENTS	RECOMMENDED COMPETENCIES
ACSM Registered Clinical Exercise Physiologist®	• Master's Degree in exercise science, exercise physiology or kinesiology from a regionally accredited college or university • Current certification as a Basic Life Support Provider or CPR for the Professional Rescuer (*available through the American Heart Association or the American Red Cross*). • Minimum of 600 clinical hours or alternatives as described in the current issue of ACSM's Certification Resource Guide. Hours may be completed as part of a formal degree program.	Demonstrate competence in the KSAs required of the ACSM Registered Clinical Exercise Physiologist®, Exercise Specialist®, Health/Fitness Instructor® and ACSM Certified Personal Trainer^SM as listed in the current edition of *ACSM's Guidelines for Exercise Testing and Prescription*.

Recommendation of hours in Clinical Practice Areas
Cardiovascular: 200
Pulmonary: 100
Metabolic: 120
Orthopedic and musculoskeletal: 100
Neuromuscular: 40
Immunological and hematological: 40

In addition, each level of certification has minimal requirements for experience, level of education, or other certifications.

ACSM also develops specialty certifications to enhance the breadth of knowledge for individuals working in a health, fitness, or clinical setting. For information on KSAs, eligibility and scope of practice for ACSM specialty certifications, visit www.acsm.org/certification or call 1-800-486-5643.

HOW TO OBTAIN INFORMATION AND APPLICATION MATERIALS

The certification programs of ACSM are subject to continuous review and revision. Content development is entrusted to a diverse committee of professional volunteers with expertise in exercise science, medicine, and program management. Expertise in design and procedures for competency assessment is also represented on this committee. The administration of certification examinations is conducted through Pearson VUE authorized testing centers. Inquiries regarding examination registration can be made to Pearson VUE at 1-888-883-2276 or on-line at www.pearsonvue.com/acsm.

For general certification questions, contact the ACSM Certification Resource Center:
1-800-486-5643
Web site: www.acsm.org/certification
E-mail: certification@acsm.org

KNOWLEDGE, SKILLS, AND ABILITIES UNDERLINING ACSM CERTIFICATIONS

Minimal competencies for each certification level are outlined below. Certification examinations are constructed based on these KSAs. For the ACSM Health/Fitness Instructor and the ACSM Exercise Specialist credentials, two companion ACSM publications, *ACSM's Resource Manual for Guidelines for Exercise Testing and Prescription, sixth edition*, and *ACSM's Certification Review Book, third edition*, may also be used to gain further insight pertaining to the topics identified here. For the ACSM Certified Personal Trainer, candidates should refer to *ACSM's Resources for the Personal Trainer, current edition* and *ACSM's Certification Review Book, third edition*. For the ACSM Registered Clinical Exercise Physiologist, candidates should refer to ACSM's Resources for Clinical Exercise Physiology, current edition and *ACSM's Resource Manual for Guidelines for Exercise Testing and Prescription, sixth edition*. Neither the *ACSM's Guidelines for Exercise Testing and Prescription* nor any of the above-mentioned resource manuals provides all of the information on which the ACSM Certification examinations are based, however. Each may prove to be beneficial as a review of specific topics and as a general outline of many of the integral concepts to be mastered by those seeking certification.

CLASSIFICATION/NUMBERING SYSTEM FOR KNOWLEDGE, SKILLS, AND ABILITIES (KSAs)

All the KSAs for a given certification or credential are listed in their entirety across a given a Practice Area or a Content Matter Area for each level of certification. Within each certification's or credential's KSA set, the numbering of individual KSAs uses a three-part number as follows:

First number–denotes Practice Area (1.x.x)
Second number–denotes Content Area (x.1.x)
Third number–denotes the sequential number of each KSA (x.x.1), within each Content Area. If there is a break in numerical sequence, it indicates that a KSA was deleted in response to the recent job-task analysis from the prior version of the KSAs. From this edition forward, new KSAs will acquire a new KSA number.

The Practice Areas (the first number) are numbered as follows:

1.x.x	General Population/Core
2.x.x	Cardiovascular
3.x.x	Pulmonary
4.x.x	Metabolic
5.x.x	Orthopedic/Musculoskeletal
6.x.x	Neuromuscular
7.x.x	Neoplastic, Immunologic, and Hematologic

The Content Matter Areas (the second number) are numbered as follows:

x.1.x	Exercise Physiology and related Exercise Science
x.2.x	Pathophysiology and Risk Factors
x.3.x	Health Appraisal, Fitness and Clinical Exercise Testing
x.4.x	Electrocardiography and Diagnostic Techniques
x.5.x	Patient Management and Medications
x.6.x	Medical and Surgical Management
x.7.x	Exercise Prescription and Programming
x.8.x	Nutrition and Weight Management
x.9.x	Human Behavior and Counseling
x.10.x	Safety, Injury Prevention, and Emergency Procedures
x.11.x	Program Administration, Quality Assurance, and Outcome Assessment
x.12.x	Clinical and Medical Considerations (ACSM Certified Personal Trainer Only)

EXAMPLES by Level of Certification/Credential

ACSM Certified Personal Trainer KSAs:

1.1.10   Have knowledge to describe the normal acute responses to cardiovascular exercise.

In this example, the Practice Area is *General Population/Core*; the Content Matter Area is *Exercise Physiology and Related Exercise Science*; and this KSA is the tenth KSA within this Content Matter Area.

ACSM Health/Fitness Instructor KSAs:

1.3.8   Skill in accurately measuring heart rate, blood pressure, and obtaining rating of perceived exertion (RPE) at rest and during exercise according to established guidelines.

In this example, the practice area is *General Population/Core*; the Content Matter Area is *Health Appraisal, Fitness, and Clinical Exercise Testing*; and this KSA is the eighth KSA within this Content Matter Area.

ACSM Exercise Specialist KSAs*:

1.7.17   Design strength and flexibility programs for individuals with cardiovascular, pulmonary or metabolic diseases, the elderly, and children.

In this example, the practice area is *General Population/Core*; the Content Matter Area is *Exercise Prescription and Programming*; and this KSA is the seventeenth KSA within this Content Matter Area. Furthermore, because this specific KSA appears in bold, it covers multiple practice and content areas.

ACSM Registered Clinical Exercise Physiologist KSAs:

7.6.1   List the drug classifications commonly used in the treatment of patients with a neoplastic, immunologic hematologic (NIH) disease, name common generic and brand names drugs within each class, and explain the purposes, indications, major side effects, and the effects, if any, on the exercising individual.

The practice area is Neoplastic, *Immunologic, and Hematologic*; the Content Matter Area is *Medical and Surgical Management*; and this KSA is the first KSA within this Content Matter Area.

A special note about ACSM Exercise Specialist KSAs:

As with the other certifications presented thus far, the ACSM Exercise Specialist KSAs are categorized by content area. Some ES KSAs, however, cover multiple practices areas within each area of content. For example, a number of them describe a specific topic with respect to both exercise testing and training, which are two distinct content areas. Rather than write out each separately (which would have greatly expanded the KSA list length) they have been listed under a single content area. When reviewing these KSAs, please note that KSAs in bold text cover multiple content areas. Each ES KSA begins with a "I" as the practice area. However, where appropriate, some KSAs mention specific patient populations (i.e., practice area). If a specific practice area is not mentioned within a given KSA, then it applies equally to each of the general population, cardiovascular, pulmonary, and metabolic practice areas. Note that "metabolic patients" are defined as those with at least one of the following: overweight or obese, diabetes (type 1 or 2), metabolic syndrome. Each KSA describes either a single or multiple knowledge (K), skill (S), or ability (A), or a combination of K, S or A, that an individual should master to be considered a competent ACSM Exercise Specialist.

The Registered Clinical Exercise Physiologist is responsible for the mastery of the ACSM Certified Personal Trainer KSAs, the ACSM Health/Fitness Instructor KSAs, the ACSM Exercise Specialist KSAs, and the following ACSM Registered Clinical Exercise Physiologist KSAs:

GENERAL POPULATION/CORE:
EXERCISE PHYSIOLOGY AND RELATED
EXERCISE SCIENCE

1.1.1   Describe the acute responses to aerobic, resistance, and flexibility training on the function of the cardiovascular, respiratory, musculoskeletal, neuromuscular, metabolic, endocrine, and immune systems.

1.1.2   Describe the chronic effects of aerobic, resistance, and flexibility training on the structure and function of the cardiovascular, respiratory, musculoskeletal, neuromuscular, metabolic, endocrine, and immune systems.

1.1.3   Explain differences in typical values for oxygen uptake, heart rate, mean arterial pressure, systolic and diastolic blood pressure, cardiac output, stroke volume, rate pressure product, minute ventilation, respiratory rate, and tidal volume at rest and during submaximal and maximal exercise between sedentary and trained persons with chronic diseases.

1.1.4   Describe the physiologic determinants of $\dot{V}O_2$, $m\dot{V}O_2$, and mean arterial pressure and explain how these determinants can be altered with aerobic and resistance exercise training.

1.1.5   Describe appropriate modifications in the exercise prescription owing to environmental conditions in individuals with chronic disease.

1.1.6   Explain the health benefits of a physically active lifestyle, the hazards of sedentary behavior, and summarize key recommendations of U.S. national reports of physical activity (e.g., U.S. Surgeon General, Institute of Medicine, ACSM, American Heart Association [AHA])

1.1.7   Explain the physiologic adaptations to exercise training that might result in improvement in, or maintenance of, health, including cardiovascular, pulmonary, metabolic, orthopedic, musculoskeletal, neuromuscular, and immune system health.

1.1.8   Explain the mechanisms underlying the physiologic adaptations to aerobic and resistance training, including those resulting in changes in, or maintenance of, maximal and submaximal oxygen consumption, lactate and ventilatory (anaerobic) threshold, myocardial oxygen consumption, heart rate, blood pressure, ventilation (including ventilatory threshold), muscle structure, bioenergetics, and immune function.

1.1.9   Explain the physiologic effects of physical inactivity, including bedrest, and methods that may counteract these effects.

1.1.10 Recognize and respond to abnormal signs and symptoms during exercise.
GENERAL POPULATION/CORE: PATHOPHYSIOLOGY AND RISK FACTORS

1.2.1 Describe the epidemiology, pathophysiology, risk factors, and key clinical findings of cardiovascular, pulmonary, metabolic, orthopedic, musculoskeletal, neuromuscular, and NIH diseases.
GENERAL POPULATION/CORE: HEALTH APPRAISAL, FITNESS AND CLINICAL EXERCISE TESTING

1.3.1 Conduct pretest procedures, including explaining test procedures, obtaining informed consent, obtaining a focused medical history, reviewing results of prior tests and physical examinations, assessing disease-specific risk factors, and presenting concise information to other health care providers and third-party payers.

1.3.2 Conduct a brief physical examination, including evaluation of peripheral edema; measuring blood pressure, peripheral pulses, and respiratory rate; and auscultating heart and lung sounds.

1.3.3 Calibrate laboratory equipment used frequently in the practice of clinical exercise physiology (e.g., motorized or computerized treadmill, mechanical cycle ergometer and arm ergometer), electrocardiograph, spirometer, and respiratory gas analyzer (Metabolic cart).

1.3.4 Administer exercise tests consistent with U.S. nationally accepted standards for testing.

1.3.5 Evaluate contraindications to exercise testing.

1.3.6 Appropriately select and administer functional tests to measure individual outcomes and functional status, including the 6-minute walk, Get Up and Go, Berg Balance Scale, Physical Performance Test, and so forth.

1.3.8 Interpret the variables that may be assessed during clinical exercise testing, including maximal oxygen consumption, resting metabolic rate, ventilatory volumes and capacities, respiratory exchange ratio, ratings of perceived exertion and discomfort (chest pain, dyspnea, claudication), electrocardiogram (ECG), heart rate, blood pressure, rate pressure product, ventilatory (anaerobic) threshold, oxygen saturation, breathing reserve, muscular strength, muscular endurance, and other common measures used for diagnosis and prognosis of disease.

1.3.9 Determine atrial and ventricular rate from rhythm strip and 12-lead ECG and explain the clinical significance of abnormal atrial or ventricular rate (e.g., tachycardia, bradycardia).

1.3.10 Identify ECG changes associated with drug therapy, electrolyte abnormalities, subendocardial and transmural ischemia, myocardial injury, and infarction, and explain the clinical significance of each.

1.3.11 Identify SA, AV, and bundle branch blocks from a rhythm strip and 12-lead ECG, and explain the clinical significance of each.

1.3.12 Identify sinus, atrial, junctional, and ventricular dysrhythmias from a rhythm strip and 12-lead ECG, and explain the clinical significance of each.

1.3.14 Determine an individual's pretest and posttest probability of coronary heart disease (CHD), identify factors associated with test complications, and apply appropriate precautions to reduce risks to the individual.

1.3.16 Identify probable disease-specific endpoints for testing in an individual with cardiovascular, pulmonary, metabolic, orthopedic, musculoskeletal, neuromuscular, and NIH disease.

1.3.17 Select and use appropriate techniques to prepare and measure ECG, heart rate, blood pressure, oxygen saturation, RPE, symptoms, expired gases, and other measures as needed before, during, and following exercise testing.

1.3.18 Select and administer appropriate exercise tests to evaluate functional capacity, strength, and flexibility in individuals with cardiovascular, pulmonary, metabolic, orthopedic, musculoskeletal, neuromuscular, and NIH disease.

1.3.19 Discuss strengths and limitations of various methods of measures and indices of body composition.

1.3.20 Appropriately select, apply, and interpret body composition tests and indices.

1.3.21 Discuss pertinent test results with other health care professionals.
GENERAL POPULATION/CORE: EXERCISE PRESCRIPTION AND PROGRAMMING

1.7.3 Determine the appropriate level of supervision and monitoring recommended for individuals with known disease based on disease-specific risk stratification guidelines and current health status.

1.7.4 Develop, adapt, and supervise appropriate aerobic, resistance, and flexibility training for individuals with cardiovascular, pulmonary, metabolic, orthopedic, musculoskeletal, neuromuscular, and NIH disease.

1.7.6 Instruct individuals with cardiovascular, pulmonary, metabolic, orthopedic, musculoskeletal, neuromuscular, and NIH disease in techniques for performing physical activities safely and effectively in an unsupervised exercise setting.

1.7.7 Modify the exercise prescription or discontinue exercise based on individual symptoms, current health status, musculoskeletal limitations, and environmental considerations.

1.7.8 Extract and interpret clinical information needed for safe exercise management of individuals with cardiovascular, pulmonary, metabolic, orthopedic, musculoskeletal, neuromuscular, and NIH disease.

1.7.9   Evaluate individual outcomes from serial outcome data collected before, during, and after exercise interventions.
GENERAL POPULATION/CORE:
HUMAN BEHAVIOR AND COUNSELING

1.9.1   Summarize contemporary theories of health behavior change, including social cognitive theory, theory of reasoned action, theory of planned behavior, transtheoretical model, and health belief model, and apply techniques to promote healthy behaviors including physical activity.

1.9.2   Describe characteristics associated with poor adherence to exercise programs.

1.9.3   Describe the psychological issues associated with acute and chronic illness, such as anxiety, depression, social isolation, hostility, aggression, and suicidal ideation.

1.9.4   Counsel individuals with cardiovascular, pulmonary, metabolic, orthopedic, musculoskeletal, neuromuscular, and NIH disease on topics such as disease processes, treatments, diagnostic techniques, and lifestyle management.

1.9.6   Explain factors that can increase anxiety before or during exercise testing and describe methods to reduce anxiety.

1.9.7   Recognize signs and symptoms of failure to cope during personal crises such as job loss, bereavement, and illness.
GENERAL POPULATION/CORE:
SAFETY, INJURY PREVENTION, AND
EMERGENCY PROCEDURES

1.10.1 List routine emergency equipment, drugs, and supplies present in an exercise testing laboratory and therapeutic exercise session area.

1.10.2 Provide immediate responses to emergencies, including basic cardiac life support, automated external defibrillator (AED), activation of emergency medical system (EMS), and joint immobilization.

1.10.3 Verify operating status of emergency equipment, including defibrillator, laryngoscope, oxygen, and so forth.

1.10.4 Explain Universal Precautions procedures and apply as appropriate.

1.10.5 Develop and implement a plan for responding to emergencies.

1.10.6 Have knowledge of advanced cardiac life support procedures.
GENERAL POPULATION/CORE:
PROGRAM ADMINISTRATION, QUALITY
ASSURANCE, AND OUTCOME ASSESSMENT

1.11.1 Describe appropriate staffing for exercise testing and programming based on factors such as individual health status, facilities, and program goals.

1.11.2 List necessary equipment and supplies for exercise testing and programs.

1.11.3 Select, evaluate, and report treatment outcomes using individual-relevant results of tests and surveys.

1.11.4 Explain legal issues pertinent to health care delivery by licensed and nonlicensed health care professionals providing rehabilitative services and exercise testing and legal risk management techniques.

1.11.5 Identify individuals requiring referral to a physician or allied health services, such as physical therapy, dietary counseling, stress management, weight management, and psychological and social services.

1.11.6 Develop a plan for individual discharge from therapeutic exercise program, including community referrals.
CARDIOVASCULAR:
EXERCISE PHYSIOLOGY AND RELATED
EXERCISE SCIENCE

2.1.2   Describe the potential benefits and hazards of aerobic, resistance, and flexibility training in individuals with cardiovascular diseases.

2.1.4   Explain how cardiovascular diseases can affect the physiologic responses to aerobic and resistance training.

2.1.5   Describe the immediate and long-term influence of medical therapies for cardiovascular diseases on the responses to aerobic and resistance training.
CARDIOVASCULAR:
PATHOPHYSIOLOGY AND RISK FACTORS

2.2.1   Describe the epidemiology, pathophysiology, rate of disease progression, risk factors, and key clinical findings of cardiovascular diseases.

2.2.2   Explain the ischemic cascade and its effect on myocardial function.

2.2.4   Explain methods of reducing risk in individuals with cardiovascular diseases.
CARDIOVASCULAR:
HEALTH APPRAISAL, FITNESS AND
CLINICAL EXERCISE TESTING

2.3.1   Describe common techniques used to diagnose cardiovascular disease, including graded exercise testing, echocardiography, radionuclide imaging, angiography, pharmacologic testing, and biomarkers (e.g., troponin, creatine kinase [CK]), and explain the indications, limitations, risks, and normal and abnormal results for each.

2.3.2   Explain how cardiovascular disease can affect physical examination findings.

2.3.4   Recognize and respond to abnormal signs and symptoms, such as pain, peripheral edema, dyspnea, fatigue, in individuals with cardiovascular diseases.

2.3.5   Conduct and interpret appropriate exercise testing methods for individuals with cardiovascular diseases.

CARDIOVASCULAR:
MEDICAL AND SURGICAL MANAGEMENT

2.6.2 Explain the common medical and surgical treatments of cardiovascular diseases.

2.6.3 Apply key recommendations of current U.S. clinical practice guidelines for the prevention, treatment, and management of cardiovascular diseases (e.g., AHA, American College of Cardiology [ACC], National Heart, Lung, and Blood Institute [NHLBI]).

2.6.4 List the commonly used drugs (generic and brand names) in the treatment of individuals with cardiovascular diseases, and explain the indications, mechanisms of actions, major side effects, and the effects on the exercising individual.

2.6.5 Explain how treatments for cardiovascular disease, including preventive care, may affect the rate of progression of disease.

CARDIOVASCULAR:
EXERCISE PRESCRIPTION AND PROGRAMMING

2.7.2 Design, adapt, and supervise an appropriate Exercise Prescription (e.g., aerobic, resistance, and flexibility training) for individuals with cardiovascular diseases.

2.7.4 Instruct an individual with cardiovascular disease in techniques for performing physical activities safely and effectively in an unsupervised setting.

2.7.5 Counsel individuals with cardiovascular disease on the proper uses of sublingual nitroglycerin.

PULMONARY (e.g., Obstructive and Restrictive Lung Diseases):
EXERCISE PHYSIOLOGY AND RELATED EXERCISE SCIENCE

3.1.1 Describe the potential benefits and hazards of aerobic, resistance, and flexibility training in individuals with pulmonary diseases.

3.1.2 Explain how pulmonary diseases can affect the physiologic responses to aerobic, resistance, and flexibility training.

3.1.3 Explain how scheduling of exercise relative to meals can affect dyspnea.

3.1.5 Describe the immediate and long-term influence of medical therapies for pulmonary diseases on the responses to aerobic, resistance, and flexibility training.

PULMONARY:
PATHOPHYSIOLOGY AND RISK FACTORS

3.2.1 Describe the epidemiology, pathophysiology, rate of disease progression, risk factors, and key clinical findings of pulmonary diseases.

3.2.3 Explain methods of reducing risk in individuals with pulmonary diseases.

PULMONARY:
HEALTH APPRAISAL, FITNESS AND CLINICAL EXERCISE TESTING

3.3.1 Explain how pulmonary disease can affect physical examination findings.

3.3.3 Have knowledge of lung volumes and capacities (e.g., tidal volume, residual volume, inspiratory volume, expiratory volume, total lung capacity, vital capacity, functional residual capacity, peak flow rate, diffusion capacity) and how they might differ between healthy individuals and individuals with pulmonary disease.

3.3.4 Recognize and respond to abnormal signs and symptoms to exercise in individuals with pulmonary diseases.

3.3.5 Describe common techniques and tests used to diagnose pulmonary diseases, and explain the indications, limitations, risks, and normal and abnormal results for each.

3.3.6 Conduct and interpret appropriate exercise testing methods for individuals with pulmonary diseases.

PULMONARY:
MEDICAL AND SURGICAL MANAGEMENT

3.6.3 Explain how treatments for pulmonary disease, including preventive care, can affect the rate of disease progression.

3.6.5 Explain the common medical and surgical treatments of pulmonary diseases.

3.6.6 List the commonly used drugs (generic and brand names) used in the treatment of individuals with pulmonary diseases, and explain the indications, mechanisms of actions, major side effects, and the effects on the exercising individual.

3.6.7 Apply key recommendations of current U.S. clinical practice guidelines (e.g., American Lung Association [ALA], NIH, NHLBI) for the prevention, treatment, and management of pulmonary diseases.

PULMONARY:
EXERCISE PRESCRIPTION AND PROGRAMMING

3.7.2 Design, adapt, and supervise an appropriate exercise prescription (e.g., aerobic, resistance, and flexibility training) for individuals with pulmonary diseases.

3.7.4 Instruct an individual with pulmonary diseases in proper breathing techniques and exercises and methods for performing physical activities safely and effectively.

3.7.5 Have knowledge of the use of supplemental oxygen during exercise and its influences on exercise tolerance.

METABOLIC (e.g., Diabetes, Hyperlipidemia, Obesity, Frailty, Chronic Renal Failure, Metabolic Syndrome):
EXERCISE PHYSIOLOGY AND RELATED EXERCISE SCIENCE

4.1.1 Explain how metabolic diseases can affect aerobic endurance, muscular strength and endurance, flexibility, and balance.

4.1.2 Describe the immediate and long-term influence of medical therapies for metabolic diseases on the responses to aerobic, resistance, and flexibility training.

4.1.3 Describe the potential benefits and hazards of aerobic, resistance, and flexibility training in individuals with metabolic diseases.
PATHOPHYSIOLOGY AND RISK FACTORS

4.2.1 Describe the epidemiology, pathophysiology, rate of disease progression, risk factors, and key clinical findings of metabolic diseases.

4.2.5 Describe the probable effects of dialysis treatment on exercise performance, functional capacity, and safety, and explain methods for preventing adverse effects.

4.2.6 Describe the probable effects of hypo- or hyperglycemia on exercise performance, functional capacity, and safety, and explain methods for preventing adverse effects.

4.2.7 Explain methods of reducing risk in individuals with metabolic diseases.
METABOLIC:
HEALTH APPRAISAL, FITNESS AND CLINICAL EXERCISE TESTING

4.3.1 Describe common techniques and tests used to diagnose metabolic diseases, and explain the indications, limitations, risks, and normal and abnormal results for each.

4.3.3 Explain appropriate techniques for monitoring blood glucose before, during, and after an exercise session.

4.3.4 Recognize and respond to abnormal signs and symptoms in individuals with metabolic diseases.

4.3.5 Conduct and interpret appropriate exercise testing methods for individuals with metabolic diseases.
METABOLIC:
MEDICAL AND SURGICAL MANAGEMENT

4.6.2 Apply key recommendations of current U.S. clinical practice guidelines (e.g., ADA, NIH, NHLBI) for the prevention, treatment, and management of metabolic diseases.

4.6.3 Explain the common medical and surgical treatments of metabolic diseases.

4.6.4 List the drugs (generic and brand names) commonly used in the treatment of individuals with metabolic diseases, and explain the indications, mechanisms of actions, major side effects, and the effects on the exercising individual.

4.6.5 Explain how treatments for metabolic diseases, including preventive care, can affect the rate of progression of disease.
METABOLIC:
EXERCISE PRESCRIPTION AND PROGRAMMING

4.7.2 Design, adapt, and supervise an appropriate Exercise Prescription (e.g., aerobic, resistance, and flexibility training) for individuals with metabolic diseases.

4.7.4 Instruct individuals with metabolic diseases in techniques for performing physical activities safely and effectively in an unsupervised exercise setting.

4.7.5 Adapt the exercise prescription based on the functional limits and benefits of assistive devices (e.g., wheelchairs, crutches, and canes).
ORTHOPEDIC/MUSCULOSKELETAL (e.g., Low Back Pain, Osteoarthritis, Rheumatoid Arthritis, Osteoporosis, Amputations, Vertebral Disorders):
EXERCISE PHYSIOLOGY AND RELATED EXERCISE SCIENCE

5.1.1 Describe the potential benefits and hazards of aerobic, resistance, and flexibility training in individuals with orthopedic or musculoskeletal diseases.

5.1.4 Explain how orthopedic and musculoskeletal diseases can affect aerobic endurance, muscular strength and endurance, flexibility, balance, and agility.

5.1.5 Describe the immediate and long-term influence of medical therapies for orthopedic and musculoskeletal diseases on the responses to aerobic, resistance, and flexibility training.
ORTHOPEDIC/MUSCULOSKELETAL:
PATHOPHYSIOLOGY AND RISK FACTORS

5.2.1 Describe the epidemiology, pathophysiology, risk factors, and key clinical findings of orthopedic and musculoskeletal diseases.
ORTHOPEDIC/MUSCULOSKELETAL:
HEALTH APPRAISAL, FITNESS AND CLINICAL EXERCISE TESTING

5.3.1 Recognize and respond to abnormal signs and symptoms to exercise in individuals with orthopedic or musculoskeletal diseases.

5.3.2 Describe common techniques and tests used to diagnose orthopedic and musculoskeletal diseases.

5.3.3 Conduct and interpret appropriate exercise testing methods for individuals with orthopedic or musculoskeletal diseases.
ORTHOPEDIC/MUSCULOSKELETAL:
MEDICAL AND SURGICAL MANAGEMENT

5.6.1 List the drugs (generic and brand names) commonly used in the treatment of individuals with orthopedic and musculoskeletal diseases, and explain the indications, mechanisms of actions, major side effects, and the effects on the exercising individual.

5.6.2 Explain the common medical and surgical treatments of orthopedic and musculoskeletal diseases.

5.6.3 Apply key recommendations of current U.S. clinical practice guidelines (e.g., NIH, National Osteoporosis Foundation, Arthritis Foundation) for the prevention, treatment, and management of orthopedic and musculoskeletal diseases.

5.6.4 Explain how treatments for orthopedic and musculoskeletal diseases can affect the rate of progression of disease.
ORTHOPEDIC/MUSCULOSKELETAL:
EXERCISE PRESCRIPTION AND
PROGRAMMING

5.7.1 Explain exercise training concepts specific to industrial or occupational rehabilitation, which includes work hardening, work conditioning, work fitness, and job coaching.

5.7.2 Design, adapt, and supervise an appropriate Exercise Prescription (e.g., aerobic, resistance, and flexibility training) for individuals with orthopedic or musculoskeletal diseases.

5.7.3 Instruct an individual with orthopedic or musculoskeletal disease in techniques for performing physical activities safely and effectively in an unsupervised exercise setting.

5.7.4 Adapt the Exercise Prescription based on the functional limits and benefits of assistive devices (e.g., wheelchairs, crutches, and canes).
NEUROMUSCULAR (e.g., Multiple Sclerosis, Muscular Dystrophy and Other Myopathies, Alzheimer's, Parkinson's Disease, Polio and Postpolio syndrome, Stroke and Brain Injury, Cerebral Palsy, Peripheral Neuropathies):
EXERCISE PHYSIOLOGY AND RELATED
EXERCISE SCIENCE

6.1.1 Describe the potential benefits and hazards of aerobic, resistance, and flexibility training in individuals with neuromuscular diseases.

6.1.4 Explain how neuromuscular diseases can affect aerobic endurance, muscular strength and endurance, flexibility, balance, and agility.

6.1.5 Describe the immediate and long-term influence of medical therapies for neuromuscular diseases on the responses to aerobic, resistance, and flexibility training.
NEUROMUSCULAR:
PATHOPHYSIOLOGY AND RISK FACTORS

6.2.1 Describe the epidemiology, pathophysiology, risk factors, and key clinical findings of neuromuscular diseases.
NEUROMUSCULAR:
HEALTH APPRAISAL, FITNESS AND
CLINICAL EXERCISE TESTING

6.3.1 Recognize and respond to abnormal signs and symptoms to exercise in individuals with neuromuscular diseases.

6.3.2 Describe common techniques and tests used to diagnose neuromuscular diseases.

6.3.3 Conduct and interpret appropriate exercise testing methods for individuals with neuromuscular diseases.
NEUROMUSCULAR:
MEDICAL AND SURGICAL MANAGEMENT

6.6.1 Explain the common medical and surgical treatments of neuromuscular diseases.

6.6.2 List the drugs (generic and brand names) commonly used in the treatment of individuals with neuromuscular disease, and explain the indications, mechanisms of actions, major side effects, and the effects on the exercising individual.

6.6.3 Apply key recommendations of current U.S. clinical practice guidelines (e.g., NIH) for the prevention, treatment, and management of neuromuscular diseases.

6.6.4 Explain how treatments for neuromuscular disease can affect the rate of disease progression.
NEUROMUSCULAR:
EXERCISE PRESCRIPTION AND
PROGRAMMING

6.7.1 Adapt the Exercise Prescription based on the functional limits and benefits of assistive devices (e.g., wheelchairs, crutches, and canes).

6.7.3 Design, adapt, and supervise an appropriate Exercise Prescription (e.g., aerobic, resistance, and flexibility training) for individuals with neuromuscular diseases.

6.7.4 Instruct an individual with neuromuscular diseases in techniques for performing physical activities safely and effectively in an unsupervised exercise setting.
NEOPLASTIC, IMMUNOLOGIC, AND
HEMATOLOGIC (e.g., Cancer, Anemia, Bleeding Disorders, Human Immunodeficiency Virus [HIV], Acquired Immunodeficiency Syndrome [AIDS], Organ Transplant, Chronic Fatigue Syndrome, Fibromyalgia):
EXERCISE PHYSIOLOGY AND RELATED
EXERCISE SCIENCE

7.1.1 Explain how NIH diseases can affect the physiologic responses to aerobic, resistance, and flexibility training.

7.1.2 Describe the immediate and long-term influence of medical therapies for NIH on the responses to aerobic, resistance, and flexibility training.

7.1.3 Describe the potential benefits and hazards of aerobic, resistance, and flexibility training in individuals with NIH diseases.
NEOPLASTIC, IMMUNOLOGIC, AND
HEMATOLOGIC:
PATHOPHYSIOLOGY AND RISK FACTORS

7.2.1 Describe the epidemiology, pathophysiology, risk factors, and key clinical findings of NIH diseases.
NEOPLASTIC, IMMUNOLOGIC, AND HEMATOLOGIC: HEALTH APPRAISAL, FITNESS AND CLINICAL EXERCISE TESTING

7.3.1 Recognize and respond to abnormal signs and symptoms to exercise in individuals with NIH diseases.

7.3.2 Describe common techniques and tests used to diagnose NIH diseases.

7.3.3 Conduct and interpret appropriate exercise testing methods for individuals with NIH diseases.
NEOPLASTIC, IMMUNOLOGIC, AND HEMATOLOGIC:
MEDICAL AND SURGICAL MANAGEMENT

7.6.1 List the drugs (generic and brand names) commonly used in the treatment of individuals with NIH disease, and explain the indications, mechanisms of actions, major side effects, and the effects on the exercising individual.

7.6.2 Apply key recommendations of current U.S. clinical practice guidelines (e.g., American Cancer Society [ACS], NIH) for the prevention, treatment, and management of NIH diseases.

7.6.3 Explain the common medical and surgical treatments of NIH diseases.

7.6.4 Explain how treatments for NIH disease can affect the rate of progression of disease.
NEOPLASTIC, IMMUNOLOGIC, AND HEMATOLOGIC:
EXERCISE PRESCRIPTION AND PROGRAMMING

7.7.1 Design, adapt, and supervise an appropriate exercise prescription (e.g., aerobic, resistance, and flexibility training) for individuals with NIH diseases.

7.7.4 Instruct an individual with NIH diseases in techniques for performing physical activities safely and effectively in an unsupervised exercise setting.

NOTE: The KSAs listed above for the ACSM Registered Clinical Exercise Physiologist are the same KSAs for educational programs in Clinical Exercise Physiology seeking graduate (master's degree) academic accreditation through the CoAES. For more information, please visit www.coaes.org.

Index

Note: Page numbers followed by *b* indicate boxes; those followed by *f* indicate figures; and those followed by *t* indicate tables.